中国科学院教材建设专家委员会规划教材
全国高等医药院校规划教材

病理学研究的基本问题

双语版 第2版

主　编　陈　莉

副主编　王桂兰　王建力

编　委　（以姓氏笔画为序）

王建力　王桂兰　付鲁渝　刘　俊
刘淑岩　孙　艳　李云龙　李杏玉
吴圆圆　何　理　羌剑锋　张丽丽
张茂娜　陈　莉　陈丹艺　陈春华
季周婧　季菊玲　周　虹　周家名
秦　婧　顾婷婷　高小娇　彭亮亮
薛玉文

科学出版社

北　京

内 容 简 介

　　双语版《病理学研究的基本问题》共 14 章，分别对病理状态下的细胞行为，如细胞凋亡、自噬、内吞，干细胞等；细胞调控，如黏附分子、细胞周期的调控、端粒与端粒酶、信号转导途径等；疾病伴随的分子现象，如上皮间质转化、肿瘤血管形成、表观遗传学改变、肿瘤微环境的组成、肿瘤浸润转移的机制；以及当下热门的为靶向治疗、精准医疗而开展的分子病理诊断进行综述。本书重点突出了病理学在医学教育、科学研究及临床医疗工作中的基础地位和桥梁作用。章节内容的编排上按引言、历史回顾、现状与进展、挑战与展望的顺序编写。每章内容既独立，又循序渐进、理论联系实际。每章最后附有重要的概念和思考题，便于对学习效果进行检测；附有主要的参考文献，旨在为读者提供足量的信息资源。中英文双语编写模式有利于医学研究生医学专业英语的训练，同时适用于来华留学医学研究生的教学。全书图片 280 余幅，大部分选自国内外医学文献，为了节约教材成本，书内均采用黑白图片，读者可通过手机扫描二维码显示原彩色图片。

　　本书在阐述本学科发展和热点中，有意引导读者了解发展动态，培养其实践能力和创新能力，为其开展科研工作打下良好的基础。因此本书可作为医学基础、临床、预防、口腔、影像、护理专业研究生、医学专业留学研究生的教材，亦可作为医学本科生、医学留学生的选修教材，或可作为病理医师、临床医师的学习参考用书。

图书在版编目（CIP）数据

病理学研究的基本问题　双语版：汉、英 / 陈莉主编. —2 版. —北京：科学出版社，2018.2

中国科学院教材建设专家委员会规划教材·全国高等医药院校规划教材

ISBN 978-7-03-056310-1

Ⅰ. ①病… Ⅱ. ①陈… Ⅲ. ①病理学–双语教学–医药院校–教材–汉、英
Ⅳ. ①R36

中国版本图书馆 CIP 数据核字（2018）第 006949 号

责任编辑：王　超　胡治国 / 责任校对：郭瑞芝
责任印制：李　彤 / 封面设计：陈　敬

科 学 出 版 社 出版
北京东黄城根北街 16 号
邮政编码：100717
http://www.sciencep.com

北京建宏印刷有限公司 印刷
科学出版社发行　各地新华书店经销

*

2018 年 2 月第　一　版　　开本：787×1092　1/16
2022 年 1 月第　二　次印刷　　印张：34
字数：920 000

定价：**158.00 元**
（如有印装质量问题，我社负责调换）

前　言

病理学是目前生命科学中发展较快的学科，病理学研究的方法和内容正是临床医学研究的手段和热点。早在 20 世纪 80 年代初，笔者开始从事病理专业，先后于香港威尔斯亲王医院、美国旧金山基因生物公司深造，曾在著名病理学专家宗永生教授、吴浩强教授的亲自指导下进行病理学研究和临床工作，受益至今。笔者从 38 年的教学和临床实践中深刻体会到基础与临床结合的重要性，特别是当今临床医学的迅猛发展迫切需要通过分子病理学的手段对临床问题进行研究和开展临床关注热点的讨论。《病理学研究的基本问题》一书将近年来病理学研究的热点，发现的问题及实验、研究和总结出来的病理学成果尽快地介绍并应用于临床，引导读者沿着医学的发展趋势，了解学科的前沿与动态，触及存在的问题与挑战，启发研究的灵感，发掘可能的创新，体现了从研究生的课程教育转向课题教育，从职业教育走向科学教育的教材编写宗旨。

本书定位于全国高等医学院校及研究机构的医学科学学位和临床专业学位的研究生教学，并不强调对某一疾病的系统、完整阐述，而是着眼于病理学领域的重大科技发现和重要病理学现象的前沿问题、争论与成果。全书 14 章内容从当代分子病理学研究的共性知识，即医学乃至整个生命科学共同关注的问题，重点突出了病理学在医学教育、科学研究及临床医疗中的基础地位和桥梁作用，突出了对学生创新意识、创新能力和批判性思维方式的培养。为使每章能兼收循序渐进、理论联系实际、顺应时代发展的功效，每章编写遵循引言、历史回顾、现状与进展、病理与临床、挑战与展望、重要的概念与思考题、参考文献的顺序进行，便于学习效果的检测和提供读者足量的信息资源以进一步查询和学习。全书采用中英文双语编写，将适用于来华留学研究生的教学；全书图片 280 余幅，大部分选自国内外医学文献，为了节约教材成本均采用黑白图片，但读者可通过手机扫描书中的二维码显示原彩色图片。

参与本书编写的作者队伍由留学归国，获得博士、硕士学位，并且活跃在教学和临床一线的骨干教师组成。他们具有丰富的教学经验，掌握国内外的教学取向，对教学改革具有敏锐的思维和莫大的积极性，他们以严谨治学的科学态度、无私奉献的敬业精神积极参加本书编写。该书的出版还得到了国家教育部来华留学生全英文病理品牌课程建设经费的资助，并作为南通大学研究生精品课程建设项目。南通大学 2016 级海外留学研究生 Gill Kainat Azeem、Gandi Deborah Shulaimite、Nazar Anaz Mohammed 等为该书的资料收集和英文校对做了大量的工作。同时我在参加科学出版社教材编写工作的 10 余年中，先后主编出版了 10 余部教材，看到了出版社编辑对教材的认真负责，在此对本书出版过程中提供帮助的所有朋友一并表示衷心的感谢。

我们正处在一个现代科学获得更大、更快发展的时代，愿这本凝聚着编者智慧与汗水的双语版《病理学研究的基本问题》能为我国研究生病理教学注入新的活力，为新一代病理医师、临床医师提供一点启发和参考，有助于他们具备更好的理论素养去迎接新的挑战。尽管在教材编写中力求尽善尽美，但由于各位编者理解的重心不一，各章节边缘内容难免有部分重叠，或多或少还存在不足与遗憾，殷切地希望得到读者的批评和指正，以在日后工作中不断改进与提高。

陈　莉

2017 年 7 月 1 日

目　　录

第一章 细胞凋亡

细胞凋亡是种系发育史中早就存在的，如在胚胎发育（embryonic development）、正常组织更新（normal tissue turnover）及在增殖淋巴细胞群体中选择适当的克隆（selection of appropriate clones）中，并有利于许多生命功能的实现。细胞凋亡不引起局部组织损伤或炎症反应，机体的凋亡机制在于维持内环境的稳定，参与免疫系统细胞的发育和克隆选择，而发挥积极的防御作用。

细胞凋亡的主要生物学意义在于以下几方面。

（1）清除多余的细胞：凋亡机制参与胚胎器官发育的过程中，以保持器官的大小与稳定状态。例如，人脑神经元在发育过程中约95%细胞发生凋亡；脊髓背根的运动神经元，当所支配的肌肉相对恒定后，约50%运动神经元凋亡；胚胎肢端发育指（趾）蹼的消失；空腔器官的管、腔、室的形成等。

（2）清除无用的细胞：在形态发育中有些遗迹随发育而凋亡、萎缩，最终消失。例如，人体发育过程中尾芽的消失；又如，人生殖腺早期无性别差异，生殖腺分化决定于生殖腺细胞膜上H-Y抗原，存在H-Y抗原时，生殖腺分化为睾丸，同时女性中肾管发生凋亡；若无H-Y抗原时分化为卵巢，男性中肾管凋亡。

（3）清除有害的细胞：在研究自身免疫性疾病、病毒感染和肿瘤机制中发现，自身反应性T、B淋巴细胞及某些病毒感染的细胞（细胞毒性靶细胞）和一些肿瘤细胞，通过凋亡得以清除。机体正是通过细胞凋亡作为自身保护的防御机制。

（4）清除衰老的细胞：在整个细胞生命周期中，细胞在分裂分化的同时，也建立了一套限制自身无限增殖和自然淘汰的机制，如人红细胞分化成熟120天后自然凋亡、结肠上皮每天更换100亿个细胞、胃黏膜上皮3~5天更新一次等。

（5）有选择性地清除细胞：在低剂量毒性刺激时（如细胞毒性药物、高温、电离辐射等），甚至极度缺氧的组织，凋亡明显发生在某类细胞，如睾丸经常暴露于放射线后精原细胞选择性的死亡、淋巴细胞增殖分化过程中的免疫选择、一些激素依赖性器官因激素撤除而引起靶细胞凋亡而萎缩（如乳腺、子宫）等。

细胞凋亡作为细胞死亡的一种形式一直是组织病理学研究的中心议题。采用什么样的标准可以比较在不同情况下、不同类型的细胞死亡呢？形态学上可以作出一个区分的标准。1972年 Kerr 根据细胞发生了与坏死（necrosis）完全不一样的死亡过程而提出了细胞凋亡（apoptosis）的概念。凋亡（apoptosis 中的 apo 为脱落，ptosis 为飘零）意味着落下（falling off）或丢掉（falling away），好像秋风落叶或头发脱落的自然凋落。

"凋亡"一词1972年开始使用，但由于检测技术的限制，这种细胞现象只停留在形态学的描述上，因此长期以来有关凋亡的研究，一直未被病理工作者重视。20世纪80年代末，随着细胞生物学、分子生物学等科学理论的发展，凋亡的检测技术也有了很大的发展，生物学家逐渐认识到细胞凋亡的特殊生物学意义，由此形成了医学研究热点，促进了凋亡理论在生物生理学各领域的广泛应用。正是由于发现了细胞凋亡的规律，三位科学家获得了2002年的诺贝尔生理学或医学奖。他们是英国的悉尼·布伦纳、美国的 H·罗伯特·霍维茨和英国的约翰·E·苏尔斯顿。

细胞凋亡的发生是由基因控制的个别细胞发生的细胞程序性死亡（programmed cell death，PCD）的表现形式，是由体内外因素触发细胞内预存的死亡程序而导致的细胞主动性死亡方式，是细胞内遗传信息程序性调控的结果。参与凋亡调控的基因又联系着细胞周期调控、细胞增殖、分化基因之间的复杂网络调节。大多数动物细胞均能自我致死，且此种普遍性的自杀程序也能由发自其他细胞的信号所激活或抑制。因此凋亡是一种能量依赖性的细胞自我销毁的主动过程。各种细胞凋亡在形态学上具有一致性，但基因或生化标记在不同细胞类型是不同的。这种由基因控制细胞有目的、有选择性的自我消亡过程是保证生命进化的基础。

细胞凋亡是否完全与 PCD 相同？现在要说明它们之间的异同还太勉强。更多的研究认为，凋亡是个形态学的概念，描述了一整套与坏死不同的形态学特征。而 PCD 侧重于功能上的描述，指细胞内特点相同的程序性表达介导的细胞死亡。细胞凋亡和 PCD 具有非常密切的关系。大多数情况下 PCD 是以凋亡的方式进行，但并不是所有 PCD 都采取凋亡的方式，如烟草蛾节间肌肉细胞、哺乳动物某些神经元和红细胞，它们的 PCD 是以非凋亡的方式进行（细胞溶解，不形成凋亡小体）。有时由外源性理化因子刺激诱发的细胞死亡，形态上似凋亡，但并不是由细胞内原装程序所引发，也不能称为 PCD（如放疗后在肿瘤组织坏死中可以看到的鬼影细胞）。

第一节　凋亡发生的机制

凋亡是哺乳动物细胞对生理性、病理性刺激做出的快速且机制复杂的反应，各种细胞外刺激如 DNA 损伤、热休克、生长因子缺乏等均可启动凋亡。

一、凋亡的生化特征

凋亡主要通过受体介导的信号途径（receptor-mediated cellular signaling pathway）诱导细胞凋亡因子或刺激因素通过第二信使系统传递信号，信号传递途径决定了细胞的命运。凋亡的生化特征主要表现为以下几方面。

（1）核小体间 DNA 双链裂解，形成180～200bp 大小及其倍数的核苷酸片段。

（2）Ca^{2+} 的堆积和重新分布。

（3）转谷氨酰胺酶的积累并激活。

（4）细胞表面糖链、植物血凝素的增加。

（5）细胞骨架的改变。

其中以下三个酶的改变最重要。

（1）核酸内切酶：该酶（endonuclease）活化能在核小体间连接区（internucleosomal linkage region）将 DNA 双链裂解，形成 180～200bp 大小及其倍数的核苷酸片段，在电泳胶上呈梯状条带（图 1-1）。

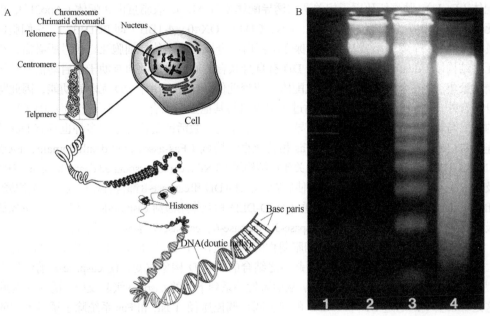

图 1-1 核酸内切酶在核小体间连接区将 DNA 双链裂解，形成 180～200bp 大小及其倍数的核苷酸片段，在电泳胶上呈梯状条带；DNA fragmentation with 180～200bp cut by endonuclease internucleosomal linkage region，DNA ladder

（2）组织转谷氨酰胺酶（tissue transglutaminase，TTG）：活化催化 ε-（γ-谷氨酰）赖氨酸交联形成僵硬而不溶性蛋白，在老化与终末分化的角化上皮中 TTG 活化形成内披蛋白（involucrin），这些蛋白可以网络住细胞内细胞器等内容物，使其不易溢出。

（3）钙依赖蛋白酶（calcium-dependent proteinase）：活化后使 Ca^{2+} 堆积和重新分布，破坏细胞骨架结构，形成细胞表面泡状突起。阻断胞质 Ca^{2+} 浓度可以抑制凋亡发生，增加胞质 Ca^{2+} 浓度可以促进凋亡。

细胞表面糖链、植物血凝素的增加和细胞骨架的改变均参与细胞凋亡的发生。

二、细胞凋亡的途径

来自细胞内外的各种信号可诱导细胞发生凋亡，但不同类型的凋亡细胞却呈现一致的特征性形态和生化改变，这些改变由半胱氨酸-天冬氨酸特异性蛋白酶（胱天蛋白酶，caspase）家族降解所造成[1]。

按启动 caspase 和信号转导机制的不同，凋亡发生有不同的途径[2]：一条为外源性途径，即死亡受体（death receptor，DR）介导途径；另一条为内源性途径，也称为线粒体介导途径。它们通过一系列分子和生物化学途径导致两个途径共同的"中央处理器"分子即 caspase 的活化，并诱导许多细胞核和细胞质内相关底物的降解。最新研究显示，内质网应激（endoplasmic reticulum stress）

途径也可以导致细胞凋亡。未折叠或错误折叠的蛋白质在内质网中过度积累，导致内质网产生应激反应从而激活保护细胞的信号通路，通常称为未折叠蛋白反应（unfolded protein response，UPR）。如果内质网收到的刺激不减弱，UPR 会恢复和保持内质网的动态平衡或者诱导细胞凋亡。

（一）外源性 DR 途径

1. 死亡配体（death ligands）结合而促发的凋亡　这些配体包括肿瘤坏死因子（TNF）、Fas 配体（FasL）、肿瘤坏死因子相关凋亡诱导配体（TRAIL）、载脂蛋白 3 配体（Apo3L），也称为死亡因子，相应的 DR 包括 TNFR、Fas、CD40、OX40、4-1BB（即 PCD137），它们胞内区都具有一约 80 个氨基酸残基组成的保守的蛋白结合域，且是传导细胞死亡信号所必需，称之为死亡结构域（death domain，DD）。DD 有自身联合的倾向，该倾向有助于在启动信号转导时的受体聚集。当受体高表达时可导致配体非依赖性信号转导。由于 DD 无酶解功能，因此除了自身结合外，它们也可直接或间接通过锚定蛋白与其他蛋白结合转导信号[3]。死亡因子以三聚体的形式与靶细胞上的 DR 结合并诱导受体三聚体化，激活的受体通过与多种也具有 DD 的受体连接蛋白或衔接蛋白，如 Fas 与 Fas 相关死亡结构域（Fas-associated death domain，FADD），TNFR（TNF receptor）1 与 TNFR 相关死亡结构域（TNF receptor-associated death domain，TRADD）及 FADD，再与 caspase-8 相互作用并使后者激活，FADD 和 caspase-8 都含有死亡效应子结构域（death effector domain，DED），它们之间通过 DED-DED 相互作用激活 caspase-8，启动 caspase 家族酶的级联反应，通过执行死亡蛋白酶 caspase-3、caspase-6、caspase-7 等导致细胞凋亡[4]。

2. Fas/FasL 系统　Fas 介导细胞凋亡的调控途径，FasL 与 Fas 结合可以导致 Fas 胞内的死亡结构域形成三聚体而活化，并引起与之结合的 FADD 构象改变，使 caspase-8 前体集聚、断裂和激活，产生有活性的 caspase-8，从而激发一系列下游的 caspase 级联反应，诱发细胞凋亡[5]。这是一条基本的通过 DD 和 FADD 的细胞凋亡调控途径。FasL 和 Fas 系统除了诱导死亡的功能外，还有导致细胞活化和增生的功能[6]（图 1-2A）。

3. 肿瘤坏死因子（tumor-necrosis factor，TNF）系统　TNF 是由 157 个氨基酸亚单位组成的同源三聚体，主要由因感染而活化的巨噬细胞和 T 细胞产生，TNF 与 TNFR1 结合诱导细胞凋亡[9]。TNF 三聚体与 TNFR1 的胞外结构域结合启动信号转导，从 TNFR1 细胞内结构域（intracellular domain，ICD）释放抑制蛋白沉默死亡结构域（silencer of death domain，SODD），结果导致聚集的 TNFR1-ICD 被衔接蛋白 TRADD 所识别，募集了其他衔接蛋白，如受体作用蛋白（receptor-interacting protein，RIP）、TNFR 相关因子-2（TNFR-associated factor-2，TRAF2）和 FADD。募集的这些蛋白是启动 TNFR1 信号转导中的关键酶[8]（图 1-2B）。

TNFR1 与 DD 和 TRADD 相互作用后，是通过 TRAF2 和 RIP 两条途径分别进行信号转导[9]。TRAF2 和受体相互作用蛋白（RIP）可以激活 NF-κB 诱导激酶（NIK），NIK 反过来又可以激活 κB 激酶复合物（IKK）的抑制剂（I-κB），导致 I-κB 降解和允许 NF-κB 转移到核内，发挥转录激活效应[10]。从 TRAF2 和 RIP 到 JNK 的途径中还涉及一个包括丝裂原激活蛋白激酶 MEKK1（MAP/Erk 激酶 1）-JNKK（JNK 激酶）-JNK 的转导通路。这样，抑制性蛋白就可以最终发挥抑制细胞凋亡的效应[11]。TNFR1 还可以和 RADD 或 CRADD（一种衔接蛋白）相互作用，RADD 通过其死亡结构域和 RIP 死亡结构域相结合或者通过胱天蛋白酶募集域（caspase recruitment domain，CARD）序列与死亡效应分子 caspase-2 结合，也可以诱发细胞凋亡产生[12]。

（二）内源性线粒体途径

启动凋亡的关键因素是线粒体功能紊乱。线粒体是含有丰富的腺嘌呤核苷酸载体（adenine nucleotide translocator，ANT）、电压依赖性阴离子通道（voltage-dependent anion channel，VDAC）、

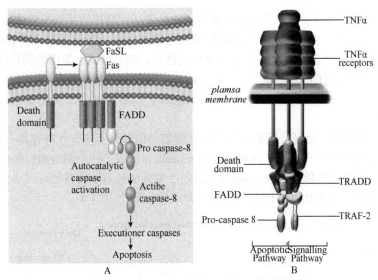

图 1-2 外源性死亡受体[Fas（A）和 TNF（B）]介导的细胞凋亡途径；FAAD：Fas-associated death domain；FasL：Fas ligand Apoptosis pathway through death receptors[Fas（A）and TNF（B）]

B 细胞淋巴瘤/白血病-2（Bcl-2）分子等的双层膜包裹的囊状结构。外膜通透性较大，容许分子量在 15kDa 以下的物质自由通过，内膜通透性小，大于 1.5kDa 物质不易通过。该双层膜通透性的改变在细胞凋亡中起重要作用，而外膜通透性改变与内膜相比更具有凋亡特征。线粒体调节细胞凋亡有 3 种机制：①线粒体电子传递与能量代谢的破坏；②细胞氧化状态的改变；③线粒体膜通透性改变导致介导细胞凋亡分子的释放。其中线粒体膜通透性改变在细胞凋亡中起重要作用。

线粒体膜通透性的改变可释放多种分子启动凋亡，主要包括 caspase 前体、细胞色素 c（Cyt-c，caspase 的激活剂）、第二个线粒体来源促凋亡的 caspase 激活剂（second mitochondria-derived pro-apoptotic activator of caspases，Smac）/低等电点的直接结合 IAP 蛋白（direct IAP-binding protein with low pI，Diablo，caspase 的协同激活剂），以及凋亡诱导因子（apoptosis inducing factor，AIF，激活核酸酶裂解 DNA 成小片段）、凋亡抑制蛋白（inhibitor of apoptosis protein，IAP，caspase 的直接抑制剂）、内切核酸酶-G（endonuclease G）等[13]。

1. 细胞色素 c 在脊椎动物细胞凋亡过程中，线粒体被认为是处于凋亡调控的中心位置，线粒体外膜的物理性损伤导致定位于线粒体的 caspase 活化物的释放，而最重要的分子是 Cyt-c。Cyt-c 是线粒体呼吸链的重要组成之一，线粒体膜通透性增高是释放 Cyt-c 的关键。

细胞损伤后，Cyt-c 从线粒体释放，并与细胞凋亡蛋白酶激活因子 1（apoptosis protease activating factor 1，Apaf-1，线虫 ced-4 的同源物）结合，并活化 caspase-9 前体，进而激活 Caspase-3，引发 caspase 级联反应，从而诱发细胞凋亡[14]（图 1-3）。

2. 凋亡体 凋亡体（apoptosome）也称为死亡复合体（death complexes），是细胞线粒体对凋

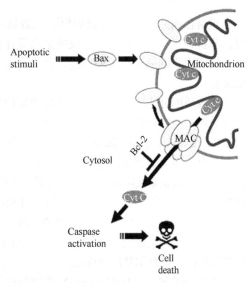

图 1-3 线粒体介导的细胞凋亡途径；Apoptosis pathway through mitochondria

亡性死亡做出反应的关键步骤，它是由线粒体通透性增高而释放的某些线粒体蛋白如 Cyt-c、Smac/Diablo 等启动的、由 Cyt-c 和 Apaf-1 形成的七聚体结构。Cyt-c 从线粒体膜间隙释放并结合胞浆中的 Apaf-1 单体，诱导其变构与 ATP 稳定连接，随后形成七聚体的凋亡体（heptameric apoptosome），再通过它的 caspase 募集域（caspase recruitment domain，CARD）募集并激活 caspase-9 前体，激活的 caspase-9 进一步激活效应因子 caspase-3、caspase-6、caspase-7，使凋亡达到了顶峰[15]。

2 条主要的细胞凋亡途径，因启动信号的亚细胞结构部位不同，各自有其一定的独特性，但在胞内凋亡信号转导中存在有广泛的串流（crosstalk），形成了一个细胞凋亡的信号转导网络。例如，在死亡受体诱导的凋亡中，caspase-8 对 Bcl-2 家族成员 Bid 的剪切可以活化线粒体途径，并使凋亡信号放大。线粒体就被作为凋亡信号的"放大器"（图 1-4）。

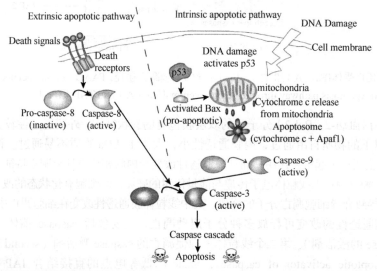

图 1-4 两个主要的凋亡信号途径；A brief overview of the extrinsic and intrinsic apoptotic pathways

（三）内质网应激途径

当新合成的蛋白质 N 端糖基化、二硫键形成及蛋白质由内质网向高尔基体转运等过程受阻时，非折叠或错误折叠的新合成的蛋白质在内质网中大量堆积，或者是 Ca^{2+} 平衡状态的打破，都会损伤内质网的正常生理功能，称为内质网应激反应（endoplasmic reticulum stress response，ESR）。

当内质网处于应激状态时，非折叠蛋白反应（unfolded protein response，UPR）可激活 3 种转录因子——IRE1/ERN1（inositol requiring 1）、PERK/PEK（PEK like ER kinase）和 ATF6（activating transcription factor 6），引起未折叠的和错误折叠的蛋白在内质网内沉积降解。IRE1 是一个内质网 I 型跨膜糖蛋白，它的 3 个功能区——胞质区的激酶域和核糖核酸酶（RNase）域、内质网腔中的氨基端区域，能感知未折叠蛋白的蓄积，并能跨过内质网膜进行 UPR 信息传递。PERK 也是一个内质网 I 型跨膜糖蛋白，ESR 时，N 端感受应激信号，免疫球蛋白重链结合蛋白质（BiP）与 PERK 的二聚化位点解离，PERK 形成寡聚体且发生自身磷酸化而被激活。ATF6 是内质网上 II 型跨膜蛋白，ESR 时，ATF6 与 BiP 分离，ATF6 以囊泡转移的方式从内质网膜转移到高尔基体，在高尔基体内被蛋白酶 S1P（site-1 protease）和 S2P（site-2 protease）切割，产生游离的 N 端片段。活化的 ATF6 N 端切割段转移到核内作为转录因子与 ESR 元件结合，激活应激元件基因启动子区域，这些基因激活分子伴侣、折叠酶和 CCAAT/增强子结合蛋白同源蛋白

[CCAAT/enhancer binding protein（C/EBP）homologous protein，CHOP]的转录（图 1-5）。

ESR 诱导细胞凋亡的 3 条主要信号途径如下。

1. CHOP 通路 生长阻滞及 DNA 损伤诱导基因 153(growth arrest and DNA-damage-inducible gene 153, CHOP/GADD153)是 ESR 特异的一个转录因子，在其启动子中能与 C/EBP 和转录因子 Fos-Jun 家族成员形成异源二聚体（heterodimer）[16]。IRE1、PERK 和 ATF6 都能诱导 CHOP 的转录，其中 PERK-eIF2α-ATF4 是 CHOP 蛋白表达主要途径[17]。CHOP 能激活 GADD34、ERO1 和 DR5 等凋亡反应蛋白。PERK 磷酸化酶 eIF2α 能诱

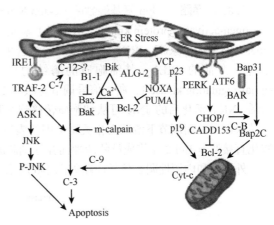

图 1-5 内质网应激途径；Protein implicated in ER stress pathways

导 ATF4、ATF3 和 CHOP 的表达，然后转录因子上调 GADD34，GADD34 通过蛋白磷酸酶(PP1)介导 eIF2α 去磷酸化，增加内质网伴侣蛋白（chaperone）的生物合成。因此在细胞应激状态时，内质网合成 chaperone 蛋白明显增加[18]，过量表达的 CHOP 能促进细胞凋亡[19]。ERO1 是一个内质网氧化酶，使内质网产生一个过氧化环境。CHOP 可减少细胞糖化，增加内质网中氧自由基（reactive oxygen species，ROS）的产生。干扰 ERO1 功能后使内质网中 ROS 减少，导致细胞的保护，表明 ERO1 是 CHOP 下游的重要凋亡效应子。DR5 编码一个能够激活 caspase 蛋白级联反应的膜表面死亡受体[20]。CHOP 能转录性下调抗凋亡蛋白 Bcl-2 和上调死亡受体家族成员 DR5，Bcl-2 和 DR5 在非内质网应激的凋亡通路中有同样的作用。CHOP 还能与 cAMP 反应元件结合蛋白（cAMP-response element-binding protein，CREBP）形成异源二聚体，能抑制 Bcl-2 蛋白的表达，这可以促进线粒体的凋亡通路。

2. caspase 通路 在 ESR 诱导的细胞凋亡中胱天蛋白酶 caspase 家族促凋亡蛋白也起关键的作用。caspase-12（一个鼠源性蛋白，大部分人不表达 caspase-12，在人类是 caspase-4 起该作用）定位于内质网外膜，是介导 ESR 凋亡的关键分子，非内质网应激性凋亡不能激活该分子，即在死亡受体和线粒体凋亡途径中是不被活化的。实验发现 caspase-12 缺陷鼠能抵抗 ESR 引起的凋亡，而对其他死亡刺激仍可发生细胞凋亡，这说明 caspase-12 与 ESR 介导凋亡的机制有关，而与非内质网应激介导的凋亡无关[21]。caspase-12 活化的机制主要有下面几个方式：①胞质钙活化蛋白酶。钙蛋白酶（calpain）是细胞质中另一 caspase 家族成员，其裂解与活化依赖于 Ca^{2+}的存在。在 ESR 状态下，细胞内 Ca^{2+}水平的升高引起细胞质中的 calpain 活化并转位到内质网膜上，剪切内质网膜上的 procaspase-12，使之活化并释放到细胞质中，同时活化的 calpain 在环状结构域剪切 Bcl-xL，使之由抗凋亡分子变为促凋亡分子。②TRAF2 依赖性机制。caspase-12 通过直接与 IRE1α 和衔接蛋白 TRAF2 的联系而主动激活，具体机制尚不清楚。在正常状态下，细胞中的 TRAF2 与 procaspase-12 形成稳定的异源二聚体，而在 ESR 状态下，TRAF2 和 procaspase-12 分离，引起 caspase-12 的活化，并同时引起 JIK-IRE1 复合物募集 TRAF2，导致 JNK 磷酸化而活化。③caspase-7 的内质网转位。ESR 时，caspase-7 转位于内质网并活化，与 caspase-12 形成复合物并剪切 procaspase-12，破坏了膜与 caspase-12 的联系，使之活化并释放到细胞质中。④葡萄糖调节蛋白 78（GRP78）、caspase-7、caspase-12 复合物途径。ESR 诱导伴侣蛋白 GRP78 表达，并在内质网膜上与 caspase-7 和 caspase-12 形成复合物，阻止 caspase-12 从内质网膜释放，dATP 可解离这种复合物，促使 caspase-12 向细胞质转位并活化。

3. JNK 通路 c-Jun 氨基端激酶（c-Jun N-terminal kinase，JNK）属于丝裂原活化蛋白激酶（mitogen-activated protein kinase，MAPK）家族或应激活化的蛋白激酶（stress-activated protein kinase，SAPK）家族。IRE1 介导的 X 盒结合蛋白 1（XBP1）剪接诱导的 UPR 能促进细胞的生存。激活的 IRE1，其细胞质的酶结构域连接接头分子 TRAF2 与 ASK1（apoptosis signal-regulating kinase 1，凋亡信号调节源激酶 1）共同形成 IRE1-TRAF2-ASK1 复合物，从而激活 JNK。活化后的 JNK 可从细胞质转移到细胞核中，通过磷酸化激活 c-Jun、c-Fos、EIk-1 等转录因子，而调节下游凋亡相关靶基因的表达。活化的 JNK 也可以留在细胞质中，通过磷酸化直接调节 Bcl-2 家族成员的活性而介导细胞凋亡的发生。

外源性和内源性凋亡信号通路如图 1-6 所示。

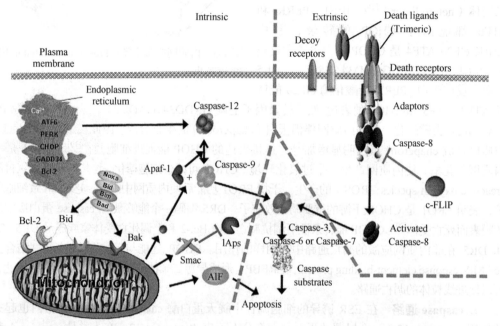

图 1-6　外源性和内源性凋亡信号通路；The extrinsic and intrinsic pathways of apoptosis signaling
外源性通路，细胞外死亡配体结合、膜受体三聚化、经由适配器招募和激活 caspase 启动子（caspase-8）。在内源性通路，应激细胞经历由 Bcl-2 家族调控的涉及线粒体和内质网渗透性的区室变化，引起 caspase 启动子的活化，包括由细胞色素 c 释放在凋亡复合体中的 caspase-9 或一系列分子相互作用之前发生钙平衡紊乱中的 caspase-12。不论外源性还是内源性通路，都通过活化启动子 caspase 和激活效应子 caspase，随后裂解分散的蛋白，引起凋亡细胞死亡；In the extrinsic pathway, extracellular death ligands bind and trimerize membrane receptors, recruit and activate initiator caspases(caspase-8). In the intrinsic pathway, cells in stress undergo compartmental changes involving the mitochondrion and endoplasmic reticulum permeability controlled by the Bcl-2 family, which cause the activation of initiator caspases, either caspase-9 in an apoptosome complex upon release of cytochrome c, or caspase-12 by disturbed calcium homeostasis prior to a series of molecular interactions. In both extrinsic and intrinsic pathways, activated initiator caspases process and activate effector caspases, which subsequently cleave divergent protein substrates and cause apoptotic cell death

除了上述 caspase 依赖的凋亡途径，还存在分子上不能较好定义的细胞死亡途径，该途径不需要 caspase 的激活。因此，不能真正定义为凋亡或坏死，而被称为"坏死样"（necrotic-like）或"凋亡样"（apoptotic-like）细胞死亡或副凋亡（parapotosis）。

三、细胞凋亡信号转导系统

细胞凋亡信号转导特点表现为多样性、耦联性、同一性、多途性。主要的凋亡信号转导通路包括：①胞内 Ca^{2+} 信号系统；②cAMP/PKA 信号系统；③Fas 蛋白/Fas 配体信号系统；④神经酰胺信号系统；⑤二酰甘油/蛋白激酶 C（PKC）信号系统；⑥酪氨酸蛋白激酶（PTK）信号系统（图 1-7）。

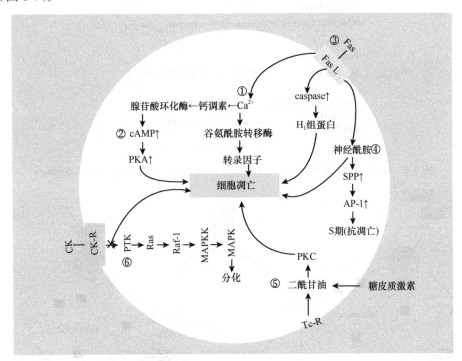

图 1-7　主要的凋亡信号转导通路；Apoptotic signal transduction system with multi-way

四、细胞凋亡调控相关基因

细胞凋亡是一个多基因调控的过程。多数抑癌基因促细胞凋亡，多数癌基因抑制细胞凋亡。

（一）Bcl-2 基因家族

首先从 t（14；18）的滤泡性淋巴瘤中发现，Bcl-2（B cell lymphoma/leukemia-2）抑制各种刺激诱发的细胞凋亡。进一步发现 Bcl-2 广泛存在于造血细胞、上皮细胞、淋巴细胞、神经细胞及多种瘤细胞，分布于线粒体内膜、细胞膜内表面、核膜及部分内质网。Bcl-2 通过抗氧化、下调促凋亡蛋白（Cyt-c、AIF）释放、下调促凋亡蛋白 Bax/Bak 的细胞毒性作用、下调凋亡蛋白酶（caspase）激活，维持细胞钙稳态，发挥抑制细胞凋亡的作用。Bcl-2 基因家族：一组 Bcl-2 的同源蛋白，含有 Bcl-2 同源结构域（Bcl-2 homology，BH）和跨膜结构域，4 个保守区具有同源结构域（BH1～4）；20 多个家族成员分为三大类（图 1-8）。其中抗凋亡成员具有 BH1 结构（Bcl-2、Bcl-xL、Bcl-w）、促凋亡成员具有 BH2（Bax、Bak、Bok、Bcl-xs）和仅有 BH3 结构的促凋亡成员（Bik、Blk、Hrk、Bim、Bnip3）和 BH4 结构的 Bid、Bad。Bcl-2 基因家族分子通过形成同源二聚体（homodimer）或异源二聚体来调节细胞凋亡。只有形成同源二聚体才能有效发挥该基因的作用。Bcl-2/Bax 的值对决定细胞凋亡的敏感性起重要作用，抑制凋亡因子与促进凋亡因子的总比率，最终决定细胞的生存或死亡（图 1-9）。

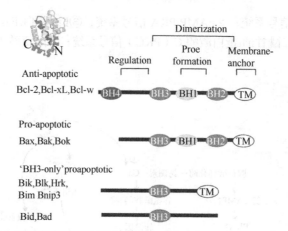

图 1-8　Bcl-2 基因家族同源结构域；Bcl-2 gene family homology（BH）domains

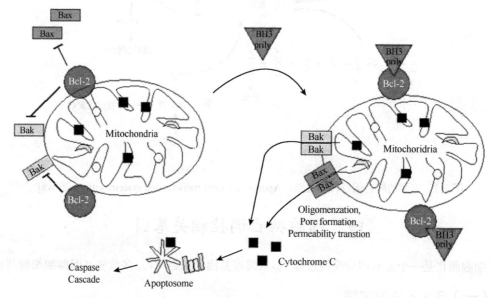

图 1-9　Bcl-2 基因家族分子通过形成同源二聚体或异源二聚体来调节细胞凋亡；The homodimers of the Bcl-2 family proteins is activation whereas the heterodimers is unactivation

1. Bcl-2 的结构　Bcl-2 是最早发现的抑制细胞凋亡的蛋白，由 Bcl-2 基因编码。Bcl-2 基因是从滤泡性淋巴瘤相关的 t（14；18）染色体易位的断裂点克隆到的。Bcl-2 基因有 2 个外显子，转录后经选择性剪切产生 2 个蛋白，分别为分子量 26kDa 的 Bcl-2α 和分子量 22kDa 的 Bcl-2β。对 Bcl-2α 的研究较多（以下简称 Bcl-2），它是定位在线粒体膜、核外膜和内质网外膜的整合蛋白，通过操控线粒体膜间隙蛋白的释放对细胞凋亡加以调控[19]。Bcl-2 的主要作用并非加速细胞分裂增殖，而是抑制细胞凋亡，延长细胞生存。Bcl-2 在成熟细胞和衰老细胞中不表达或低表达。

2. Bcl-2 在正常组织中的表达

（1）在成人的上皮组织中，Bcl-2 的表达可分为两大类：一类受内分泌控制，在激素作用下的上皮中出现了 Bcl-2 的不同表达与定位；另一类不受内分泌控制。在后一类中，Bcl-2 主要表达在增殖状态的细胞内，如皮肤、咽、气管黏膜的基底细胞及肠隐窝细胞。

（2）在成人的前列腺中，Bcl-2 主要表达在不依赖雄激素的细胞内如基底细胞，而对雄激素敏感的分泌细胞则不表达 Bcl-2。这一发现对临床治疗可能有指导作用，因为 Bcl-2 表达阳性的前列腺癌对激素治疗不敏感。

（3）增生状态的子宫内膜腺体中 Bcl-2 表达强阳性，这使内膜细胞在月经周期开始时能够存活，随着月经周期的进行，蛋白的表达量逐渐减少。

（4）Bcl-2 在乳腺小叶上皮中的表达最强，其表达水平在月经期末也会减少。

（5）在骨髓的前体细胞中 Bcl-2 表达阳性，而在成熟的细胞中表达阴性。

3. Bcl-2 在肿瘤中的表达与肿瘤发生的相关性 Bcl-2 在多种肿瘤中的表达，如造血系统肿瘤（白血病、淋巴瘤）、乳腺癌、神经母细胞瘤、鼻咽癌、前列腺癌、肺鳞癌、肺腺癌等。Bcl-2 阳性的肿瘤要比 Bcl-2 阴性的肿瘤预后差。在 85% 的滤泡型恶性淋巴瘤，存在 t（14；18）（q32；q21）。这一染色体易位使位于 14 号染色体长臂的免疫球蛋白重链基因和位于 18 号染色体的 Bcl-2 基因的转录活性位点拼接，造成 Bcl-2 基因的过度表达，使 B 淋巴细胞免于凋亡而长期存活，并可能附加其他基因的突变而发展成淋巴瘤。Bcl-2 的免疫染色最常用于区别反应性滤泡性淋巴瘤。阳性染色位于细胞质。在滤泡性淋巴瘤的滤泡中出现 Bcl-2 表达强阳性，而反应性滤泡增生只在滤泡中心的单个细胞内出现阳性（大多数是 T 细胞）。染色上的这一区别并非由于 Bcl-2 mRNA 的下调或减少，而主要是因为翻译后机制导致蛋白水平下降。此时，Bcl-2 免疫染色不能用于区别不同类型的淋巴瘤（图 1-10）。

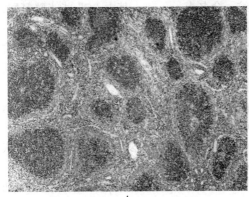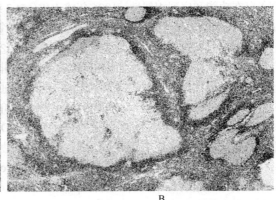

A B

图 1-10 Bcl-2 免疫染色区别（滤泡性）淋巴瘤（A）和反应性滤泡增生（B）；Bcl-2 immunostaining most commonly used to distinguish between follicular lymphoma（A）and reactive proliferation（B）

现在已经发现 Bcl-2 既是抗凋亡基因，又是一种新型的耐药基因。单独 Bcl-2 蛋白的表达增多不足以引发肿瘤状态。因为 Bcl-2 能够增强细胞的生存能力，但 Bcl-2 可能与某些癌基因和病毒产生协同作用，Bcl-2 和 c-myc 的协同作用已经在这两种基因的转基因小鼠中得到证实，这种包含 Bcl-2 和 c-myc 两种基因的小鼠比缺少其中任何一种基因的小鼠能够更快地发生肿瘤。

4. Bcl-2 家族的其他成员

（1）Bcl-xL 是一个重要的抑制细胞凋亡的蛋白，由 Bcl-x 基因编码。

Bcl-x 基因在人类有 2 种 cDNA 形式，Bcl-xL 和 Bcl-xs。Bcl-xL 蛋白在大小、结构上均与 Bcl-2 极为相似；相反，Bcl-xs 蛋白则缺乏与 Bcl-2 高度同源的 63 个氨基酸。Bcl-xs 与 Bcl-2、Bcl-xL 不同，它具有促进细胞凋亡的作用，转染 Bcl-xs cDNA 的细胞，可使 Bcl-2 丧失抑制细胞凋亡的作用。

（2）Bax 是应用免疫共沉淀方法获得的，分子量 21kDa 的促进凋亡因子，在保守区 BH1、BH2、BH3 都与 Bcl-2 同源。Bax 高表达，能促进和加速细胞凋亡，增加细胞对凋亡信号的敏感性。野生型的 P53 蛋白可以诱导 Bax 的合成，而促使 DNA 受损的细胞进入凋亡。

（3）Bak 是另一促凋亡因子，与 Bax 相似，在适当的刺激下，Bak 促进细胞凋亡，增加细胞凋亡的敏感性；与 Bax 不同的是，Bak 在 EB 病毒转化的细胞株中抑制细胞凋亡。另有报道，它还能抑制由细胞毒性试剂——维生素 K_3 诱导的凋亡。

5. Bcl-2 家族成员的相互作用 细胞内 Bax 高表达时，细胞对死亡信号敏感，加速细胞凋亡，当 Bcl-2 高表达，细胞则长期存活；Bcl-2 可与 Bax 形成异源二聚体，抑制细胞凋亡。所以 Bcl-2/Bax 的值对决定细胞凋亡的敏感性起重要作用，抑制凋亡因子与促进凋亡因子的总比值，最终决定细胞的的生存或死亡。

Bcl-2 过度表达不能影响 Bax 的表达，但是可以抑制细胞质中的 c-myc 的蓄积和 caspase-3 的活性，进而促进神经元的存活[20]。Bcl-2 可通过抑制氧自由基而发挥抗细胞凋亡作用。正常情况下 Bcl-2 和 Bax 在细胞内保持平衡，Bcl-2 家族能调节线粒体膜的通透性，下调 Bcl-2 或过度表达 Bcl-2 家族中促凋亡基因 Bax 均能增加线粒体膜的通透性。研究大鼠模型时发现应用西洛他唑清除羟氧基和氧自由基，可以减少缺血区的 Bax 蛋白表达水平，相应地提高 Bcl-2 蛋白表达和抑制 Cyt-c 的释放，减少缺血脑组织梗死体积，从而抑制细胞凋亡和氧化。

（二）caspase 家族

1993 年发现 ced-3 基因和哺乳动物 ICE（interleukin-1β-converting enzyme，白介素 1β 转化酶）存在功能和序列相似性；1996 年将 ICE/ced-3 统一命名为 caspase。其中"C"指半胱氨酸，"aspase"指天冬氨酸，即该酶的作用部位都在天冬氨酸残基后的位点上。因此 caspase 家族是一组蛋白酶，其特征为：①都是半胱氨酸蛋白酶；②作用部位都在天冬氨酸残基后（Asp）的位点被切断后从酶原转换成活性蛋白酶。caspase 以非活化的蛋白酶前体形式存在于胞质中，必须经过剪切形成活性亚单位才能发挥作用。当它们通过一定的途径被活化后，依据一定的顺序，裂解一些重要的蛋白底物，在即将死亡的细胞中介导高效而特异的蛋白水解，其将裂解 DNA 酶的抑制剂，使得 DNA 酶被激活，进一步降解 DNA 至 180～200bp 的片段。因此 caspase 在细胞凋亡的启动和完成中起重要作用，是细胞凋亡的执行者。至今已发现有 14 种 caspase，依结构和功能的不同可分为 3 组。其中具有 large-prodomain 的 caspase-2、caspase-8、caspase-9，是细胞凋亡的起始 caspase，而具有 prodomain 的 caspase-3、caspase-6、caspase-7，则主要与细胞凋亡的最终执行有关，是效应 caspase。这两组 caspase 在细胞凋亡中缺一不可。另一组由 caspase-1、caspase-5 组成，该组与细胞凋亡的关系不是很密切，可能与多种炎症因子的成熟有关。最近发现 caspase-4（caspase-12）与内质网应激介导的凋亡有关。激活的 caspase 主要功能：通过灭活凋亡抑制物、水解活性效应蛋白和水解结构蛋白，导致凋亡细胞产生一系列的形态和生物化学的改变（图 1-11）。

凋亡细胞独特的形态特征与活化的 caspase 裂解一系列的蛋白底物有关。细胞凋亡过程一旦启动，就有不同的蛋白被裂解。目前，已知的底物如下。

（1）与基因组功能相关的酶，如 PARP（poly ADP-ribose polymerase，多腺苷二磷酸核糖聚合酶），依赖 DNA 的蛋白激酶 460kDa 的催化亚基，组成 DNA 复制复合物的 140kDa 的多肽等。

（2）结构蛋白（核和细胞质骨架）如核层蛋白、肌动蛋白等，细胞凋亡时核骨架和细胞质骨架的分解被易化。

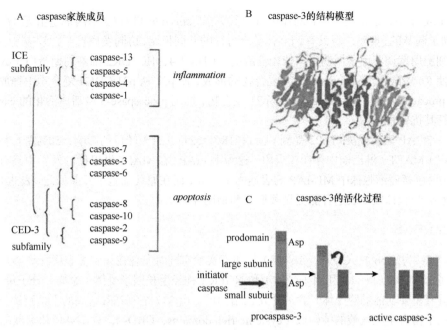

图 1-11 caspase 家族（A），结构（B），活化（C）；caspase family（A），structure（B），and activation（C）

（3）核有丝分裂相关蛋白，如 NuMA、D4G 等。

（4）DNA 断裂因子（DFF）复合物中的 45kDa 多肽水解后，DFF 活化引起 DNA 断裂。

（三）IAP 家族

IAP 构成第三类调节蛋白。IAP 结合并抑制 caspase。它们同样具有泛素连接酶的功能，促进与之结合的 caspase 降解。IAP 以具有 BIR（baculoviral IAP repeat）结构域为特点。人类细胞中存在 9 个 IAP 家族成员，包括 XIAP（hILP，MIHA，ILP-1），cIAP1（MIHB，HIAP-2），cIAP2（HIAP-1，MIHC，API2），NAIP，ML-IAP，ILP2，livin（KIAP），apollon 和 survivin。尽管如此，并不是所有的 BIR 包含蛋白都是抑制凋亡的，它们中的一些同样具有功能而不是抑制 caspase。IAP 被 Smac/Diablo 所抑制。在细胞凋亡过程中，该蛋白随 Cyt-c 从线粒体释放，促进 caspase 的活化，结合并抑制 IAP。有研究表明，以上蛋白的过表达，都可以不同程度地抑制多种细胞凋亡。作用强度为 XIAP>cIAP2>cIAP1>survivin。

IAP 家族蛋白 survivin 的表达具有高度的肿瘤特异性。它存在于大多数人类肿瘤但不存在于正常的组织。在神经母细胞瘤中，它的表达与侵袭性更强、预后不良有关。但是，尽管 survivin 具有 BIR 结构域，其是否直接作为凋亡抑制因子尚不清楚。survivin 对细胞周期的完成也是必须的。然而，在某些情况下，survivin 的过表达会抑制凋亡：在转基因小鼠皮肤中表达 survivin 使抗凋亡功能较其在细胞分裂中的功能更为显著。在体内外，survivin 均可抑制 UVB 诱导的凋亡，却不影响 CD95 引起的细胞死亡。survivin 非磷酸化突变体的表达引起 Cyt-c 的释放及细胞死亡。在异种肿瘤移植物模型中，这种突变可以抑制肿瘤的生长并减少肿瘤播散。有报道说，survivin 与肿瘤细胞的抗药性、肿瘤转移过程中的血管生成有关。

体外实验表明，survivin 特异性地结合于细胞死亡蛋白酶的终末阶段分子 caspase-3 和 caspase-7，而不是起始阶段的 caspase-8，并由此对于暴露于多种凋亡刺激因素如 Fas（CD95）、Bax、caspases 及化疗药物的细胞起到抑制 caspases 活性和细胞死亡的作用[22]。caspase-3 是死亡受体途径及线粒体途径介导的凋亡过程中必需的死亡因子，在细胞中，caspase-3 通过与线粒体中 p21 或与 IAP 家族成员 ILP 的作用可使其失活。*survivin* 和 *bcl-2* 基因都是由无 TATA 富含 GC 启动子调节的，推测二者具有调节转录流行性的共同机制，协同发挥抗凋亡效应[22]。survivin 作用于细胞周期调节因子周期蛋白依赖性激酶（CDK）4，使 CDK2/细胞周期蛋白（cyclin）E 活化并使 Rb 磷酸化。survivin/ CDK4 复合物的形成，使 p21 从 p21/CDK4 复合物中释放出来并作用于 procaspase-3，形成 procaspase-3/p21 复合物，抑制 procaspase-3 激活成活化的 caspase-3，从而发挥其抗凋亡作用。

另一个 IAP 家族成员 cIAP2 受到 t（11；18）（q21；q21）转位的影响，50% 左右黏膜相关淋巴组织（MALT）淋巴瘤中存在该现象。这说明 cIAP2 在 MALT 淋巴瘤的发生中具有一定的作用。在黑色素瘤细胞株中 ML-IAP 的表达水平很高，而在原代细胞中并非如此。表达 ML-IAP 的黑色素瘤细胞株较不表达者能更显著抵抗药物诱导的凋亡。

（四）Fas

Fas 也称为 Apo-1、CD95，是 1989 年两家实验室同时发现在细胞株表面介导凋亡的蛋白分子，属于 NTFR（肿瘤坏死因子受体）和 NGFR（神经生长因子受体）家族，分子量 45kDa，是一种具有重要功能的膜受体，含一个死亡结构域。由 317 个氨基酸组成的 I 型跨膜糖蛋白，胞外有三个富含半胱氨酸的结构域（cysteine-rich domains，CRDs），具 TNFR 超家族的特点。Fas 配体（Fas ligand，FasL）是主要由免疫系统表达的配体，为 T 淋巴细胞上 Fas 的天然配基（ligant），又称为 CD95L。FasL 为 II 型膜蛋白，是 TNF 家族成员。FasL 与表达 Fas 的细胞结合，即导致后者走向凋亡。

在许多肿瘤细胞有广泛的 Fas 抗原表达，如结肠癌、乳腺癌、肝癌、肾细胞癌、膀胱癌、前列腺癌、恶性胶质瘤等[23]。Fas 能抑制肿瘤细胞增殖，诱导凋亡。许多耐药与复发的肿瘤中 CD95 和 FasL 突变，尤其在淋巴瘤、白血病和肠癌患者中常有 Fas 的表达，对预后有一定影响。抗肿瘤的免疫活性细胞如细胞毒性 T 细胞（cytotoxic T lymphocyte，CTL）介导肿瘤细胞死亡的机制中有凋亡作用，主要是通过渗透性溶解的凋亡方式，即在诱导肿瘤细胞凋亡中多个穿孔素在肿瘤细胞膜聚集成小管道，颗粒酶进入肿瘤细胞，引起肿瘤细胞 DNA 切割、细胞凋亡。同时 CTL 细胞也可以释放一些细胞因子，诱导肿瘤细胞上调凋亡抗原 Fas，后者与 CTL 细胞上的 FasL 结合激活肿瘤细胞中 DNA 核酸内切酶使细胞凋亡。反之，肿瘤细胞也可以引起 CTL 细胞的凋亡，有些肿瘤细胞高表达 FasL，可以激活 CTL 细胞上的 Fas，导致 CTL 细胞凋亡。

（五）p53

1979 年 Lane 等在 SV40 感染的小鼠细胞中发现了 p53 基因，对 p53 的认识分 3 个阶段：在 20 世纪 80 年代初一经发现就认为是一种肿瘤基因，后来发现主要表现在癌中所以称为癌基因，经过相当一段时间后，随着对凋亡研究的深入，1989 年才证明 p53 为抑癌基因。p53 基因定位于染色体 17p13.1。编码的正常 P53 蛋白（野生型）存在于核内，是一种核结合蛋白。正常细胞内存在野生型 p53（WT p53）对细胞增殖有抑制作用。研究发现，当细胞停滞在 G_1 期或发生细胞凋亡时细胞表达 p53。野生型 p53 基因在维持细胞生长、抑制细胞恶性增殖中起重要作用，因此 p53 被誉为基因卫士和分子警察（molecular policeman）（图 1-12）。

在静止细胞和终末期细胞中诱导细胞凋亡是困难的，因为细胞内不出现凋亡分子，所以细胞凋亡分子不会在所有的细胞类型和内环境稳定的条件下出现。当细胞中 DNA 损伤时，可以激活凋亡基因（如 WT p53）来抑制细胞周期激酶（cyclin-dependent kinase，CDK，该酶使细胞从 G_1 期进入 S 期），使进入增殖周期的细胞停留在 $G_1 \rightarrow S$ 期之间，容许细胞修复 DNA、避免突变。如修复成功，细胞进入 S 期；如修复失败，则通过活化 Bax 基因使细胞进入凋亡，以保证基因组的遗传稳定。

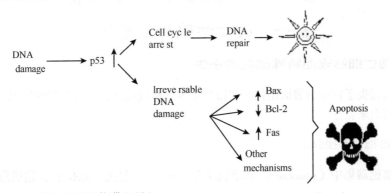

图 1-12　上调 p53 使细胞周期停滞和凋亡；Upregulation of p53 leads to cell-cycle arrest and apoptosis

在应激诱导的凋亡中，p53 是一个重要的分子。通过翻译后机制对各种形式的应激做出反应使 p53 迅速发挥作用。通过 ARF 或 MDM2 直接磷酸化使 MDM2 失活后可以稳定并活化 p53。增殖信号诱导 ARF，该分子由 CDKN2A（细胞周期依赖性激酶抑制基因）基因位点内的可选择性读码框架所编码，周期素依赖性蛋白激酶抑制子 INK4A 也是由其编码。p53 被 MDM2 所抑制，MDM2 是一种泛素连接酶，通过蛋白酶体靶向作用于 p53，MDM2 与 ARF 结合后失去活性。ARF 和泛素连接酶 MDM2 相互作用，阻止其结合 p53，引起蛋白酶体的靶向破坏。p53 的上调引起细胞周期停滞和细胞凋亡。此外，很多翻译后修饰可以增强 p53 的转录活性，包括磷酸化、SUMOYLATION（SUMO 为小泛素相关修饰物，SUMO 修饰其底物即 SUMOYLATION 过程）和乙酰化。p53 的转录活性对其功能的发挥是非常重要的。p53 可以诱导线粒体途径中一些蛋白的表达，如 Bax、NOXA、PUMA 和 p53AIP1 及死亡受体途径中蛋白质的表达（如 CD95、TRAIL-R1 和 TRAIL-R2）。除此之外，p53 的转录非依赖活性介导了一些促凋亡效应，包括蛋白质和蛋白质之间的相互作用、线粒体中的直接效应和细胞表面死亡受体的重新分布。

在许多肿瘤细胞有 p53 的缺失和突变则凋亡过程减弱。p53 基因发生突变后，因空间结构的变化影响其转录活化功能，从而丧失野生型 p53 抑制肿瘤的作用，而具备癌基因的功能。50% 以上的人类肿瘤中发现有 p53 基因的突变，尤其在结肠癌、肺癌、乳腺癌和胰腺癌的突变更为多见。p53 基因异常方式包括纯合缺失和点突变。在大多数肿瘤，两个 p53 等位基因均有失活。具有遗传性的一个 p53 基因突变的患者，如 Li-Fraumeni 综合征，发生第二次突变产生恶性肿瘤的可能性高于 p53 基因正常的人群 25 倍，主要发生肉瘤、乳腺癌、白血病等。近来还发现某些 DNA 病毒，如人乳头瘤病毒（HPV）和猿猴空泡病毒 40（SV-40），其致癌作用是通过它们的癌蛋白与活化的 Rb 蛋白或 P53 蛋白结合而使得转录因子 E2F 活化实现的。消化道上皮因最易受到食物中所含致癌物质的影响而受损或恶变。为维持正常功能，上皮每 3～5 天更新一次，主要以凋亡方式进行。凋亡过程中常有抑癌基因（p53、Rb 等）的激活和表达。因此，一旦消化道肿瘤发生，则常伴有癌基因表达，包括突变型 p53 基因、Rb 基因、DCC（deleted in colorectal carcinoma）基因、FAP（家族性息肉病）基因、MCC（mutated in colorectal carcinoma）基因和 nm23 转移抑制基因等。

第二节 凋亡细胞的形态特征

一、凋亡细胞的形态学

（一）凋亡细胞表面特殊结构的丧失

凋亡细胞丧失了特殊的表面结构（如微绒毛等）和接触区，形成光滑的轮廓，容易从周围活细胞中分离出来。

（二）细胞体积缩小

①胞质细胞器集中（squeeze）；②胞膜出芽（bud）或起泡（bleb）；③胞质致密；④细胞皱缩（shrinkage）。

（三）保持细胞器完整性

凋亡细胞中①线粒体不肿胀，内膜不破裂；②短暂滑面内质网（SER）扩张，扩张间隙与细胞表面融合；③有时有聚集排列的半结晶状核糖体；④可有与细胞表面平行的微丝束。

（四）核内染色质结构改变

凋亡细胞最具特征性的改变在于细胞核。①核质固缩（condensation）；②染色质边集（margination）；③核质紧实（compaction）；④核膜皱褶（fold）。在透射电镜下，染色质浓缩在一起呈颗粒状、半月形蘑菇状，或完整的念珠形；核孔集中于少数区域，浓缩的染色质并不贴附在核膜上；转录复合物（transcriptional complexes）从核仁中脱落到核质中呈一簇嗜锇酸小体。残留的核仁蛋白核心转移到周围染色质特征性部位。核扭曲、断裂呈若干片段，所有片段开始时均有核膜包绕。

（五）形成凋亡小体

凋亡细胞胞质芽突并脱落形成若干个由质膜包绕的小体，称为凋亡小体（apoptotic body）。凋亡小体中可含有细胞器的成分和细胞核碎片。

二、凋亡细胞被清除的过程

凋亡细胞或凋亡小体迅速被邻近的实质细胞（通常为同类细胞）或吞噬细胞识别（图 1-13），被噬于吞噬细胞体内形成吞噬体（phagosome），所以凋亡小体最常见于细胞异吞噬体中（heterophagosome），经溶酶体消化后形成溶酶体残余小体（lysosomal residual bodies），最终被降解。偶尔凋亡小体逃避被吞噬，如凋亡的导管上皮可以掉入导管腔中，这种凋亡小体最终丧失其密度、膜断裂。细胞凋亡被吞噬后留下的空隙由周围细胞填充，不留痕迹。

（1）凋亡发生早期细胞体积缩小（<50%）、密度增加、胞质细胞器保留完整，说明细胞是有选择性地丧失了水和电解质，而较致密的结构成分得以保留下来，这种水分的迅速输出可能在内质网，使之在与细胞表面融合前呈短暂性扩张。

（2）细胞质、细胞核冒泡的机制还不十分清楚，Fesus 发现在这个时相中，TTG 的活性可在受损细胞中检测到，TTG 是交联蛋白酶，能使蛋白质变质而不被溶解，在凋亡细胞膜下构成一层由 TTG 诱导的交联蛋白质形成的僵硬壳，引起凋亡细胞的形态改变。因此 TTG 与凋亡细胞体积缩小和不溶解性有关。

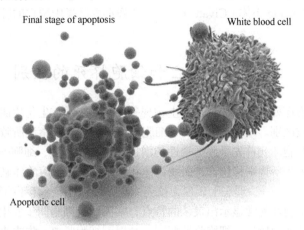

图 1-13　扫描电镜下白细胞吞噬凋亡小体；The leukocyte phagocytosis apoptotic body under the scanning electron microscopy

（3）凋亡细胞、凋亡小体被邻近吞噬细胞或其他细胞识别与吞噬，这需要一种特殊的非免疫性识别机制。近期研究显示，人体巨噬细胞通过巨噬细胞玻连蛋白受体（vitronectin receptor）与凋亡的中性粒细胞或其他凋亡细胞上的相关配体相连接，巨噬细胞玻连蛋白是整合素家族的一个成员，属于细胞黏附分子（cell adhesion molecule，CAM），分子量为 75kDa，分布于血浆和组织中。至于受体识别凋亡细胞表面配体后发生连接的性质还有待于进一步研究。

除了巨噬细胞吞噬凋亡细胞外，上皮细胞、肿瘤细胞也有这一功能，最近发现吞噬细胞上至少有 3 类受体（植物凝集素、磷脂酰丝氨酸受体和血栓连接素），凋亡细胞上出现有相应的配体，介导两者相互应答反应。

（4）吞噬细胞的识别机制

1）凋亡细胞表面膜结构改变，表面糖蛋白失去唾液酸侧键，使原来处于隐蔽状态的单糖暴露出来，与吞噬细胞表面的植物凝集素结合被吞噬。

2）细胞膜内侧的磷脂酰丝氨酸翻露到细胞外，被吞噬细胞表面相应的受体识别并吞噬[24]。

3）吞噬细胞可以分泌血小板反应蛋白（thrombospoudin），也是细胞外基质成分，存在于血小板、巨噬细胞、内皮细胞、成纤维细胞中，可黏附纤维连接蛋白（纤连蛋白，FN）、纤维蛋白原和糖蛋白。

4）介导多种细胞的相互作用或细胞表面的蛋白多糖、硫酸脂等受体，也可与凋亡小体表面的相应成分结合而有利于凋亡小体被吞噬。

（5）定时电动摄像研究发现，凋亡发生开始得很突然，受到死刺激后不久，被攻击的细胞突然皱缩、冒泡并凋亡，这时期仅仅持续数分钟，然后产生皱缩的凋亡小体。凋亡小体一旦形成，停留在组织中被辨认出来的时间为 4～9 小时，这段时间与巨噬细胞在体内吞噬大生物结构完全被降解的时间相符，由于这一过程很短，因此在组织切片中，所见到的凋亡小体即便是少量的增加，也可能隐藏着较大的细胞丧失率。例如，在历经 3 天细胞数已丧失一半的萎缩组织中，在光镜下见到的凋亡小体数还不到 5%。凋亡发生迅速，在短期内即完成细胞死亡阶段（dying process）和细胞被清除阶段（elimination process）。凋亡细胞迅速被吞噬，其空隙由周围细胞来填充，凋亡小体的完整膜使之周围缺乏炎症反应，因此不留痕迹。

（6）尽管凋亡对细胞死亡来说是非常有意义的生物学行为，但至今为止凋亡表现在不同组织中仍有不同的名称，如①存在于淋巴滤泡生发中心中的含有凋亡淋巴细胞或其他细胞碎片的巨噬细胞，称为可染色的巨噬细胞（tingible body macrophages）；②银屑病中的凋亡性角化细胞称为胶样小体或 Civatte 小体（Civatte body）；③病毒性肝炎中凋亡的肝细胞称为康西耳曼体（Councilman body）。

三、细胞凋亡和细胞坏死的区别

细胞凋亡与细胞坏死是不同的过程与生物现象。在形态学、生化代谢、分子机制、结局和意义等方面都有本质区别。坏死常常是由于细胞外环境条件严重紊乱所致，并伴有不可控制的细胞肿胀和破裂，细胞坏死首先是膜通透性的增加、渗透性改变、细胞外形发生不规则变化、内质网扩张、核染色质不规则移位，进而线粒体和细胞核肿胀、溶酶体破坏、细胞膜破裂、胞质外溢、周围引起炎症反应，形态上表现为核固缩、碎裂、溶解。坏死的细胞内 ATP 和蛋白的合成受抑与终止。细胞坏死常显示出被杀的特点，常为成组细胞同步发生。

凋亡细胞的特征如前所述，细胞收缩变圆，与周围细胞脱离，失去表面结构，胞质浓缩，内质网扩张与膜融合，线粒体无明显变化。核染色质密度增加并凝聚于核膜下，核仁裂解，进而细胞膜内陷将细胞自行分割为多个具膜包裹的凋亡小体，这种细胞死亡过程不发生溶酶体、线粒体及细胞膜破裂，没有细胞内含物的外泄，故不引起炎症反应，不影响局部微环境和周围组织的次级损伤。凋亡时 ATP、某些 mRNA 和蛋白质的合成仍在进行，细胞第二信使系统仍能活动。发生凋亡的细胞有蛋白质和 RNA 合成的功能，有某些特殊基因的表现，显示主动自杀性特点。从形态学方面鉴别凋亡与坏死见表 1-1 和图 1-14。

表 1-1　凋亡与坏死主要鉴别

指标	凋亡	坏死
细胞形态	细胞膜出芽、冒泡但完整性好，活组织中个别细胞死亡	细胞完整性破坏 成片细胞死亡，破坏组织结构
过程	核固缩，胞质浓染，细胞脱离，形成凋亡小体	细胞肿胀，核淡染，凝固性坏死，无膜性小体
细胞器	细胞器未遭破坏，胞质浓缩	细胞器肿胀、溶解
染色质	染色质致密、凝集或边集浓染	染色质疏松变性、粗糙
溶酶体	完整	损伤
线粒体	浓缩，跨膜电位受损，Cyct-c 释放等	肿胀、破裂，能量生成受损
染料排斥试验	开始被排斥	染料掺入（膜破裂或通透性增加）
DNA 破坏机制	核酸内切酶作用核酸 DNA，裂解为 200bp 或其倍数片断（核孔裂开）	随机降解，弥漫 ATP 膜损伤，氧自由基损伤
蛋白质	caspase 活化	非特征性降解
底物	特异性降解	非特异性水解
对 ATP 要求	必需	无需
组织分布	单个细胞	细胞群体
结局	凋亡小体可被同种或异种细胞识别吞噬	吞噬细胞吞噬细胞碎片、溶解
组织反应	不引起炎症反应，迅速退化，无整个组织瓦解，不诱发组织的再生与修复，细胞生长增殖→凋亡	引起炎症反应，继发性组织损伤，诱发组织再生与修复，形成瘢痕，坏死→补偿性增生→细胞增殖

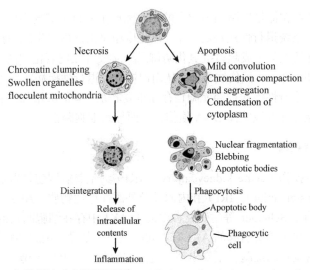

图 1-14　细胞凋亡和坏死的区别；Differences between necrosis and apoptosis

第三节　疾病中凋亡的研究

一、诱发细胞凋亡的因素

（1）诱导性因素：①激素和生长因子失衡，如在部分生理性萎缩与退化中有凋亡机制参与，凋亡在正常周期性刺激的上皮（包括人体子宫内膜表皮等）细胞更新中与核分裂相平衡。临床使用大量糖皮质激素时可导致淋巴细胞凋亡。②射线、高温、酸、碱、乙醇、抗癌药物等理化因素。在有些情况下凋亡明显表现为某些细胞具有选择性，如睾丸经放射或暴露于放射性药物后，精原细胞选择性死亡，而间质细胞却保留着（使性功能、性特征保留，但生育能力降低）。③免疫性因素，如 CTL 分泌穿孔素在靶细胞膜聚合，使释放粒酶能够进入靶细胞。粒酶活化靶细胞中的 caspase。此外，粒酶 B 可能直接剪切 Bcl-2 家族成员 Bid 以活化线粒体死亡途径，导致靶细胞凋亡；微生物学因素，如艾滋病 HIV 感染使 CD4$^+$细胞凋亡等。

（2）抑制性因素：包括有细胞因子（IL-2/NGF）和激素（促肾上腺皮质激素、睾酮、雌激素）。一旦细胞因子释放减少或信号转导及受体障碍，就会引起效应细胞的凋亡发生，如前列腺、肾上腺皮质在靶器官激素减少后（由于手术或药物的作用），哺乳后的乳腺的生理萎缩与退化，结扎主导管后腮腺的萎缩等，部分由上皮细胞凋亡而介导。其他因素有金属阳离子(Zn^{2+})、药物（苯巴比妥、半胱氨酸酶抑制剂）、病毒（EB 病毒、牛痘病毒）等。

二、细胞凋亡异常增加

（一）神经系统退行性疾病

神经系统退行性疾病是一类严重影响人类健康的常见病，神经元死亡是一些神经系统退行性疾病的共同特征，其中包括较少数病程进展较快（2~3 年）的肌萎缩性侧索硬化症及病程较长（20 年或更长）的如帕金森病（Parkinson disease，PD）、阿尔茨海默病（Alzheimer disease，AD）、亨廷顿病（Huntington disease，HD）等，某些导致这些疾病的发病机制现已得到基本确认，其中线粒体功能失调及由线粒体介导的神经细胞凋亡在退行性疾病发生、发展中起了重要作用。现普遍认为线粒体是控制细胞凋亡的中心和产生氧自由基的主要场所，线粒体功能失调可以导致许多神经系统退行性疾病的发生。氧化应激是指活性氧生成与抗氧化防御系统之间的不平衡状态，可在活性氧生成超过抗氧化防御系统时或者在抗氧化剂活性降低时发生，导致线粒体能量代谢失调，进一步损伤线粒体，从而促进神经退行性疾病的发生、发展。例如，AD中线粒体氧化应激与退行性疾病神经元凋亡存在重要联系，其能够增加线粒体膜的通透性、抑制线粒体呼吸链功能和导致线粒体 DNA 损伤，从而导致细胞凋亡。

（二）损伤性疾病

临床上，急性肾损伤（acute kidney injury，AKI）的主要病因包括败血症、缺血再灌注损伤（ischemia reperfusion injury，IRI）和内源性及外源性毒性物质。AKI 的主要病理学改变为肾小管损伤。1992 年，Schumer 等的研究首次证实 AKI 中存在细胞凋亡的现象[25]，而缺血再灌注损伤和毒性物质如顺铂所引起的 AKI 有不同的发病机制导致细胞凋亡[26, 27]。在 AKI 中，肾皮质和肾髓质都有凋亡的细胞，主要出现在近曲和远曲小管上皮细胞。多种肾脏保护药物，如米诺环素（minocycline），均能通过减少肾小管上皮细胞凋亡以减轻 AKI。最新研究显示，针对 caspase-3 的裸小干扰 RNA 能够保护猪的离体肾脏冷缺血造成的损伤[23]。尽管多种类型的病因导致的 AKI 中都有细胞凋亡的证据，但是引起凋亡的上游信号通路各有不同。研究表明，缺氧条件下培养的肾小管上皮细胞，缺氧直接导致线粒体外膜通透性（mitochondrial outer membrane permeabilization，MOMP）的改变，导致 Cyt-c 的释放，结合于 Apaf-1 进一步激活 caspase-9，即内源性凋亡通路。该通路中，Bcl-2 蛋白家族成员 Bak 和 Bax 能够促进细胞凋亡，而这两个基因的敲除能够减轻 AKI[26]。缺血和败血症所引起的 AKI 中，死亡受体 TNF-α、Fas 和配体相结合后募集适体蛋白，然后激活 caspase-8，即外源性凋亡通路[28]。TNF-α受体敲除的小鼠能够抵抗顺铂造成的 AKI[29]。内质网应激激活 caspase-12 也是小管细胞凋亡通路[30]。

（三）感染性疾病

病毒感染导致的细胞死亡多数属于细胞凋亡，可能引起凋亡的病毒包括腺病毒、人类免疫缺陷病毒（HIV）、肝炎病毒等。人类免疫缺陷病毒 1 型（HIV-1）感染可使被感染者体内 CD4+ 细胞数量减少，最终导致艾滋病。细胞凋亡为 HIV-1 诱导细胞死亡的一个重要机制。HIV 可直接诱导细胞凋亡，也可以通过活化作用，同源被感染的细胞的介导，以及 CD8+ T 细胞诱导细胞凋亡。且细胞因子在 HIV 诱导细胞凋亡的过程中发挥着重要的作用。HIV 编码的蛋白质可以通过各种不同的机制诱导感染和未被感染的细胞发生凋亡。HIV 感染伴随着被感染和未被感染 HIV 的 CD4+ T 细胞中凋亡的增多。HIV-1 表达的 Vpr 蛋白除通过使 CD4+T 细胞周期停止在 G2 期而诱导细胞凋亡外，还可直接导致线粒体膜通透性增加激活内源性凋亡途径诱导细胞死亡。HIV 病毒的外膜糖蛋白 gp120 与 CD4+ T 细胞的交叉结合引起对 Fas 介导的杀伤作用敏感性的升高。在已激活的 CD4+ T 细胞中，gp120 的交叉结合引起细胞凋亡（可能由 IFN、TNF 或两者同时介导），Bcl-2 表达的下调，以及 caspase-3 的活化。另外，Tat 还被视为在未被感染的 T 细胞中的细胞凋亡的诱导者，它可能是通过依赖于 Fas 的机制，或过氧化物歧化酶的抑制作用，或者细胞周期依赖性蛋白激酶（CDK）的活化作用诱导细胞死亡。由于 Nef 在 HIV 病毒的致病性中是必需的，所以 HIV 编码的 Nef 已经被视为一个潜在的细胞凋亡的中介体。HIV 蛋白酶直接裂分 caspase-8，并且通过对抗凋亡蛋白质 Bcl-2 的蛋白水解酶的降解作用改变细胞对凋亡的易感性，而 HIV 蛋白酶不能影响未感染细胞的死亡。CTL 介导的靶细胞凋亡：CTL 活化后大量表达并分泌 FasL，释放颗粒酶，可借助穿孔素构筑的小孔穿越靶细胞膜，激活另一个起始性 caspase-10，引发 caspase 级联反应，导致靶细胞凋亡。

在病毒性肝炎中，由于机体对病毒发生免疫反应，而引起肝细胞的凋亡，表现为嗜酸性小体的形成，甚至肝细胞碎屑状坏死中也有凋亡机制的作用。

（四）缺血性损伤

心肌缺血-再灌注损伤性损伤中①缺血早期以凋亡为主；②梗死灶周边以凋亡为主；③轻度缺血区以凋亡为主④发生缺血-再灌注损伤较单纯缺血凋亡严重。

心力衰竭时由于氧化应激/压力、容量负荷增加/神经-内分泌失调/TNF/缺血/缺氧引起心肌细胞凋亡。引起凋亡的机制：①氧化应激，SOD 可减轻；②受体 Fas 上调，FasL 反应；③p53 激活。缺血性脑病有相似的情况。

三、细胞凋亡过度减少

以细胞凋亡不足为特征的疾病包括肿瘤、自身免疫疾病和某些病毒感染疾病等。细胞凋亡不足，导致细胞群体失稳态，病变细胞异常增多或凋亡减少，影响器官功能。

（一）自身免疫性疾病

淋巴细胞发育成熟过程中，约有95%的细胞发生凋亡，T 细胞受体（T cell receptor，TCR）基因发生重排时，TCR 基因某一连接点上发生等位基因无意义突变，不能产生或产生不正确的 TCR 分子，细胞即走向凋亡。即使产生正确 TCR 分子，细胞还必须经过进一步的严格选择机制，使可能导致自身免疫性疾病的细胞凋亡，这就是胸腺的阴性选择机制。

淋巴细胞发育成熟过程中，约有95%的细胞发生凋亡，自身免疫病最主要的特征是自身抗体或致敏 T 淋巴细胞攻击含有自身抗原的细胞，造成器官组织损伤。正常情况下，免疫系统在发育过程中通过细胞凋亡可将针对自身抗原的免疫细胞有效清除。胸腺通过阳性选择（positive selection）将具有与非己抗原——主要组织相容性复合体（MHC）抗原结合的 TCR 的单阳性细胞选择性保留和存活下来，并进入外周 T 细胞库。这样可以确保阳性选择的 T 细胞不会针对自身抗原而仅针对非己抗原产生免疫反应。胸腺通过阴性选择（负选择，negative selection）将具有与自身抗原——MHC 抗原有高度亲和力的 TCR 的双阳性细胞选择性去除（即在自身抗原与胸腺上皮细胞膜的 MHC 分子共同作用下，通过细胞凋亡而清除）。如果胸腺功能异常，负选择机制失调，那些针对自身抗原的细胞就可存活并增殖，进而攻击自身组织，产生自身免疫病，如多发性硬化症、胰岛素依赖型糖尿病、慢性甲状腺炎等。在淋巴细胞中调节细胞凋亡的一个重要细胞表面受体为 Fas。病毒感染或抗原刺激能诱导 T 淋巴细胞产生 FasL。FasL 与靶细胞表达的 Fas 结合能引起靶细胞的凋亡。B 细胞的发育过程与 T 细胞相似，编码免疫球蛋白的基因片段要经过基因重排，才能在细胞表面产生独特的个体型免疫球蛋白的受体。发育成熟的 B 淋巴细胞表面免疫球蛋白，在抗原的刺激下引起克隆消除，从而把可能引起自身反应性的 B 细胞清除掉，这就是 B 细胞的阴性选择机制。成熟的白细胞的寿命以天计算，死一批，生一批，互相交替，非常严格有序，若细胞凋亡障碍，就会导致白细胞堆积而引起白细胞增生症。如果 B 细胞的发育过程发生错误重组，表面免疫球蛋白就不能正常表达，对自身抗原反应的细胞该死亡的不死亡，发生自身免疫性疾病。60%的系统性红斑狼疮（systemic lupus erythematosus，SLE）患者外周血中存在可溶性 Fas，它能竞争性地抑制 Fas 和 FasL 的相互作用，结果减少了 Fas 介导的凋亡而加速了自身免疫细胞的增生。Bcl-2 过量表达的转基因小鼠亦通过影响 B 淋巴细胞的凋亡而出现 SLE 类似症状。此外，Bcl-2 过量表达也与自身免疫性糖尿病有关。因此，从细胞凋亡角度看，自身免疫病的发病是由于细胞凋亡不足，未能有效清除自身免疫性淋巴细胞所致。迄今为止，糖皮质激素仍是治疗自身免疫性疾病的有效药物之一，其主要机制就是诱导那些异常存活的自身免疫性 T 细胞凋亡。

（二）感染性疾病

生物因素引起的组织损伤称为感染，炎症是感染的主要形式。炎症的基本病变中，渗出是最重要的，没有渗出就不称为炎症。炎症时，从血管渗出的中性粒细胞在病灶中完成抗炎任务后，不能重回血管，需要启动细胞凋亡的机制，使炎症终止。创口修复中的肉芽组织，成纤维细胞增生与胶原分泌，以及随后成纤维细胞转变为纤维细胞，及瘢痕形成，凋亡机制也可能参与愈合。

肿瘤相关病毒 EB 病毒（Epstein–Barr virus，EBV）和人疱疹病毒 8（HHV8 或者卡波西肉瘤相关疱疹病毒）编码 Bcl-2 同源性蛋白。来自 EBV 的 BHRF1 和来自 HHV8 的 KSbcl-2(vBcl-2)均具有抗凋亡功能并能增强感染细胞的存活。由此看来，在病毒感染后，它们有助于肿瘤的形成并使肿瘤抵抗治疗。病毒感染（腺病毒、疱疹病毒、痘病毒等）与细胞凋亡之间关系密切，表现在病毒基因及其表达产物对细胞凋亡具有显著的调节作用。病毒感染，通过其特定基因组的表达，抑制或促进细胞凋亡，与病毒形成长期潜伏感染、致正常细胞的恶性转化、调节免疫功能、自身免疫疾病的发病等有着极为密切的关系。病毒的靶目标是宿主活细胞，它需要利用宿主细胞的物质和能量系统来复制自己，完成自身的生活周期。病毒的侵入对细胞造成的损害，以及为病毒复制需要而表达的病毒蛋白，都会激发宿主细胞的凋亡机制。这对周围未感染细胞和机体是一种保护，但对病毒的大量复制则是不利的。经过选择和进化的病毒具有抑制细胞凋亡的能力，病毒通过自身抗凋亡基因的表达或者激活宿主细胞的抗凋亡基因的表达以阻止细胞凋亡、完成病毒的复制和生活周期。例如，猿猴病毒 40(SV40)的 T 抗原和人乳头瘤病毒（HPV）的 E6 蛋白通过灭活 p53 而抑制细胞凋亡。因此在病毒感染的局部常呈增生性改变，如尖锐湿疣等。部分病毒则是肿瘤发生的诱因，如 EBV、HPV、乙型肝炎病毒（HBV）、丙型肝炎病毒（HCV）等。在 EB 病毒阳性的伯基特淋巴瘤细胞株中，Fas 相关性死亡结构域蛋白样白介素转化酶抑制蛋白（FLIP）和 caspase-8 比例的升高与对 CD95 介导的凋亡的抵抗相关。FLIP 的病毒类似物称为病毒性 FLIPs(v-FLIP)由一些肿瘤病毒编码，包括 HHV8。在潜在感染 HHV8 的细胞中，v-FLIP 的表达水平较低，而在进展期卡波西肉瘤中其表达增加，这种情况也出现在体外培养的淋巴瘤细胞中。因此，v-FLIP 可能赋予了 v-FLIP 编码病毒的持续性和致瘤性。虽然 FLIP 的表达通过死亡受体途径阻碍凋亡，但它并不抑制由穿孔素/粒酶、化疗药物或放疗诱导的细胞死亡。在小鼠模型中它介导了肿瘤的免疫逃逸。在体内，穿孔素/粒酶途径存在的情况下，FLIP 表达水平高的肿瘤逃避了 T 细胞介导的免疫。因此，FLIP 水平高的肿瘤细胞具有选择优势。FLIP 过表达也可以通过穿孔素缺乏的 NK 细胞防止肿瘤的抵抗。此外，人黑色素瘤和鼠科 B 细胞淋巴瘤细胞株表达高水平 FLIP，它在死亡受体水平干扰凋亡。

（三）肿瘤性疾病

在多细胞器官的细胞和组织中，有效的生理机制控制细胞增殖和内环境的稳定。很多这种生长调控机制都和凋亡相关：在不当部位的过度增殖或生长会引起细胞凋亡。目前认为细胞增殖和分化异常是肿瘤发病的途径之一，而凋亡受抑、细胞死亡不足是肿瘤发病的另一途径。肿瘤细胞对凋亡的抵抗可能是癌症发生的基本特征。肿瘤的形成中过表达生长促进的癌基因如

c-myc、E1A 或者 E2F1 的细胞是对凋亡敏感的细胞。除了表达促进细胞增殖的蛋白，肿瘤的发生发展还需要抗凋亡蛋白的表达或者必要的凋亡前体蛋白失活。

许多人类恶性肿瘤细胞对生理刺激做出凋亡反应的能力显著下降。肿瘤细胞通过表达抗凋亡蛋白，或者下调或突变促凋亡蛋白，获得对凋亡的抵抗力。多种肿瘤组织（如前列腺癌、结肠癌等）中 Bcl-2 基因的表达显著高于周围正常组织，提示这些肿瘤与细胞凋亡减少有关。肿瘤细胞可以通过不同的机制获得对凋亡的抗性，这些机制在不同水平干扰凋亡信号。其中一种机制是抗凋亡基因的过表达。滤泡型 B 细胞淋巴瘤的普遍特点是染色体易位 t（14；18），偶联 Bcl-2 基因至免疫球蛋白重链，导致 Bcl-2 表达增强。Bcl-2 和癌蛋白 c-Myc 或者急性前髓细胞性白血病中的前髓细胞性白血病视黄酸受体（PML-RAR）融合蛋白协同作用，由此导致肿瘤的形成。一些研究证实了高水平 Bcl-2 表达和人类肿瘤恶性程度相关。此外，体内实验和体外实验表明 Bcl-2 的表达引起机体对多种化疗药物和放疗的抵抗。在一些类型的肿瘤中，高水平 Bcl-2 的表达与对化疗的低反应性相关，并可能预示较短的无瘤生存率，如乳腺作为激素控制的靶器官，乳腺细胞凋亡受激素控制,细胞凋亡调控异常是乳癌发生的原因之一。雌激素（ER）或孕激素（PR）（+）的乳腺癌抗雌激素治疗，或采用内分泌干预能使瘤细胞发生凋亡。Bcl-2 阳性乳腺癌产生耐药主要机制是抑制化疗药物多柔比星诱发细胞凋亡的作用。同样前列腺癌是男性激素依赖性肿瘤，随着前列腺特异性抗原（prostatic specific antigen，PSA）的应用，新发现的前列腺癌增多。雄激素依赖型前列腺癌（androgen dependent prostatic carcinoma，ADPC）Bcl-2（-）时，性腺切除、雄激素拮抗剂的治疗有效，其机制是对雄激素敏感的癌细胞在缺乏雄激素后凋亡。雄激素非依赖型前列腺癌（androgen independent prostatic carcinoma，AIPC）Bcl-2（+）时，上述治疗效果差。转移性前列腺癌 70%患者只有短暂疗效，3 年内复发转变为 AIPC。

除了过表达抗凋亡基因，肿瘤可以通过下调或突变促凋亡分子获得对凋亡的抗性。在某些类型的癌症中，促凋亡 Bcl-2 家族成员 Bax 突变。两种较常见的突变是移码突变（导致表达丢失）和 BH 功能域的突变（导致功能丧失）。发生移码突变的肿瘤细胞株对凋亡更具有抵抗力。Bax 的表达下降与对化疗的反应性差相关，并在某些情况下缩短了存活率。除此以外，其他研究表明野生型 Bax 的失活在肿瘤的克隆演变中赋予其很强的优势。给裸小鼠注入野生型或突变型 Bax 克隆，在这两种情况下，均可产生肿瘤。

大约 60%的肿瘤中有 p53 的突变。当 p53 基因突变或缺失时，细胞凋亡减弱，机体肿瘤的发生率明显增加。例如，在非小细胞肺癌中 p53 基因突变率为 50%以上，小细胞肺癌甚至高达 80%。许多肿瘤凋亡指数（apoptotic index，AI）与肿瘤进展、预后有关。在基底细胞癌中，就癌细胞异型性和分化程度应为高度恶性的肿瘤，但其生物学行为为低度恶性表现，仅为局部浸润、很少转移。研究发现，该肿瘤中细胞凋亡明显，这对降低肿瘤浸润与转移有一定关系。

在不同的癌细胞株中可以观察到促凋亡蛋白 XAF1（XIAP 相关因子）的表达下降。XAF1 与 XIAP 结合，从而在 caspases 水平抵抗其抗凋亡功能。

转移性黑色素瘤可以通过另外一种途径逃避线粒体依赖的凋亡。这些肿瘤往往不表达 APAF1，该分子可以形成凋亡体，并且 APAF1 基因座具有很高的等位基因丢失率。剩余的等位基因通过基因甲基化发生转录失活。APAF1 阴性的黑色素瘤不能对化疗发生反应，这种状况在该类型肿瘤中较为常见。

此外，在很多肿瘤中死亡受体下调或失活。死亡受体 CD95 在一些肿瘤细胞中是减少的。例如，与它们的正常组织相比，在肝癌、结肠癌、黑色素瘤和其他一些肿瘤中表达减少。或许，通过转录下调引起的 CD95 的丢失是抗药性和免疫逃逸的原因。致癌性 Ras 可能下调 CD95，并且在 CD95 表达缺失的肝癌中伴有 p53 的异常。几种 CD95 基因突变已报告在骨髓瘤和 T 细胞白血病中。突变包括 CD95 胞质死亡功能域中的点突变及可以导致死亡受体缩短的染色体缺失。CD95 的这些突变形式可能通过明显相反的途径干扰由其诱导的凋亡。在遗传性 CD95 突变的家族中，常导致自身免疫淋巴细胞增生综合征（autoimmune lymphoproliferative syndrome, ALPS），在肿瘤中，同样也观察到了死亡受体 TRAIL-R1 和 TRAIL-R2 的缺失和突变。在头颈部癌症和非小细胞肺癌中染色体 8p21-22 的缺失影响 TRAIL-R2 基因。TRAIL-R1 或 TRAIL-R2 的外结构域或死亡结构域中发现有突变。进一步的突变导致这些 TRAIL 受体缩短或其他抗凋亡形式。

肿瘤干扰死亡受体介导的凋亡的另外一种机制可能是作为死亡配体诱饵的可溶性受体的表达。两个可溶性受体——可溶性 CD95（sCD95）和诱饵受体 3（DcR3）竞争性抑制 CD95 信号途径。sCD95 在不同的恶性肿瘤中都有所表达，在癌症患者的血清中其水平增高。在黑色素瘤患者中，高 sCD95 血清水平与预后较差相关。DcR3 和 CD95L 及 TNF 家族成员 LIGHT（一种与淋巴细胞毒素同源的细胞因子，呈诱导性表达，与单纯疱疹病毒（HSV）糖蛋白 D 竞争与疱疹病毒调节子（HVEM，一种 T 细胞表达的受体）结合并抑制 CD95L 诱导的凋亡。在一些肺癌和结肠癌患者中，它能通过遗传学放大；在一些腺癌、神经胶质瘤细胞株和恶性胶质瘤中过表达。在大鼠神经胶质瘤模型中，DcR3 的异位表达引起免疫细胞浸润减少，提示 DcR3 与恶性胶质瘤的免疫逃逸相关。最终，肿瘤细胞不仅通过死亡受体途径，还通过干扰穿孔素/粒酶途径来抵抗细胞毒性淋巴细胞的杀伤。丝氨酸蛋白酶抑制剂 PI-9/SPI-6 的表达可以抑制粒酶 B，导致肿瘤细胞对细胞毒性淋巴细胞的抵抗，引起免疫逃逸。

大部分肿瘤依靠 PI3K/AKT（磷酸肌醇 3-激酶/蛋白激酶 B）途径改变的生存信号而不依赖于能防止正常细胞死亡的生存信号。致癌基因如 Ras 或 BCR-ABL 可以增强 PI3K 的活性。在卵巢癌中 PI3K 的催化亚单位得到增强。PTEN 是 PI3K 的细胞性抵抗物，在进展期肿瘤中常缺失。在不同的癌症类型中可以发现 PTEN 的突变率较高。

在神经母细胞瘤中，N-myc 致癌基因被放大。在该肿瘤中，启动子 caspase-8 常由于基因缺失或甲基化而失活。caspase-8 缺失的神经母细胞瘤细胞可以抵抗死亡受体介导的凋亡和多柔比星介导的凋亡。

在机体与肿瘤细胞的对抗中，细胞凋亡具有十分重要的生物学意义。一方面，机体利用细胞凋亡机制，主动出击、围剿、清除肿瘤细胞，实现机体的抗肿瘤作用；另一方面，肿瘤细胞利用细胞凋亡机制，清除衰老细胞或正常细胞，维持肿瘤细胞高速增长。肿瘤的形成、恶化或消退是相互制约、相互对抗的结果。增加癌细胞的凋亡能干扰肿瘤的生物学过程。

四、细胞凋亡不足与过度并存

人类组织器官通常由不同种类的细胞构成，如心脏的主要细胞是心肌细胞和心肌间质细胞，血管则以内皮细胞和平滑肌细胞为主。由于细胞类型的差异，各种细胞在致病因素的作用下，有些细胞可以表现为凋亡不足，而另一些细胞则可表现为凋亡过度，因此在同一疾病或病理过程中两种情况可同时并存。动脉粥样硬化（atherosclerosis, AS）的粥样斑块中，内皮细胞凋亡，而平滑肌细胞的增殖始终占主导地位，使 AS 的血管壁变厚、变硬。研究表明，当血管平滑肌增殖活性升高的同时，伴随的细胞凋亡活动也有所增强，试图维持平滑肌细胞数的动态平衡。正常情况下血管平滑肌细胞也有低水平（约 0.06%）凋亡存在，在 AS 过程中血管平滑肌细胞的凋亡大幅度升高。有人定量地测定冠状动脉粥样硬化病灶内凋亡的平滑肌细胞可达29%。显然，平滑肌细胞的凋亡是为了抗衡平滑肌增殖活动的增强，是一种防止血管壁增厚的保护性反应。有学者在实验性经皮腔内冠状动脉成形术（PTCA）后再狭窄模型中发现，在内皮损伤后第 9 天，平滑肌细胞增殖与凋亡均达到峰值，但细胞凋亡数仅为增殖数的 75%。因此，增殖与凋亡相抵后平滑肌细胞数的净增殖仍然增加。最近有学者提出促进平滑肌细胞凋亡防止其过度增殖是抗 AS 的新思路。

此外，细胞凋亡机制在其他许多疾病如骨质疏松、胰岛素依赖型糖尿病、白血病、胶原病、皮肤病、肝脏疾病、胃肠道疾病等的发生和发展中均具有重要作用。对细胞凋亡的研究必将为上述疾病的防治开辟新的领域。

五、针对细胞凋亡的治疗策略

目前临床上所采用的各种抗肿瘤的治疗方法如化学治疗、放射治疗、物理治疗、生物治疗、促细胞分化治疗甚或基因治疗多是通过诱导细胞凋亡，以求达到治疗肿瘤的目的。抗癌药物分为 DNA 损伤剂、抗代谢药、有丝分裂抑制剂、核苷酸类似物或拓扑异构酶抑制剂。用这些药物进行治疗或者放疗能引起细胞应激并最终导致细胞死亡。但在肿瘤治疗中癌细胞的耐药则是化疗中最棘手的问题。

（1）合理利用凋亡因素：如中、小剂量放疗引起的细胞凋亡而不引起坏死（坏死对组织损害较大）。低剂量照射使急性 T 细胞性白血病发生细胞凋亡；TNF-α 可在体外引起白血病细胞株 U937 凋亡；高温（43℃）时肿瘤细胞发生凋亡；神经生长因子（NGF）可防止 AD，激素依赖性肿瘤治疗中配合内分泌干预等。

（2）干预凋亡信号转导：如化疗药物多柔比星通过促进靶细胞中 Fas/FasL 表达增加使肿瘤细胞凋亡。

（3）调节凋亡相关基因：肿瘤细胞的凋亡中，p53 是一关键的分子，如通过基因转移将 WT p53 导入 p53 基因突变肿瘤细胞抑制肿瘤增生；利用核酸干扰技术或反义寡核苷酸技术下调突变型 p53、Bcl-2、IAP（如 survivin）的活性与表达，减弱其对细胞凋亡的抑制；使异常表达癌基因失活、修复突变基因或向肿瘤细胞导入细胞凋亡活化基因，如 caspase、Bax、Bad 等，使其过表达可诱导细胞凋亡。导入药物敏感基因，有助于细胞凋亡。如上所述，p53 被 MDM2 所抑制，但 MDM2 与 ARF 结合后失去活性。由放疗或化疗引起细胞应激，或者通过抑制 MDM2 直接活化 p53 而诱发，或者间接地由 ARF 活化引起 MDM2 失活。ARF 可以被增殖癌基因如 Ras 所诱导。活化的 p53 反式激活凋亡前体基因，包括 Bax、NOXA、CD95 和肿瘤坏死因子相关凋亡诱导配体受体 1（TRAIL-R1）以促进凋亡（图 1-15）。化疗药物（如核苷酸类似物氟尿嘧啶，5-FU）通过转录调节的 p53 依赖性机制诱导 CD95 的产生。它们同样参与 SAPK/JNK 途径，最终导致 CD95L 的上调。CD95 和 CD95L 的上调引起细胞自杀或杀伤邻近细胞。显然，这不是化疗药物引起细胞死亡的唯一途径。很多药物直接通过线粒体途径发挥作用。除此以外，细胞的死亡并不一定需要 caspase 的激活。化疗药物是否具有单独的主要效应途径值得怀疑。也许，这种途径有赖于应激刺激、细胞类型、肿瘤环境和许多其他因子。由于化疗和放疗主要通过诱导凋亡发挥作用，可以想象对凋亡信号途径中关键分子的调节能够直接影响治疗引起的肿瘤细胞死亡。此外，抗凋亡 Bcl-2 家族成员也参与了肿瘤对凋亡的抵抗。例如，在细胞株中，Bcl-xL 可以引起对多种凋亡诱导途径的抵抗，并且在体外构成性活化的突变表皮生长因子受体（EGFR）能使其表达上调。MCL1（髓细胞白血病序列 1）同样也能赋予细胞株对化疗的抵抗。在一些白血病的患者中，MCL1 的表达在复发时增加，提示可以针对具有较高水平 MCL1 的白血病细胞选择一些靶向性抗癌药物。穿孔素在靶细胞膜聚合，使粒酶能够进入细胞。粒酶活化靶细胞中的 caspase。此外，粒酶 B 可能直接剪切 Bcl-2 家族成员 Bid 以活化线粒体死亡途径。

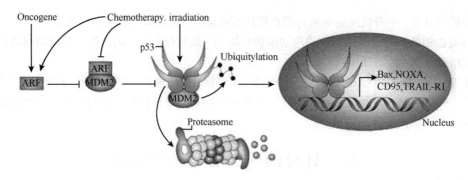

图 1-15　由放疗或化疗、抑制 MDM2 引起细胞应激，或者通过活化 ARF 间接引起细胞应激进而激活 p53 促进细胞凋亡；Cellular stress induced by chemotherapy or irradiation, by inhibition of MDM2, or indirectly by activation of ARF activates p53 to promote apoptosis

（4）控制凋亡相关酶的活性：如提高核酸内切酶和 caspases 的活性；Ca^{2+} 载体可使核酸内切酶活性增加，相反 Ca^{2+} 阻断剂使核酸内切酶活性降低。增加 Zn^{2+} 水平使 caspases 活性降低。

（5）防止线粒体跨膜电位的下降：如环孢素 A、N-methyl-Val-Cyclosporin（环孢素 A 的衍生物）等。

（6）肿瘤的疗效判定应考虑到以下几方面。

1）是否经过治疗后发生凋亡，这是肿瘤化疗效果好坏的关键之一。

2）增加 AI 与细胞增殖（proliferation index，PI）的比值（AI/PI）已成为新的治疗目标。

3）能否同时诱导细胞凋亡已成为筛选抗癌药物的新标准。

4）诱导细胞凋亡的治疗将是对肿瘤治疗方法的重要补充与革新。

第四节　凋亡的检测方法

1972 年 Kerr 提出细胞凋亡的概念，1980 年用电泳检测细胞凋亡，并证实了 DNA 断裂的特征，即 DNA 断折成相等大小 180～200bp 或倍数大小的片断，电泳呈梯度。1986 年在秀丽隐杆线虫（Caenorhabditis elegans）中观察 1090 个体细胞，其中 131 个细胞在发育过程中通过凋亡而消失，并找到 ced-3、ced-4 两个基因，它们的表达与细胞凋亡密切相关，故称为死亡基因。因此细胞凋亡的检测经历以下几个过程：从单纯形态学辨认→形态与生化结合→形态、生化、分子生物学技术相结合的多种手段联合研究。

一、凋亡检测要解决的问题

（1）被研究体系中是否有凋亡发生，即定性。

（2）凋亡的发生率，这显示群体细胞的量度。当然这还是一个相对的概念，应同时结合细胞群体的增殖率来分析则更客观、更能反映细胞群体的生长状态。

（3）了解细胞凋亡的严重度，以反应凋亡的阶段。

二、检　测　方　法

主要方法包括电镜、荧光显微镜、琼脂糖凝胶电泳、TUNEL（terminal deoxynucleotidyl

transferase mediate dUTP-biotin nick end labeling）检测、流式细胞检测（FCM），以及 RT-PCR、RT-QPCR、ELISA 法和 Western blot 分别检测凋亡相关基因 mRNA 和蛋白水平等。

（一）形态学观察

这是认识凋亡的基本方法，在拥有众多检测手段的今天仍有其特定的价值，因为各种检测细胞凋亡的结果，必须与组织学比较，其结果分析才具有实际意义。

光学显微镜下可以看见胞膜起泡现象和凋亡小体，被认为是最方便简捷的方法，但凋亡细胞的形态学变化大多发生在超微结构水平，透射电镜可清楚地观察到细胞结构在凋亡不同时期的变化。电镜形态学观察是迄今为止判断凋亡最经典、最可靠的方法，被认为是确定细胞凋亡的金标准。缺点：①只能定性，不能定量；②标本处理过程复杂，设备相对昂贵，操作技术水平要求较高，不适于大批量标本的检测；③在组织切片上进行电镜观察时，凋亡与正常细胞有丝分裂有时难鉴别，因为两种情况下都可出现染色质浓聚。如同时进行免疫组织化学和免疫荧光（immunohistochemistry and immunofluorescence）检测，可弥补电镜检查的不足[31]。检测细胞凋亡的各种形态学方法比较见表 1-2。

表 1-2 检测细胞凋亡各种形态学方法比较

检查方法	可鉴定凋亡细胞的特征
光学显微镜（LM）	细胞体积缩小、核浓缩、细胞周围透明圈
相差显微镜（PCLM）	细胞鼓泡、凋亡小体
透射电镜（TEM）	微绒毛消失、核染色质沿核膜分布、新月体形成、凋亡小体
激光共聚焦（CLSM）	凋亡细胞固缩染色质及核碎片定位
扫描电镜（SEM）	细胞表面泡状突起
流式细胞仪（FCM）	低前向散射光（FSC）、高侧向散射光（SSC）
缩时摄影术（TLP）	凋亡细胞的形成过程

（二）annexin Ⅴ-FITC 单染法

在正常的活细胞，磷脂酰丝氨酸（phosphatidylserine，PS）位于细胞膜的内侧，但在凋亡早期 PS 从细胞膜的内侧翻转到细胞膜的表面，可通过一种与带负电荷磷脂高度亲和的蛋白——annexin Ⅴ 来检测。annexin-Ⅴ（膜联蛋白-Ⅴ）是一种分子量为 35～36kDa 的 Ca^{2+} 依赖性磷脂结合蛋白，能与 PS 高亲和力结合。因此将 annexin-Ⅴ 进行荧光素（如 FITC、PE）或生物素（biotin）标记作为探针，利用流式细胞仪或荧光显微镜可检测细胞早期凋亡的发生（图 1-16）。

（三）流式细胞检测[PI（碘化丙啶）染色法]

利用细胞内 DNA 能够和荧光染料 PI 结

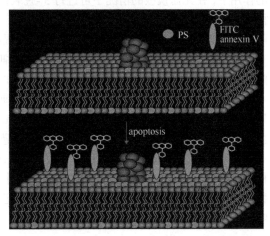

图 1-16 annexin Ⅴ-FITC/PI 双染流式细胞检测细胞早期凋亡；Early apoptotic annexin Ⅴ-FITC/PI double staining in flow cytometry

合的特性检测细胞各个时期，由于其 DNA 含量不同从而结合的荧光染料不同，流式检测的荧光强度也不一样。

$G_2 \sim M$ 期 DNA 含量是 $G_0 \sim G_1$ 的两倍，而 S 期介于两者之间。

在细胞凋亡中 DNA 含量较少，因而可以在细胞 $G_0 \sim G_1$ 期前面有一个亚二倍体峰（从而认为是凋亡细胞）。但是由于死亡的细胞本身其 DNA 含量也是减少的，因而非常难于区分凋亡和死亡的细胞。经典的流式检测资料给出的图是认为凋亡的细胞是紧挨着 $G_0 \sim G_1$ 期峰的一个峰，死亡的细胞峰离 $G_0 \sim G_1$ 期峰较远，但是这种典型的结果很难获得。

（四）核酸电泳检测细胞凋亡（DNA 片段检测细胞凋亡）

细胞凋亡和坏死时，细胞中 DNA 发生断裂，小分子 DNA 片断增加，高分子 DNA 减少，胞质内出现 DNA 片段。凋亡细胞的 DNA 断裂是由内源性的内切酶作用，断点都是规律性的发生在核小体之间，因此出现 $180 \sim 200 bp$ 及其倍数的 DNA 片段；而坏死细胞的 DNA 片断是无特征的杂乱片段。提取细胞或组织 DNA 后琼脂糖凝胶电泳检测，在凝胶电泳中出现的特征性的泳带（DNA Ladder）可以判断存在凋亡细胞。其优点是简单、成本低。但这方法缺乏定位特性，无法确定哪个细胞发生凋亡，出现 DNA Ladder 的结果比较难。

（五）caspase 活性检测

将 caspase-3 序列特异性的多肽偶联至发色基团（DEVD-pNA）。当该底物被 caspase-3 剪切后，发色基团（pNA）即游离出来，可通过酶标仪或分光光度计（$\lambda = 405 nm$ 或 $400 nm$）测定其吸光值，考察 caspase-3 的活化程度。根据处理组与空白对照组的倍增关系来反应组织 caspase-3 活性的高低。根据组织 caspase-3 活性的高低可在一定程度上反映处理因素有无诱发体内细胞凋亡[32]。

（六）DNA 片断原位标记

原位标记的原理：细胞凋亡中 DNA 断裂是内切酶作用，其断端 3'端的羟基（—OH）暴露，这是凋亡细胞 DNA 断裂的特征，以此区别细胞坏死 DNA 断裂。在末端脱氧核苷酸转移酶（TdT）的作用下，在无需模板的情况中可进行 3'-脱氧核苷酸合成。如果在反应体系中加入标记的脱氧核苷酸，则在 3'端出现带有标志物的寡核苷酸，通过荧光或其他显色反应，可以在原位较特异的显示发生凋亡的细胞。1993 年 Wifsman 等提出 DNA 片段末端标记（ISNT）法，Fehsel 等 1994 年提出 TUNEL 检测的方法，该法与流式细胞技术相结合可定量凋亡细胞的百分比；与免疫组织化学结合可进行形态学分析。这些方法的提出把凋亡研究带进了新阶段，特别是这些技术发展为原位凋亡检测试剂盒，在基础和临床研究方面得到了广泛的应用。TUNEL 的敏感性远高于 ISNT，尤其是对早期凋亡的检出 TUNEL 更为适用。这两种方法还可以同时进行细胞表面标志检测，以明确多细胞组成的组织或细胞悬液中发生凋亡的细胞种类。缺点：①坏死细胞亦有 DNA 裂点，无规则，其中也有少数细胞出现了 3'端—OH 暴露，也可呈现 TUNEL 反应阳性，因而特异性较差。据报道，TUNEL 反应中坏死细胞的标记量比凋亡细胞的标记量少一个数量级。②TUNEL 结合免疫组化检测时，固定过程对检测的影响较大，切片的薄厚会直接影响到固定效果，从而产生结果的差异。

三、凋亡检测的注意点

截至目前，凋亡检测的方法已有许多种，但任何一种方法都有自身的缺点和应用的局限性，可能影响检测结果的判断和意义分析。

（1）因为凋亡是多因素、多通路参与的过程，不能根据单一指标来判断细胞凋亡，所以需进行多指标同时检测。

（2）由于凋亡细胞在不同时间出现的凋亡事件不同，而每个指标维持有一个时间段，所以需要在不同的时间点进行采样，以保证检测结果的准确性。

（3）实验需要合理设定阳性和阴性对照，建立正常时该体系的凋亡状态，设置正常对照组，以判断检测组凋亡是生理性，还是病理性的。

（4）考虑如何定量与排除其他干扰。

挑战与展望

（一）小结

虽然发现细胞凋亡的现象已经半个多世纪，已经明确凋亡是多步骤、多途径的细胞死亡过程，是机体每个细胞所固有的。凋亡过程受到各种蛋白的严格调控，很多控制细胞增殖和组织内环境稳定的生理性生长调控机制都与凋亡有关，其中 caspase 均被活化，它剪切细胞底物引起特征性的生化和形态学改变。同样也存在 caspase 非依赖性细胞死亡。但细胞凋亡仍然是当今生命科学研究的重要议题，在细胞凋亡研究中还有许多问题未得到解决。

（1）细胞发育过程中，细胞凋亡究竟是何时，又是如何开始的（时间与方式）？

（2）机体是如何决定一个细胞将要走向死亡的？

（3）在细胞有丝分裂和成熟之间有没有能激活细胞凋亡的开关点基因（switch point gene）存在？

（4）机体内有没有真正的杀手基因（killer gene）存在？死亡相关基因是如何调控的？

（5）是否有活命基因（survival gene）的存在？

（6）如何选择凋亡相关基因并干预其表达以达到减轻疾病过程中组织损伤的目的？

（二）问题

（1）凋亡是多步骤、多途径的细胞死亡过程，是机体每个细胞所固有的。在癌中，凋亡与细胞分裂比值发生改变，导致恶性组织生成。

（2）凋亡的启动或者通过死亡受体途径或者通过线粒体途径。在两种途径中，caspase 均被活化，它剪切细胞底物引起特征性的生化和形态学改变。凋亡过程受到各种蛋白的严格调控。同样也存在 caspase 非依赖性细胞死亡。

（3）很多控制细胞增殖和组织内环境稳定的生理性生长调控机制都与凋亡有关。因此，肿瘤细胞对凋亡的抵抗可能是癌症发生的基本特征。

（4）免疫细胞（T 细胞和自然杀伤细胞）通过颗粒胞吐途径或死亡受体途径杀死肿瘤细胞。肿瘤细胞对凋亡的抵抗可能导致其对免疫监视的逃避并影响免疫治疗的有效性。

（5）化疗和放疗杀死靶细胞的癌症疗法主要通过诱导凋亡。因此，凋亡信号关键成分的修饰直接影响治疗诱导的肿瘤细胞死亡。

（6）通过表达抗凋亡蛋白，或者下调或突变促凋亡蛋白，肿瘤细胞可以获得对凋亡的抵抗力。

（7）p53 途径的改变也会影响肿瘤细胞对凋亡的敏感性。此外，大多数肿瘤细胞是生存信号非依赖性的，因为其 PI3K/AkT 途径是上调的。

（三）展望

如果能发现凋亡特异性的基因或其产物，或其他特异性的标志物，就可能成为检测凋亡的指标。目前对凋亡的认识是它一个连续的过程，进一步研究也许会发现凋亡存在不同的阶段，而不同阶段可能会出现不同的标志物，从而发现凋亡阶段性标志物。凋亡机制在细胞生长、发育过程中所具有的独特的生物学效应，可以通过增加或降低某些特定的细胞对凋亡的敏感性来发展治疗疾病的新方法和药物。阻断凋亡可能有利于艾滋病的治疗，某些神经激素的基因替代疗法可能对中枢神经系统的退行性病变有益。在肿瘤治疗中多数抗癌药物是促进细胞凋亡的，而癌细胞的耐药是化疗中最棘手的问题。从凋亡角度来研究肿瘤的耐药性，可能找到新的解决方法。应该承认，对细胞凋亡的研究还有许多哑区有待探索，还有很多工作要做。例如，如何利用分子生物学和细胞生物学等当代最新技术，从分子水平上深入揭示细胞凋亡的启动、发生和发展规律，为研究胚胎发生、发展、个体形成、器官的细胞平衡稳定、自身免疫性疾病、肿瘤形成的原因等增加新的理论内容，并以此来指导医疗实践。随着对细胞凋亡机理的深入研究将对一些重大疾病如肿瘤、免疫系统疾病、心脑血管疾病等的治疗产生重大的突破。

思 考 题

1. 本章基本概念：凋亡（apoptosis），细胞程序性死亡（programmed cell death，PCD），凋亡小体（apoptotic body），内质网应激反应（endoplasmic reticulum stress response，ESR），Bcl-2，P53。

2. 阐述细胞凋亡的形态学改变。

3. 阐述调节细胞凋亡的主要途径及相互关系。

4. 细胞凋亡调节中有哪些重要的酶，分别发挥什么作用？

5. 细胞凋亡调控的相关基因有哪些？

6. 阐述细胞凋亡和细胞坏死的区别。

7. 列举 5 种细胞凋亡的检测方法。

8. 在你关注的疾病中如何进行凋亡的研究？

9. 细胞为什么要"自杀"？

参 考 文 献

[1] Degterev A，Boyce M，Yuan J. A decade of caspases [J]. Oncogene，2003，22（53）：8543-8567.

[2] Kumar S，Vaux D L. Apoptosis. A cinderella caspase takes center stage [J]. Science，2002，297（5585）：1290-1291.

[3] Grassmé H，Gulbins E. CD95/CD95 ligand interactions on epithelial cells in host defense to Pseudomonas aeruginosa [J]. Science，2000，290（5491）：527-530.

[4] Wajant H. The Fas signaling pathway：more than a paradigm [J]. Science，2002，296（5573）：1635-1636.

[5] Stewart J H，Nguyen D，Chen G A，et al. Induction of apoptosis in malignant pleuralmeso thelioma cells by activation of the Fas（Apo-1/CD95）death signal pathway [J]. The Journal of Thoracic and Cardiovascular Surgery，2002，123（2）：295-302.

[6] Grassme H，Kirschnek S，Riethmueller J，et al. CD95/ CD95 ligand interactions on epithelial cells in host defense to Psedomonas aeruginosa [J]. Science，2000，290（5491）：527-530.

[7] Lm D O P，Garcia S，Lecoeur H，et al. Increased sensitivity of T lymphocytes to tumor necrosis factor receptor 1（TNFR1）- and TNFR2-mediated apoptosis in HIV infection：relation to expression of Bcl-2 and active caspase-8 and caspase-3[J]. Blood，2002，99（5）：1666-1675.

[8] Chen G，Goeddel D V. TNF-R1 signaling：a beautiful pathway [J]. Science，2002，296（5573）：1634.

[9] Park K J，Choi S H，Koh M S，et al. Hepatitis C virus core protein potentiates c-Jun N-terminal kinase activation through a signaling

complex involving TRADD and TRAF2[J]. Virus Research，2001，74（1）：89-98.

[10] Gupta S. Molecular steps of tumor necrosis factor receptor mediated apoptosis [J]. Current Molecular Medicine，2001，1（3）：317-324.

[11] Sartorius U，Schmitz I，Krammer P H. Molecular mechanisms of death-receptor-mediated apoptosis [J]. Chembiochem A European Journal of Chemical Biology，2001，2（1）：20-29.

[12] Shearwin-Whyatt L M，Harvey N L，Kumar S. Subcellular localization and CARD-dependent oligomerization of the death adaptor RAIDD[J]. Cell Death & Differentiation，2000，7（2）：155-165.

[13] Brenner C，Kroemer G. Apoptosis. Mitochondria-the death signal integrators [J]. Science，2000，289（5482）：1150-1151.

[14] Herr I，Debatin K. Cellular stress response and apoptosis in cancer therapy [J]. Blood，2001，98（9）：2603-2604.

[15] Goodsell D S. The molecular perspective：Bcl-2 and apoptosis [J]. Stem Cells，2002，20（4）：355-356.

[16] Oyadomari S，Mori M. Roles of CHOP/GADD153 in endoplasmic reticulum stress [J]. Cell Death & Differentiation，2004，11（4）：381-389.

[17] Fels D R，Koumenis C. The PERK/elF2 alpha/ATF4 module of the UPR in hypoxia resistance and tumor growth [J]. Cancer Biology & Therapy，2006，5（7）：723-728.

[18] Ron D，Habener J F. CHOP，a novel developmentally regulated nuclear protein that dimerizes with transcription factors C/EBP and LAP and functions as a dominant-negative inhibitor of gene transcription [J]. Genes & Development，1992，6（3）：439-453.

[19] McCullough K D，Martindale J L，Klotz LO，et al. Gadd153 sensitizes cells to endoplasmic reticulum stress by down-regulating Bcl2 and perturbing the cellular redox state. Molecular and Cellular Biology，2001，21（4）：1249-1259.

[20] Yamaguchi H，Wang H G. CHOP is involved in endoplasmic reticulum stress-induced apoptosis by enhancing DR5 expression in human carcinoma cells. Journal of Biological Chemistry. 2004，279（44）：45495-45502.

[21] Nakagawa T，Zhu H，Morishima N，et al. Caspase-12 mediates endoplasmic-reticulum-specific apoptosis and cytotoxicity by amyloid-beta [J]. Nature，2000，403（6765）：98-103.

[22] Wei Q，Dong G，Chen J K，et al. Bax and Bak have critical roles in ischemic acute kidney injury in global and proximal tubule-specific knockout mouse models [J]. Kidney International，2013，84（1）：138-148.

[23] Yang C，Zhao T，Zhao Z，et al. Serum-stabilized naked caspase-3 siRNA protects autotransplant kidneys in a porcine model [J]. Molecular Therapy the Journal of the American Society of Gene Therapy，2014，22（12）：1817-1828.

[24] Schlegel R，Williamson P. Phosphatidylserine，a death knell [J]. Cell Death & Differentiation，2001，8（6）：551-563.

[25] Schumer M，Colombel M C，Sawczuk I S，et al. Morphologic，biochemical，and molecular evidence of apoptosis during the reperfusion phase after brief periods of renal ischemia[J]. American Journal of Pathology，1992，140（4）：831-838.

[26] Havasi A，Borkan S C. Apoptosis and acute kidney injury [J]. Kidney International，2011，80（1）：29-40.

[27] Linkermann A，Bräsen J H，Darding M，et al. Two independent pathways of regulated necrosis mediate ischemia-reperfusion injury[J]. Proceedings of the National Academy of Sciences of the United States of America，2013，110（29）：12024-12029.

[28] Ashkenazi A，Dixit V M Death receptors：signaling and modulation. Science，1988，281：1305-1308.

[29] Ramesh G，Reeves W B. Inflammatory cytokines in acute renal failure [J]. Kidney International Supplement，2004，66（91）：S56-61.

[30] Nakagawa T，Zhu H，Morishima N，et al. Caspase-12 mediates endoplasmic-reticulum-specific apoptosis and cytotoxicity by amyloid-beta [J]. Nature，2000，403（6765）：98-103.

[31] Mirakian R，Nye K，Palazzo F F，et al. Methods for detecting apoptosis in thyroid diseases [J]. Journal of Immunological Methods，2002，265（1-2）：161-175.

[32] Kischkel F C，Lawrence D A，Chuntharapai A，et al. Apo2L/TRAIL-dependent recruitment of endogenous FADD and caspase-8 to death receptors 4 and 5 [J]. Immunity，2000，12（6）：611-620.

（吴圆圆 羌剑锋 陈 莉）

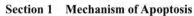

Chapter 1　Apoptosis

Section 1　Mechanism of Apoptosis
　1. Biochemical Changes of Apoptosis
　2. Apoptosis Pathways
　3. Signal Transduction of Apoptosis
　4. Regulating Apoptosis Related Genes
Section 2　Morphology of Apoptosis
　1. Morphological Changes of Apoptotic Cells
　2. Elimination Process
　3. Difference Between Apoptosis and
　　Necrosis (Table 1-1 and Fig. 1-14)
Section 3　Apoptosis and Diseases
　1. Etiology
　2. Excessive Apoptosis Relating Diseases
　3. Insufficient Apoptosis Relating Diseases
　4. Insufficient and Excessive Apoptosis
　　Coexist Diseases
　5. Therapeutic Induction of Apoptosis
Section 4　Detection Methods of Apoptosis
　1. Apoptosis Detection Solved Follow Problems
　2. Methods
　3. Precautions in Apoptosis Detection
Challenges and Prospects

Apoptosis is to ensure individual development, maturation, and is necessary to maintain the normal physiological processes. (Cell mass——has a complex structure of tissues and organs). ①To maintain a stable internal environment; Selectively remove excess, abnormal, completed task, damaged, aging and mutation, useless and harmful cells. ②Immune system cells involved in the development and clonal selection.③To play an active role in defense.

Under certain physiological or pathological conditions, cells follow its own procedures by the death process of gene regulation.

Conception: Apoptosis is a distinct type of cell death (cell suicide). It usually involves single cells, or cluster of cells. It is thought to be responsible for numerous physiologic events as well pathologic including the programmed destruction of cells during embryogenesis.

Programmed cell death (PCD): is a cell self-destructive way of gene guidance.

Apoptosis is an important mechanism in multicellular organisms to eliminate cells that are either in excess or potentially dangerous.

Sydney Brenner Noel, Robert Horvitz and John Sulston were awarded the Nobel Prize in Physiology and Medicine in October 7, 2002, in terms of the genetic regulation of programmed cell death and organ development studies.

Section 1　Mechanism of Apoptosis

1. Biochemical Changes of Apoptosis

(1) Internucleosomal linkage region DNA duplexes cleavage form 180-200bp size and multiple times nucleotide fragments

(2) Accumulation and redistribution of Ca^{2+}

(3) Accumulation and activation of transglutaminase

(4) Increasing cell surface sugar chains and lectins

(5) Changing cytoskeleton

Three Important Enzymes in Regulating Apoptosis

Primarily, the signaling pathways determine the fate of cells.A variety of endogenous and exogenous stimuli through receptor-mediated cellular signaling pathways induce apoptosis factor or the second messenger system transfer signals, increase calcium ion concentration intracellularly, leading to the cascade of intracellular degradation

(1) Endonuclease 180-200bp DNA fragmentation(DNA ladder) internucleosomal linkage region (Fig. 1-1).

(2) Tissue tranglutaninase (TTG): TTG activation forms a sheath protein (involucrin) under cellular membrane through cytoplasmic protein cross linkage, which can make a network of the organelles and other intracellular contents, and avoid overflow and lead to cell shrinkage.

(3) Calcium-dependent protease:Activation of protease destroys the cytoskeleton structure and forms bubble-like protrusions on the cell surface leading to cell budding

2. Apoptosis Pathways

Based on the start of different caspase enzymes (Cysteine protease family) and signal transduction mechanisms, the regulatory pathways of apoptosis are divided into two ways: extrinsic pathway: the death receptors (DR) mediated pathway; extrinsic signal activated transmembrane receptors. Intrinsic pathway: also known as the mitochondria-mediated pathway causing stress signaling, DNA damage and defects in initiation.

(1) Extrinsic Pathway, Death Receptor-Mediated Signal Transduction

1) Death ligands(death factor):TNF, FasL, TRAIL, Apo3L

2) Death receptor: TNF-R, Fas, CD40, OX40, 4-1BB

3) Death domain(DD)   There are about 80 amino acid residues conserving protein binding domain in apoptotic intracellular area, which are necessary for signal transduction cell death.

Death-inducing signaling complex (DISC): Homotrimeric body (FasL, Fas/CD95 receptor), Binding protein, FADD (Fas-associated death domain protein, also known as MORT1), Pro-caspase8.

Death receptors (DR) are the members of the tumor-necrosis factor (TNF) receptor superfamily and comprise a subfamily that are characterized by an intracellular domain — the death domain.

Death receptors are activated by their natural ligands, the TNF family. When ligands bind to their respective death receptors — such as CD95, TRAIL-R1 (TNF-related apoptosis-inducing ligand-R1) or TRAIL-R2---the death domains attract the intracellular adaptor protein FADD which, in turn, recruits the inactive pro-forms of certain members of the caspase protease family.

The caspases that are recruited to this death-inducing signaling complex (DISC) -caspase-8 and caspase-10function as 'initiator' caspases. At the DISC, procaspase-8 and procaspase-10 are cleaved and yield active initiator caspases (Fig. 1-2).

Binding of death ligands (CD95L is used here as an example) to their receptor leads to the formation of the death-inducing signalling complex (DISC). In the DISC, the initiator procaspase-8 is recruited by FADD (FAS-associated death domain protein) and is activated by autocatalytic cleavage. Death-receptor-mediated apoptosis can be inhibited at several levels by anti-apoptotic proteins: CD95L can be prevented from binding to CD95 by soluble 'decoy' receptors, such as soluble CD95 (sCD95) or DCR3 (decoy receptor 3). FLICE-inhibitory proteins (FLIPs) bind to the DISC and prevent the activation of Caspase-8; and inhibitors of apoptosis proteins (IAPs) bind to and inhibit caspases. FLIPL and FLIPS refer to long and short forms of FLIP, respectively.

(2) Intrinsic Pathway/ Mitochondrial Pathway

In some cells, the amount of active Caspase-8 is too small and mitochondria are used as 'amplifiers' of the apoptotic signal. Activation of mitochondria is mediated by the Bcl-2 family member Bid. Bid is cleaved by active Caspase-8 and translocates to the mitochondria to activate Caspase-9 to achieve the mitochondrial pathway.

After activation by an apoptotic stimulus, mitochondria release cytochrome *c (Cyt-c)*, AIF (apoptosis inducing factor) and other apoptogenic factors from the intermembrane space to the cytosol. Concomitantly, the mitochondrial transmembrane potential drops. According to one model, mitochondrial membrane permeability involves the permeability transition pore complex (PTPC), a multiprotein complex that consists of the adenine nucleotide translocator (ANT) of the inner membrane, the voltage-dependent anion channel of the outer membrane and various other proteins. Bcl-2 proteins might interact with the PTPC and regulate its permeability (Fig. 1-3).

According to another model, BH3-only proteins serve as 'death sensors' in the cytosol or cytoskeleton. Following a death signal, they interact with members of the Bax subfamily. After this interaction, Bax proteins undergo a conformational change, insert into the mitochondrial membrane, oligomerize and form protein-permeable channels. Anti-apoptotic Bcl-2 proteins inhibit the conformational change or the oligomerization of Bax and Bak.

The localization of the pro-apoptotic Bcl-2 family member Bad is regulated by phosphorylation. Only non-phosphorylated Bad is capable of antagonizing anti-apoptotic Bcl-2 or Bcl-XL on the mitochondrial membrane. Bad phosphorylation results in its redistribution to the cytosol and its sequestration by 14-3-3 proteins.

Chemotherapy, radiation and other stimuli can initiate apoptosis through the mitochondrial (intrinsic) pathway. Pro-apoptotic Bcl-2 family proteins - for example, Bax, Bid, Bad and Bim- are important mediators of these signals. Activation of mitochondria leads to the release of Cyt-c into the cytosol, where it binds apoptotic protease activating factor 1 (APAF1) to form the apoptosome. At the apoptosome, the initiator caspase-9 is activated. Apoptosis through mitochondria can be inhibited on different levels by anti-apoptotic proteins, including the anti-apoptotic Bcl-2 family members Bcl-2 and Bcl-XL and inhibitors of apoptosis proteins (IAPs), which are regulated by SMAC/DIABLO (second mitochondria-derived activator of caspase/direct IAP binding protein with low pI). Another way is through survival signals, such as growth factors and cytokines that activate the phosphatidylinositol 3-kinase (PI3K) pathway. PI3K activates AKT, which phosphorylates and inactivates the pro-apoptotic Bcl-2-family member Bad.

A Brief Overview of Two Main Apoptosis Signaling Pathways

Apoptosis can be initiated by two alternative pathways: either through death receptors on the cell surface (extrinsic pathway) or through mitochondria (intrinsic pathway). In both pathways, induction of apoptosis leads to activation of an initiator caspase: caspase-8 and possibly caspase-10 for the extrinsic pathway; and caspase-9, which is activated at the apoptosome, for the intrinsic pathway. The initiator caspases then activate executioner caspases. Active executioner caspases cleave the death substrates, which eventually results in apoptosis. There is the crosstalk between these two pathways. For example, cleavage of the Bcl-2family member BID by caspase-8 activates the mitochondrial pathway after apoptosis induction through death receptors, and can be used to amplify the apoptotic signal (Fig. 1-4).

Once the initiator caspases are activated, they cleave and activate 'executioner' caspases, mainly caspase-3, caspase-6 and caspase-7. The active executioner caspases then cleave each other and, in this way, an amplifying proteolytic cascade of caspase activation is started.

Eventually, the active executioner caspases cleave cellular substrates — the 'death substrates' —

which leads to characteristic biochemical and morphological changes. Cleavage of nuclear LAMINS is involved in chromatin condensation and nuclear shrinkage. Cleavage of the inhibitor of the DNase CAD (caspase-activated deoxyribonuclease, DFF40), ICAD (also known as DNA fragmentation factor, 45 kDa; DFF45), causes the release of the endonuclease, which travels to the nucleus to fragment DNA. Cleavage of cytoskeletal proteins such as actin, plectin, Rho kinase 1 (ROCK1) and gelsolin leads to cell fragmentation, blebbing and the formation of apoptotic bodies. After exposure of 'eat me' signals (for example, exposure of phosphatidylserine and changes in surface sugars), the remains of the dying cell are engulfed by phagocytes.

1) The major inducers of apoptosis include specific death ligands (TNF and Fas ligand), withdrawal of growth factors(GF) or hormones, and injurious agents (e.g., radiation). Some stimuli (such as cytotoxic cells) directly activate execution caspases. Others are acted by way of adapter proteins and initiator caspases, or by mitochondrial events involving Cyt-c.

2) The regulation of apoptosis is influenced by members of the Bcl-2 family, which can either inhibit or promote the cell's death.

3) Executioner caspases activate latent cytoplasmic endonucleases and proteases that degrade nuclear and cytoskeletal proteins. This results in a cascade of intracellular degradation, including fragmentation of nuclear chromatin and breakdown of the cytoskeleton proteins.

4) The end is formation of apoptotic bodies containing intracellular organelles and other cytosol components. These bodies also express new ligands for binding and uptake by phagocytic cells.

(3) Endoplasmic Reticulum Stress Response (ESR)

Whenever post-translational modifications such as the N-linked glycosylation, disulfide bond formation or translocation to Golgi apparatus of newly synthesized peptides is restrained, the resulting unfolded or misfolded proteins accumulate on endoplasmic reticulum (ER). Additionally, in higher eukaryotes ER serves as the majorintracellular Ca^{2+} store and therefore, alteration of Ca^{2+} concentration may lead to ER stress. Accordingly, metazoan cells react rapidly to ER dysfunction through a set of adaptive pathways known collectively as the ER stress response (ESR).

During ER stress, 3 transcription factors: IRE1/ERN1 (inositol requiring 1), RERK/PEK (PEK like ER kinase) and ATF6 (activating transcription factor 6) can be activated, resulting in unfolded protein response (UPR) （Fig1-8）. As a consequence, unfolded or misfolded proteins accumulate on endoplasmic reticulum (ER).IRE1, a type IER transmembrane protein, consists of an N-terminal luminal domain and cytoplasmic C-terminal serine/threonine kinase and endonuclease domains. Under ER stress conditions unfolded or misfolded proteins accumulate inside the ER and titrate Kar2p away from Ire1p. The removal of Kar2p permits the oligomerization of Ire1p through its luminal domain and the subsequent activation of Ire1p by trans-autophosphorylation via the C-terminal kinase domain. PERK is another type I ER transmembrane protein. It is believed that the excess unfolded protein that accumulates during ER stress, competes with mammalian IRE1 and PERK for BiP binding, allowing IRE1 or PERK to homodimerize and self-activate by trans-autophosphorylation. Consistent with this model, the displacement of BiP from IRE1or PERK is correlated with the appearance of activated PERK and IRE1, and over-expression of BiP attenuates their activation. ATF6 is a type II ER transmembrane protein. During ER stress, continued accumulation leads to translocation of ATF6 to the Golgi compartment where it undergoes regulated intramembrane proteolysis by proteases S1P and S2P, yielding a free cytoplasmic domain that triggers transcriptional up regulation of several ER resident proteins. The free cytoplasmic domain translocates to nucleus and combined with ER stress respond element, activating the related promoters, which could further activate the transcription of chaperone, foldase and CHOP (Fig. 1-5).

ER stress leads to cells apoptosis through 3 major pathways:

1) CHOP Pathway

CHOP/GADD153 (Growth Arrest and DNA-Damage-inducible gene 153) is a bZIP transcription factor that contains an ER stress response element in its promoter, which can form heterodimers with members of the C/EBP and fos-jun families of transcription factors and likely contributes to the regulation of many genes in orchestrating the transcriptional component of the ESR. CHOP is transcription ally up regulated by IRE1, RERK and ATF6. During ER stress, PERK phosphorylates eIF2α, which induces the expression of ATF4, ATF3, and CHOP. These transcription factors then upregulate GADD34, which mediates the dephosphorylation of eIF2α by PP1. Therefore, synthesis of endoplasmic reticulum chaperone proteins increases. CHOP can also transcriptionally downregulate the antiapoptotic protein Bcl-2 and upregulate DR5, a member of the death receptor protein family, two effectors that function in non-ER forms of cell death as well. Interestingly, CHOP also leads to a depletion of cellular glutathione and an increase of reactive oxygen species (ROS) in the ER, due in part to its induction of ERO1α, an ER oxidase. Interfering withERO1α function reduces the accumulation of ROS in the stressed ER, leading to cytoprotection. This implies thatERO1α may be an important apoptotic effector downstream of CHOP that can form heterodimers with cAMPresponse elementbinding protein CREB. The complex could downregulate Bcl-2 expression level, further inducing mitochondrial apoptotic pathway.

2) Caspase Pathway

The caspase family of proapoptotic cysteine proteases also plays a critical role in ER stress-induced apoptosis. Caspase-12, a murine protein (in the murine system; most human do not express caspase-12, and in humans, caspase-4 may play this role) associated with the cytosolic side of the ER membrane, is activated by ER stress-induced apoptosis, but not by non-ER stimuli, and is required for cell death in response to both pharmacological ER stress and ER-targeted Bim (Pro-apoptotic BH3-only proteins). Caspase-12 can be activated by ER stress in several ways: ① The cytoplasmic calcium-activated protease calpain can cleave and activate caspase-12 in response to calcium flux from the ER, which is often triggered by ER stress. Calpain can also cleave Bcl-xL, making it proapoptotic molecule from antiapoptotic protein. Caspase-12 can also auto activate through adirect association with IRE1α and the adaptor protein TRAF2 (TNF receptor-associated factor 2), though how the formation of this complex is regulated by ER stress is not yet clear. Under normal condition, TRAF2 can form stable heterodimer with procaspase-12, but ER stress can trigger the disassociate of them, which activate caspase-12. ② At the same time, the complex JIK-IRE1 recruit TRAF2, followed by JNK phosphorylation. ③ In addition, caspase-7 translocates to the ER in response to some apoptotic stimuli, and it has been proposed thatcaspase-7 can directly activate caspase-12. However, other experiments suggest that caspase-12 cleavage precedescaspase-7 cleavage under ER stress conditions, implying that the order of activation may be the opposite. ④ GRP78/BiP interacts with caspase-7 [requiring the adenosine triphosphate (ATP)–binding domain and caspase-12], preventing activation of caspase-12, but this inhibition is relieved byATP. Although the upstream activation of this pathway is not certain, one candidate is the triggering of c-Jun N-terminal kinase activation by IRE1, via TRAF2 and ASK1.

3) JNK Pathway

C-Jun N-terminal kinase (JNK) are mitogen-activated protein kinases (MAPKs) or stress-activated protein kinase (SAPKs also known as JUN-N-terminal kinase or JNK) that are activated in response to a variety of stresses, including inflammatory cytokines, osmotic stress, radiation, and excitotoxicity.TRAF-2 is recruited to IRE1 and mediates JNK activation through apoptosis signal-regulating kinase (ASK-1). JNK-1 phosphorylation of Bcl-2 inhibits its survival function. Beyond the transcriptional and post-translational mechanisms that impinge on Bcl-2 family members on ER stress-induced apoptosis, select members of this family can functionally interact with the ER by regulating Ca^{2+} homeostasis and IRE1 activation.

The SAPK pathway is activated in response to chemotherapy. SAPKs, which are members of the MAPKs family, can regulate the activity of AP-1 transcription factors. Known pro-apoptotic target genes for AP-1 are CD95L and TNF-a. Moreover, oxidative stress triggered by the production of reactive oxygen intermediates and glutathione depletion can also induces CD95L expression.

The best-defined mechanism by which therapy-induced cellular stress eventually leads to the death of tumor cells—particularly liver tumor cells—involves the CD95 system. Chemotherapeutic drugs (for example, the nucleotide analogue 5-fluoruracil, 5-FU) induce CD95 by a transcriptionally regulated, p53-dependent mechanism. They also engage the SAPK/JNK pathway, which eventually leads to upregulation of CD95L. Upregulation of CD95 and CD95L then allows the cells to either commit suicide or kill neighbouring cells.

Besides these prototypic caspase-dependent apoptosis pathways, there are also molecularly less-well-defined cell-death pathways that do not require caspase activation. These pathways share some, not all, characteristics of apoptotic classical pathways. Therefore, they cannot be readily classified as apoptosis or necrosis and have been called 'necrotic-like' or 'apoptotic-like' cell death or paraptosis.

The extrinsic and intrinsic pathways of apoptotic signaling (Fig. 1-6)

3. Signal Transduction of Apoptosis

Two major apoptotic pathway, due to structural parts of the start signal subcellular different and each has its uniqueness, but in intracellular signal transduction of apoptosis there is broad convergence (crosstalk), to form a cell wither death of the signal transduction networks. Apoptotic signal transduction system with multi-way: ① Intracellular Ca^{2+} signaling system; ② cAMP / PKA signaling system; ③ Fas protein/Fas ligand signaling system; ④Ceramide signaling system; ⑤ Diacylglycerol / PKC signaling system; ⑥ Tyrosine kinase (PTK) signaling system (Fig. 1-7).

4. Regulating Apoptosis Related Genes

Apoptosis is a multi-step, multi-pathway cell-death programme that is inherent in every cell of the body. The apoptotic process is tightly controlled by various proteins. There are also other caspase-independent types of cell death. Many physiological growth-control mechanisms that govern cell proliferation and tissue homeostasis are linked to apoptosis.

(1) Bcl-2 Genes Family

Bcl-2: B2cell lymphoma/ leukemia-2. From the t (14; 18) of follicular lymphoma was found to inhibit apoptosis induced by various stimuli.

The members of the Bcl-2 family, which regulate apoptosis at the mitochondrial level. They is an important class of regulatory proteins. It can be divided into anti-apoptotic (Bcl-2, Bcl-XL, Bcl-w, MCL1, A1/BFL1, BOO/DIVA, NR-13) and pro-apoptotic proteins(Bax, Bak, Bok/MTD, Bcl-XS, Bid, Bad, Bik/NBK, Blk, Hrk/DP5, Bim/BOD, NIP3, NIX, NOXA, PUMA, BMF) according to their function. Bcl-2 family proteins influence the permeability of the mitochondrial membrane.

Most anti-apoptotic members contain the Bcl-2 homology (BH) domains 1, 2 and 4, and transmembrane domains, whereas the BH3 domain seems to be crucial for apoptosis induction. The pro-apoptotic members can be subdivided into the Bax subfamily (Bax, Bak, Bok) and the BH3-only proteins (for example, Bid, Bad and Bim). 4 conserved region having homology domain (BH1- 4) more than 20 members divided into three categories (Fig.1-8)

These molecules widely present in hematopoietic cells, epithelial cells, lymphocytes, nerve cells and a variety of tumor cells are located in the inner mitochondrial membrane, cell membrane surface portion of the inner nuclear membrane and endoplasmic reticulum. Homodimers and the form of heterodimers by the Bcl-2 family proteins can promote or inhibit apoptosis (Fig. 1-9)

Bcl-2/Bax ratio determines sensitivity to apoptosis play an important role in inhibition of apoptosis factor / promote overall rate of apoptotic factors, the final decision cell survival or death.

In more common malignancies, Bcl-2 expression has often positive: such as, hematopoietic malignancies (leukemia, lymphoma), breast cancer, neuroblastoma, nasopharyngeal carcinoma, prostate cancer, lung squamous cell carcinoma, adenocarcinoma, and so on. Bcl-2-positive tumors are poorer prognosis than the Bcl-2-negative tumors.

Tumor cells can acquire resistance to apoptosis by various mechanisms that interfere at different levels of apoptosis signaling. One mechanism is the overexpression of anti-apoptotic genes. A common feature of 85% follicular B-cell lymphoma is the chromosomal translocation t (14;18), which couples the Bcl-2 gene to the immunoglobulin heavy chain locus and leads to enhanced Bcl-2 expression. Bcl-2 cooperates with the oncoprotein c-Myc or, in acute promyelocytic leukaemia and the promyelocytic leukaemia–retinoic-acid-receptor- (PML–RAR) fusion protein, thereby they contribute to tumorigenesis. Some studies have shown a correlation between high levels of Bcl-2 expression and the severity of malignancy of human tumors. Bcl-2 immunostaining commonly used to distinguish between the reactive proliferation and follicular lymphoma (Fig. 1-10).

Moreover, it has been shown in in vitro and in vivo models that Bcl-2 expression confers resistance to many kinds of chemotherapeutic drugs and irradiation. In some types of tumors, a high level of Bcl-2 expression is associated with a poor response to chemotherapy and seems to be predictive of shorter, disease-free survival. The tumor-associated viruses Epstein–Barr virus (EBV) and human herpesvirus 8 (HHV8 or Kaposi's sarcoma-associated herpesvirus) encode proteins that are homologues of Bcl-2. Both proteins — BHRF1 from EBV and KSbcl-2 (vBcl-2) from HHV8 — have an anti-apoptotic function and enhance survival of the infected cells. In this way, they might contribute to tumor formation after virus infection, and to resistance of these tumors to therapy.

In addition, other anti-apoptotic Bcl-2 family members also seem to be involved in resistance of tumors to apoptosis. For example, Bcl-XL can confer resistance to multiple apoptosis-inducing pathways in cell lines and seems to be upregulated by a constitutively active mutant epidermal growth factor receptor (EGFR) in vitro. myeloid cell leukemia sequence 1(MCL1) can also render cell lines resistant to chemotherapy. In some leukemia patients, MCL1 expression is increased at the time of relapse, which indicates that some anticancer drugs might select for leukemia cells that have elevated MCL1 levels.

(2) Caspase Family

It is a set of important regulators of apoptosis. Caspase family is a group of proteases, by which efficient and specific proteolysis is mediated by dying cells. It is the executor of apoptosis. A total of 14 key members, including caspase-2, 3, 6, 7, 8, 9, 10 are mainly involved in apoptosis and others are involved in inflammation (Fig. 1-11).

Caspase proteolytic enzyme has two characteristics: ①all are cysteine proteases; ② All the sites of action, after spartic acid residues (Asp) sites. are cut off after being converted from the zymogen into the active protease. For example cascase 3 structural model and its activation process

Caspase family protein is an inactive zymogen present in the cytoplasm manner, when they are activated by certain way, according to a certain order, some important protein cleavage substrate, which result in a series of apoptosis morphological and biochemical changes.

(3) IAP Family

The IAPs (inhibitor of apoptosis proteins) as regulatory proteins bind to and inhibit caspases. They also might function as ubiquitin ligases, promoting the degradation of the caspases by binding. IAPs are characterized by a domain termed the baculoviral IAP repeat (BIR). Nine IAP family members — including XIAP (hILP, MIHA, ILP-1), cIAP1 (MIHB, HIAP-2), cIAP2 (HIAP-1, MIHC, API2), NAIP, ML-IAP, ILP2, KIAP, apollon and survivin — have been identified in human cells. However, not all BIR-containing proteins have been shown to suppress apoptosis, and some of them might also have functions other than caspase inhibition. IAPs are inhibited by a protein named SMAC/DIABLO (second mitochondria-derived activator of caspase/direct IAP binding protein with low pI), which is released from mitochondria along with cytochrome c during apoptosis and promotes caspase activation by binding to, and inhibiting, IAPs.

Studies have shown that over-expression of the above protein can inhibit a variety of different degrees of apoptotic cells. Intensity is XIAP> c-IAP2> c-IAP1> survivin

Expression of the IAP-family protein survivin is highly tumor specific. It is found in most human tumors but not in normal adult tissues. In neuroblastoma, expression correlates with a more aggressive and unfavourable disease. But although survivin has a BIR domain, it is not clear whether it directly acts as an apoptosis inhibitor, for example by binding to caspase-9 or interacting with SMAC/DIABLO. Survivin might also be necessary for completion of the cell cycle. Nevertheless, overexpression of survivin counteracts apoptosis in some settings: in transgenic mice that express survivin in the skin, its anti-apoptotic function was more prominent than its role in cell division. Survivin that is inhibited in UVB-induced apoptosis in vitro and in vivo, whereas it did not affect CD95-induced cell death. Expression of a non-phosphorylatable mutant of survivin induces *Cyt-c*release and cell death. In xenograft tumor models, this mutant suppressed tumor growth and reduced intraperitoneal tumor dissemination.

Most tumors are independent on the survival signals that protect normal cells from death by neglect. This is achieved by alterations in the PI3K/AKT pathway. Oncogenes such as RAS or BCR–ABL can increase PI3K activity. The catalytic subunit of PI3K has been shown to be amplified in ovarian cancer.

Another IAP family member, cIAP2, is affected by the translocation t(11;18)(q21;q21), which is found in about 50% of marginal cell lymphomas of the mucosa-associated lymphoid tissue (MALT). This indicates a role for cIAP2 in the development of MALT lymphoma. ML-IAP is expressed at high levels in melanoma cell lines, but not in primary melanocytes. Melanoma cell lines that express ML-IAP are significantly more resistant to drug-induced apoptosis than those that do not express ML-IAP.

(4) Fas

Also known as APO-1 (CD95), while in 1989 the two laboratories found that a protein molecule surface-mediated apoptosis in cell lines, which belonged to NTFR family, and its molecular weight was 45,000, cell membrane antigen, can inhibit tumor cell proliferation and induce apoptosis, Fasl and CD95 mutated in many tumor drug resistance and relapse, especially in lymphoma, APO-1 expression of Fas leukemia and cancer patients often have a certain influence on the prognosis. Fasl of T lymphocytes natural Fas ligand (ligant), Fasl and binding to cells expressing Fas that cause the latter events to apoptosis.

Another mechanism, by which tumors interfere with death-receptor-mediated apoptosis, might be the expression of soluble receptors that acts as decoys for death ligands. Until now, two distinct soluble receptors-soluble CD95 (sCD95) and decoy receptor 3 (DcR3) — have been shown to competitively inhibit CD95 signaling. sCD95 is expressed in various malignancies, and elevated levels can be found in the sera of cancer patients. High sCD95 serum levels were associated with poor prognosis in melanoma patients.

DcR3 binds to CD95L and the TNF family member LIGHT (a cytokine that is homologous to lymphotoxins, exhibits inducible expression and competes with herpes simplex virus (HSV) glycoprotein D for herpesvirus entry mediator (HVEM), a receptor expressed by T cells) and inhibits CD95L-induced apoptosis. It is genetically amplified in several lung and colon carcinomas and is overexpressed in several adenocarcinomas, glioma cell lines and glioblastomas. Ectopic expression of DcR3 in a rat glioma model results in decreased immune-cell infiltration, which indicates that DcR3 is involved in immune evasion of malignant glioma.

(5) p53: (Molecular Policeman)

Wild-type p53 gene plays an important role in the maintenance of cell growth, cell malignant proliferation inhibition (Fig. 1-12). After the p53 gene mutation, promote cells carcinogenesis. A key element in stress-induced apoptosis is p53. Rapid induction of p53 function is achieved in response to most forms of stress through post-translational mechanisms. p53 can be stabilized and activated through the inactivation of MDM2, either by ARF, or by direct phosphorylation of MDM2.Proliferative signals induce ARF, the product encoded by an alternative reading frame within the CDKN2A tumor-suppressor gene locus, which also encodes the cyclin-dependent kinase inhibitor INK4A. p53 is inhibited by MDM2, an ubiquitin ligase that targets p53 for destruction by the proteasome. MDM2 is inactivated by binding to ARF.ARF interacts with the ubiquitin ligase MDM2, and prevents it from binding p53 and targeting it for destruction in the proteasome. Upregulation of p53 leads to cell-cycle arrest and apoptosis.In addition, many post-translational modifications of p53 have been shown to enhance its transcriptional activity in response to stress, including phosphorylation, sumolation and acetylation. The transcriptional activity of p53 is important for its pro-apoptotic function. p53 can induce the expression of proteins involved in the mitochondrial pathway — such as Bax, NOXA, PUMA and p53AIP1—and in the death receptor pathway—such as CD95, TRAIL-R1and TRAIL-R2.Moreover, transcriptionally independent activities of p53 mediate some of their pro-apoptotic effects, including protein–protein interactions, direct effects in the mitochondria and relocalization of death receptors to the cell surface.

After the p53 gene mutation, due to changes in the spatial structure affects its transcriptional activation, thus the loss of wild-type p53 tumor suppression, and have the function of oncogenes.

The presence of p53 mutations in more than 50% of malignant tumors lead to different CML apoptosis genes downstream of Bcr-abl, APL in PML-RARa, inhibition of apoptosis.

Section 2   Morphology of Apoptosis

1. Morphological Changes of Apoptotic Cells

Microvilli on the cell surface disappear; the cells show dehydration, condensation, budding, blebbing, nuclear squeeze, shrinkage, chromatin condensation and margination, then they form apoptotic bodies.

2. Elimination Process

Apoptotic cells and apoptotic bodies are recognized and quickly engulfed by homogeneous or heterogeneous cells (macrophage, etc). They form phagosomes, and undergo further degeneration and digestion in lysosomes. They sometimes present either lysosomal residual bodies or occasionally escape, such as duct epithelial apoptosis falls into the lumen.

Apoptosis involves rapid DNA damage, possibly due to activation of endogenous endonucleases and early condensation and fragmentation of chromatin, followed by cell lysis. The fragmented "apoptotic bodies" may be phagocytosed by adjacent macrophages (Fig.1-13)and same cell types. There are some explanations: ①Selective loss of water and electrolytes in apoptotic cells. ②The mechanism of cytoplasm and nucleus bubbling is related to the damage of cytoskeletal proteins. ③The stiff shell of protein under membrane is related to apoptotic cell shrinkage and insolubility. ④Receptors on the phagocytes and ligands on apoptotic cells respond each other resulting in the eliminating process. ⑤The mutual response happens suddenly, and it sustains for several minutes, in about 4 to 9 hours it is recognized out from tissues.

They have different names in different tissues: ① Tingible body macrophages in reactive hyperplasia of lymph nodes; ② Civatte bodies; ③ Councilman bodies in hepatitis

3. Difference Between Apoptosis and Necrosis (Table 1-1 and Fig. 1-14)

Table 1-1   Difference Between Apoptosis and Necrosis

	Apoptosis	Necrosis
Cause	Physiological or pathological	Pathological changes or severe injury
Scope	Scattered single cell	Large organizations or groups of cells
Membrane	Intact until the formation of apoptotic bodies	Damaged
Chromatin	In the nuclear membrane condensed half-shaped	flocculent
Organelles	No significant change	Swelling, endoplasmic reticulum disintegration
Cell volume	Condensation smaller	Swelling increases
Apoptotic bodies	Yes, there was engulfed neighboring cells or macrophages	No, cell autolysis, residual debris phagocytosis by macrophages
Genomic DNA	There controlled degradation, electrophoresis pattern showed ladder	Random degradation, electrophoresis pattern was spreadable
Protein synthesis	Have	No
Adjustment process	By gene regulation, proactively	Passive conduct
Inflammation	No, does not release the cell contents	Yes , the release of the contents

Section 3   Apoptosis and Diseases

1. Etiology

(1) Various damaging factors are not sufficient to cause cell death

(2) Certain viral infections

(3) Some atrophy lesions

(4) Tumor progression

(5) TCL induced cell death

(6) Some mitochondrial apoptosis and necrosis in injury.

2. Excessive Apoptosis Relating Diseases

(1) Neurodegenerative Diseases: Alzheimer's disease (AD)

①β- amyloid protein / calcium overload / oxidative stress / NGF ↓ → neuronal apoptosis (Alzheimer Disease, AD); ②Parkinson's disease; ③Multiple sclerosis; ④Retinitis pigmentosa

(2)Acute kidney injury(AKI) , Heart Failure (Hypoxic-ischemic Encephalopathy)

Oxidative stress / pressure, volume overload ↑ / nerve - endocrine disorders / TNF / ischemia / hypoxia → myocardial apoptosis

(3) AIDS HIV -Infection→ CD4$^+$cell apoptosis;

Liver Lesions: viral hepatitis and alcoholic hepatitis

(4)Myocardial Ischemia - Reperfusion Injury

Early ischemic or surrounding the infarct areas, ischemic - reperfusion injury serious than a simple ischemic apoptosis

Mechanism: ① oxidative stress: SOD reduce, ② Fas receptor upregulation: FasL reaction, ③ p53 activation

(5) Myelodysplastic Syndrome: Pernicious anemia

3. Insufficient Apoptosis Relating Diseases

(1) Autoimmune diseases - thymus negative selection mechanism disorders

Autoimmune diseases, viral infection of autoreactive T, B lymphocytes, for some virus-infected cells, the cytotoxicity of the target cells, and some tumor cells by apoptosis way to clear and subsided.

(2) Various infect diseases during basic lesions of inflammation, exudate is the most important, no exudation does not account for inflammation. After the neutrophils from the vascular leak to complete the anti-inflammatory function in lesions inflammation, it cannot return to the blood vessels, so there is a need to start the mechanism of apoptosis, so that inflammation is terminated. Wound granulation tissue repair, and fibroblast proliferation and collagen secretion, and subsequently fibroblasts into fibroblasts, and scar formation, apoptotic mechanisms may be involved in healing.

The tumor-associated viruses Epstein–Barr virus (EBV) and human herpesvirus 8 (HHV8 or Kaposi's sarcoma-associated herpesvirus) encode proteins that are homologues of Bcl-2. Both proteins - BHRF1 from EBV and KSbcl-2 (vBcl-2) from HHV8 - have an anti-apoptotic function and enhance survival of the infected cells. In this way, they might contribute to tumor formation after virus infection, and may resist these tumors to therapy.

In EBV-positive Burkitt's lymphoma cell lines, an increased FLIP:caspase-8 ratiocorrelated with resistance to CD95-mediated apoptosis. Viral analogues of FLIP, called viral FLIPs (v-FLIPs), are encoded by some tumorigenic viruses, including HHV8. In cells that are latently infected with HHV8, v-FLIP is expressed at low levels, but its expression is increased in advanced Kaposi's sarcomas or on serum withdrawal from lymphoma cells in culture. Therefore, v-FLIPs might contribute to the persistence and oncogenicity of v-FLIP-encoding viruses. Although FLIP expression prevents apoptosis induction through death receptors, it does not inhibit cell death induced by perforin/granzyme, chemotherapeutic drugs or g-irradiation. Nevertheless, it mediates the immune escape of tumors in mouse models. Tumors with high expression levels of FLIP were shown to escape from T-cell-mediated immunity in vivo, despite the presence of the perforin/granzyme pathway, so tumor cells with elevated FLIP levels seem to have a selective advantage. FLIP overexpression also prevents rejection of tumors by perforin-deficient NK cells. Moreover, human melanomas and a murine B-cell lymphoma cell line are shown to express high levels of FLIP, which interfere with apoptosis induction at the level of the death receptors.

(3) Tumors   In cells and tissues of multicellular organisms, potent physiological mechanisms govern cell proliferation and homeostasis. Many of these growth-control mechanisms are linked to apoptosis. Excessive proliferation or growth at inappropriate sites induces apoptosis in the affected cells. Tumors can proliferate beyond these constraints, which limit growth in normal tissue. Therefore, resistance of tumor cells to apoptosis is an essential feature of cancer development.

Over expression of growth-promoting oncogenes in tumor formation-such as c-Myc, E1A or E2F1 — sensitizes cells to apoptosis. Besides the expression of proteins that promote cell proliferation,tumor progression requires the expression of anti-apoptotic proteins or the inactivation of essential pro-apoptotic proteins.

Some studies have shown Bcl-2 expression confers resistance to many kinds of chemotherapeutic drugs and radiation. In some types of tumors, a high level of Bcl-2 expression is associated with a poor response to chemotherapy and seems to be predictive of shorter, disease-free survival.

Another mechanism, by which tumors interfere withdeath-receptor-mediated apoptosis, might be the expression of soluble receptors that acts as decoys for death ligands. Until now, two distinct soluble receptors — soluble CD95 (sCD95) and decoy receptor 3 (DcR3) — have been shown to competitively inhibit CD95 signaling. sCD95 is expressed in various malignancies, and elevated levels can be found in the sera of cancer patients. High sCD95 serum levels are associated with poor prognosis in melanoma patients.DcR3 binds to CD95L and the TNF family member LIGHT (a cytokine that is homologous to lymphotoxins, exhibits inducible expression and competes with herpes simplex virus (HSV) glycoprotein D for herpesvirus entry mediator (HVEM), a receptor expressed by T cells and inhibits CD95L-induced apoptosis. It is genetically amplified in several lung and colon carcinomas and is overexpressed in several adenocarcinomas, glioma cell lines and glioblastomas. Ectopic expression of DcR3 in a rat glioma model results in decreased immune-cell infiltration, which indicates that DcR3 is involved in immune evasion of malignant glioma. Finally, tumor cells resist killing by cytotoxic lymphocytes not only by blocking the death-receptor pathway, but also by interfering with the perforin/granzyme pathway. Expression of the serine protease inhibitor PI-9/SPI-6, which inhibits granzyme B, results in the resistance of tumor cells to cytotoxic lymphocytes,leading to immune escape.

Besides overexpression of anti-apoptotic genes, tumors can acquire apoptosis resistance by downregulating or mutating pro-apoptotic molecules. In certain types of cancer, the pro-apoptotic Bcl-2 family member Bax is mutated. Frameshift mutations that lead to loss of expression, and mutations in the BH domains that result in loss of functions, are common. Tumor cell lines with frameshift mutations are more resistant to apoptosis. Reduced Bax expression is associated with a poor response rate to chemotherapy and shorter survival in some situations.

Moreover, others showed that inactivation of wild-type Bax confers a strong advantage during clonal evolution of the tumor. Injection of clones with either wild-type or mutant Bax into nude mice led to outgrowth of tumors that did not express Bax in both situations.

Metastatic melanomas have found another way to escape mitochondria-dependent apoptosis. These tumors often do not express APAF1, which forms an integral part of the apoptosome, and the APAF1 locus shows a high rate of allelic loss. The remaining allele is transcriptionally inactivated by gene methylation. APAF1-negative melanomas fail to respond to chemotherapy- a situation that is commonly found in this type of tumor.

The N-Myc oncogene has been amplified.in neuroblastomas, the gene for the initiator caspase-8 is frequently inactivated by gene deletion or methylation. Caspase-8-deficient neuroblastoma cells are resistant to death-receptor- and DOXORUBICIN-mediated apoptosis.

Moreover, death receptors are downregulated or inactivated in many tumors. The expression of the death receptor CD95 is reduced in some tumor cells- for example, in hepatocellular carcinomas, neoplastic colon epithelium, melanomas and other tumors -compared with their normal counterparts. Loss of CD95, probably by downregulation of transcription, might contribute to chemoresistance and immune evasion.Oncogenic Ras seems to downregulate CD95, and in hepatocellular carcinomas loss of CD95 expression is accompanied by p53 aberrations.

Several CD95 gene mutations have been reported in primary samples of myeloma and T-cell leukaemia. The mutations include point mutations in the cytoplasmic death domain of CD95 and a deletion that leads to a truncated form of the death receptor. These mutated forms of CD95 might interfere in a dominant-negative way with apoptosis induction by CD95. In families with germ-line CD95 mutations, which usually result in autoimmune lymphoproliferative syndrome (ALPS), the risk of developing lymphomas is increased.

Deletions and mutations of the death receptors TRAIL-R1 and TRAIL-R2 have also been observed in tumors. The frequent deletion of the chromosomal region 8p21-22 in head and neck cancer and in non-small-cell lung cancers affects the TRAIL-R2 gene. Mutations have been found in the ectodomain or the death domain of TRAIL-R1 or TRAIL-R2. Further mutations result in truncated forms of these TRAIL receptors or other anti-apoptotic forms.

Finally, reduced expression of the pro-apoptotic protein XAF1 (XIAP-associated factor 1) can be observed in various cancer cell lines. XAF1 binds to XIAP and antagonizes its anti-apoptotic function at the level of the caspases.

Most tumors altered survival signaling and are independent on the survival signals that protect normal cells from death by neglect. This is achieved by alterations in the PI3K/AKT pathway. Oncogenes such as Ras or BCR–ABL can increase PI3K activity. The catalytic subunit of PI3K has been shown to be amplified in ovarian cancer. PTEN, the cellular antagonist of PI3K, is frequently deleted in advanced tumor s, and a significant rate of PTEN mutations can be found in various cancer types.

4. Insufficient and Excessive Apoptosis Coexist Diseases

Such as Atherosclerosis

5. Therapeutic Induction of Apoptosis

Cancer treatment by chemotherapy and -irradiation kills target cells primarily by the induction of apoptosis. Anticancerdrugs are classified as the following: DNA-damaging agents, antimetabolites, mitotic inhibitors, nucleotide analogues or inhibitors of topoisomerases.Treatment with these agents or with-irradiation causes cellular stress and finally cell death. However, few tumors are sensitive to these therapies, and the development of resistance to therapy is an important clinical problem. Patients who have tumor relapse usually present with tumors that are more resistant to therapy than the primary tumor. Failure to activate the apoptotic programme represents an important mode of drug resistance in tumor cells.

Clearly, this is not the only pathway of chemotherapy-induced cell death. Many drugs seem to initiate the mitochondrial pathway directly. Moreover, cell death might not even require caspase activation. It is questionable whether a single predominant effector pathway of chemotherapy can be identified at all. Probably, the engagement of pathway depends on the stress stimulus, the cell type, the tumor environment and many other factors. However, because chemotherapy and irradiation exert their effects primarily by apoptosis induction, it is conceivable that modulation of the key elements of apoptosis signaling directly influences therapy-induced tumor-cell death.

Induced apoptosis in cancer therapy: ① Stimulating some apoptosis-inducing genes activity: ② inhibitingp53 mutation and weaken Bcl-2 to inhibit apoptosis; ③ The application point mutation technology, inactiving or repairing the abnormal expression and mutation of oncogenes; ④ Import drug sensitivity gene helps apoptosis.

p53 is a key element in apoptosis induction in tumor cells. As discussed above,p53 is inhibited by MDM2. MDM2 is inactivated by binding to ARF. Cellular stress, including that induced by chemotherapy or irradiation, activates p53 either directly, by inhibition of MDM2, or indirectly by activation of ARF. ARF can also be induced by proliferative oncogenes such as Ras. Active p53 transactivates pro-apoptotic genesto promote apoptosis. (Fig.1-15). Chemotherapeutic drugs (for example, the nucleotide analogue 5-fluoruracil, 5-FU) induce CD95 by a transcriptionally regulated, p53-dependent mechanism. They also engage the SAPK/JNK pathway, which eventually leads to upregulation of CD95L. Upregulation of CD95 and CD95L then allows the cells to either commit suicide or kill neighbouring cells. Clearly, this is not the only pathway of chemotherapy-induced cell death. Many drugs seem to initiate the mitochondrial pathway directly. Moreover, cell death might not even require caspases activation. It is questionable whether a single predominant effector pathway of chemotherapy can be identified at all. Probably, the engagement of pathway depends on the stress stimulus, the cell type, the tumor microenvironment and many other factors. However, because chemotherapy and irradiation exert their effects primarily by apoptosis induction, it is conceivable that modulation of the key elements of apoptosis signaling directly influences therapy-induced tumor-cell death.

Perforin target cell membrane polymerization that granzyme is able to enter the cell. Grainactivating target cells caspases. In addition, granzyme B may be directly cut Bcl-2family members BID to activate mitochondrial death pathway.

Cancer treatment effects should take into account:① Whether have apoptosis after treatment, because it is a key of chemotherapy effects; ② Apoptosis Index and proliferating Index ratio(AI / PI); ③ At the same time can induce apoptosis has become a new standard for screening anti-cancer drugs; ④Induced apoptosis in tumor therapy would be an important complement and innovation.

Section 4   Detection Methods of Apoptosis

1. Apoptosis Detection Solved Follow Problems

(1) Whether there is apoptosis in research system or not, namely qualitative.

(2) The incidence of apoptosis is shown in all population of cells. This is a relative concept, the analysis combining with the proliferation rate of the cell population, is more objective, more reflecting of the growth state of the cell population.

(3) Learning apoptosis severity to reflect the stage of apoptosis.

The methods include morphology, biochemistry, molecular biology technology such as electron microscopy, fluorescence microscopy, agarose gel electrophoresis, Tunel (terminal deoxynucleotidyl Transferase mediate dUTP Nick End Labeling) in situ detection of apoptosis, flow cytometry (FCM), etc.

2. Methods

(1) Morphology Methods: Light microscope, Transmission electron microscope,Scanning electron microscope, Laser confocalmicroscope, Imunohistochemistry and Imunofluoresence,etc.

(2) Annexin V-FITC Staining: In normal living cells, phosphatidylserine（ PS ）is positioned inside the cell membrane，but in the early apoptotic PS flip from the inside of the cell membrane to the surface of the cell membrane can it be detected by a negatively charged phospholipids with high affinity protein——Annexin V Annexin- V is a molecular weight of 35-36KD Ca^{2+} dependent phospholipid binding protein, and it binds to PS with high affinity. Therefore Annexin-V luciferase (such as FITC, PE) or biotin (Biotin) is labeled as a probe by flow cytometry or fluorescence microscopy to detect the occurrence of early apoptotic cells.（ Fig. 1-16 ）.

(3) Flow Cytometry [PI (propidium iodide) staining]: Using the cell DNA binding properties of the fluorescent dye PI to detect each of the cells because of its different DNA content, thus combining different fluorescent dyes, fluorescent intensity is not the same flow cytometry.

$G_2 \sim M$ phase DNA content is twice the $G_0 \sim G_1$, and S phase in between.In apoptosis less DNA content, which can be in front of the cell $G_0 \sim G_1$ phase has a diploid peak (thus considered to be apoptotic cell).However, due to its DNA content, cell death itself is reduced, which makes it very difficult to distinguish between apoptosis and death。The classic test data flow diagram is given that the apoptotic cells are next to a peak $G_0 \sim G_1$ phase peak, peak cell death from the G_0-G_1 phase peak is far, but the typical result is difficult to get.

(4) Nuclear DNA Fragments Detection(DNA Ladder): After extracting the cells or tissue DNA agarose gel electrophoresis

Benefits of this method are simple and low cost. But the results appear more difficult

(5) Caspase Activity Assay: The caspase-3 sequence-specific peptides conjugate to the chromophore (DEVD- pNA). When the substrate cuts caspase-3, the chromophore (pNA) that is freed，absorbance values can be measured by a microplate reader or spectrophotometer(λ=405nm or 400nm), to examine the degree of activation of caspase-3. To multiply the relationship with the control group treated to reflect the level of organization of caspase-3 activity. Caspase-3 activity level in tissue may, to some extent, reflect the presence or absence of treatment factors inducing apoptosis in vivo.

(6) TUNEL(Terminal deoxynucleotidyl transferase-mediated dUTP nick-end-labeling): By the end of the DNA transferase tagged dNTP (mostly dUTP) indirectly (through digoxin) or directly to the 3'-OH DNA fragment ends, and then by enzyme-linked chromogenic or fluorescence detection quantitative analysis. It is in situ apoptosis detection to carry out in cell suspensions or tissue paraffin slides.

The shortcoming of TUNEL follows:

1) Necrotic cell's DNA also splits point form, but also presents TUNEL-positive, and therefore has poor specificity。

2) TUNEL immunohistochemical detection, influences the process of testing a larger fixed size slices, thickness will directly affect the fixed effect, resulting in differences in the results。

3. Precautions in Apoptosis Detection

(1) Because apoptosis is a multi-factorial, multi-step process,the results cannot be judged based on a single apoptotic indicator, so there is a need for the simultaneous detection of multiple indicators

(2) Because apoptotic events and apoptotic cells appear different at different times, and each indicator has a period of time to maintain, so they need to be detectedat different time points of samples to ensure the accuracy of test results.

(3) Experiments need to set positive and negative controls, to avoid false positive or false negative.

(4) Considering how to quantity and remove the other interferes。

Challenges and Prospects

1. Summary

(1) Apoptosis is a multi-step, cell-death programme pathway that is inherent in every cell of the body. In cancer, the apoptosis: cell-division ratio is altered, which results in a net gain of malignant tissue.

(2) Apoptosis can be initiated either through the death-receptor or the mitochondrial pathway. Caspases that cleave cellular substrates leading to characteristic biochemical and morphological changes are activated in both pathways. The apoptotic process is tightly controlled by various proteins. There are also other caspase-independent types of cell death.

(3) Many physiological growth-control mechanisms that govern cell proliferation and tissue homeostasis are linked to apoptosis. Therefore, resistance of tumor cells to apoptosis might be an essential feature of cancer development.

(4) Immune cells (T cells & natural killer cells) can kill tumor cells using the granule exocytosis pathway or the death-receptor pathway. Apoptotic resistance of tumor cells might lead to escape from immunosurveillance and might influence the efficacy of immunotherapy.

(5) Cancer treatment by chemotherapy and -irradiation kills target cells primarily by inducing apoptosis. Therefore, modulation of the key elements of apoptosis signaling directly influences therapy-induced tumor-cell death.

(6) Tumor cells can acquire resistance to apoptosis by the expression of anti-apoptotic proteins or by the downregulation or mutation of pro-apoptotic proteins.

(7) Alterations of the p53 pathway also influence the sensitivity of tumor cells to apoptosis. Moreover, most tumors are independent of survival signals because they have upregulated the phosphatidylinositol 3-kinase (PI3K)/AKT pathway.

2. Problems

(1) Is there apoptosis in the process of cell development (time and manner, at which point gene exists)?

(2) Whether the real killer genes exist in the body or not? How do the death related genes regulate?

(3) Which signal transduction pathways of apoptosis are exactly working?

(4) Can the therapeutic purposes of diseases and disorders be achieved through regulating apoptosis?

(5) What is the relationship between apoptosis and senescence? Does survival gene exist?

Consider/Questions

1. Basic concepts in this chapter

Apoptosis, programmed cell death(PCD), apoptotic body, Endoplasmic reticulum stress response (ESR), Bcl-2, p53.

2. What is the difference between necrosis and apoptosis?

3. What morphological changes occur in the cell apoptosis?

4. What are the ways for regulating apoptosis?

5. Which three important enzymes are regulating apoptosis?

6. How many apoptosis-related genes are there?

7. List five methods of detecting apoptosis.

8. How do you research cell apoptosis in your focus on the disease?

9. Why should a cell commit"suicide" ?and what makes a cell decide to coumit"suicide" ?

第二章 细胞自噬

细胞有多种死亡形式，其主要有三种类型：凋亡即 I 型细胞程序性死亡、自噬即 II 型细胞程序性死亡和细胞坏死。

自噬是一种溶酶体降解途径，以双层膜自噬囊泡的形成为特点。从粗面内质网的无核糖体附着区或线粒体脱落的双层膜包裹的自噬小泡又被称为自噬体，其可吞没部分细胞溶质、受损的细胞器、蛋白质聚集体及细菌等。自噬囊泡通常是沿着微管运输定位到细胞核周围。随后自噬囊泡的外膜与溶酶体融合，形成自噬溶酶体，降解其所包裹的内容物和内膜，以实现细胞自身代谢的需要和某些细胞器的更新[1, 2]。

自噬是一种进化保守的细胞内自卫机制[3]，其中细胞器和蛋白质被隔离到自噬小泡内，随后自噬小泡通过与溶酶体融合后被降解，因此细胞可以预防一些损伤或不必要的成分的毒性积累，也可以回收这些成分来维持体内代谢平衡。

2016 年诺贝尔生理学或医学奖得主是日本工业大学的 Yoshinori Ohsumi，获奖理由：他的研究阐明了细胞自噬的分子机制和生理功能，帮助人们认识到自噬不仅仅是耗损细胞元件的一个垃圾处理系统，还是一种必不可少的细胞功能。这一研究促进了对自噬的分子生物学机制及自噬的生理功能的认识。他还是首批撰写酵母中自噬信号通路相关蛋白名单的研究人员之一。

第一节 细胞自噬的形态学和发生过程

一、自噬的形态学特点

Ashford 和 Porten 于 1962 年用电子显微镜在人的肝细胞中最早观察到自噬现象。因此通过透射电镜检测细胞超微结构的形态学一直被认为是检测自噬发生的"金标准"，典型的自噬超微结构改变包括细胞器肿胀、出现空泡状双层膜结构，以及出现双层膜结构环绕的自噬体和不能完全降解的残体等[4]（图 2-1）。

二、自噬泡的形成及融合方式

当自噬发生初期，细胞质中可见到游离的大量膜性结构即前自噬泡。

前自噬泡逐渐延展，构成一种膜性小泡，其内包裹着受损的细胞器和变性的大分子物质，这种膜性小泡就是自噬泡（autophagic vesicle，AV）或称自噬体（autophagosome）。

在自噬过程中，自噬泡形成后其外膜与溶酶体膜相互融合，在溶酶体内水解酶作用下，自噬泡内膜与其中包裹的物质进入到溶酶体腔，被分解为氨基酸、核苷酸及游离脂肪酸等，可被细胞再利用以组成细胞成分。自噬体与溶酶体融合成自噬溶酶体（图 2-2）。

在真核细胞中自噬发生的分子机制具有高度保守性，包括独特的自噬囊泡产生的步骤，即启动，成核，自噬囊泡成熟，以及在溶酶体自噬囊泡内容物的融合与降解（图 2-3）。在启动期，新生的自噬泡（AV）膜有多种来源（包括隔离膜、内质网或线粒体外膜），形成一个与自噬机制相关的，包

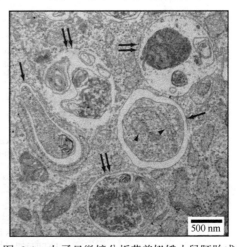

图 2-1 电子显微镜分析营养饥饿小鼠胚胎成纤维细胞；Electron microscopic analysis of nutrient-starved mouse embryonic fibroblasts
箭号表示自噬体，双箭号表示自噬溶酶体/自噬内涵体，箭头指示内质网内的自噬体的碎片；Arrows indicate autophagosomes and double arrows indicate autolysosomes/amphisomes. Arrowheads indicate fragments of endoplasmic reticulum inside the autophagosome

括与微管相关蛋白 LC3 的动力学变化有关的杯样结构的自噬体。在应激和（或）泛素化底物积累诱导的自噬中，放大杯样自噬体结构，能测序底物，其中包括泛素蛋白或细胞器及饥饿诱导自噬中的可溶性胞质。新生的 AV 中双膜封闭形成成熟的 AV，然后靶向性地与溶酶体融合。在溶酶体中水解酶消化 AV 内容物和内膜。通过细胞质招募其他新的 AV 使自噬机制（如 LC3）再循环。

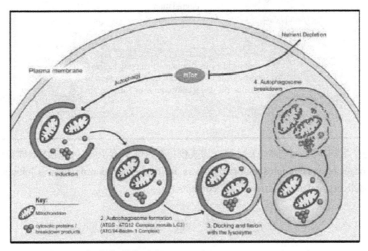

图 2-2 自噬泡形成过程；Autophagosome forming process

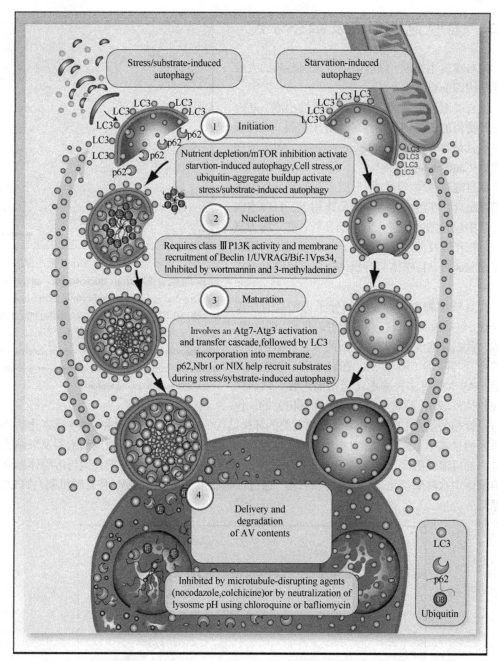

图 2-3 自噬囊泡产生的步骤，包括：①启动；②成核；③自噬囊泡成熟；④在溶酶体自噬囊泡内容物的融合与降解；Autophagy occurs through a multistep process, including four control points: ①initiation; ②nucleation; ③maturation; ④delivery and degradation of AV contents

三、自 噬 分 类

根据底物进入溶酶体途径的三种不同类型的自噬被广泛研究[5]（图 2-4）。

（1）巨自噬（macroautophagy）：细胞质中的物质通过形成小泡的方式转运到溶酶体中，巨自噬主要降解细胞内老化的或损坏的细胞器和蛋白质。

隔离膜包封部分细胞质或细胞器形成自噬体。随后自噬体外膜与溶酶体融合，溶酶体脱颗粒使自噬体中内容物被降解。在酵母中自噬体产生的前自噬体结构（PAS），在哺乳动物细胞尚未确定。值得注意的是，锂可能通过激活西罗莫司靶蛋白 mTOR 抑制自噬。迄今为止被确认在隔离膜中的 Atg 蛋白，包括 ULK1/2、Atg5、Beclin-1、LC3、Atg12、Atg13、Atg14、Atg16L1、FIP200、Atg101（图 2-5）。

（2）微自噬（microautophagy）：由溶酶体直接内吞细胞物质并降解。

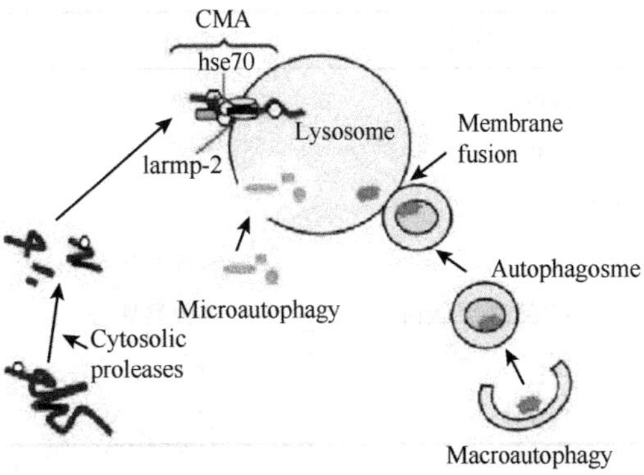

（3）分子伴侣介导的自噬（chaperone-mediated autophagy，CMA）：细胞中可溶性蛋白直接通过分子伴侣进入到溶酶体中被降解。

图 2-4　三种类型的自噬；Three types of autophagy

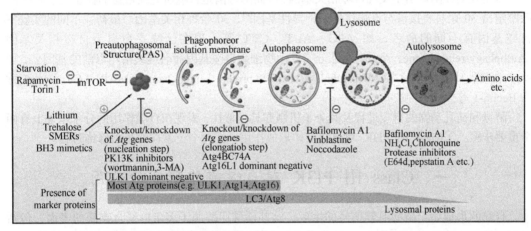

图 2-5　巨自噬的过程；The process of macroautophagy

三种自噬方式比较见表 2-1。

表 2-1　三种自噬方式比较

特点	巨自噬	微自噬	分子伴侣介导的自噬
活化方式	压力与应激	组成性	压力与应激
机制			
内吞	是	是	否
膜来源	非溶酶体	溶酶体	/
受体介导	不需要	不需要	需要
参与成分			
ATP	需要	需要	需要
GTP 和 GTPastes	需要	需要	否
细胞骨架	需要	不需要	未知
分子伴侣	未知	未知	需要
囊泡酸性 pH	是	是	否

续表

特点	巨自噬	微自噬	分子伴侣介导的自噬
膜电位	未知	是	是
PI3K	需要	未知	不需要
底物			
细胞器	各种类型	各种类型	无
可溶性胞质蛋白	各种类型	各种类型	含一种靶向序列五肽（KFERQ）的可溶性蛋白
蛋白去折叠	否	否	是
选择性	部分	部分	总是

第二节　自噬相关基因

最初人们在酵母菌中发现自噬相关基因，因而酵母菌是自噬研究最常见的模型。迄今为止，已鉴定出 30 余种直接参与自噬作用的特异性基因[6]，50 余种相关基因。最初在不同的实验室自噬基因有不同的命名，如 APG、AUT、CVT 等，现在已统一命名为自噬相关基因（Autophagy-related gene，Atg）。而部分哺乳动物细胞自噬基因命名继续沿用以前的基因名，如 Atg8 在哺乳动物称为 LC3（Microtubule-associated protein 1 light chain 3，MAP1-LC3），Atg6 称为 Beclin-1 等。

酵母和哺乳动物的自噬过程及其分子机制亦具相似性；表现在自噬作用的分子水平上有两个重要步骤：①Class Ⅲ PI3K 对自噬前体形成作用；②两个泛素样的蛋白修饰过程。

一、Class Ⅲ PI3K 对自噬前体形成的作用

自噬的形成始于磷酸肌醇信号的生成，这些磷酸肌醇源于多蛋白复合物膜的表面，包括 PI3K、Vps34 及 Beclin-1[7, 8]。Beclin-1 是 Liang 等在研究 Bcl-2 相关基因时发现的一种蛋白。

Beclin-1 是介导其他自噬蛋白定位于前自噬体的关键因子，参与调控哺乳动物自噬体的形成，是细胞自噬过程中最重要的正性调节因子[9]。

Beclin-1 是自噬泡形成所需的 PI3K 的一部分，也是自噬过程中一个重要基因，能招募自噬降解的胞质蛋白质或提供膜成分的自噬通路[10]，Beclin-1 在胚胎发育阶段及抑制肿瘤的过程中通过调节自噬活性而发挥中重要作用[11-13]。Beclin-1 失活增加了小鼠肿瘤的发生。Beclin-1 在多种人类肿瘤中异常表达。人黑色素瘤、结肠癌、卵巢和脑肿瘤[14-17]，在肝细胞癌、乳腺癌、卵巢癌和前列腺癌中有高频率的 Beclin-1 单等位基因缺失[18-21]。因此，在肿瘤发生中 Beclin-1 可能扮演肿瘤抑制基因角色，其表达下降可能导致人类癌症的发生。

二、自噬相关基因 LC3

LC3 作为自噬标志物最初被确定为微管相关蛋白 1A 和 1B 的一个单元，它是哺乳动物与自噬体膜紧密相关的酵母 Atg8 的同系物。LC3 不仅对自噬体的形成至关重要，而且也决定了自噬活性。

LC3 前体被合成、加工、修饰后其羧基端甘氨酸残基（Gly-）暴露于细胞质中形成可溶性的 LC3-Ⅰ，再被 Atg7、Atg3 活化[22]，以 LC3-Ⅱ膜结合的形式而定位于前自噬体和自噬体内

外膜上[23]（图 2-6）。

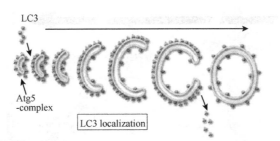

图 2-6　LC3 在自噬体内外膜定位后，Atg 复合物从膜上脱离继续参与下次自噬泡形成；After LC3s fix their positions in the autophagosome inner and outer membrane，Atg complexes away from the membrane continue to be involved in autophagosome formed next time

　　一旦 LC3 整合到双层膜上，它会产生载体连接蛋白即自噬受体，如 p62、Nbr1、NIX[24]。这些蛋白可从胞质招募载体以促进自噬囊泡的关闭。然后这些自噬囊泡被运输到溶酶体，在溶酶体中被水解酶降解。溶酶体水解酶会释放这些降解产物到胞质以便重复使用。没有被溶酶体水解酶降解的自噬泡成分会由多种外膜 Atg9、Atg2、Atg18 及 Atg21 组成的系统来实现其再循环。自噬体也可能与质膜融合，并且释放它们的内容物。

　　由于 LC3-Ⅱ始终存在于自噬体形成到自噬体与溶酶体融合的整个过程中，直到自噬体与溶酶体融合后 LC3-Ⅱ才被溶酶体中的酸性水解酶降解，因而 LC3-Ⅱ成为自噬体的标志性分子。在癌症中，自噬不仅具有肿瘤抑制剂的作用，也是维持肿瘤生存的机制之一。目前通过评估 LC3 在肿瘤标本中的表达代表细胞自噬活性，并将其结果与患者的临床病理参数联系起来进行综合研究。

三、两个泛素样的蛋白修饰过程

　　自噬作用有两个重要步骤即自噬过程中的两个泛素样蛋白加工修饰（图 2-7）。

　　（1）Atg12 首先被 Atg7 活化[25]，然后在 Atg10 的作用下形成偶联[26]，Atg12 与 Atg5 由共价键连接成异源二聚体，多个 Atg12-Atg5 复合物再与 Atg16 形成一更大的复合物[27]，从而形成自噬体前体（autophagosomal precursor）。

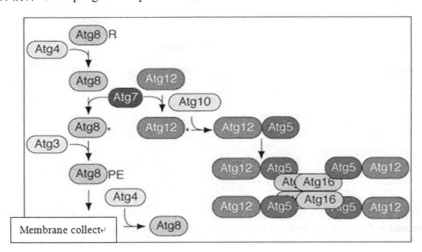

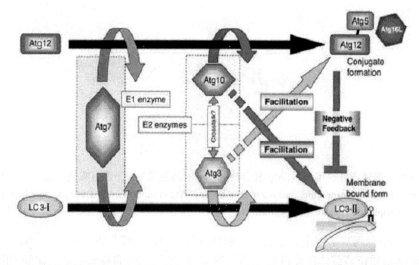

图 2-7 两个泛素样的蛋白修饰过程；Two ubiquitin-like protein modification process

（2）通过泛素样蛋白共轭级联，LC3 可以发生酯化（其涉及 Atg7、Atg3），随后由 caspase 裂解（Atg4）。

检测或干扰自噬过程中的重要基因 Beclin-1 和 LC3 可以了解细胞自噬的水平（图 2-8）。

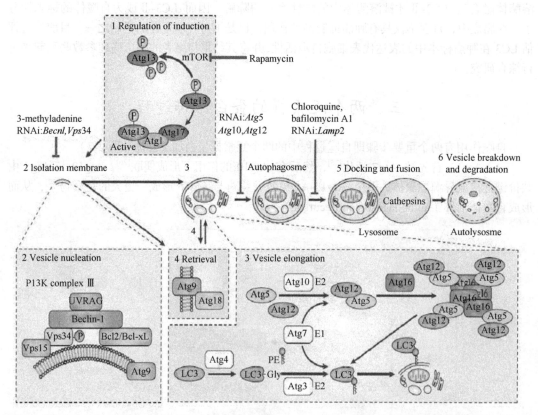

图 2-8 检测或干扰自噬过程中的重要基因 Beclin-1 和 LC3 可以了解细胞自噬的水平；Cell autophagy levels tested by detecting and interfering important genes Beclin-1 and LC3 at autophagy process

第三节 自噬与其他细胞事件的关系

自噬几乎是所有存活细胞的基本能力以维持细胞的功能，如蛋白质和细胞器转化。当细胞需要细胞内营养物质及能量，如在饥饿和生长因子摄取或有高能量需求时，自噬会上调。除此之外，在应激状态，如需清除聚合的蛋白质、受损的细胞器或细胞内病毒体时自噬也会上调。许多信号通路与自噬系统交织在一起，这种交互作用允许一个严格调控和动态的自噬以应对相应环境的变化。

一、自噬与吞噬的联系与区别

自噬是基于对细胞内物质的清除，吞噬则是对细胞外物质的清除（图 2-9 ）。

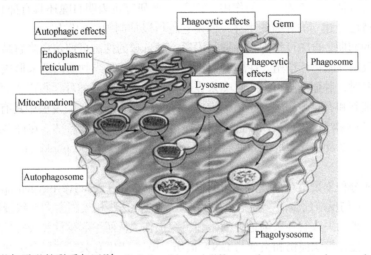

图 2-9 自噬与吞噬的联系与区别；Relationship and difference between autophagy and phagocytosis

二、自噬与凋亡

凋亡，即 I 型细胞程序性死亡依赖 caspase 参与，具有染色体浓聚、细胞皱缩、DNA 降解和凋亡小体形成等特征，其细胞的残余部分最终被巨噬细胞清除。

自噬性细胞死亡，即 II 型细胞程序性死亡，以自噬体的出现为特征，不依赖于 caspase 的参与，自噬体和其内的成分最终通过自身的溶酶体系统清除[28, 29]。因此，自噬和凋亡无论在生化代谢途径，还是形态学方面都有显著的区别。

凋亡和自噬也可共存于同一细胞内，两者间的作用和功能相互影响、制约和平衡（图2-10 ）。

作为两种不同形式的程序性细胞死亡方式，自噬与凋亡之间的关系一直是近年来研究的热点。目前的研究表明自噬与凋亡之间的关

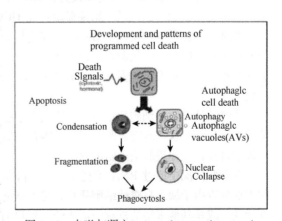

图 2-10 自噬与凋亡；Autophagy and apoptosis

系分为三类。

（1）自噬为凋亡所需：此时自噬通常早于凋亡发生，进而启动凋亡。

（2）自噬抑制凋亡保护细胞：自噬对线粒体的分隔可防止促凋亡因子如细胞色素和凋亡诱导因子的扩散。避免凋亡因子进入胞质，保护细胞。

（3）自噬和凋亡共同促进细胞死亡：抑制一种细胞死亡途径将激活另一种细胞死亡途径。

三、自噬与癌症

自噬通过降解细胞中的细胞器和蛋白质导致细胞死亡，它是一个在进化上保守并且能够高度调控一些重要细胞功能的过程。自噬的调节异常会使正常的生理过程紊乱，并且与各种疾病的发生有关，包括癌症[30]。在癌症中自噬的作用具有环境依赖性。许多证据表明在代谢应激和缺氧时自噬具有维持肿瘤细胞生存的作用，相反，一些研究也表明自噬还具有抑制肿瘤的作用，即自噬可以支持已经建立的肿瘤的生存，但是它也可以抑制肿瘤的发展。

肿瘤发生的初期，自噬可作为一种抑制因素，对自噬的抑制可使蛋白降解减少，合成代谢增加，最终导致癌细胞持续增殖。在肿瘤生长过程中，尤其是当肿瘤内还未形成足够的血管为其扩增提供营养时，肿瘤细胞可通过自噬来克服营养缺乏和低氧的环境得以生存。

正常小鼠细胞和有自噬缺陷的小鼠细胞比较结果显示自噬在肿瘤发展中具有抑制作用。有自噬缺陷的小鼠积累泛素化角蛋白、自噬载体连接物 p62 和异常线粒体。在许多组织和肿瘤中的高水平 p62[31]，以及在乳腺组织和肿瘤中的磷酸化角蛋白 8（phosphokeratin 8）都是自噬缺陷的潜在指标。

受损细胞成分积累聚集在自噬内含物的过程常与活性氧（reactive oxygen species，ROS）的产生、DNA 损伤反应的激活、细胞损伤及死亡有关，这些相关因素会导致慢性炎症。自噬介导细胞垃圾处理的失败会导致渐进性细胞和组织损伤，从而引起变性和炎症性疾病，可能会引起癌症[32-35]。慢性组织损伤和炎症与 DNA 损伤、ROS 产生有关，并且会引起细胞突变。这些突变可以引起癌症并促进其进展。

自噬必需基因 Beclin-1 的等位基因缺失的老鼠可以改变蛋白质体内平衡（泛素化蛋白质和 p62 的累积）引起组织损伤的形态学改变，这些损伤（尤其是发生在肝脏的）会加速肝细胞癌的发病率[36]。这些发现表明自噬刺激物也许能预防这些退行性疾病和由于慢性组织损伤和炎症所引起的癌症如肝细胞癌。

笔者研究了 Beclin-1 表达和人类肝细胞癌（HCC）增殖、凋亡、微血管密度（MVD）和临床病理变化及预后的关系。结果显示：在 HCC 组织中 Beclin-1 阳性率明显低于相邻的组织（72.8%和89.5%）。在 HCC 中 Beclin-1 表达与肝硬化背景、Edmondson 分级、血管侵犯、增殖细胞核抗原（PCNA）、抗凋亡蛋白 Bcl-2 和微血管密度（MVD）均呈负相关，而与促凋亡蛋白表达呈正相关。单变量和多变量 Cox 回归分析显示，Beclin-1 表达是 HCC 患者预后的独立指标之一[37]。

自噬的诱导与癌细胞死亡有关，这是由于癌细胞通过自噬而死亡，这也被称为伴有自噬特征的细胞死亡。这一研究强调了当自噬体存在时，重点在于查明自噬的功能性作用。在肿瘤微环境中自噬也能促进肿瘤细胞的存活。

在有些情况中通过 RNA 干扰使关键的自噬基因沉默可以提高癌症患者的生存率。生存率的增加是否由于缺乏自噬性细胞死亡，或是防止了由致命性自我消耗所致的自噬细胞死亡的过度活跃，或是其他未知的机制所造成的，到目前为止还不清楚。

在有些情况下，自噬性细胞死亡仅限于体外条件，并不在机体内表现。但是，体内结果更为重要。在体内自噬多是由细胞应激所诱导，包括营养物质、生长因子、缺氧，以及维持正常细胞、小鼠肿瘤细胞生存的功能。当体外模型中的压力应激完全对应于体内时，自噬对于维持细胞生存的作用更明显。例如，有自噬缺陷的肿瘤细胞在经历代谢应激（如局部缺血）时与具有自噬能力的细胞相比会表现出较弱的生存力。此外，在肿瘤缺氧区，自噬基因消失会促进这些代谢应激细胞的选择性死亡。因此，在这个意义上自噬能维持肿瘤的生存。

自噬能够在应激状态下维持正常细胞和肿瘤细胞生存的机制并不清楚。在氧化应激下受损蛋白质和细胞器（尤其是线粒体）能通过活性氧含量来限制细胞损伤和死亡[38]。当营养物质限制时自噬可以通过胞内代谢循环维持细胞新陈代谢和提高细胞生存能力。

总的来说，肿瘤中自噬作用有至关重要的三个关键点。

（1）癌基因激活和肿瘤抑制基因失活在决定肿瘤细胞自噬水平和功能中的作用。

（2）在靶向治疗中自噬激活的作用。

（3）蛋白酶体、内质网应激反应和自噬调节网络的交互作用；通过免疫系统、肿瘤间质和血管对细胞外自噬的调控；网络激酶信号、蛋白质代谢和自噬之间的相互作用。

自噬作为真核细胞中一种溶酶体依赖性的降解系统，在机体病理和生理过程中都能见到，关于其所起的作用是负面还是正面的目前尚未完全阐明，同样对肿瘤具有保护和杀伤的双重作用，与肿瘤的发生和发展有重要关系。

第四节　针对自噬的药物靶点

不管自噬是如何在应激下增加生存率，但协同自噬抑制可能会改善癌症治疗的结果。细胞毒性抗癌疗法可以诱导自噬，其最可能的机制是通过损伤 DNA、细胞蛋白质和细胞器来实现的。在临床前实验中抑制自噬能够提高肿瘤对烷化剂的反应性，这表明抑制自噬可以提高肿瘤对化疗的敏感性。自噬在癌症中的功能以促进细胞存活为主，肿瘤细胞可通过自噬而对抗细胞毒性物质的干扰，这可能是放化疗耐受的机制之一。因而，抑制自噬可作为提高肿瘤放化疗敏感性的一种方法。所谓自噬开关就是指可以调整体内从抑制自噬过渡到增强自噬的过程。抑制自噬对于肿瘤形成的初期很重要，而增强自噬会导致恶性进展。理解这些复杂的过程有利于发展合理的肿瘤治疗性策略。

但也有研究发现癌症靶向治疗通过模拟饥饿信号或其信号分子促进自噬，特别是mTOR的抑制剂是自噬的强效催化剂，未来一个重要的研究方向是研究肿瘤治疗中激活自噬的功能性作用。

一、自噬控制点

（1）自噬启动与 mTORC1 活性下调有关。通过 Atg13 的高磷酸化来活化 mTORC1，降低 Atg1/ULK1 的相互影响[39]，并通过控制自噬效应物如 Beclin-1 复合物的磷酸化来抑制自噬。

蛋白质组学研究 mTORC1 的抑制途径是如何控制自噬的结果表明，在核心共轭、脂质激酶和回收复合物中并没有明显的变化，当自噬途径活化时翻译后修饰可能涉及自噬囊泡的积累，这对于控制自噬或许是一个潜在的方法。

（2）自噬囊泡成核代表了第二个自噬控制点，涉及 Vps34、Beclin-1 和 p150 的相互作用[40]。干扰 Vps34 膜成分的药物可能有效地（尽管非特异性）作为自噬抑制剂[41, 42]，这些药物包括渥曼青霉素和 3-甲基腺嘌呤（3-methyladenine，3-MA）。

Vps34 的直接抑制剂和某些可单独去除 Beclin-1 的药物也将用于抑制自噬。许多 PI3K/Beclin-1 复合物会涉及哺乳类动物的自噬。

3-MA 抑制自噬后通过激活 caspase-3 诱导肝癌细胞发生凋亡，引起 caspase 依赖的细胞凋亡。3-MA 与化疗药物联用可增加化疗敏感性[43]。自噬的特异性抑制剂可能成为肿瘤化疗的增敏剂。

（3）泛素蛋白与 Atg 家族蛋白是自噬囊泡成熟的中央调节器，是第三个自噬控制点，LC3 是被最广泛研究的 Atg8 家族成员。LC3 由 Atg4 所降解，且与 PE（磷脂酰乙醇胺）共轭，由 Atg3 和 Atg7 依赖激酶和级联传递，使 LC3 可以与这些协调自噬囊泡生成和载体连接的膜融合。载体连接涉及 LC3 表面表达并与载体连接结合蛋白的基序相互作用，这些基序的突变会使载体连接适配器蛋白质，如 p62、Nbr1、NIX 减少与 Atg8 的绑定，并且干扰自噬囊泡载体连接向溶酶体的转移，Nbr1 和 p62 除了包含能与 LC3 相互作用的一些基序外还包含有泛素结合域[44, 45]，从而允许这些适配器蛋白质将泛素蛋白载体与 LC3 及少量的胞质内容物结合起来。LC3 膜包围少量的胞质内容物使泛素蛋白载体紧密封存。同样，这些载体适配器蛋白 NIX 会招募线粒体到含有 LC3 的膜上[46, 47]，使载体直接通过与载体适配器蛋白的相互作用结合起来，从而决定在自噬中的载体类型。

（4）自噬囊泡内容物的运输和降解代表着第四个自噬控制点，因为自噬囊泡和溶酶体沿着微管移动，一些能干扰微管移动的药物如诺考达唑、秋水仙碱、紫杉烷、长春花生物碱等会抑制自噬囊泡与溶酶体融合从而引起自噬囊泡累积。Rab GTP 酶很可能在囊泡成熟和与溶酶体融合的过程中起作用。

溶酶体是酸性细胞器，其消化水解酶依赖低 pH。因此一些药物如巴佛洛霉素、氯喹衍生物可干扰液泡型氢离子 ATP 酶酸化溶酶体，这些药物会阻止自噬进展，从而导致自噬囊泡的累积。

自噬抑制剂的药物效应动力学分析见图 2-11。

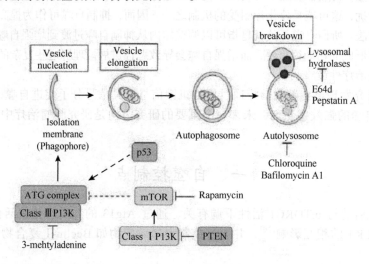

图 2-11　自噬抑制剂的药物效应动力学分析；Pharmacodynamic assay for autophagy inhibition

自噬又是一种辅助性细胞死亡机制。抑制自噬，使自噬对肿瘤细胞死亡的辅助性介导作用下调，具有潜在的促进肿瘤生长作用，这一安全性问题又限制了其在肿瘤治疗中的应用。

二、自噬、免疫和癌症

有些慢性炎症导致成年人癌症发病率升高。肿瘤微环境是以无序状态为特点，这种无序状态与缺氧、糖酵解、自噬和合成坏死相关[48]。最近研究强调了肿瘤细胞代谢、自噬、免疫耐受性是密切联系在一起的。研究集中在高度保守的核内蛋白高迁移率族蛋白 B1（HMGB1）的作用上。自噬刺激物能够促进胞质线粒体异位和细胞外释放 HMGB1。作为一种胞质因子，HMGB1自身就可以促进自噬，增加 ATP 产生，并限制细胞凋亡。细胞外 HMGB1 作为一种损伤相关模式分子（DAMP），可以使晚期糖基化终末产物（RAGE）受体与 Toll 样受体（TLR）相互作用以产生炎症细胞并聚集在损伤部位[49]。因此，HMGB1 是将细胞新陈代谢、细胞死亡及免疫力联系起来的重要分子[50-52]。

三项随机调查表明免疫疗法有利于治疗最难治的癌症。对肿瘤组织和免疫细胞中自噬的研究发现，癌症患者具有全身自噬综合征，即癌细胞中自噬增加，免疫细胞中自噬则受到抑制[53]。因此改善宿主和肿瘤自噬反应之间失衡的方法有 T 细胞疗法、树突细胞（DC）疫苗、抗体制剂及人类重组细胞因子（如 IL-2）等，只有改善了宿主免疫细胞和肿瘤细胞自噬之间的失衡才能对免疫疗法抱有希望。

DC 疫苗首先是对患者的抗原提呈细胞（APC）的分离，之后进行体内基因治疗或针对与肿瘤相关的靶点及特异性抗原（TAA、TSA），随后重新引入成熟的 DC，以活化的 CD8⁺T 细胞来促进抗肿瘤的免疫反应。在特异性抗原提呈细胞内部，抗原加工并运输到 MHC-Ⅰ 和 MHC-Ⅱ 的过程是在蛋白酶体和自噬引导下进行的[53]。肿瘤的细胞外基质中存在自噬载体，这些自噬载体则是作用于 T 细胞启动抗原 DC 的良好刺激物。在适应性免疫中，早期自噬的系统性诱导也许可以预防免疫耐受，并且在抗原存在下来自体内的自噬诱导可以提高细胞免疫疗法的疗效。

将来的方法包括体内诱导 DC 中的自噬和系统性自噬的抑制，在辅助治疗时传输和刺激细胞毒性效应，将有利于促进通过 DC 传输来提高的抗肿瘤免疫，并且增加激活免疫系统的抗肿瘤功效。自噬失衡导致癌症患者的免疫耐受见图 2-12。

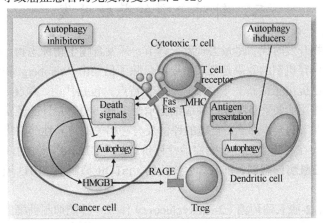

图 2-12　自噬失衡导致癌症患者的免疫耐受；Imbalance of autophagy leads to immune tolerance in cancer patients
增加肿瘤细胞自噬可防止免疫效应细胞介导细胞毒性。此外，压力诱导释放的损伤相关模式分子 HMGB1 诱发保护性自噬，一旦释放到细胞外基质，招募调节性 T 细胞（Treg）导致过敏。DC 中抑制自噬能限制有效启动抗原呈递细胞毒性 T 细胞。同时或随后用药物诱导 DC 中自噬和肿瘤细胞的自噬抑制能较好地扭转这种失衡，增强抗肿瘤免疫；Heightened autophagy in tumor cells prevents immune effector cell–mediated cytotoxicity. In addition, stress-induced release of the damage-associated molecular pattern molecule HMGB1 induces cytoprotective autophagy and, once extruded into the extracellular matrix, recruits regulatory T cells (Treg) resulting in anergy. Suppressed autophagy in DCs limits effective priming of antigen presentation that trains cytotoxic T cells. Simultaneous or sequential pharmacologic induction of autophagy in DCs and autophagy inhibition in the tumor cell would ideally reverse this imbalance and enhance antitumor immunity

一旦效应 T 细胞和自然杀伤细胞（NK）被活化杀伤肿瘤，自噬抑制会增加这些细胞的细胞毒性，这一概念类似于自噬限制了化疗和放疗的有效性。近期，在联合抗癌治疗的难治性恶性肿瘤患者中，用羟氯喹实现自噬抑制。在许多组织学不同的临床前肿瘤模型中自噬抑制能够增加抗癌药物的疗效。文献报道在体内有效地抑制自噬可以通过抗疟药氯喹（CQ）来实现，在此基础对于有晚期恶性肿瘤的患者来说，临床试验是可行的。在过去的 60 年间，CQ 衍生物已经确定用于疟疾，类风湿关节炎及 HIV 感染的临床治疗。这些药物都是较经济的口服药，能够穿过血脑屏障。由单一药片误食导致婴儿死亡的案例报道表明高浓度的 CQ 能导致显著的毒性。相反，羟氯喹（HCQ）不会导致意外死亡，表明 HCQ 在癌症患者中可以适当安全地增加剂量。通过试管内的研究发现这两种药物抑制自噬的作用是相等的。用 HCQ 结合 IL-2 形成的自噬抑制剂在小鼠肿瘤模型中实验，并准备快速应用到多种肿瘤的临床实验。

对恶性胶质瘤的患者放疗和卡莫司汀治疗时加或不加 CQ 联合治疗的比较中，发现在 CQ 和安慰剂治疗的患者中间的总生存期是 1 年 11 个月。单因素研究未发现生存的显著差异，但通过安全地添加低剂量的 CQ 损害 DNA 的治疗。从药理学角度来说，HCQ 有长半衰期，常几周才能达到峰浓度，对低效力药物而言，需要其微摩尔浓度抑制自噬，因此 HCQ 和低效力药物的药理学特点会限制其作为患者的自噬抑制剂发挥作用。为了解决这一问题，由美国脑肿瘤联盟所开始的对恶性胶质瘤患者采取药物治疗和放疗进行 HCQ 试验，包括药物效应动力学（PD）和药物代谢动力学（PK）分析，以及评估患者总生存期。通过使用一种新颖的电子显微镜分析连续血液单核细胞得到 HCQ 剂量依赖性自噬抑制的 PD 证据，所以关于 HCQ 联合抗肿瘤作用的信息包括总体生存期应该很快就可以获得。

目前，包括 HCQ 在内已超过 20 种试验对癌症患者进行治疗，他们中许多人都有初步的抗肿瘤疗效的证据。通过 PD、PK 获得的结果和在这些研究中用到的预测生物标志物将会引导更有效和特异性自噬抑制剂的研发，这些自噬抑制剂是通过学术界和工业界联合来研制。

三、针对自噬的药物开发

在靶向性的药物开发时代，尽量去理解、调节、开发自噬生物标志物，检测其作为肿瘤细胞承受压力的一种生存机制的效果是极其重要的。除了最初由 Weinberg 和他的同事所提出的癌症标志物之外，已提出了最新关于癌细胞的基本特点，包括代谢、氧化、DNA 损伤、有丝分裂及蛋白毒性的作用。如果自噬允许肿瘤细胞承受多种压力，并且已经发现在临床试验中开发的许多药物可以调节自噬。那么，自噬的评估及与它相关的特异性药物将很可能有助于提高疗效。事实上，以前在制药公司或者癌症治疗评价计划（CTEP）开发的许多药物可以调节自噬，包括组蛋白脱乙酰酶抑制剂、抗血管生长药物、mTOR 抑制剂、BH3 域模拟药、糖酵解抑制剂。

在临床试验中，2-脱氧葡萄糖（2-deoxyglucose）作为一种能抑制糖酵解的经典药物，可克服并减少在外周血单核细胞中诱导自噬调节蛋白 p62 的作用[54, 55]。临床前研究表明 2-脱氧葡萄糖诱导与调节自噬，可以增加细胞毒性[56]，这一点支持了通过药物可以诱导自噬的假设。因此 2-脱氧葡萄糖的进一步研究应结合自噬抑制剂进行试验。

迄今为止，一项综合研究还未能比较出不同种类的抑制剂在相同模型中诱导自噬的差别。

除了将研究方向集中于确定哪一种抗癌治疗并存抑制自噬外，人们更感兴趣的是开发出新的能够通过化学库、高效筛选（HTS）来识别新的在各个点控制和抑制自噬的候选化合物用于癌症治疗。

目前已经发现了一些化合物能够抑制自噬，如 2-PES 是一个小分子热休克蛋白 70（HSP70）

的抑制剂，能够导致许多溶酶体蛋白的错误折叠。对药物开发至关重要的试验进展表明，这些试验从针对诱导或抑制自噬反应的药效可以转变为预测自噬的生物标志物。随着其他标志物的出现，在先前开始自噬标志物的研究中，初步的数据支持通过免疫化学评估 Beclin-1 可以作为衡量自噬水平的指标，并且可以直接通过电子显微镜观察或通过 LC3、P62 的水平去评估自噬囊泡的数量将其作为自噬调节的标志。

考虑到在不同癌症和治疗诱导的应激中，自噬作为细胞生存机制的生物学的重要性，一场在实验室和临床研究之间的探索正在进行。对于确定在肿瘤晚期中抑制自噬或在早期诱导自噬作为化疗策略十分必要。

自噬在生存、适应及整个生理过程中有着重要作用，其作用的广度表明了自噬有多种模式，这些模式可以定位，也可以是细胞间的特定成分及组织间的特异性来判断。因此，抑制或诱导自噬的治疗策略需要根据不同原因所引起的自噬做出相应的调整，进一步分析生理条件下各种自噬亚型及进一步选用特异性诱导剂和抑制剂所针对特有的自噬途径来指导调节自噬用于癌症治疗。

自噬是肿瘤治疗的一个新的靶点，然而，很多分子机制还有待于进一步阐明，自噬在肿瘤治疗方面的研究仍处于起步阶段，相关报道有限，如何进行进一步的临床应用关键是依赖于自噬机制及自噬与凋亡等过程相关理论的完善。

第五节 研究自噬的方法

一、自噬诱导剂与抑制剂

正常培养的细胞自噬活性很低，不适于观察，因此，必须对自噬进行人工干预和调节，主要的工具药如下。

1. 自噬诱导剂

（1）Bredeldin A / Thapsigargin / Tunicamycin：模拟内质网应激。

（2）卡马西平（carbamazepine）/L-690，330/氯化锂（lithium chloride）：IMP 酶抑制剂（Inositol monophosphatase，肌醇单磷酸酶）。

（3）Earle's 平衡盐溶液：制造饥饿。

（4）N-Acetyl-D-sphingosine（C2-神经酰胺）：Ⅰ型 PI3K 通路抑制剂。

（5）西罗莫司（rapamycin）：mTOR 抑制剂。

（6）Xestospongin B/C：IP3R 阻滞剂。

2. 自噬抑制剂

（1）3-MA：（Ⅲ型 PI3K）hVps34 抑制剂。

（2）巴佛洛霉素（bafilomycin）A1：质子泵抑制剂。

（3）羟氯喹（hydroxychloroquine）：溶酶体腔碱化剂。

在研究中除了选用上述工具药外，一般还需结合遗传学技术对自噬相关基因进行干预，包括 RNA 干扰技术（knockdown）、突变株筛选、外源基因导入等。

二、自噬的检测方法

通常检测自噬的方法有直接形态学观察与分子生物学检测。

1. 直接形态学观察

（1）透射电子显微镜（TEM）观察：迄今认可的研究自噬的金标准。

（2）激光共聚焦显微镜观察细胞自噬。

（3）标记蛋白免疫荧光检测。

在哺乳动物细胞中鉴别自噬，检测自噬体中的 LC3 已被证明是一个有用的和敏感的标志。已有报告在食管、胃和胰腺癌中 LC3 高表达。值得注意的是高表达 LC3 与胰腺癌预后差有关。

（4）单丹（磺）酰戊二胺（MDC）染色法：是一种特异的检测自噬体方法。

自噬体形成过程中，自噬相关蛋白 Atg8 定位于自噬体膜上，能够与荧光染料 MDC 相结合，通过荧光染色，在荧光显微镜下可见核周区域阳性。

（5）免疫组化

2. 分子生物学检测手段 LC3 为自噬发生的特异标志物，检测 LC3 水平是评价自噬的常用方法。另外作为酵母 Atg6 基因的同源物，哺乳动物中的 Beclin-1 也可反应细胞自噬的活性。

（1）实时荧光定量 RT-PCR 检测自噬相关基因 Beclin-1、Atg5、Atg7 和 Atg12 的表达。

（2）检测长寿蛋白的降解：自噬是真核细胞内降解胞质细胞器和长寿蛋白的一种溶酶体途径，它与降解短寿蛋白的泛素依赖蛋白酶体系统一起在细胞的新陈代谢中发挥着至关重要的作用。

与蛋白质聚集相关的疾病，尤其是神经变性疾病（PD、AD、HD、DLB）可被归类为蛋白质构象紊乱症（protein conformational disorders），也称蛋白性状调控障碍性疾病（protein quality disease）。研究表明，自噬-溶酶体途径（ALP）在清除与疾病相关的错误折叠和突变的易聚集蛋白方面起着关键作用。

（3）Western blot 检测自噬相关蛋白。

（4）间接自噬体检测法：检测自噬溶酶体及其不能降解的产物——残体，主要是显微观察脂褐素颗粒。

挑战与展望

自噬机制就好比是细胞自身净化和实现自动环保的一条运输线。它将细胞内代谢废物及一些过期无用或有损伤的细胞零件，装到其独特的运输工具——自噬体中，然后沿着特定路线，送到"垃圾加工厂"——溶酶体中进行回收和废物再利用。

自噬机制还能在细胞能量匮乏时开启紧急运输通道，以供应能量。因此，自噬机制是细胞内庞大运输网络体系中非常重要的一部分，它对于维系细胞基本的生存需求与平衡是不可或缺的。

自噬几乎是在所有存活细胞的基本能力，以开展维持自我平衡的功能如蛋白质和细胞器转化。当细胞需要细胞内营养物质及能量如在饥饿和生长因子摄取或有高能量需求时，自噬会上调。除此之外，在应激状态如需清除聚合的蛋白质、受损的细胞器或细胞内病毒体时自噬也会上调。许多信号通路与自噬系统交织在一起，这种交互作用允许一个严格调控和动态的自噬以应对相应的环境变化。

自噬是胞质内的一种进化保守过程，通过隔离细胞器和蛋白质到自噬泡（自噬体），进而与溶酶体融合形成自噬溶酶体导致囊泡内成分的降解。自噬处于复杂的细胞应激反应网络的中心，维持细胞内稳态和解压需要的自噬与多种疾病密切相关，如神经退行性病变和免疫功能缺陷。

肿瘤抑制效应包括：①防止染色体稳定性降低及致癌突变积累；②限制氧化应激；③减轻

瘤内坏死和局部炎症。当发生自噬障碍时可使肿瘤细胞对增殖抑制信号反应迟钝、凋亡障碍、无限增殖、产生血管生长因子、转移而致组织侵袭、逃避免疫监视、增加合成代谢。同时使肿瘤细胞对低氧代谢、分化诱导和治疗性应激反应减弱。因此，自噬障碍是肿瘤细胞的基本特征之一。

　　药物调节自噬是抗肿瘤治疗的有效工具，一方面，化学药物诱导自噬可能用于肿瘤的预防；在治疗方面，联合自噬抑制可增加疗效，减少常规药物副作用。但由于抑制自噬后，又具有保护肿瘤细胞的潜能，而对该方法的临床应用有所限制。因此，自噬对肿瘤细胞作用的分子机制及用于治疗的安全性等问题尚需进一步探讨。进一步阐明自噬对肿瘤影响的分子机制及整体效应，对辅助放化疗及发展新疗法将产生深远的影响。

　　虽然在癌症发生、发展，以及在判断治疗的反应中自噬被看作是一把双刃剑，但越来越多的证据表明，自噬的主要作用是促进癌细胞的生存和抗细胞凋亡，有助于癌症的形成。总之有关自噬与肿瘤的复杂关系还有待更深入的研究。

思　考　题

　　1. 本章基本概念：自噬（autophagy），巨自噬（macroautophagy），微自噬（microautophagy），分子伴侣介导的自噬（chaperone-mediated autophagy，CMA），自噬开关（autophagic switch），蛋白质构象紊乱病（protein conformational disorders），Beclin-1，LC3。

　　2. 简述自噬发生的过程。

　　3. 比较三种自噬方式。

　　4. 阐述自噬与吞噬的联系与区别。

　　5. 比较自噬与凋亡。

　　6. 阐述何为自噬控制点。

　　7. 简述常见的自噬检测方法。

参 考 文 献

[1] Fader C, Sanchez D, Furlan M, et al. Induction of autophagy promotes fusion of multivesicular bodies with autophagic vacuoles in K562 cells[J]. Traffic, 2008, 9（2）：230-250.

[2] Yu L, Mcphee C K, Zheng L, et al. Termination of autophagy and reformation of lysosomes regulated by mTOR.[J]. Nature, 2010, 465（7300）：942-946.

[3] Esclatine A, Chaumorcel M, Codogno P. Macroautophagy signaling and regulation[J]. Current Topics in Microbiology & Immunology, 2009, 335：33-70.

[4] Yläanttila P, Vihinen H, Jokitalo E, et al. Monitoring autophagy by electron microscopy in Mammalian cells.[J]. Methods in Enzymology, 2009, 452：143-164.

[5] Mizushima N, Levine B, Cuervo A M, et al. Autophagy fights disease through cellular self-digestion[J]. Nature, 2008, 451（7182）：1069-1075.

[6] Geng J, Baba M, Nair U, et al. Quantitative analysis of autophagy-related protein stoichiometry by fluorescence microscopy [J]. Journal of Cell Biology, 2008, 182（1）：129-140.

[7] 杨永华，包勇，姜小筱. 自噬与肿瘤防治新策略[J]. 中国药理学与毒理学杂志，2015（2）：179-190.

[8] Sahni S, Merlot A M, Krishan S, et al. Gene of the month：BECN1[J]. Journal of Clinical Pathology, 2014, 67（8）：656-660.

[9] Mizushima N, Levine B, Cuervo A M, et al. Autophagy fights disease through cellular self-digestion[J]. Nature, 2008, 451（7182）：1069-1075.

[10] Cao Y, Klionsky D J. Physiological functions of Atg6/Beclin 1：a unique autophagy-related protein [J]. Cell Research, 2007, 17（10）：839-849.

[11] Han Y，Xue X F，Shen H G，et al. Prognostic significance of Beclin-1 expression in colorectal cancer：a meta-analysis[J]. Asian Pacific Journal of Cancer Prevention，2014，15（11）：4583-4587.

[12] Sun Y，Liu J H，Jin L，et al. Inhibition of Beclin 1 expression enhances cisplatin-induced apoptosis through a mitochondrial-dependent pathway in human ovarian cancer SKOV3/DDP cells[J]. Oncology Research，2014，21（5）：261-269.

[13] Wang S M，Li X H，Xiu Z L. Over-expression of Beclin-1 facilitates acquired resistance to histone deacetylase inhibitor-induced apoptosis[J]. Asian Pacific Journal of Cancer Prevention，2014，15（18）：7913-7917.

[14] Li B X，Li C Y，Peng R Q，et al. The expression of beclin 1 is associated with favorable prognosis in stage IIIB colon cancers[J]. Autophagy，2009，5（3）：303-306.

[15] Miracco C，Cevenini G，Franchi A，et al. Beclin 1 and LC3 autophagic gene expression in cutaneous melanocytic lesions[J]. Human Pathology，2010，41（4）：503-512.

[16] Nitin K，Vivek S，Deobrat D，et al. Bicyclic triterpenoid Iripallidal induces apoptosis and inhibits Akt/mTOR pathway in glioma cells[J]. BMC Cancer，2010，10（1）：328.

[17] Wang Z H，Xu L，Duan Z L，et al. Beclin 1-mediated macroautophagy involves regulation of caspase-9 expression in cervical cancer HeLa cells[J]. Gynecologic Oncology，2007，107（1）：107-113.

[18] Liang X H，Jackson S，Seaman M，et al. Induction of autophagy and inhibition of tumorigenesis by beclin 1 [J]. Nature，1999，402（6762）：672-676.

[19] 徐凌凡. 自噬基因 Bedin-1 在前列腺癌组织中的表达及意义[D]. 安徽医科大学，2015.

[20] Aita V M，Xiao H L，Murty V V V S，et al. Cloning and Genomic Organization of Beclin 1，a Candidate Tumor Suppressor Gene on Chromosome 17q21 [J]. Genomics，1999，59（1）：59-65.

[21] Gajewska M，Gajkowska B，Motyl T. Apoptosis and autophagy induced by TGF-B1 in bovine mammary epithelial BME-UV1 cells.[J]. Journal of Physiology & Pharmacology，2005，Suppl 3：143-157.

[22] Tanida I，Tanidamiyake E，Komatsu M，et al. Human Apg3p/Aut1p homologue is an authentic E2 enzyme for multiple substrates，GATE-16，GABARAP，and MAP-LC3，and facilitates the conjugation of hApg12p to hApg5p[J]. Journal of Biological Chemistry，2002，277（16）：13739-13744.

[23] Kabeya Y，Mizushima N，Ueno T，et al. LC3，a mammalian homologue of yeast Apg8p，is localized in autophagosome membranes after processing[J]. EMBO Journal，2000，19（21）：5720-5728.

[24] Pankiv S，Clausen T H，Lamark T，et al. p62/SQSTM1 binds directly to Atg8/LC3 to facilitate degradation of ubiquitinated protein aggregates by autophagy[J]. Journal of Biological Chemistry，2007，282（33）：24131-24145.

[25] Shintani T，Mizushima N，Ogawa Y，et al. Apg10p，a novel protein-conjugating enzyme essential for autophagy in yeast[J]. The EMBO Journal，1999，18（19）：5234-5241.

[26] Shintani T，Mizushima N，Ogawa Y，et al. Apg10p，a novel protein-conjugating enzyme essential for autophagy in yeast[J]. EMBO Journal，1999，18（19）：5234-5241.

[27] Mizushima N，Noda T，Ohsumi Y. Apg16p is required for the function of the Apg12p–Apg5p conjugate in the yeast autophagy pathway[J]. The EMBO Journal，1999，18（14）：2888-3896.

[28] Gozuacik D，Kimchi A. Autophagy and cell death[J]. Current Topics in Developmental Biology，2007，78（4）：217-245.

[29] Bialik S，Kimchi A. Autophagy and tumor suppression：recent advances in understanding the link between autophagic cell death pathways and tumor development[J]. Advances in Experimental Medicine and Biology，2008，615：177-200.

[30] Shintani T，Klionsky D J. Autophagy in health and disease：A double-edged sword[J]. Science，2004，306（5698）：990-995.

[31] Ichimura Y，Komatsu M. Selective degradation of p62 by autophagy[J]. Seminars in Immunopathology，2010，32（4）：431-436.

[32] Degenhardt K，Mathew R，Beaudoin B，et al. Autophagy promotes tumor cell survival and restricts necrosis，inflammation，and tumorigenesis[J]. Cancer Cell，2006，10（1）：51-64.

[33] Kang R，Livesey K M，Iii H J Z，et al. HMGB1 as an autophagy sensor in oxidative stress[J]. Autophagy，2011，7（8）：904-906.

[34] Scherzshouval R，Elazar Z. Regulation of autophagy by ROS：physiology and pathology[J]. Trends in Biochemical Sciences，2011，36（1）：30-38.

[35] Yang S，Wang X，Contino G，et al. Pancreatic cancers require autophagy for tumor growth[J]. Genes & Development，2011，25（7）：717-729.

[36] Levine B，Kroemer G. Autophagy in the pathogenesis of disease[J]. Cell，2008，132（1）：27-42.

[37] Qiu D M，Wang G L，Chen L，et al. The expression of beclin-1，an autophagic gene，in hepatocellular carcinoma associated with clinical pathological and prognostic significance[J]. BMC Cancer，2014，14（1）：327.

[38] Menrad H，Werno C，Schmid T，et al. Roles of hypoxia-inducible factor-1α（HIF-1α）versus HIF-2α in the survival of hepatocellular tumor spheroids [J]. Hepatology，2010，51（6）：2183-2192.

[39] Chang H J，Ro S H，Jing C，et al. mTOR regulation of autophagy[J]. FEBS Letters，2010，584（7）：1287-1295.

[40] Ryter S W, Cloonan S M, Choi A M. Autophagy: a critical regulator of cellular metabolism and homeostasis[J]. Molecules and Cells, 2013, 36 (1): 7-16.

[41] Kim J, Kim Y C, Fang C, et al. Differential regulation of distinct Vps34 complexes by AMPK in nutrient stress and autophagy[J]. Cell, 2013, 152 (1-2): 290-303.

[42] Wei Y, Zou Z, Becker N, et al. EGFR-Mediated Beclin 1 phosphorylation in autophagy suppression, tumor progression, and tumor chemoresistance[J]. Cell, 2013, 154 (6): 1269-1284.

[43] Chen N, Debnath J. Autophagy and tumorigenesis [J]. FEBS Letters, 2010, 584 (7): 1427-1435.

[44] Krikin V, Lamark T, Sou Y S, et al. A role for NBR1 in autophagosomal degradation of ubiquitinated substrates[J] Molecular Cell 2009, 33 (4): 505-516.

[45] Kirkin V, Lamark T, Johansen T, et al. NBR1 cooperates with p62 in selective autophagy of ubiquitinated targets[J]. Autophagy, 2009, 5 (5): 732-733.

[46] Aerbajinai W, Giattina M, Lee Y T, et al. The proapoptotic factor Nix is coexpressed with Bcl-xL during terminal erythroid differentiation[J]. Blood, 2003, 102 (2): 712-717.

[47] Schweers R L, Zhang J, Randall M S, et al. NIX is required for programmed mitochondrial clearance during reticulocyte maturation[J]. Proceedings of the National Academy of Sciences of the United States of America, 2007, 104 (49): 19500-19505.

[48] Nyberg P, Salo T, Kalluri R. Tumor microenvironment and angiogenesis[J]. Frontiers in Bioscience, 2008, 13 (17): 6537-6553.

[49] Tang D, Kang R, Rd Z H, et al. Masquerader: high-mobility group box 1 and cancer[J]. Clinical Cancer Research, 2007, 13 (10): 2836-2848.

[50] Wen H Q, Luo Y, Chen R F, et al. Protective effect of HMGBl gene silence on astrocyte injury caused by oxygen-glucose deprivation/reoxygenation[J]. Medical Journal of Chinese Peoples Liberation Army, 2014, 39 (4): 302-306.

[51] Rong-Jian X U, Wang F G, Dang W, et al. Influences of laser treatment on the expressions of the plasma vascular endothelial growth factor and basic fibroblast growth factor in children cutaneous hemangioma[J]. Journal of Shandong University, 2013, 51 (4): 96-99.

[52] Xiao J H, Wang Y P, Zhu H Y, et al. Expression of serum HMGB1 and MMP-9 in early gastric cancer patients and its clinical significance[J]. Journal of Shandong University, 201351 (10): 70-73.

[53] 夏朋延, 王硕, 范祖森. 细胞自噬与免疫研究进展[J]. 生命科学, 2016, 28 (2): 208-215.

[54] Wangpaichitr M, Savaraj N, Maher J, et al. Intrinsically lower AKT, mammalian target of rapamycin, and hypoxia-inducible factor activity correlates with increased sensitivity to 2-deoxy-D-glucose under hypoxia in lung cancer cell lines[J]. Molecular Cancer Therapeutics, 2008, 7 (6): 1506-1513.

[55] Moscat J, Diazmeco M T. Feedback on fat: p62-mTORC1-autophagy connections[J]. Cell, 2011, 147 (4): 724-727.

[56] Krishna S, Low I C, Pervaiz S. Regulation of mitochondrial metabolism: yet another facet in the biology of the oncoprotein Bcl-2[J]. Biochemical Journal, 2011, 435 (3): 545-551.

（李云龙　彭亮亮　陈　莉）

Chapter 2　Cell Autophagy
——"Self-Eating"

There are three major types of cell death: Apoptosis is type I of programmed cell death, autophagy is the type II of programmed cell death and cellular necrosis.

Autophagy is a lysosomal degradative pathway characterized by the formation of double-membrane from the rough endoplasmic reticulum without ribosomes attached area or mitochondrial membrane packaged autophagic vesicles (AV), also known as autophagosomes, which engulf portions of the cytosol, damaged organelles, protein aggregates, and bacteria. AVs are typically transported along microtubule tracks to a perinuclear location. The outer membrane of the AV subsequently fuses with the lysosome to form autophagic lysosome, resulting in degradation of the AV contents and inner membrane.

Cell autophagy is a kind of common and important eukaryotic cell life phenomenon, is a programmed intracellular degradation mechanism. Its main function is to clear and degradation of their damaged organelles and redundant biological macromolecules, provide the energy recovery and using the degradation products to achieve the metabolism of the cells themselves needs, and updated some proteins and organelles, maintain metabolic balance.

Autophagy is an evolutionary conserved, intracellular self-defense mechanism in which organelles and proteins are sequestered into autophagic vesicles that are subsequently degraded through fusion with lysosomes. Cells, thereby, prevent the toxic accumulation of damaged or unnecessary components, maintaining the steady state of cells. but also recycle these components to sustain metabolic homoeostasis.

Yoshinori Ohsumi. The former professor of research center at Tokyo Instiute of Technology, was awarded the Nobel Prize in Physiology and Medicine in October 3, 2016 because of his studies on autophagy promote to understand the molecular biological mechanism and physiological functions ofautophagy.

Section 1 Morphology and Process of Cell Autophagy

1. Autophagy Morphology

Autophagy phenomenon was first observed with an electron microscope in human hepatocytes by Ashford and Porten in 1962. Autophagy detected in cell ultrastructure morphological examination by transmission electron microscopy has been considered is a "gold standard". Typical autophagy ultrastructural changes include organelle swelling, vacuole-like bilayer membrane structure, or autophagosome with double membrane structure, and isn't completely biodegradable residues (Fig. 2-1).

2. Formation of Autophagic Vacuoles

When the initial autophagy occurs, the cytoplasm can be seen in the large number of free membrane structure is former preautophagosome. Preautophagosome gradually extends to form a membranous vesicles, which is wrapped around the damaged cells and degenerating macromolecular substances, this membranous vesicles are the autophagosome (known as AV).

In the autophagy process, after the formation of autophagic vacuoles its outer membrane fusion with lysosomal membrane, under the effect of lysosomes hydrolysis enzyme, preautophagosome endometrium and parcel of these substances into the lysosomes body cavity, is decomposed into amino acids, nucleotides and free fatty acids, etc, used by cells to form cellular components. Autophagosome in nuclear fusion to autophagolysosome (Fig.2-2).

The anatomy, physiology, and molecular machinery of autophagy are highly conserved among eukaryotic cells. They include distinct steps for AV production and turnover, including ①initiation, ②nucleation, ③maturation of AVs, and ④fusion and degradation of AV contents in lysosomes (Fig.2-3).

During initiation, nascent AV membranes derived from multiple potential sources (including isolated membranes, ER, or mitochondria outer membranes) form a cup-like structure onto which autophagosomal machinery, including LC3, dynamically associates. As the cup-like structure enlarges, it sequesters substrate, which includes ubiquitinated proteins or organelles in the case of stress and/or ubiquitinated substrate accumulation-induced autophagy, and soluble cytoplasm in the case of starvation-induced autophagy. The double membrane comprising the nascent AV then closes to form the mature AV, which then targets and fuses with the lysosome. In the lysosome, hydrolytic enzymes digest the contents and inner membrane of the AV, with autophagic machinery (i.e., LC3) recycled through the cytoplasm for recruitment to other nascent autophagosomes.

3. Fusion Patterns of Autophagy

According to the different substrates into the lysosomal pathway: macroautophagy, microautophagy and chaperone-mediated autophagy (CMA).Themacroautophagy in three types is the most extensively studied (Fig.2-4).

1) Macroautophagy: The substances of cytoplasm transit themselves to lysosomes by way of the formation of vesiclesfor degrading intracellular aging or damaged organelles and proteins.

A portion of cytoplasm, including organelles, is enclosed by a phagophore or isolation membrane to form an autophagosome. The outer membrane of the autophagosome subsequently fuses with the lysosome, and the internal material is degraded in the autolysosome. In yeast, autophagosomes are generated from the preautophagosomal structure (PAS), which has not yet been identified in mammalian cells. Notably, lithium may also inhibit autophagy through mTOR activation. Atg proteins that have thus far been identified on isolation membranes include ULK1/2, Atg5, Beclin 1, LC3, Atg12, Atg13, Atg14, Atg16L1, FIP200, and Atg101（Fig.2-5）.

2) Microautophagy：Directly endocytosis and degradation cells substance by the lysosome.

3) CMA(chaperone-mediated autophagy)：Intracellular soluble proteins through molecular chaperones directly go into the lysosomes to be degraded.

Comparison chart of three autophagy patterns is shown in table 2-1.

Table 2-1　Comparison chart of three autophagy patterns

characteristic		macroautophagy	microautophagy	chaperone-mediated autophagy
activation mechanism		Pressure and stress	constitutive	Pressure and stress
participant	endocytosis	yes	yes	not
	membrane Sources	Non lysosomal	lysosomal	
	Receptor-mediated	not required	not require	require
	ATPs	require	Require	require
	GTP and GTPases	require	require	not
	cytoskeleton	require	not require	unknown
	molecular chaperone	unknown	unknown	require
	Acid vesicles PH	yes	yes	not
	membrane chaperone	unknown	yes	yes
	Kinase of P13	require	unknown	not require
substrate	cell organelle	Variety of types	Variety of types	none
	Soluble cytoplasmic protein	Variety of types	Variety of types	KFERQ-label
	Protein unfolding	not	not	yes
	selectivity	part	part	always

Section 2　Autophagy Associated Genes

Autophagy-related genes (Atg) are originally found to be in yeast, thus yeast is the most common model to the study of autophagy. So far, more than 30 species specific genes have been identified that directly involved in autophagy, more than 50 kinds of related genes. Originally in different laboratories, autophagy genes have different names such as APG, AUT, CVT and etc, but now autophagy related gene is universal naming. While some mammalianAtg still used the previous gene name, such as Atg8 in mammals called LC3（Microtubule-associated protein 1 light chain 3, MAP1-LC3）, Atg 6 called Beclin 1.

Process and its molecular mechanism of autophagy in yeast and mammals also have similarities; Performance at the molecular level of autophagy has two important steps: ①Class III PI3K contribution to the preautophagosome; ②Two ubiquitin - like protein modification process.

1. Beclin-1

AV formation begins with the generation of phosphoinositide signals on the surface of source membranes by multiprotein complexes that include the class III phosphoinositide 3-kinase (PI3K) Vps34 and Beclin1. Beclin-1 expression analysis in edothelial cells is under hypoxia microenvironment: Beclin-1 was found during a research that Liang and others discovered a protein in the study of Bcl-2 gene. Beclin-1 plays an important role in the process of embryonic development as well as suppress tumor through regulating autophagic activity.

Beclin-1, the mammalian counterpart of the yeast Atg6 gene, is an essential autophagy gene and part of a type III phosphatidylinositol 3-kinase complex required for autophagic vesicle formation. recruiting proteins from the cytoplasm for autophagic degradation or in supplying the autophagic pathway with membrane components Inactivation of Beclin-1has been demonstrated to result in increased tumorigenesis in mice. Abnormal expression of Beclin-1 has been found in human melanoma, colon, ovarian and brain cancers, hepatocellular carcinoma. Allelic loss of Beclin-1 is found in human breast and ovarian cancers with high frequency. Therefore, Beclin-1 could play a role as a tumor suppressor and its decreased expression may contribute to the development of human cancer.

2. LC3

Autophagymarker light chain 3 (LC3), is originally identified as a subunit ofmicrotubule-associated proteins 1A and 1B, is a mammalian homologue of the yeast Atg8 that becomes lapidated and tightly associated with the autophagosomal membranes. LC3 is essential for autophagosome formation and is indicative of autophagic activity. In cancer, autophagy has been shown to act both as a tumor suppressor and as a mechanism to sustain survival. The present study investigated autophagy activity in tumor by assessing the expression of LC3 in tumor samples and correlated the results with clinical and pathological characteristics of patients

LC3 precursors are synthesized, processed, modified to its carboxyl - terminal Glycine Residues (Gly-) exposure in the cytoplasm to form LC3-I of a soluble modality. Then they are activated by Atg7, Atg3, and located in the preautophagsome and autophagy inner and outer membrane by LC3-II membrane-bound form (Fig. 2-6).

Once LC3 is integrated into the bilayer, it recruits cargo adaptor proteins (also known as autophagy receptors), such as p62, Nbr1, or NIX. These proteins, in turn, recruit cargo from the cytoplasm to promote AV closure. AVs are then delivered to lysosomes in which their luminal and inner membrane constituents are broken down by lysosomal hydrolases. Lysosomal permeases then release the degradation products into the cytosol for reuse. AV components not exposed to lysosomal hydrolases are recycled via a system involving multiple components of the outer membrane Atg 9, Atg 2, Atg 18, and Atg 21. Alternatively, autophagosomes may also fuse with the plasma membrane and release their contents.

Because LC3-II are always present in autophagic form to the whole process that autophagy and lysosomal fusion, until after the autophagy and lysosome fusion that LC3-II was degraded by lysosomal acid hydrolases. Thus became a symbol molecules of autophagy.

3. Two Ubiquitin -Like Protein Modification Process

The molecular level of autophagy has two important steps and ubiquitin-like protein processing modification in the process ofautophagy

1) Atg12 first is activated by Atg7, and then forming a coupling under the effect of Atg10. Atg12 to Atg5 are heterodimer which connected by covalent bond (Atg12-Atg5 Complex). Multiple Atg12-Atg5 Complex with Atg16 to form a complex that more large, thus the formation of autophagosomes precursors.

2) Lipidation of LC3 occurs by a ubiquitinlike protein (UBL) conjugation cascade involving an

E1-like enzyme (Atg 7) and E2-like enzyme (Atg 3), following cleavage by a cysteine protease (Atg 4) (Fig.2-7).

The results of interfere important genes Beclin-1and LC3 at autophage process (Fig 2-8)

Section 3   Relationship of Autophagy and Other Cellular Events

Autophagy occurs at basal levels in virtually all cells, carrying out homeostatic functions such as protein and organelle turnover. Autophagy is upregulated when cells require intracellular nutrients and energy, such as during starvation and growth factor withdrawal or in the context of high bioenergetic demand.

Additionally, autophagy is upregulated under other stress conditions, such as when there is a need to clear aggregated proteins, damaged organelles, or intracellular pathogens. A number of signaling pathways intersect with the autophagy system. This intersection allows a tightly regulated and dynamic autophagic response to environmental perturbations.

1. Autophagy and Phagocytosis (Fig.2-9)

2. Autophagy and Apoptosis

Apoptosis, namely Type I programmed cell death, with the participation of caspase - dependent, chromosome concentration, cell shrinkage, DNA degradation and formation of apoptotic body and other characteristics. Remnants of their cells ultimately cleared by macrophages.

Autophagic cell death, the type II of programmed cell death, is characterized by the emergence of autophagosome and are not depended on the involvement of caspase. Autophagy and its internal components eventually cleared through its own lysosome system. Therefore, there is a significant differences in biochemical metabolic pathway or morphological of autophagy and apoptosis.

Apoptosis and autophagy coexist in the same cell, their roles and functions between them are interaction, checks and balances (Fig. 2-10).

Autophagy and apoptosis always retains a hot research point in recent years.

Three types follows:

(1) Autophagy is necessary for apoptosis. Autophagy always early occur to apoptosis, furthermore initiate apoptosis.

(2) Autophagy inhibits apoptosis to protect the cells: Separation of autophagy on mitochondria can prevent the pro-apoptotic factors such as cytochrome C and apoptosis inducing factors proliferating, avoid apoptosis factors into the cytoplasm, and protect cells.

(3) Autophagy and apoptosis work together to promote cell death: At this point, inhibit a death pathway will be converted to another death pathway.

3. Roles for Autophagy in Cancers

Autophagy, the type II programmed cell death that degrades cellular organelles and proteins from the cells, is an evolutionarily conserved and highly regulated process that contributes to an array of vital cellular functions. Dysregulation of autophagy disrupts normal physiological processes and is associated with various diseases including cancer. The role of autophagy in cancer has been shown to be context dependent. Many lines of evidence support a role for autophagy in maintaining tumor cell survival in response to metabolic stress and hypoxia. In contrast to the cancer-promoting effect of autophagy, studies have also indicated a role of autophagy in tumor suppression.

Autophagy suppresses tumor development while supporting survival of established tumors.Initial autophagy in tumorigenesis may serve as a disincentive to the inhibition of autophagy protein degradation can be reduced, increase anabolism, eventually leading to the original cancer cells continue to multiply.

In the course of tumor growth，especially when the tumor has not yet formed sufficient blood vessels provide nutrition for amplification, tumor cells can survive by overcome nutritional deficiencies and low oxygen environment through autophagy.

Comparison of normal and autophagy-defective mice and cells has illuminated the role of autophagy in suppression of tumor development. Mice with autophagy defects accumulate ubiquitinated keratins, the autophagy cargo adaptor p62, and abnormal mitochondria. High levels of p62 in many tissues and tumors and phosphokeratin 8 in mammary tissues and tumors are potential biomarkers for autophagy defects.

These damaged cellular components accumulate usually in large aggregates or inclusions, and are linked to reactive oxygen species (ROS) production, activation of the DNA damage response, cell damage, and death that can lead to a chronic inflammatory state. Progressive cell and tissue damage due to failure of autophagy-mediated cellular garbage disposal provokes degenerative and inflammatory diseases and may contribute to cancer. Chronic tissue damage and inflammation is associated with DNA damaging ROS production, contributing to mutations that can initiate cancer and promote tumor progression.

Mice with allelic loss of the essential autophagy gene beclin1 display defective autophagy, altered protein homeostasis (accumulation of ubiquitinated proteins and p62), and gross morphologic tissue damage that is particularly striking in liver where there is also an accelerated incidence of hepatocellular carcinoma. These findings suggest that autophagy stimulators may prevent both degenerative diseases and cancers arising from chronic tissue damage and inflammation, such as hepatocellular carcinomas.

We investigated the significance and relationship between Beclin-1 expression and cell proliferation, apoptosis, microvessel density (MVD) and clinical pathological changes or prognosis in human hepatocellular carcinoma (HCC).Results: The positive rate of Beclin-1 was significantly lower in HCC tissues than adjacent tissues. Beclin-1 expression negatively relate to HCC differentiated (Edmondson grade) and vascular invasion Univariate and multivariate Cox regression analysis revealed that Beclin-1 expression was an independent indicator for overall survival in HCC patients.

Although autophagy induction can be associated with cancer cell death, this may be due to a futile attempt of the cancer cells to survive through autophagy, also known as cell death with autophagic features. This finding underscores the importance of interrogating the functional role of autophagy when autophagosomes are present Autophagy clearly plays a role in promoting the survival of tumor cells within the tumor microenvironment.

In some cases, knockdown of essential autophagy genes by RNA interference (RNAi) enhances survival. Whether this increased survival is due to the absence of autophagic cell death and prevention of overactivation of autophagy and cell death by fatal self-consumption or another unknown mechanism is not yet known.

In other situations, autophagic cell death is limited to in vitro conditions and not manifested in vivo. The most prevailing and convincing evidence, however, is that in vivo, autophagy is induced by cellular stress, including nutrient, growth factor, and oxygen deprivation, and functions to maintain survival of normal cells, mice, and also tumor cells. When in vitro models incorporate stresses commonly encountered in vivo, autophagy's contribution to cell survival becomes clearer. For example, autophagy defective tumor cells undergoing metabolic stress (ischemia) (are showed impaired survival in comparison with autophagy-proficient cells. Furthermore, autophagy localizes to hypoxic regions within tumors, and genetic ablation of autophagy promotes the selective death of those metabolically stressed cells.

The mechanism by which autophagy enables survival of normal or tumor cells in stress is not known. In oxidative stress the clearance of damaged proteins and organelles, particularly mitochondria, may limit cellular damage and death through ROS production. When nutrients are limiting, autophagy may promote viability by maintaining cellular metabolism through intracellular recycling

Three additional areas of intense focus critical to understand the role of autophagy in cancer are:

The role of commonly activated oncogenes and inactivated tumor suppressor genes in: ①Determining autophagy levels and function within the tumor cell; ②The role of activation of autophagy by targeted therapies;③Network interactions among the proteasome, the ER stress response, and autophagy; And extracellular control of autophagy by the immune system, tumor stroma, and vasculature. Network interactions between kinase signaling, protein metabolism, and autophagy.

Autophagy as a lysosome dependent degradation system in eukaryotic cells, in pathological and physiological processes of the body can be seen. Whether its role negative or positive is not yet fully elucidated. Also it has the dual function of protection and kill tumor and has important relation with tumor occurrence and development.

Section 4   Pharmacologic Targets to Autophagy System

Regardless of how autophagy increases survival in stress, concurrent inhibition of autophagy may improve outcomes in cancer therapy. Cytotoxic cancer therapeutics induce autophagy, most likely by causing damage to DNA, cellular proteins, and organelles. Inhibition of autophagy in preclinical models improves the response of tumors to alkylating agents, suggesting that autophagy promotes survival. Targeted cancer therapies also stimulate autophagy, often by mimicking signaling of starvation or factor deprivation. Inhibitors of mTOR, in particular, are potent activators of autophagy, yet the functional consequences of this activation in cancer therapy are not fully understood. An important future direction is to establish the functional consequence of autophagy stimulation by cancer therapeutics.

Main Functions of autophagy in order to promote cell survival, tumor cells can interfere to cell toxic substances through autophagy. This is probably one of the mechanisms of tolerance to chemotherapy. Thus, inhibition of autophagy may be used as a way to improve the sensitivity of radiotherapy and chemotherapy of tumor.

"Autophagic switch" mediates the transition from suppressed autophagy. Toinhibit autophagy is important early in neoplasia, the enhanced autophagy will cause malignant progression, is critical to understanding this complicated process and to developing rational therapeutic strategies.

1. Major Autophagy Control Points

(1) Autophagy initiation is associated with downregulation of mTORC1 activity. Activated mTORC1 inhibits autophagy through hyperphosphorylation of Atg 13to reduce its interaction with Atg 1/ULK1, and by controlling phosphorylation of autophagy effectors such as Beclin-1 complex.

Proteomic studies investigate how inhibition of the mTORC1 pathway affects the global features of autophagy, the control shows no large-scale changes in core conjugation, lipid kinase, and recycling complexes. This finding implies that post-translational modifications may be involved in AV accumulation when the autophagy pathway is activated and may be a potential means to control autophagy.

(2) AV nucleation represents a second major autophagy control point, involving Vps34 and interacting partners Beclin-1 and p150. Drugs that are interfered with recruitment of Vps34 to membranes, including

wortmannin and 3-methyladenine, are powerful (although nonspecific) proximal inhibitors of autophagy.

Direct inhibitors of Vps34 and drugs that sequester or free up Beclin-1 may also be deployed for autophagy inhibition. Multiple PI3K/Beclin-1 complexes may be involved in mammalian autophagy.

3-MA (autophagy inhibitor) combines with chemotherapy drugs that can increase the sensitivity to chemotherapy. After 3-MA inhibiting autophagy by activated caspase-3 induced hepatoma cells apoptosis and caused caspase-dependent cells apoptosis. Specific inhibitor of autophagy may be a tumor chemotherapy sensitizer.

(3) UBL-containing Atg 8 family proteins are central coordinators of AV maturation and represent a third autophagy control point. LC3, the most widely studied Atg8 family member

LC3 is cleaved by Atg 4 and conjugated to PE by an Atg7- and Atg3-dependent activation and transfer cascade. In this manner, LC3 is incorporated into the membrane where it or chestrates AV growth and cargo recruitment. Cargo recruitment involves a conserved surface on LC3, interacting with motifs in cargo-binding proteins. Mutations in these motifs reduce the binding of cargo adaptor proteins, such as p62, Nbr1, and Nix, to Atg8 proteins and disrupt transfer of AV cargo to lysosomes. Nbr1 and p62 contain ubiquitinbinding domains in addition to the motif that interacts with LC3. This characteristic allows these adaptor proteins to bind both ubiquinated cargo and LC3, enabling tight sequestration of ubiquinated cargo by surrounding LC3-containing membranes, with little cytosolic content included. The cargo adaptor protein NIX similarly recruits mitochondria to LC3-containing membranes. Atg8 family members, such as LC3, dictate cargo binding through cargo adaptor interaction, thereby determining the type of cargo sequestered during autophagy.

(4) Delivery and degradation of AV contents represents a fourth autophagy control point. Because AVs and lysosomes move along microtubules, drugs that disrupt microtubules, such as nocodazole, colchicines, taxanes, and vinca alkaloids, inhibit AV fusion with lysosomes, resulting in AV accumulation.

Rab GTPases likely play a role in vesicle maturation and fusion with lysosomes. Lysosomes are acidic organelles, with their digesting hydrolases dependent on low pH. Consequently, agents such as bafilomycin or chloroquine derivatives, which disrupts the vacuolar H ATPase responsible for acidifying lysosomes, block autophagy in its final step, resulting in the accumulation of AVs. Pharmacodynamic assay for autophagy inhibition (Fig. 2-11).

But the autophagic is a kind of auxiliary cell death mechanisms. Inhibiting autophagy makes effect down-regulation of autophagic on tumor cell death which is mediated by supporting. It has potentially cancer-promoting effects. This security issue restricted its application in tumor therapy.

2. Autophagy, Immunity and Cancers

Cancer in adults, but not in children, arises in the setting of chronic inflammation. The tumor microenvironment is characterized by a disordered state associated with hypoxia, glycolysis, perpetual autophagy, and resultant necrosis under conditions of heightened stress.

A good example of how intimately linked tumor cell metabolism, autophagy, and immune tolerance can be is highlighted by recent studies focused on the pleiomorphic functions of the highly conserved nuclear protein high mobility group B1 (HMGB1). Autophagic stimuli promote cytosolic and mitochondrial translocation and extracellular release of HMGB1. As a cytosolic factor, HMGB1 itself promotes autophagy, enhances ATP production, and limits apoptosis. Extracellular HMGB1 serves as a damage-associated molecular pattern molecule (DAMP), which interacts with the receptor for advanced glycation end products (RAGE) and toll-like receptors to recruit inflammatory cells to the site of damage. Thus HMGB1 represents one of likely many molecules that critically link cellular metabolism, cell death decisions, and immunity.

Recently, 3 random studies have shown survival benefits for immunotherapy in refractory cancers. These limited successes come on the heels of decades of failures. Studies of autophagy in tumor tissue and immune cells suggest that cancer patients are suffering from a systemic autophagic syndrome in which autophagy is pathologically increased within the cancer cell and suppressed in the immune cells. Adoptive transfer of T cells, dendritic cell (DC) vaccines, administration of antibodies, or administration of human recombinant cytokines, such as interleukin 2 (IL-2), only hold promise for immunotherapy if the imbalance between host and tumor autophagic response can be ameliorated.

DC vaccines involve isolation of the patient's antigen presenting cells (APC), followed by a procedure of ex vivo gene therapy or incubation with targeted tumor associated and specific antigen (TAA, TSA), and subsequent reintroduction of the matured DCs so that they may mediate a highly specific antitumor immune response facilitated by DC-activated CD8$^+$Tcells. Within professional APCs, antigen processing and delivery to MHC class I and class II molecules is directed by the proteasome and autophagy. Autophagic cargo, which can be extruded into the extracellular matrix from tumor cells, should be superior sources from which DCs can derive antigen for T-cell priming.

Thus, systemic induction of autophagy early in the course of adaptive immunity may prevent the emergence of immune tolerance, and ex vivo induction of autophagy in the presence of antigen may improve the efficacy of cellular immunotherapies.

Autophagy inhibition may augment the cytotoxicity of effector T cells and natural killer (NK) cells once they have been activated to lyse the tumor, similar to the notion that autophagy limits the effectiveness of chemo- and radiation therapy. Currently, autophagy inhibition with hydroxychloroquine (HCQ) in combination with IL-2 is being tested in a murine tumor model and is poised to be rapidly translated into a multiinstitution clinical trial.

Future approaches may include combination of ex vivo induction of autophagy in DCs and systemic autophagy inhibition, delivered at the time of adjunctive treatment and designed to stimulate cytotoxic effectors. This approach may facilitate improved antitumor immunity with DC delivery and enhanced antitumor efficacy of the activated immune system (Fig. 2-12).

Autophagy inhibition with hydroxychloroquine in combination anticancer regimens for patients with refractory malignancies. Autophagy inhibition augments the efficacy of anticancer agents in a variety of tumor histologies in multiple preclinical models. On the basis of reports that effective autophagy inhibition can be achieved in vivo with the antimalarial drug chloroquine (CQ), clinical trials for patients with refractory malignancies were undertaken. For the past 60 years, CQ derivatives have been prescribed for malaria, rheumatoid arthritis, and HIV. They are inexpensive oral drugs that cross the blood-brain barrier. Case reports of infant deaths associated with single tablet ingestions suggest high peak concentrations of CQ may result in significant toxicity. In contrast, suicide attempts involving HCQ did not result in fatalities, suggesting HCQ can be safely dose escalated in cancer patients. In vitro studies indicate these two drugs are equipotent at autophagy inhibition.

A phase III trial in glioblastoma patients treated with radiation and carmustine with or without daily CQ found a median overall survival of 24 and 11 months in CQ- and placebo-treated patients, respectively. This single in stitution study was not adequately powered to detect a significant difference in survival, but established the safety of adding low dose CQ to DNA damaging therapy. Key issues remain that the pharmacology of HCQ (characterized by a long half-life resulting in weeks to achieve peak concentration) and the low potency of the drug (micromolar concentrations are required to inhibit autophagy) may limit its efficacy as an autophagy inhibitor in patients. To address these concerns, a phase I-II trial of HCQ with temozolomide and radiation for glioblastoma patients was launched through the American Brain Tumor Consortium and included pharmacodynamic (PD) and pharmacokinetic (PK) analyses. PD evidence of HCQ dose-dependent autophagy inhibition was observed using

Currently, more than 20 trials involving HCQ are accruing cancer patients nationwide, and many of them have evidence of preliminary antitumor activity. The knowledge gained from the PD, PK, and predictive biomarkers in these studies will guide the development of more potent and specific autophagy inhibitors that are being developed by academic and industry discovery programs.

3. Future Drug Development of Autophagy Modulators

In the era of targeted drug development, efforts to understand, modulate, and develop biomarkers of autophagy as a survival mechanism used by tumor cells to tolerate stress are critically important. As an addition to the hallmarks of cancer originally proposed by Weinberg and colleagues, new basic hallmarks of cancer cells were recently highlighted and included the ability to tolerate metabolic, oxidative, DNA damage, mitotic, and proteotoxic stresses. Given that autophagy can allow tumor cells to tolerate these multiple stresses, and many novel agents under development in clinical trials have been found to modulate autophagy, the assessment of autophagy and its relevance to a particular agent will likely help improve effectiveness.

In fact, multiple agents under development within pharmaceutical companies or the Cancer Therapy Evaluation Program (CTEP; http://ctep.cancer.gov/branches/idb/default.htm) have been shown to modulate autophagy, including histone deacetylase inhibitors, antiangiogenic agents, mTOR inhibitors, BH3 domain mimetics, and glycolytic inhibitors.

In a phase I clinical trial, 2-deoxyglucose, a prototypical agent that inhibits glycolysis, was well tolerated and reduced p62 in peripheral blood mononuclear cells consistent with induction of autophagy. Preclinical studies with 2-deoxyglucose show that induction of autophagy, and modulation of autophagy increased cytotoxicity, supporting the hypothesis that further studies of agents such as 2-deoxyglucose that induce autophagy should be tested in combination with autophagy inhibition.

So far, a no comprehensive study has been compared multiple classes of inhibitors for their ability to induce autophagy in the same model system.

In addition to focusing research efforts on identifying which anticancer therapeutics are most limited by therapy induced autophagy, interest is growing in developing more potent and specific autophagy inhibitors. Academic and industry efforts are underway to develop tools that will enable high-throughput screening of chemical libraries to identify novel candidate compounds that inhibit autophagy at various points of control described above.

Compounds have been found that unexpectedly inhibit autophagy such as 2-phenylethynesulfonamide (PES), a small molecule heat shock protein 70 (HSP70) inhibitor that results in misfolding of a number of lysosomal proteins. A critical component to drug development is the development of assays that can be translated into PD and predictive biomarkers of response to autophagy induction and inhibition.

Although studies of biomarkers of autophagy are early in development with additional markers emerging, preliminary data support the ability to measure Beclin1 by immunohistochemistry as a measure of autophagy competence, and the measurement of AV number directly by electron microscopy, LC3, and p62 levels as markers of autophagy modulation.

Given the basic biological importance of autophagy as a cellular mechanism of survival during multiple forms of cancer and therapeutic-induced stress, an ongoing dialogue between emerging laboratory and clinical research will be imperative to address autophagy as a targetable resistance mechanism in advanced disease and the induction of autophagy as chemoprevention strategy in early phase disease.

The breadth of autophagy's crucial roles in survival, adaptability, and overall physiology suggests multiple subtypes of autophagy that are location and cargo specific within the cell, and tissue specific within the organism. Thus, therapeutic strategies for inhibiting or inducing autophagy need to be tailored toward stress- versus starvation-induced autophagy. Further analysis of the physiologic conditions under which different subtypes of autophagy are used, and further clarification of which autophagy pathway is targeted by specific inducers or inhibitors will guide development of autophagy modulators in cancer therapeutics.

Autophagy is a new target for tumor therapy. However, many molecular mechanism remains to be further clarified, autophagy in cancer therapy research is still in its infancy, reports is still very limited, further applications of the key depends on the perfection of the mechanism of autophagy theory and the relationship between autophagy and Apoptosis process.

Section 5   Studying Methods of Autophagy

1. Autophagy Inhibitors and Inducers

Autophagic activity of normal cultured cells is very low, not to be seen. Therefore, the need for manual intervention and regulation of autophagy, the tools of medicine has reported:

(1) Autophagy Inducers

1) Bredeldin A / Thapsigargin / Tunicamycin ： Simulation of endoplasmic reticulum stress

2) Carbamazepine/ L-690，330/ Lithium Chloride：IMPase inhibitor（Inositol monophosphatase）

3) Earle's balanced salt solution：Manufacture of hunger

4) N-Acetyl-D-sphingosine（C2-ceramide）：Class I PI3K Pathway inhibitor

5) Rapamycin：mTOR inhibitor

6) Xestospongin B/C：IP3R retarder

(2) Autophagy Inhibitors

1) 3-Methyladenine（3-MA）：（Class III PI3K）hVps34 inhibitor

2) Bafilomycin A1：proton pump inhibitor

3) Hydroxychloroquine：Lysosomal lumen alkalizer

In addition to these drug tools, generally combined with genetics techniques on autophagy-related genes are needed to intervene: including antisense RNA interference technology (Knockdown), mutant strain screening, introducing exogenous gene and etc.

2. Detection Methods of Autophagy

Detection of autophagy usually has a direct morphological observation and molecular biological detection methods.

(1) Direct Morphological Observation

1) By using TEM (Transmission Electron Microscope) to observe: So far approved research is the gold standard of autophagy.

A novel electron microscopy assay on serial blood mononuclear cells. Overall survival is the primary endpoint for this phase I-II trial, so information about the antitumor activity of this combination should be forthcoming.

2) By using confocal laser scanning microscopy to observe.

3) Immunofluorescence Detection of Marker proteins

The detection of LC3 in autophagosomes has been shown to be a useful and sensitive marker for distinguishing autophagy in mammalian cells. High expression of LC3 has been reported in esophageal, gastric, and pancreatic cancers. Notably, high LC3 expression was associated with poor survival in pancreatic cancer.

4) MDC staining method: In the Autophagy occurs process, a specific detection method of autophagy to analysis of molecular mechanism.

During the formation of autophagosomes, autophagy-related protein Atg 8 located in the membrane of autophagosome, can be combined with fluorescent dyes MDC, by fluorescence staining, can see the positive Color rendering in perinuclear region.

5) Immunohistochemistry

(2) Molecular biological detection methods: LC3 is specific markers for autophagy. Detection of LC3 level is also commonly used method to evaluate autophagy. In addition as a homologue of yeast Atg 6 gene and Beclin-1 in the mammalian autophagy can also be reaction activity.

1) Real-Time fluorescence quantitative RT-PCR and Western Blot detecting Autophagy-related protein expressions. β-actin as the internal reference.

2) Detecting bulk degradation of long-lived protein

Autophagy is a lysosomal pathway which degrades the cytoplasmic organelle and long-lived proteins in the eukaryotic. It and the ubiquitin-dependent proteasome system-degradation of short-lived proteins, together play an important role in cellular metabolism.

At present, diseases associated with the protein aggregation, in particular the neurodegenerative disease (PD, AD, HD, DLB) can be categorized as a large class of Protein Conformational Disorders, also known as Protein Quality Disease. Recent studies have shown that Autophagy-lysosome pathway (ALP) plays a key role in clear associated with the disease misfold and accumulation proteins of mutations, especially in the occurrence and development process of neurodegenerative diseases play an important role.

3) Western blot detecting autophagy related proteins. Analysing the expression of Beclin- 1 in endothelial cells under hypoxic microenvironment.

4) Indirect autophagy detection method: Autophaglysosome and its products-residues not be degraded, mainly on microscopic observation of lipofuscin granules.

Challenges and Prospects

Autophagy mechanism is like cells themselves purification and realize automatic environmental protection a transit. It will carry the waste material in the cell and some overdue, useless or damage parts of cells, to its unique transport-autophagosome, then along the specific route, to the "garbage processing factory"–lysosome to recovery and recycling.

Autophagy mechanism can open emergency transport corridor when cell energy shortage, in order to supply energy. Accordingly, the mechanisms of autophagy is very important part of huge transportation network system in the cells.It is indispensable to maintain cell basic survival needs and balance.

Autophagy is almost a basic ability in all living cells, to carry out to maintain homeostatic functions such as proteins and organelles transform. When cells need nutrients and energy, such as hunger and absorbing growth factors or having a high energy demand, autophagy go up. In addition, in a stress state if removing protein aggregation, damaged organelles or virus inside body, the autophagy also increase. Many signaling pathways intertwined to the autophagy system, this interaction allows a strict control and dynamic autophagy to accordingly response the environmental changes.

Autophagy is an evolutionarily conserved process through which organelles and proteins are sequestered into autophagic vesicles (autophagosomes) within the cytosol. These vesicles fuse with lysosomes to form autolysosomes leading to degradation of intracellular contents. Autophagy is in the center of the complex cellular stress response network. Autophagy is required for cellular homeostasis and its deregulation is closely related to a variety of diseases, such as neurodegeneration and impaired immunity.

The tumor - suppressing effects include: ①To prevent to decrease the stability of chromosomes and cancer-causing mutations accumulate; ②Limit oxidative stress; ③Reduce local inflammation and intratumor necrosis.

Autophagy disorder make tumor cells slow to react to the proliferation inhibitory signals, obstacles of apoptosis, unlimited proliferation, prodection of vascular endothelial growth factor, metastasis, lead to tissue invasion and escape immunosurveillance, increasing anabolism. While make tumor cells have a weak responses to low oxygen metabolism, differentiation induction and treatment of stress. Therefore, autophagy disorder is one of the basic characteristics of tumor cell.

Drug regulation of autophagy is an effective tool for anti-tumor therapy. On one hand, autophagy induced by chemical substances may be used for cancer prevention. In the area of treatment, combined with inhibition of autophagy can increase the efficacy and reduce the side effects of conventional drugs. But due to inhibition of autophagy, it has the potential to protect tumor cells that limit the clinical application of the method. Therefore, the molecular mechanism of autophagy in tumor cells and the treatment security and other problems need to further study. Further clarification that autophagy affects the molecular mechanism of tumor, its overall effect, can have far-reaching consequences for adjuvant radiotherapy and chemotherapy and the development of new therapies.

Although autophagy is regarded as a double-edged sword in cancer development, progression, and responses to treatment, increasing evidence indicates that autophagy primarily promotes cancer cell survival and resistance to apoptosis. Autophagy contributes to the pathogenesis of cancer. The complex relationship between autophagy and the tumor remains to be furthermore studied.

Consider/Questions

1. Basic concepts in this chapter

autophagy, macroautophagy, microautophagy, chaperone－mediated autophagy (CMA), Autophagic switch, Protein Conformational Disorders, Beclin1, LC3.

2. Briefly Summarize the process of autophagy.

3. Comparison of three kinds of autophagy ways.

4. Explain the relationship and difference between autophagy and phogcytosis.

5. Comparison between autophagy and apoptosis.

6. Which major autophagy control points are there?

7. Give 5 kinds of autophagy detection methods.

本章彩图

第三章 细胞内吞

　　在细胞新陈代谢过程中，不断有各种物质进出细胞，这些物质包括一些离子、小分子物质、大分子物质及一些颗粒物质。大分子物质及颗粒性物质不能穿过细胞膜，以一种特殊方式进行跨细胞膜转运，即物质在进出细胞的转运过程中都是由膜包裹，形成囊泡并与膜融合或断裂使细胞外物质进入细胞内，这就是目前公认的生物体摄取生物大分子的主要途径——内吞作用（endocytosis）[1]。

　　目前的研究发现内吞作用的异常可能参与了某些疾病的发生机制，如与糖尿病、神经性疾病有关，也与细胞的恶性转化密切相关。因此细胞内吞在疾病发生中的意义日益受到重视。随着这一领域的深入研究，将有助于我们认识这些疾病，从而发现新的治疗方法。

　　2013 年诺贝尔生理学或医学奖授予 Randy Schekman、James Rothman 和 Thomas Südhof 三位科学家，获奖理由是他们发现了细胞内的主要运输系统——囊泡运输的调节机制。细胞内外的分子通过包封的囊泡被传递。其中 Randy Schekman 发现了囊泡传输所需的一组基因；James Rothman 阐明了囊泡是如何与靶蛋白融合并传递；Thomas Südhof 则揭示了信号是如何引导囊泡精确地释放其运输物质。

　　本章就细胞的内吞途径、调控机制及内吞相关蛋白和内吞作用的意义做一介绍。

第一节　内吞作用的类型和机制

　　根据摄取的物质主要由液体和溶质组成或是由大颗粒物质组成，内吞机制大致可以分为两类，前者为胞饮作用（pinocytosis），后者为吞噬作用（phagocytosis）。胞饮作用根据其产生的机制不同进一步分为发动蛋白依赖性（dynamin depentent）内容，包括网格蛋白依赖的（clathrin mediated）内吞和小凹蛋白依赖的（caveolin dependent）内吞，发动蛋白非依赖性（dynamin independent）内吞，包括网格蛋白、小凹蛋白非依赖的（non clathrin- caveolin dependent）内吞、脂筏介导的（lipid mediated）内吞和巨胞饮作用（macrophocytosis）[2]（图 3-1）。

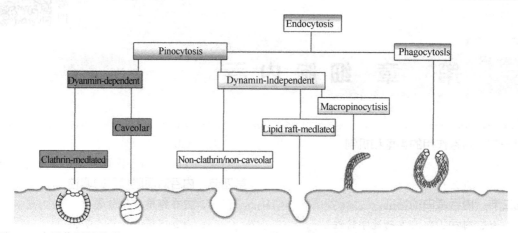

图 3-1 内吞作用的类型；Types of endocytosis Figure adapted from Mercer and Helenius，2009. Reprinted with permission of Nature Cell Biology

细胞内吞途径中转运物质主要的细胞器有早期内体、晚期内体、循环内体和溶酶体。早期内体是拥有管和空泡域的复杂细胞器。空泡域分解其中的内容物，并通过微管介导的发动蛋白依赖性转运到核周区域。它们成熟后为晚期内体，彼此融合，最终与溶酶体融合产生内吞溶酶体。在早期内体、晚期内体、循环内体的水平上，内吞途径经囊泡运输或在内吞溶酶体水平的内吞回收隔室（endocytic recycling compartment，ERC）被连接到反面高尔基网（trans-Golgi network，TGN）和高尔基复合体上进行[3]（图 3-2）。

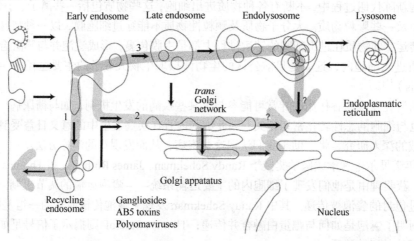

图 3-2 细胞内吞途径的转运；Trafficking in the endocytic pathway

图中显示主要的运输途径由单（或复合）神经节苷脂（1）、AB5 毒素（2），以及多瘤病毒（3）标明；The main trafficking pathways are emphasized for mono- or paucivalent gangliosides（1），AB5 toxins（2），and polyomaviruses（3）

已知颗粒和溶质可以通过多种途径进入细胞而引起不同类型的细胞内吞，不同类型的细胞内吞具有不同的机制[4]（图 3-3）。

一、吞 噬 作 用

吞噬作用是指内吞大颗粒物质（＞250 nm），它为宿主提供了消化外源性物质的直接途径，是最重要的免疫防御机制之一。在哺乳动物体内吞噬作用只能由特化的吞噬细胞来完成，如巨噬细胞和中性粒细胞。吞噬细胞通过免疫球蛋白的 Fc 受体、补体受体分别识别病原体上的免疫球蛋白 Fc 段及补体，并与之结合。当细胞膜表面受体与相应配体结合后即可启动下游信号

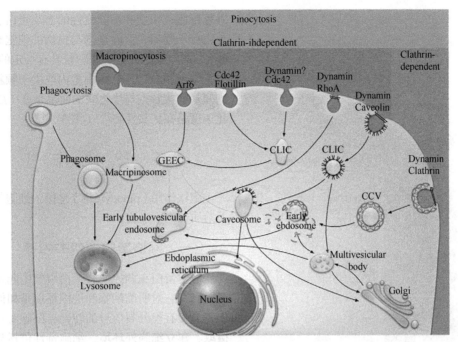

图 3-3 不同内吞的机制；Different mechanisms of endocytosis

在所有情况下，细胞内吞作用首先从吞噬物质通过细胞质膜进入细胞内囊泡开始，而后通过内吞体对吞噬物进行分类。最终吞噬物被运送到目的地溶酶体，再循环到细胞外环境或跨细胞传递

CCV：网格蛋白包被小泡；CLIC：网格蛋白非依赖性载体；GEEC：GPI 锚定富集蛋白成分；In all cases the initial stage of endocytosis proceeds from the plasma membrane portals of cellular entry and involves engulfment of cargo into intracellular vesicles. The second stage often involves sorting of the cargo through endosomes. It is followed by the final stage during which the cargo is delivered to its final destination，recycled to extracellular milieu or delivered across cells

CCV，clathrin coated vesicles；CLIC，clathrin-independent carriers；GEEC，GPI-anchored protein-enriched compartment；GPI，glycophosphatidylinositol；MVB，multivesicular body

转导，引起摄入部位质膜下肌动蛋白（actin）聚合，肌动蛋白收缩使吞噬细胞的质膜突出形成伪足包绕病原体，伪足融合形成囊泡，将病原体吞入。在胞质内，发动蛋白（dynamin）在囊泡颈部装配成环，并水解与其结合的 GTP，发动蛋白收缩使囊泡自颈部与细胞膜断离形成吞噬体，吞噬体再与溶酶体融合形成吞噬溶酶体，溶酶体脱颗粒，使其中的酸性水解酶对病原体进行消化（图 3-4）。除吞噬病原体外，巨噬细胞还能通过配体-受体模式吞噬异物；识别和杀伤

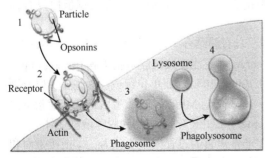

图 3-4 吞噬细胞吞噬颗粒；Stages of phagocytosis of particles

①颗粒通过血液中调理作用识别，如蛋白质的吸附[免疫球蛋白（Ig）G 和 M，补体成分（C3、C4、C5）；血清蛋白（包括层粘连蛋白，纤连蛋白等）]；②调理素化的颗粒，通过存在于吞噬细胞上的表面受体附着在细胞膜上；③这些颗粒被整合入吞噬体；④吞噬体成熟并与溶酶体融合、酸化从而导致颗粒在富含酶的吞噬溶酶体中降解；① Particles undergo recognition in the bloodstream through opsonization i.e. adsorption of proteins [immunoglobulins（Ig）G and M]，complement components（C3，C4，C5）；blood serum proteins（including laminin，fibronectin，etc.）.②Opsonized particles attach onto the cell membrane through receptors present on the cell surface of a phagocyte. ③The particles are ingested into phagosomes. ④The phagosomes mature，fuse with lysosomes and become acidified，leading to the enzyme-rich phagolysosomes where the particles are prone to degradation

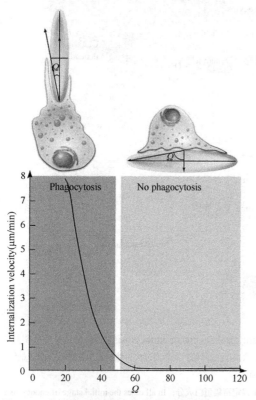

8
7
6
5
4
3
2
1
0

Phagocytosis   No phagocytosis

Internalization velocity(μm/min)

0   20   40   60   80   100   120
Ω

图 3-5 吞噬作用中颗粒的几何效应；Effect of particle geometry on phagocytosis

颗粒经历内化时 $\Omega \leq 45°$，当角度超过临界值（$\approx 45°$）时内化速度为零，巨噬细胞将失去包裹颗粒的能力，并开始在颗粒上伸展；The internalization velocity is positive at $\Omega \leq 45°$, which indicates that the particle undergoes internalization. As the angle exceeds critical value ($\approx 45°$), the internalization velocity is zero, the macrophages lose the ability to entrap particles and start spreading over the particles

肿瘤细胞；识别和清除变性的血浆蛋白、脂类等大分子物质；清除衰老与损伤的细胞和细胞碎片。巨噬细胞吞噬病原颗粒具有一定的条件，一个纳米颗粒进入巨噬细胞内取决于颗粒与细胞膜最初接触点与线之间的曲率角度（Ω），内化速度是在正 $\Omega \leq 45°$[4]（图 3-5）。

二、胞饮作用

胞饮作用（pinocytosis）是摄入细胞外液体及溶质的内吞过程。

（一）网格蛋白依赖的内吞

网格蛋白在调控质膜蛋白组成中起重要作用，研究它对明确细胞和周围环境是如何相互作用、促有丝分裂信号的转导、细胞对营养的摄取、建立细胞外环境、细胞特性包括与免疫系统的作用和维持细胞内环境的稳定有重要的意义。

一旦一个细胞表面受体被它的特异性配体或物质激活，胞内衔接蛋白和网格蛋白在膜受体上装配形成网格蛋白包被小孔，而后形成网格蛋白有被小泡（clathrin-coated vesicle，CCV）。网格蛋白介导的内吞作用（clathrin-mediated endocytosis，CME）有四个主要步骤[5, 6]（图 3-6）。

网格蛋白（clathrin）是包被液泡外面骨架蛋白，网格包被液泡直径在 100～150nm，存在于所有真核生物细胞中，它们是蛋白质和脂类、其他营养物质、抗体和生长因子等从质膜运到胞内的方式，也是蛋白质和脂类从反面高尔基网到核内体的载体。网格蛋白形似蜘蛛，由 3 根链在顶部聚合而成，称为三脚蛋白复合体（triskelion）[1]。

衔接蛋白（adaptin，AP）位于包被液泡的内部，具有膜结合与定位、识别分类信号（sorting signal）和肌醇磷酸化的功能，既能连接"货物"（cargo），还能连接质膜磷脂头簇（headgroup）。现已发现 4 种衔接蛋白（AP1～AP4）分别由一对 100～130 kDa 亚单位组成。这些亚单位分别能识别甘露糖-6-磷酸受体（mannose -6-phosphate receptor，MPR）、转铁蛋白、低密度脂蛋白和表皮生长因子受体（epidermal growth factor receptor，EGFR）、蛋白酶和脱唾液酸受体。

CME 的作用机制 网格蛋白从招募到解离是非常短暂的过程，主要分为：①衔接蛋白和网格蛋白的招募：在质膜受体胞质尾区分类信号和停靠蛋白质（docking protein）的作用下，招募 AP2 复合体到高活性、可饱和、易酶解的位点，启动质膜上形成网格蛋白有被小泡（CCV）[7]。②网格蛋白有被小泡的内陷、缢缩和液泡的芽殖：在离体没有核酸和胞质条件下，网格蛋白平面网格能转型为弯曲的小窝；在活体内，网格蛋白有被小泡也有不同程度的弯曲。内陷可

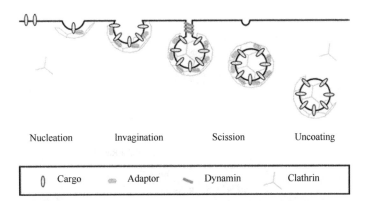

图 3-6 网格蛋白介导内吞作用的示意图；Schematic diagram of clathrin-mediated endocytosis

四个主要步骤：①成核，物质将被聚集到形成的小凹内。②内陷，小凹向内凹陷。③分离，CCV 从质膜切断。④脱壳，去除网格蛋白被膜，新生的小泡释放；The four main stages of clathrin-mediated endocytosis（CME）are shown. ①Nucleation, where cargo is gathered into the forming pit. ②Invagination, where the pit curves inwards. ③Scission, where the CCV is severed from the plasma membrane. ④Uncoating, where the clathrin coat is removed and the nascent vesicle is freed

能是由于网格蛋白在晶格内或网格蛋白间组装时结构的改变和重排所引起。网格蛋白有被小泡的芽殖需要含有 GTP 酶的发动蛋白。该蛋白在体外形成指环形或管形，它是小泡从膜上解离的"扳机"。③网格蛋白有被小泡的脱壳：这是一个耗能过程，需要热休克蛋白（HSC70）、辅助蛋白（auxilin）和 ATP。网格蛋白的大链有两个位点与衔接蛋白和 HSC70 相互作用。HSC70与网格蛋白相互作用能破坏网格蛋白与衔接蛋白间的作用。过表达 HSC70 突变型能阻断运铁蛋白受体的循环，使"装配-拆卸"平衡向装配方向移动。在体外 HSC70 介导网格蛋白从包被液泡上解离，但不解离衔接蛋白。衔接蛋白在网格蛋白脱壳的过程中起重要作用。衔接蛋白不仅具有招募 HSC70 到网格蛋白有被小泡的活性，还可刺激 HSC70 ATP 酶的活性。

内吞作用始于质膜，跨膜蛋白如受体及其他膜相关蛋白簇陷入网格蛋白包被小窝（clathrin-coated pits，CCP）。这簇蛋白依赖于由衔接蛋白（如 AP2）复合体的适当载体蛋白的识别，AP2也负责招募网格蛋白包被亚基以形成囊泡。诸如 GTP 酶发动蛋白被招募到芽泡的颈部，从而促进膜断裂，囊泡从细胞膜释放。一旦释放，网格蛋白包被就从囊泡上解离，使囊泡和早期内体（EE）靶区膜相互作用。小 GTP 酶 Rab5 通过效应蛋白促进物质运送到早期内体，效应蛋白通过 SNARE 复合体激活膜融合作用。在 Rab4 或 Rab11 介导的机制下物质可以从早期内体回到细胞表面再利用。未回收的物质残留在内体从而获得 Hrs 标记。蛋白质如 ESCRT（转运必需内体分选复合物）被招募到内体，促进腔内囊泡（intraluminal vesicle，ILV）的出芽和断裂，形成晚期内体/多泡体（multivesicular body，MVB）。MVB 与含有蛋白酶、脂肪酶等消化酶的溶酶体融合最终导致物质降解[8, 9]（图 3-7）。

（二）小凹蛋白依赖性内吞

小凹（caveolae）/小凹蛋白（caveolin）介导了许多物质的内吞，是非网格蛋白依赖的内吞途径的主要形式。早在 1950 年，日本学者 Yamada 用透射电子显微镜首次观察到细胞质膜上存在一些小凹。小凹是细胞表面特异性内陷结构，亦称细胞质膜微囊。由小凹蛋白包被形成的小泡直径在50～100nm，主要由脂类和蛋白质组成。这些囊泡单个或成串出现以内陷的形式连接在细胞质膜上，呈现典型的脂质双层结构[7]。目前认为小凹是信号转导中心，许多与信号转导有关的受体、激酶和连接蛋白在小凹区域高度富集。在小凹内吞作用的调节过程中酪氨酸激酶依赖信号的激活是一个重要步骤。经磷酸酶抑制剂处理后的细胞中小凹蛋白依赖性内吞作用明显增强[5]（图 3-8）。

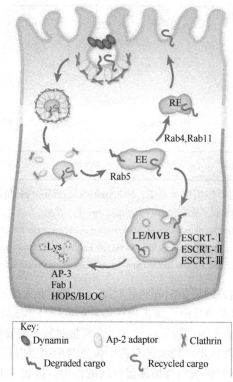

图 3-7 囊泡运输和内吞途径中的关键因子；Vesicle trafficking and key players in the endocytic pathway

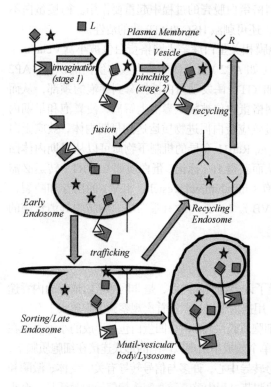

图 3-8 小凹蛋白依赖的内吞的转运过程；Caveolin dependent endocytic trafficking processes

局部区域质膜内陷(阶段 1),然后质膜断裂形成囊泡(阶段 2)。囊泡含有先前的细胞外物质[包括细胞外域的配体(L)和受体(R)复合物],而面对胞质囊泡面所含的物质，及先前暴露在胞质的物质，包括胞质受体尾(△)与衔接蛋白或靶蛋白结合(绿色)。内化囊泡与较大的早期核内体融合。然后内化物被转运到管状泡样晚期核内体，一方面可回收核内体或再循环回到细胞表面，另一方面或被进一步内化，形成多泡体进入溶酶体降解；A small area of the plasma membrane invaginates(stage 1), and then it is pinched off into a vesicle(stage 2). The vesicle lumen contains previously extracellular material [including ligands（L）bound to the receptor（R）extracellular domains]. While the vesicle surface that faces the cytoplasm contains the material, previously exposed into cytosol（including the cytoplasmic receptor tails（△）with bound adaptor or target proteins. The internalized vesicle fuses with larger, early endosomes. The internalized material is then trafficked to tubulovesicular sorting endosomes. From here, material can either be taken to recycling endosomes and thus back to the cell surface, or be re-internalized, creating a multi-vesicular body destined for lysosomal degradation

溶酶体降解的泛素化膜蛋白：泛素化过程中靶蛋白借由 26S 蛋白酶体降解后标记。泛素化通常以单一形式存在或短链泛素修饰（如在许多情况下 K63-键）导致膜蛋白的内吞作用。早期内体中非泛素化蛋白可以再循环回到质膜或被引导至其他细胞内隔室。相反，泛素化蛋白被分类进入多泡体最终到溶酶体中被降解。去泛素化酶（de-ubiquitinating enzymes，DUBs）可逆转泛素化过程。去泛素化在通过转运必需的内体分选复合物（the endosomal sorting complexes required for transport，ESCRT）途径发挥调节细胞内运输的重要作用，在某些情况下还可确保回收内化转运到质膜中的物质（图 3-9）[10]。

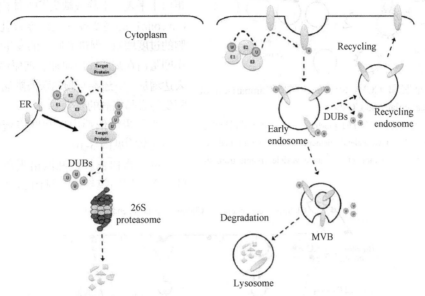

图 3-9　真核细胞中泛素依赖性蛋白降解的主要途径；Major pathways for ubiquitin-dependent protein degradation in eukaryotic cells

小凹蛋白的生物学特性　小凹蛋白是小凹的主要表面标志蛋白，即修饰于小凹内表面的膜整合蛋白，分子量 21～25kDa，它由 N 端、跨膜区和 C 端组成。N 端和 C 端均面向胞质面，其肽链似发夹状结构，主要存在于膜上的囊泡、高尔基体和部分可溶性脂蛋白复合物中。在小凹的组装过程中小凹蛋白及胆固醇起关键作用，是许多信号分子的支架蛋白和负性调节蛋白，属于高度保守的完整膜蛋白家族[11]。Frank 等[12]通过实验证实了 Caveolin1 是小凹胞吞作用的关键分子。如果敲除小凹蛋白基因，就不能形成小凹。迄今为止，在哺乳动物已发现小凹蛋白 4 种异构体：Caveolin1α、Caveolin1β、Caveolin2 和 Caveolin3。它们是不同基因编码的产物，大多数细胞主要表达 Caveolin1 和 Caveolin2，二者形成稳定的异源寡聚体复合物，尤以终末分化的细胞，如脂肪细胞、内皮细胞和成纤维细胞中含量丰富。小凹作为信号分子发挥作用的平台，参与信号转导（signal transduction），Caveolin1 则处于这些平台中各个信号通路的中心位置。小凹蛋白在正常信号转导通路中抑制信号分子的激酶活性，作为信号分子的支架蛋白和负性调节蛋白。Caveolin2 在骨架区无抑制活性，可能 Caveolin2 存在其他信号分子活性抑制区。Caveolin1 与胆固醇具有极强的亲和力，因此小凹中胆固醇的含量远高于其他生物膜，参与胆固醇平衡（cholesterol homeostasis）。研究表明，缺乏小凹结构可能最终导致泡沫细胞的产生，提示小凹和 Caveolin1 可以将过多的脂蛋白来源的胆固醇清除，保持细胞胆固醇的平衡。而 Caveolin3 主要存在于各种肌细胞（如心肌细胞、骨骼肌细胞及横纹肌细胞）中，与该细胞合成密切相关[13]。在肌细胞中 Caveolin3 参与能量代谢。在外周血细胞和神经细胞中未见小凹蛋白的表达，也未见小凹结构。

　　小凹蛋白与肿瘤的相关性已成为肿瘤生物学研究的热点之一，其中，对 Caveolin1 与肿瘤发生、转移关系的研究最为深入。Caveolin1 基因定位于可疑肿瘤抑制位点（D7S522；7q31.1），此位点在多种肿瘤中（如肝癌、卵巢癌、乳腺癌、子宫肌瘤、胃腺癌等）出现缺失或断裂[14]。此外，用反义 Caveolin1 诱导的正常 NIH3T3 细胞移植到裸鼠体内见肿瘤形成，表明 Caveolin1 具有肿瘤抑制因子的功能。在许多癌症和转染活化癌基因的细胞中，Caveolin1 mRNA 和蛋白水平表达下降或缺失[15]。体内实验证实 Caveolin1 的突变或缺失能导致乳腺上皮细胞的过度增殖，促进乳腺癌的发生[16]。此外，小凹蛋白在高胆固醇血症、糖尿病等疾病中表达增加[17]，还参与阿尔茨海默病[18]、肌肉病变与心肺疾病的发生。

小凹蛋白依赖内吞和网格蛋白依赖的内吞比较[5]见图 3-10。

网格蛋白依赖性和网格蛋白非依赖性的内吞作用的膜系统[19]见图 3-11。

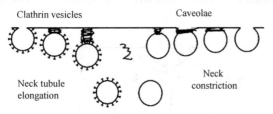

图 3-10 小凹和 CCVs 断裂的比较；Comparison of scission in caveolae and CCVs

细胞骨架元体与发动蛋白介导的 pinchase 激活被认为是诱导囊泡从膜分离的因素；Cytoskeletal elements and dynamin-mediated "pinchase" activity are thought to induce vesicle fission from the membrane

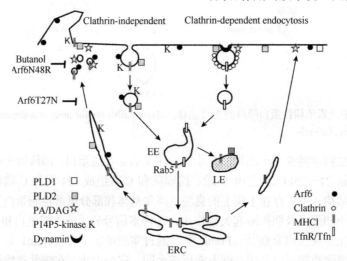

图 3-11 网格蛋白依赖性和网格蛋白非依赖性的内吞作用的膜系统；Model of PLD and clathrin-dependent and clathrin-independent endocytosis membrane systems

网格蛋白依赖性内吞作用内化物如转铁蛋白受体（TfnR）依赖于发动蛋白（dynamin）。这些内体随后与早期内体（EE）融合，转铁蛋白受体可通过核旁内吞回收隔室（endocytic recycling compartment，ERC）再循环到质膜（PM）。网格蛋白非依赖性内吞内化，如 MHCI 进入细胞不依赖于发动蛋白。MHCI 与 EE 融合也可以再循环到质膜，但管式膜载体（PLD）缺乏转铁蛋白受体。在质膜的 PLD1 与晚期内体相关。在 HeLa 细胞中观察到 PLD2 在 PM 也与网格蛋白非依赖性内体相关。磷脂酸和 DAG 生成的可能位点（星）；Clathrin-dependent endocytosis internalizes cargo such as the transferrin receptor（TfnR）and is dependent upon dynamin. These endosomes subsequently fuse with the early endosome（EE）and transferrin receptor can be recycled back to the PM via the juxtanuclear endocytic recycling compartment（ERC）. Clathrin-independent endocytosis internalizes cargo such as MHCI into cells independently of dynamin. These endosomes fuse with EE and MHCI can also recycle back to the PM but in distinct tubular membrane carriers devoid of transferrin receptor. PLD1 is shown associated with late endosomes and also at the PM. PLD2 is shown at the PM and also associated with clathrin-independent endosomes observed in HeLa cells. Possible sites of PA and DAG generation（stars）

（三）巨胞饮

在某些因素刺激下，伸展细胞边缘的细胞膜皱褶形成大且不规则的原始内吞小泡，即巨胞饮体。巨胞饮体大小不一，直径一般为 0.5～2μm。巨胞饮（macropinocytosis）在巨噬细胞和树突状细胞中发挥主要作用，在许多肿瘤细胞中也存在巨胞饮[19]。

巨胞饮体没有网格蛋白或小凹蛋白包被，其在早期形成阶段与肌动蛋白密切相关，为非选择性内吞细胞外营养物质和液相大分子提供了一条有效的途径。巨胞饮受到多种蛋白调节，如肌动蛋白、Scar 蛋白、AP21 连接复合体，RabB。细胞膜皱褶形成的程度不同，导致巨胞饮产生的速率不同。例如，从吸收不同大小的镍颗粒（Ni_3S_2）可分别通过巨胞饮作用和（或）网格蛋白介导的内吞作用使其在囊泡转化为二价镍离子（Ni^{2+}）并释放到胞质与多种生物分子作用或随囊泡进入细胞核，Ni^{2+} 聚集在核膜中（图 3-12）。Ni^{2+} 可以导致多种效应，包括 DNA 的凝聚和表观遗传标记的 G 改变，包括 DNA 甲基化增加和 H2A、H2B、H3 和 H4 中组蛋白乙酰化的丢失，H3K9 二甲基化作用，H3K4 三甲基化作用，H2A 及 H2B 泛素化增加。

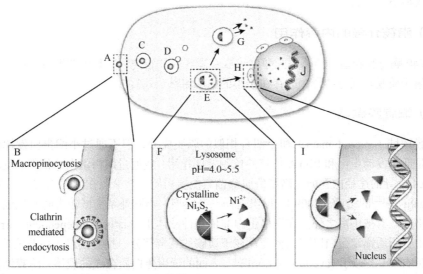

图 3-12　吸收镍颗粒（Ni_3S_2）的模型；Proposed Model of particulate nickel uptake

晶体状的 Ni_3S_2 黏附在细胞表面（A）、推测这些颗粒是通过巨胞饮作用和（或）网格蛋白介导的内吞作用进入细胞，其中吸收形式的不同可能与颗粒的大小有关（B）；在巨胞饮作用中膜首先皱褶形成然后摄取，这是在细胞内吞 Ni_3S_2 中常可观察到的特征。在网格蛋白介导的内吞作用下膜通过内陷发生形态变化从而形成一种"膜孔"。一些蛋白质参与网格蛋白介导的内吞作用，图中显示有网格蛋白的蛋白稳定小凹的弯曲度和发动蛋白形成聚集体在开口处裂解之前。内吞微粒通过某些形式囊泡（特殊的形式可根据内吞作用有所不同，如巨胞饮体或网格蛋白有被小泡的形式）跳跃式的向核运动（C）。然后在溶酶体攻击的过程中溶酶体与囊泡相互作用（D），这些相互作用常导致其与溶酶体融合（E）。一旦融合，质子泵作用导致囊泡酸化和 Ni_3S_2 结晶体的溶解从而改变囊泡的 pH。此过程中产生高浓度的 Ni^{2+}（F）。在某些情况下 Ni^{2+} 出囊泡进入细胞质，从而与生物分子相互作用（G）。在另一些情况下囊泡能继续向细胞核运动最后聚集在核膜（H）这些聚集在核膜表面的物质能促进 Ni^{2+} 转运入细胞核（I）[2]；The nickel particle, crystalline Ni_3S_2 affixes at the cell surface（A）. We hypothesize that the particle enters via macropinocytosis and/or clathrin mediated endocytosis-where the different forms of uptake may be related to the size of the particle（B）. In macropinocytosis the membrane exhibits ruffling prior to uptake, a feature that was frequently observed during Ni_3S_2 endocytosis. In clathrin-mediated endocytosis the membrane undergoes a morphological change via invagination and forms a membrane pit. A number of proteins are involved in CME, pictured here are the clathrin proteins that stabilize the pit curvature and the dynamin that aggregates at the neck prior to scission. The endocytized particle moves via saltatory motion towards the nucleus inside some form of vesicle（the specific form will vary in accordance with the form of endocytosis-macropinosome or clathrin coated vesicle）（C）. Lysosomes then interact with the vesicle in a process of lysosomal attack（D）. These interactions often lead to lysosomal fusion（E）. Once fused, the pH of the vesicle may be altered through proton pumps leading to acidification of the vesicle and the dissolution of the crystalline Ni_3S_2 particle. This process produces high concentrations of Ni^{2+}（F）. In some cases the Ni^{2+} may exit the vesicle into the cytoplasm where they can interact with biomolecules（G）. While in other cases the vesicles will continue to travel towards the nucleus where they will aggregate at the nuclear membrane（H）. Those aggregated at the membrane will promote the transfer of Ni^{2+} ions into the nucleus（I）

巨胞饮发生的机制 细胞松弛素 D 和秋水仙碱能显著抑制巨胞饮体的形成,提示微管和微丝在这个过程中扮演重要角色。其机制可能为多种因素的刺激下,相应的酪氨酸激酶受体被激活,激活的受体快速磷酸化。磷酸化的残基招募三磷酸肌醇(PI3)激酶并激活之,活化的 PI3k 促使 Rac1 的激活,后者可能通过两条途径引起微丝的重构:第一,活化的 Rac1 激活蛋白激酶(PAK)1 调节肌球蛋白轻链的磷酸化状态,进一步调节肌球蛋白与肌动蛋白的相互作用。肌球蛋白与肌动蛋白相互作用促进微丝的重构,细胞膜皱褶的产生,巨胞饮的形成。第二,活化的 Rac1 结合到其靶蛋白 IRSp53 的 N 端,IRSp53 C 端的 SH₃ 区域与 WAVE 结合形成三分子复合体[20],后者激活 WAVE 蛋白,进一步激活肌动蛋白相关蛋白(actin related protein, Arp)2/3 复合体,刺激微丝成核使微丝重构,形成细胞膜皱褶产生巨胞饮[21]。更深入的调节机制还需进一步深入研究。

(四)脂筏介导的内吞作用

如 SV40 病毒颗粒通过招募胆固醇以形成膜微区或"脂筏"使膜内凹形成,同时病毒改变自身形状附于质膜与细胞结合,或存在于小的内凹中[3](图 3-13)。

(五)细胞膜微域

细胞膜微域(microdomain)和小凹有相似的脂质成分,但不通过小凹蛋白发挥作用。细胞膜微域是通过发动蛋白和 Rho A 依赖的机制发挥作用,或通过网格蛋白非依赖、发动蛋白非依赖、Cdc4 介导的途径内吞糖化磷脂酰肌醇锚定的蛋白质。该途径在内吞 IL-2 中发挥作用。根据 Bhagatji 等[22]的结论(2009),提出这样一个模型,当胞外结构域较大时脂质锚定蛋白被排除在网格蛋白有被小窝之外。在网格蛋白非依赖性载体 1(clathrin-independent carrier 1)的内吞作用中,脂质锚定蛋白以相同密度存在于质膜的其余部分。推测网格蛋白非依赖性载体 2 中,由嵌在质膜(类似于 caveolin 或 flotillin)表面的低聚蛋白质合成的载体,跨膜结构域被排除在外,可能导致胞膜小叶外对脂质锚定蛋白的选择性,而与这类蛋白积聚的浓度无关[23](图 3-14)。

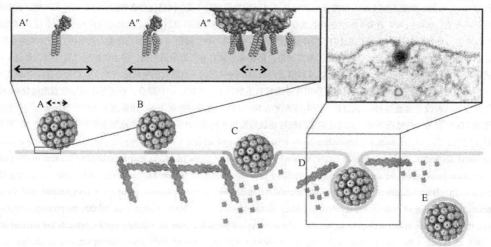

图 3-13 SV40 脂筏介导的内吞作用;Steps in SV40 Lipid mediated endocytosis

(A)与质膜结合,在质膜上平行运动。(B)薄膜微区"脂筏"形成和肌动蛋白依赖的固定。(C)质膜内陷。(D)非依赖性发动蛋白(肌动蛋白 α)招募,依赖酪氨酸激酶内化的膜机械断裂。(E)胞内运输。(插图)(左)GM1 在膜上的流动性。单个神经节苷脂分子在不含胆固醇的膜上快速扩散(A0),并被瞬时限制在胆固醇表面的纳米级域(A00)。当 SV40 结合质膜,扩散速度大大降低(A000)和 SV40-GM1-络合物可能招募胆固醇以形成膜微区的"脂筏"(右);(A)Binding to plasma membrane and lateral motion in the plane of the plasma membrane,(B)formation of a membrane microdomain "lipid raft" and actin-dependent immobilization，（C）invagination of the plasma membrane，（D）recruitment of dynamin-independent scission machinery（actin?）and tyrosine kinase-dependent internalization，and（E）intracellular transpor（Insets）（Left）GM1 mobility in membranes. Individual GM1 molecules undergo fast diffusion in cholesterol-free membranes（A0），but are transiently confined in nanoscopic domains in the presence of cholesterol（A00）.When SV40 binds to plasma membrane，diffusion speed is greatly reduced（A000）and the SV40-GM1-complex likely recruits cholesterol to form a membrane microdomain or "lipid raft"（Right）

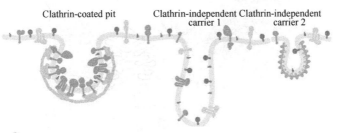

图 3-14　胞外结构域的大小决定了脂质锚定蛋白的细胞内吞途径；Ectodomain size determines the endocytic pathway for lipid-anchored proteins

　　细胞膜微域途径和网格蛋白依赖的内吞作用比较[22]如图 3-15 所示。

　　事实上，各种形状的微粒可以利用多种途径进入细胞[4]，包括 CME、胞膜小凹介导的内吞、巨胞饮作用。微粒的形状似乎对调节其进入细胞的速度是至关重要。立方体形的微粒可利用多种途径进入细胞，但主要是巨胞饮作用（图 3-16）。

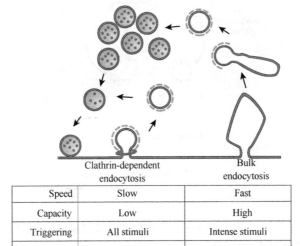

	Clathrin-dependent endocytosis	Bulk endocytosis
Speed	Slow	Fast
Capacity	Low	High
Triggering	All stimuli	Intense stimuli
When active?	During&Alter	During
Generates	SVs directly	SVs via endosome
Molecules involved	Well characterised	Little characterisation

图 3-15　细胞膜微域途径和网格蛋白依赖的内吞作用比较；Comparison of bulk endocytosis with clathrin-dependent endocytosis

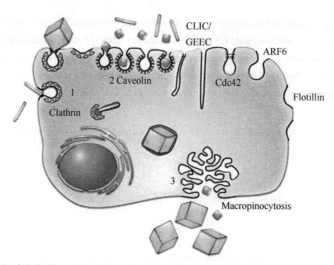

图 3-16　各种形状的纳米微粒可通过多种途径进入细胞；Cellular entry of nanoparticles of all shapes utilize multiple pathways to gain cellular entry

CLIC：网格蛋白非依赖性运载体；GEEC：GPI 锚定富集蛋白成分；CLIC, clathrin-independent carriers；GEEC, GPI-anchored protein-enriched compartment

　　在不同的情况中，对外源性物质（如多聚物阻断剂）的内吞作用可分别通过小凹蛋白依赖的内吞途径、小凹蛋白非依赖的内吞途径或由网格蛋白依赖的内吞途径（图 3-17）。

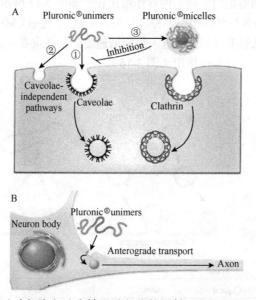

图 3-17　多聚物阻断剂进入上皮细胞（A）和神经元（B）的机制；The entry mechanisms of Pluronic® block copolymers in（A）epithelial cells and（B）neurons

A. ①多聚物阻断剂单体可直接通过胞膜小凹介导的内吞作用进入细胞；②在缺乏小凹的细胞中多聚物单体可以通过小凹非依赖性途径进入细胞；③一旦多聚物浓度增加形成多聚物胶粒，则可通过网格蛋白依赖的内吞途经（CME）进入细胞，在此条件下，多聚物胶粒能抑制小凹介导的内吞作用。B. 在初级神经元（亦缺乏小凹）多聚物单体可顺行转运到轴突/树突进入胞体；A. ①In cells displaying the caveolae pathway Pluronic® unimers enter through caveolae-mediated endocytosis. ②In cells devoid of caveolae，the block copolymer unimers can also enter through caveolae-independent pathways. ③Once the concentration of the block copolymer increases above the CMC the micelles are formed，which enter through the CME. Under these conditions the block copolymer inhibits the caveolae-mediated endocytosis. B. In primary neurons(also devoid of the caveolae)the Pluronic® unimers enter the cell body from where they undergo anterograde trafficking to the axons / dendrites

第二节 内吞蛋白的特征

在内吞途径中囊泡运输的各种步骤由特定蛋白质的活性相互调控。

一、内吞蛋白的生物能学特性

内吞蛋白的主要功能与神经递质的内吞有关。内吞蛋白在 C 端有一个独特结合功能 SH$_3$ 结构域[24]，可与一些特殊功能的蛋白质如发动蛋白相互作用并结合，从而影响其他蛋白的功能。N 端则参与细胞膜的内凹形成囊泡。2002 年有人建议命名为内吞蛋白 A1、内吞蛋白 A2、内吞蛋白 A3，如亨廷顿蛋白（huntingtin）属于内吞蛋白 A1 的结合蛋白，它与 huntingtin 连接蛋白 40（HAP40）组成的复合物抑制微管依赖的早期内体运动，增加了早期内体和肌动蛋白的连接[25]。此后又发现了一类新的成员，后者命名为内吞蛋白 B。

二、内吞蛋白相关的信号转导

由于内吞蛋白与多种蛋白质相互作用，因此涉及细胞内多条细胞信号传导通路。

1. 与细胞膜受体相互作用 内吞蛋白主要分布于细胞质和细胞膜上，如 β_1 肾上腺素能受体。内吞蛋白还参与磷脂信号通路，许多内吞蛋白都含有肌醇 4，5-二磷酸（PIP2）的结合位点。PIP2 的降解是完成内吞所必需的。用免疫荧光蛋白标记 PIP2 连接域，跟踪观察其在活细胞内吞时的运动，发现 PIP2 在细胞膜表面形成许多小斑块，这些斑块逐渐移入了细胞内，研究证实这一内移就是内吞作用。PIP2 的消失与磷酸肌醇磷脂酶的募集相吻合，因此推测后者降解前者。而当 PIP2 的降解受阻时，环绕在膜斑块上的剪切机器失灵导致异常的内陷，而不能完成内吞，因此，PIP2 的降解是内吞囊泡剪切的关键步骤。内吞囊泡形成的时间和蛋白质修饰的构件[26]。

2. 神经递质回收 它实质上也是一种细胞的内吞过程，先由网格蛋白与 AP2 或 AP180 和细胞膜类脂相互作用形成网格蛋白有被小泡。其形成过程正是内吞蛋白 A1 驱动凹陷膜囊泡颈部结构与细胞膜断裂，内吞蛋白 A1N 端的 LPAAT 可催化溶血磷脂酸（LPA）和花生四烯酰辅酶 A 形成磷脂酸（PA），LPA 呈倒锥体形结构，PA 呈锥体形，前者结构有利于膜的正向突出，后者有利于膜的负向凹陷，正是这种 PA 的转变驱动了囊泡和细胞膜的断裂。因此内吞蛋白突变后，将严重影响突触颗粒回收机制[27]。

3. 内吞以外的作用 内吞蛋白 A2 还参与吸收营养和生长因子、病原体和受体内吞等多种功能，参与多种所谓的膜交通机制。而内吞蛋白 B1 细胞内定位主要在细胞膜部分，它的功能主要与细胞膜的动力学有关。如果内吞蛋白缺失，凋亡受体 Fas / CD95 就不能正确地定位于细胞膜上，从而导致细胞凋亡机制受抑制。

第三节 内吞通路中的关键蛋白

一、发动蛋白

发动蛋白（dynamin）是一个 100kDa 的 GTP 酶，它的 N 端 GTP 酶区域能结合并水解 GTP，PH（pleckstrin homology）区可与膜结合，介导发动蛋白之间的聚合，C 端的 PRD（praline arginine rich）区则介导其他蛋白之间的相互作用。另外，dynamin 还有一个小的 GTP 酶效应子（GTPase effector，GED）区，它在水解 GTP 时是必需的。在网格蛋白介导的细胞内吞中也是必需的[28]，并在部分网格蛋白非依赖内吞途径中也发挥重要作用。剪切和囊泡的形成都离不开 dynamin 的作用。dynamin-1 通过和配体（amphiphysin1）结合，在周期蛋白依赖性激酶 5（CDK5）的调控下，即在发动蛋白依赖的内吞中发挥关键的作用。dynamin-1 依赖的内吞发生迅速，通常只要几秒钟，而 dynamin-2 介导的内吞则较慢，需要 10 分钟左右。

dynamin 通过机械和化学特异性作用挤压扭转形成内吞囊泡[29]。在内吞早期，dynamin 位于内吞囊泡的颈部，这表明 dynamin 利用 GTP 水解释放的能量直接挤压细胞膜形成囊泡。dynamin 在体外管化脂质，使小管脱离胞膜。而 Sandy Schmid 提出调控性 GTP 酶的模型[30]：dynamin 并不是在水解 GTP 时被活化，而是与 GTP 相结合中发挥作用，GTP 需与其他蛋白相结合来完成缢缩。GTP 引起的挤压、收缩和分割需要纵向的拉力。在哺乳动物体内，dynamin 位于较短的内吞囊泡颈部，皮质肌动蛋白（cortactin）可能是拉力的来源。这种拉力可使肌动蛋白自由地挤压扭转内吞囊泡。

dynamin 既具有内在 GTP 酶活性，又是小脑激酶 Dyrk1A 的底物，具有自身聚集倾向的基本特性，可以帮助新生的内膜上突起的囊泡从细胞膜上分离。发动蛋白通过 pH 结构与 epsin 的 ENTH（epsin NH$_2$-terminal homology）结构域参与成管。野生型 dynamin 则阻止管化，从而调控网格蛋白有被小泡和其他内吞介质的内陷程度。

二、肌动蛋白

肌动蛋白（actin）是微丝的主要构成成分。微丝参与细胞形态和极性的维持、内吞作用、胞内运输、细胞收缩及运动、细胞分裂等众多功能。actin 有两种形式：G-actin 和 F-actin。通过使用肌动蛋白-单体-分离药物 latrunculin A 可以清楚地表明 F-actin 在内吞中的重要性：添加该药物 5 分钟内，actin 斑块消失，内吞停止。此时，酵母菌的 Las17p 和Ⅰ型肌球蛋白（Myo3p and Myo5p）开始活化 Arp2/3 复合物来核化肌动蛋白丝。这组蛋白被称为"肌动蛋白网络生长机器（actin network growth machinery）"。研究者用荧光显微镜和全反显微镜（TIRF）技术观察人体活细胞内陷小凹的内化。Merrifield 等发现肌动蛋白的暂时性募集与囊泡内陷相吻合，同时还观察到网格蛋白小凹募集 Arp2/3 复合物。pH 敏感探针的使用使研究者观察到网格蛋白有被小泡内吞物质的过程，并分辨出内陷和剪切的界限。内陷中 actin 的募集为被膜小窝的内陷提供动力[31]。actin 在内吞位点核化后，actin 丝被加帽成束，才有足够的力量使膜内陷产生囊泡。

膜的原始曲率由网格蛋白和额外的内吞蛋白（如包含 Syp1 的 F-BAR）所产生。Syp1 能抑制 WASP/Las17-Arp2/3 调控 actin 的装配，在 CME 早期可能有助于保持 actin 聚合过程中的抑制性。随着膜凹过程的进展，膜曲率可由 BAR 结构域蛋白的改变，如 Bzz1 与其他内吞蛋白一起被招募到靶部位进行调控 Arp2/3[32]（图 3-18）。

断裂是由囊泡颈部的收缩来完成，驱动性 BAR 蛋白驱使膜变形，脂质相分离产生 actin 应力和 Sjl2p 线性张力。囊泡断裂后，PAN1 复合物蛋白 Sla1p、Pan1p 和 End3p，由 Ark1p/Prk1p 磷酸化，导致其分离。Ark1p/Prk1p 还负责结束 actin 聚合，允许 Cof1p/Aip1p/Crn1p 裂解 actin 细丝。Sjl2p 负责 PIP2 的去磷酸化，减少 Sla2p 和 Ent1/2p 对囊泡的亲和力。ARF3p、Gts1p 和 Lsb5p 一起参与了 PAN1 复合物的解离[26]（图 3-19）。

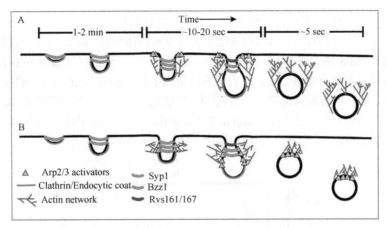

图 3-18　内吞作用中 actin 装配的主要模型；Major models for actin assembly during endocytosis

在模型 A 中，actin 激活 Arp2/3 形成 actin 网络核离开质膜。内吞包被蛋白既连接膜与 actin 网络，又提供了物质进一步内陷进入细胞内的力。神经元突触前膜蛋白 Rvs161 和 Rvs167 能驱动膜断裂。在模型 B 中 actin 是沿着膜小管的侧面形成 actin 网络核，可能是对缺失 Syp1 的反应及招募 Bzz1 的结果。actin 倒刺状末端推动着膜小管的生长，挤压膜小管，在膜破裂过程中驱动小管伸长，协助神经元突触前膜蛋白作用。在此模型中，actin 网络作为驱动囊泡从膜释放后运动的位点。哺乳动物 CME 期间如何利用 actin 聚合的最佳模式类似于 B 模型；In model A, a ring of actin activates Arp2/3 which nucleates an actin network that flows away from the plasma membrane. Proteins of the endocytic coat link the membrane to this flowing network and this provides the force to invaginate further into the cell. The amphiphysin proteins, Rvs161 and Rvs167, drive membrane scission. In model B, actin is nucleated along the sides of the membrane tubule, perhaps in response to the loss of Syp1, and the recruitment of Bzz1, which can promote actin nucleation. The growing barbed ends of the actin push on the membrane tubule, squeezing it, driving elongation and assisting the amphiphysin proteins during membrane scission. In this model, the actin network is in a position to drive movement after the vesicle has been freed from the membrane. The best models for how actin polymerization is utilized during CME in mammals are similar to the model presented in B

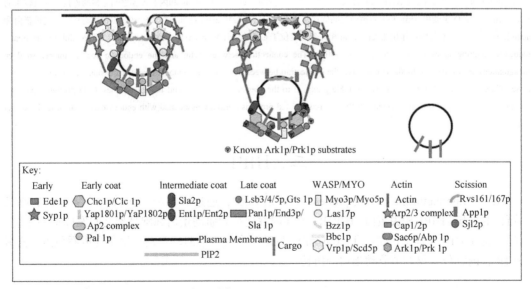

图 3-19　断裂和内吞囊泡脱壳；Scission and uncoating of endocytic vesicles

目前已知囊泡剪切涉及两种酵母菌双载蛋白（amphiphysin），Rvs161p 和 Rvs167p。这些蛋白含有 BAR 结构域，与细胞膜结合并参与成管现象，小管的形成促进了剪切过程；actin 及其相关蛋白具有募集 amphiphysin 的作用。如果 amphiphysin 缺失，会导致囊泡颈部的延长最终挤压断离。在 actin 的调控基因突变时，经常可以看到延长的囊泡颈部，表明 actin 在剪切过程中可能也起着重要的作用。剪切后囊泡脱去被膜和内体融合。actin 在这个过程可能有两种作用：囊泡沿着 actin 轴索移动；actin 在囊泡表面核化更易于囊泡在细胞内的移动。剪切后，这些肌动蛋白从内吞位点解聚。最具代表性的解聚因子是 cofilin。cofilin 是哺乳动物内吞作用所必需，但其具体作用机制尚需进一步研究[33]。在细胞膜内陷的过程中还需要 Sac6p/微丝结合蛋白/丝束蛋白（fimbrin）的参与，Sac6p 缺失时，actin 虽然可以在内吞位点聚集，却不能使膜内陷[34]。影响 actin 聚合的内吞突变体的作用[26]如图 3-20 所示。

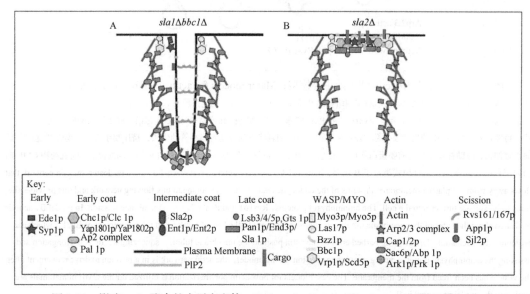

图 3-20　影响 actin 聚合的内吞突变体；Endocytic mutants affecting actin polymerization
A. 在 sla1D bbc1D 突变中，Las17p 抑制性大大降低，导致过度的 actin 聚合。actin 和内吞被膜之间完整的连接，形成较深的内陷。B. 在 sla2D 突变中 actin 和内吞被膜之间的连接缺失，导致长带状 actin 尾部不断装配靠近质膜和扁平膜。包被蛋白和 actin 留在质膜，而所有与内吞作用相关的 actin 相关蛋白定位于 actin 尾部；A. In sla1D bbc1D mutants，Las17p inhibition is greatly reduced，resulting in excessive actin polymerization. The connection between actin and the endocytic coat is intact，so deep invaginations are formed. B. In sla2D mutants，the connection between actin and the endocytic coat is missing，resulting in long，treadmilling actin tails that continuously assemble proximal to the plasma membrane，and flat membranes. Coat proteins and actin remain at the plasma membrane whereas all the actin-associated proteins normally associated with endocytosis localize to the comet tails

三、HIP1

HIP1（huntingtin-interacting protien 1）激活 Cdc4，通过 N-WASP 和 Arp2/3 复合物加速肌动蛋白的聚集。HIP1 相关蛋白（HIP1R）也在内吞途径和肌动蛋白细胞骨架之间发挥重要作用。有趣的是在 HIP1R 缺失的情况下肌动蛋白、发动蛋白和皮质肌动蛋白仍聚集在内吞位点，表明 HIP1R 在内吞位点仅调节肌动蛋白的扭转。

四、PCH/F-BAR

PCH（pombe Cdc15 homology）/F-BAR 是作用于内吞途径和肌动蛋白细胞骨架之间的另一家族蛋白。这些蛋白的 BAR 域与磷酸肌醇相结合，在体外能使脂质体包膜管化。FBP17 是 PCH

蛋白家族的一员，含有 PCH 结构域和 EFC 结构域（extended FC domain）。EFC 结构域与 BAR 结构域的同源性不强，其与磷脂酰丝氨酸及磷脂酰肌醇-4，5-二磷酸[PI（4，5）P2]紧密结合使细胞膜变形，并使脂质体成管状。大多数 PCH 蛋白含有 SH3 结构域，和发动蛋白结合后募集 N-WASP 到细胞膜上，含有 EFC 结构域的 FBP17 就是通过与发动蛋白和 N-WASP 结合这种机制参与胞膜的内陷和肌动蛋白聚合，敲除 FBP17 会使内吞受损，说明 FBP17 是发动蛋白依赖性内吞作用所必需[35]。

五、Rab 蛋白

Rab 蛋白是内吞的重要调控因子，属于小 GTP 酶。其中 Rab5 与成管相关，在内吞途径中的作用已较清楚。Rab5 蛋白有三个异构体，分别为 Rab5A、Rab5B 和 Rab5C，在多种组织中均有表达。Rab5 蛋白主要存在于质膜、网格蛋白覆盖的囊泡和早期内体上，调节内吞物质在胞膜与早期内体间的运输，并帮助囊泡沿微管运动，调控囊泡融合和囊泡再循环。Rab5 蛋白在发挥功能时不断进行 GTP/GDP 循环，作为囊泡运输的分子开关，当与 GTP 结合时处于活性状态称之为"开"，当与 GDP 结合时处于非活性状态称之为"关"。HAP40 是 Rab5 有效的调节因子，Rab5 必须在 HAP40 存在的情况下才能增加内体与肌动蛋白的连接；Young 等发现 Rab5A 蛋白与 α-突触核蛋白（α-synuclein）内吞相关[36]。α-synuclein 与帕金森病、Lewy 小体痴呆和 AD 等多种中枢神经疾病有关。Young 通过研究 Rab5A GTP 酶突变体，发现此突变体可引起 α-synuclein 的内吞减少，同时 Lewy 小体样细胞中包含体生成减少，继而减少细胞毒性。一旦免疫系统出现缺陷 Rab5A 蛋白过表达可引起巨噬细胞对病原体的吞噬减慢，病原体降解速率下降，使 IFN-C（干扰素 C）介导的吞噬作用减弱。

受体介导内吞作用由网格蛋白有被小泡产生，由 Rab5 和 Rab21 调控，使内化物被传输、并分配到内体中。分子可以从这里通过专门的回收内体和不同的 Rab GTP 酶或快或慢地经回收途径返回到质膜。新合成的质膜蛋白从高尔基体外侧传递到内体再循环，而溶酶体水解酶经由两个甘露糖-6-磷酸受体被传递到早期和晚期内体中。从早期内体到高尔基体的重吸收取决于 Rab6，同时 Rab9 控制从晚期内体到高尔基体外侧的运输。Rab7 是多个降解途径中的关键 Rab GTP 酶，它促进后期内体，吞噬体和自噬体与溶酶体的融合，这些溶酶体与特异性 Rab GTP 酶相关。Rab7 与 Rac1 结合后在上皮细胞和神经元中降解钙黏着蛋白，并在破骨细胞的骨吸收中发挥作用[37]。

六、PTEC 受体、巨蛋白及其相关的分子

在近端小管上皮细胞（PTEC）的顶膜上，各种分子参与受体介导的内吞的过程。在此过程中巨蛋白（megalin）与其他膜蛋白如 CUBAM 复合物（cubilin-amnionless complex）、NHE3、ClC5 结合发挥关键作用。巨蛋白和 CUBAM 直接与不同的配体结合，而 NHE3 和 ClC5 参与内体酸化，这对进一步处理内吞蛋白十分重要。巨蛋白还与细胞内衔接蛋白，如 ARH、DAB2 和 GIPC 相互作用。DAB2 与发动蛋白、肌球蛋白Ⅵ和非肌肉肌球蛋白Ⅱ型重链 A（NMHC ⅡA）结合，通过肌动蛋白微丝分子复合物介导内吞转运。巨蛋白的胞质尾区经 γ-分泌酶作用从膜上释放，参与细胞内信号转导[38]（图 3-21）。

第四节 内吞对质膜信号的调控

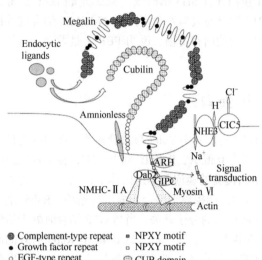

图 3-21 在 PTEC 的顶膜上巨蛋白和其相关分子参与受体介导的内吞作用；Megalin and its associated molecules involved in receptor-mediated endocytosis in PTEC

在内吞作用中研究较多的是配体介导的 Notch 信号通路[39]。

一、内吞作用后信号衰减

受体酪氨酸激酶（RTK）或 G 蛋白偶联受体（GPCR）的配体诱导激活信号效应器介导受体招募，促进信号从质膜到磷酸化的 RTK，或当 Gα 亚基被绑定到的 GTP 时，与 GPCR 相关的 G 蛋白被激活（图 3-22，步骤 1）。GPCR 的信号既可以由 GTP 结合的 Gα 亚基介导，也可以由 Gβ-Gγ 复合亚基介导。受体招募到包被小凹（图 3-22，步骤 2），在质膜上分隔基板和（或）介质使网格蛋白依赖的内吞作用信号衰减（图 3-22，步骤 3）。一些受体在内吞作用后转运到溶酶体被蛋白酶水解，信号进一步衰减（图 3-22，步骤 4）[40]。

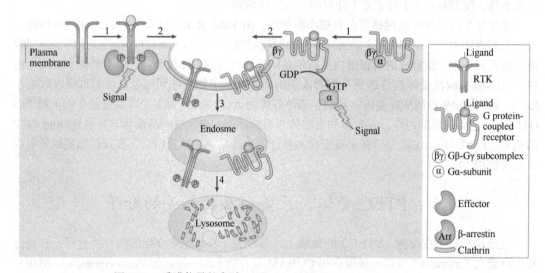

图 3-22 质膜信号的衰减；Schematic depicting signal attenuation

二、内吞中信号通路的切换

一些 GPCR 激活三聚体 G 蛋白（图 3-23，信号 1，步骤 1）的能力在通过受体磷酸化和 β-抑制（图 3-23，步骤 2）的内吞作用之前就已经衰减。这些脱敏的 β-抑制-受体复合物浓缩成网格蛋白有被小泡后（图 3-23，步骤 3）被内吞进入酸性（H⁺）内体（图 3-23，步骤 4），促进了配位体（取决于受体和细胞型）β-抑制和磷酸酶催化的去磷酸化的解离或破坏（图 3-23，步骤 5）。再循环使受体恢复到细胞表面，为细胞进行下一轮信号的再致敏做准备（图 3-23，步骤 6）。在某些情况下，GPCR 把受体重复插入含不同 G 蛋白偶联环境中（图 3-23，步骤 7），这将在一系列下游受体激活后，产生特异性信号通路（图 3-23，信号 2，步骤 8）[40]。

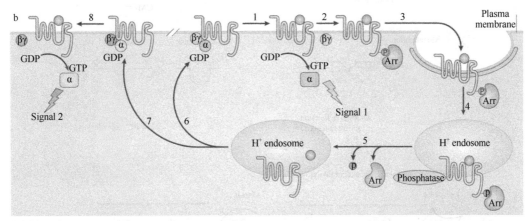

图 3-23　内吞作用对信号脱敏、再循环和通路切换；Schematic depicting signal desensitization, re-sensitization and pathway switching

第五节　内吞作用的意义

一、对细胞有丝分裂的影响

（一）细胞有丝分裂中内吞的抑制

在有丝分裂过程中 CME 停滞有四个机制：①有丝分裂磷酸化。CME 蛋白在基层或第二层的重要分子通过有丝分裂激酶磷酸化后无法与其他分子相互作用，从而推迟 CME。②改变膜的张力。在细胞 CME 作用中，机械力必须克服三种力：双层平面的张力（TM）、膜和细胞骨架之间的相互作用力（γ）及弯曲膜的硬度（B）；B 依附于内陷膜的半径上。在细胞分裂间期 CME 的机械力可以轻易克服这些力的总和，但在有丝分裂过程中 CME 的机械力并不能克服这些力的总和。③有丝分裂的其他作用。与第一种机制不同的是在有丝分裂过程中还有不一定涉及有丝分裂磷酸化的另一种关键蛋白能延迟 CME 的途径。④有丝分裂纺锤体依赖性抑制作用。微管网络的重组和有丝分裂过程中相关发动蛋白能抑制 CME 的后期阶段[6]（图 3-24）。

（二）内吞转运中调节分裂细胞的表面积

在细胞分裂间期，膜经过持续的内化和再循环回到细胞表面，此时再循环被阻止，内化物积聚在细胞内体中，减少了细胞的表面积，为细胞分裂做准备，一旦该过程停止，即开始下一个细胞周期。细胞进入分裂期，细胞内吞作用主要发生在纺锤体两极附近。回收的内体堆积在中间区并快速向增大的胞质分裂沟提供大量的膜原料[41]（图 3-25）。

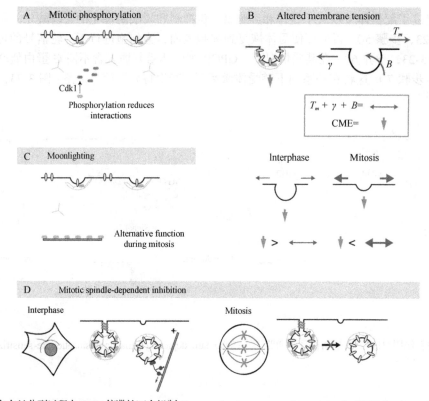

图 3-24 在有丝分裂过程中 CME 停滞的四个机制；Four mechanisms proposed to account for CME shutdown during mitosis
A. 有丝分裂磷酸化；B. 膜张力的改变；C. 有丝分裂的其他作用；D. 有丝分裂纺锤体依赖性抑制作用；A. Mitotic phosphorylation；B. Altered membrane tension；C. Mitotic moonlighting；D. Mitotic spindle-dependent inhibition

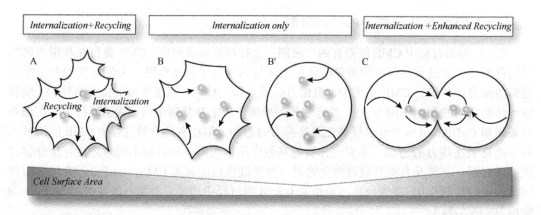

图 3-25 内吞转运作用调节分裂细胞的表面积；Endocytic trafficking regulates the surface area of dividing cells
在细胞间期（A），膜经过持续的内化（虚线箭头）和再循环回到细胞表面（实线箭头），为细胞分裂做准备（B 和 B′），再循环被阻止和内化物积聚在细胞内体中，减少细胞的表面积，终止其他过程并使内化物聚集。在细胞分裂期（C），细胞内吞作用主要发生在纺锤体两极附近。回收的内体堆积在中间区域并快速向增大的胞质分裂沟提供大量的膜原料；In interphase cells（A），membranes undergo continuous internalization（dotted arrows）and recycling back to the cell surface（solid arrows）.（B and B′）as cells prepare for division，recycling is shut down and internalized material accumulates in endosomal compartments. As a consequence，cells decrease their surface area，retract their processes and round up. During cytokinesis（C），endocytosis occurs mainly close to the spindle poles. Recycling endosomes accumulate in the midzone region to rapidly deliver large amounts of membrane material to the ingressing cytokinesis furrow

（三）细胞周期依赖于内吞相关蛋白的定位

在细胞不对称性分裂中，细胞周期依赖于内吞衔接蛋白 Numb 的定位。在细胞分裂间期的整个细胞皮质中能检测到 Numb 和其结合配体 Pon。PAR6、aPKC 与 Lgl 在细胞皮层顶端形成三聚体复合物。随着细胞进入有丝分裂前期，有丝分裂激酶 Aurora A（AurA）和 Polo 被激活。PAR6 被定位于细胞后皮层并被 AurA 磷酸化。结果，Lgl 从膜释放，PAR6、aPKC 和 PAR3 形成新复合物。后者能使 aPKC 磷酸化 Numb，并使其从细胞后皮层释放。另外，Pon 经 Polo 磷酸化促进 Pon 和 Numb 定位于细胞前皮层[41]（图 3-26）。

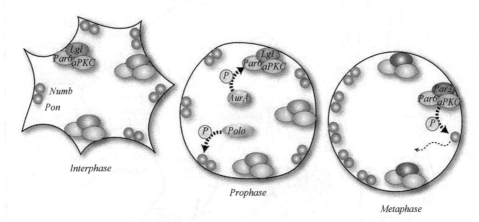

图 3-26　在细胞不对称性分裂中细胞周期依赖于内吞衔接蛋白 Numb 的定位；Cell cycle dependent localisation of the endocytic adapter protein Numb in asymmetrically dividing sensory precursor cells

二、对细胞极性的调节

由于内吞作用蛋白质由质膜进入细胞，通过内吞途径运输，或在溶酶体中降解，或再循环返回到质膜。由肌动蛋白和 Rab5 控制关键的极性调节剂（如 Cdc42、PAR 蛋白），发挥正性或负性调节蛋白质从质膜到内体的运输，以保持上皮细胞极性[9]。

（1）内吞作用控制上皮细胞极性的可能模式：①在内吞作用发生之前，合成的顶端蛋白质首先从高尔基体内网递送到基底侧膜，进行分类后输送到膜顶端，此过程称为胞吞转运（transcytosis）。通过细胞-细胞连接分隔顶膜与基底外侧膜。当细胞内吞作用被阻断，这些原本该转运到顶部的靶蛋白异常地积聚在基底侧面，破坏了顶端-基底极性。②假设主要的极性调控因子在细胞表面通过内吞作用可以保持正常水平。当细胞内吞作用被阻断，这些调控因子堆积在细胞表面导致细胞极性紊乱。③内在的胞吐错误或膜结构域之间的横向扩散偶尔会导致基底极性蛋白错误定位于细胞顶端表面，阻止了细胞内吞作用和溶酶体降解。因此细胞内吞作用的紊乱将导致细胞内完全的传输错误和随后的极性紊乱[9]。

（2）非上皮细胞中极性蛋白和内吞调控子之间的调节：在线虫胚胎的不同区域，阻遏性 PAR 蛋白包括 PAR6 和 PAR2 均不同。发动蛋白促进细胞内吞作用在前皮质区的富集。PAR6 保持发动蛋白在前皮质区和早期内体中富集。PAR6/Cdc-42 可经由早期内体协同作用而内化和转运。这些极性物质可迅速从早期内体回收，或与循环利用的早期内体一起重吸收回到前（后）皮质区。据推测与高尔基体相关的 PAR6/Cdc-42 和发动蛋白可在此处参与囊泡的断裂。另一假设认为发动蛋白依赖性内吞作用是通过促进 PAR2 清除和重吸收进入后皮质区防止 PAR2 扩散到前皮质区来保持非上皮细胞的极性[9]。

三、肿瘤形成中内吞的意义

许多肿瘤中出现内吞转运多个步骤被阻断的现象（图 3-27）。许多肿瘤抑制基因在物质内化过程中随吞噬物一起进入内体或与泛素依赖的降解物进入 MVB 被降解，导致肿瘤上皮结构的缺失及生长失控。许多人类肿瘤的发生过程中均出现主要内吞作用调节因子的紊乱[42]。

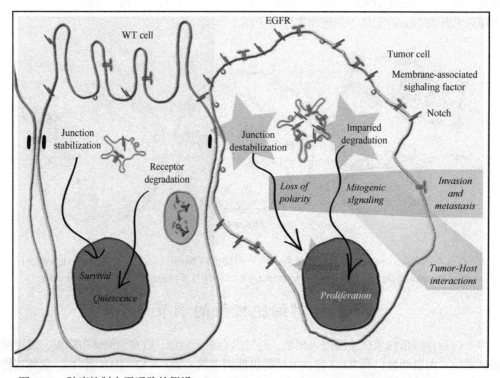

图 3-27　肿瘤抑制内吞通路的假设；Speculative model of endocytic tumor suppression circuitry

WT 上皮细胞正常内吞作用确保适当的受体降解和细胞间连接的稳定，保持细胞的活性或静止（左）。在肿瘤细胞中（右），由于内体系统中有多种受体的积累，增加了促有丝分裂的信号，有助于获得自主的生长信号。此外，由于内吞作用受损，细胞间连接的不稳定导致上皮细胞极性丧失和潜在的对抗生长信号的不敏感。连接的丧失也可能减弱细胞间的接触抑制，导致凋亡通路的激活。此外，增加促有丝分裂的信号，增加细胞增殖可能有助于肿瘤细胞免于凋亡清除。最终，失去极性和增加促有丝分裂信号的作用共同促进肿瘤细胞的侵袭性和转移性的生物学行为；In WT epithelial cells, normal endocytic function ensures proper receptor degradation and cell–cell junction stabilization promoting survival and quiescence（left）. In tumor cells（right）, increased mitogenic signaling, due to accumulation of multiple receptors in the endosomal system, contributes to acquire self-sufficiency in growth signaling. In addition, junction destabilization, due to impaired endocytic trafficking, results in loss of epithelial polarity and potential insensitivity to antigrowth signals. Loss of junctions might also relieve contact inhibition, leading to activation of apoptotic pathways. Moreover, increased mitogenic signaling and increased proliferation might help tumor cells escape apoptotic elimination. Finally, loss of polarity and increase mitogenic signaling cooperate to promote invasive and metastatic behavior in tumor cells

利用细胞的内吞机制开发抗肿瘤药物的传输系统，如细胞穿透肽（cell-penetrating peptide, CPP）与细胞膜相互作用，可促进载药脂质体通过细胞内吞作用进入肿瘤细胞（图 3-28），利用一种交联胶粒（crosslinked-micelle）可抑制肿瘤细胞间连接的丧失等[4]（图 3-29）。

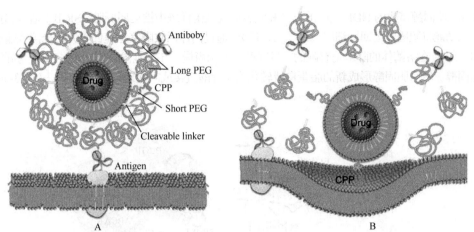

图 3-28　刺激敏感的双靶脂质体靶向肿瘤细胞；Targeting of stimuli-sensitive double-targeted liposome to tumors

A. 加载药物脂质体的表面由细胞穿透肽（CPP）修饰与相对短的 PEG 链连接。利用这种肽对 pH 的敏感性可裂解并连接锚定在脂质体表面长 PEG 链使其屏蔽。这些长 PEG 链修饰针对特定肿瘤抗原的抗体，屏蔽长 PEG 链后使该抗体暴露，可以与肿瘤细胞表面抗原结合。B. 在肿瘤内酸性微环境中长 PEG 链和抗体螯合物从脂质体脱离使 CPP 暴露。CPP 与细胞膜相互作用，促进载药脂质体通过细胞内吞作用进入肿瘤细胞；A. The surface of the drug-loaded liposome is modified with a cell-penetrating peptide（CPP）attached via relatively short PEG chains. This peptide is masked by long PEG chains anchored to the liposome surface via pH-sensitive cleavable links. Some of the long PEG chains are decorated with the antibody specific to the tumor antigen. The antibody is exposed and can bind with the antigen at the tumor cell surface. B. Inside the acidic microenvironment of the tumor the long PEG chains and the antibody conjugates are detached from the liposome resulting in exposure of the CPP. The CPP interacts with the cell membrane and facilitates endocytosis of the drug-loaded liposomes into tumor cells

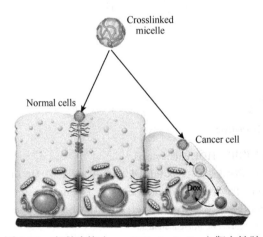

图 3-29　交联胶粒（crosslinked-micelles）靶向性肿瘤传输途径；Pathways of intracellular trafficking of crosslinked-micelles（cl-micelles）in normal and cancer

epithelial cells

交链胶粒携带一种药物（多柔比星，Dox）在正常上皮细胞胞膜顶端面通过紧密连接（TJS）隔绝外物质进入。然而，癌细胞中 TJS 丢失使癌细胞通过细胞质膜小凹内化交联胶粒，进入细胞的交联胶粒被转运到溶酶体，溶酶体通过 pH 依赖性机制释放药物，使药物进入细胞核并聚集在细胞核内杀死癌细胞；The cl-micelles carrying a drug, doxorubicin（Dox）, in normal epithelial cells were shown to sequester at the apical surface of the cell membrane near the junctions. However, during cancer progression the junctions are lost. As a result the cancer epithelial cells internalize the cl-micelles through caveolae. The cl-micelles are then routed to the lysosomes where the drug is released through a pH-dependent mechanism. The released drug accumulates in the nucleus and kills the cancer cells

四、其 他

（1）高密度脂蛋白的内吞作用：由肝脏和小肠分泌的载脂蛋白 A-Ⅰ（ApoA-Ⅰ）转运磷脂和胆固醇，具有防止动脉粥样硬化的保护作用。ApoA-Ⅰ和高密度脂蛋白（HDL）必须经内皮细胞运送到巨噬细胞来源的泡沫细胞中。ApoA-Ⅰ在内皮细胞中的转胞作用必需 ATP 结合盒转运体 A1（ABCA1）的协助。清道夫受体 B 类 I 型（SR-BI）、ATP 结合盒转运 G_1（ABCG1）和外生 F1-ATP 酶促进 HDL 的运输。通过 ABCA1 将巨噬细胞中过剩的游离胆固醇转运到 ApoA-Ⅰ或通过 SR-BⅠ转运到 HDL 中。HDL 逆向内吞作用将介导胆固醇流出。ABCG1 主要在细胞内胆固醇转运中发挥作用。胆固醇富集的 HDL 经由淋巴管和滋养血管从粥样斑中被运回肝脏。SR-B I 通过选择性脂质摄取功能将胆固醇运回肝细胞。内吞后，HDL 通过内体回收隔室迅速回收并重分泌或输送到多泡体。HDL 在溶酶体的降解是有限的，且降解速度相当慢。在细胞内吞作用中，HDL 与肝细胞交换胆固醇。然后胆固醇形成新的脂蛋白或转化为胆汁酸直接或间接地分泌入胆汁[43]（图 3-30）。

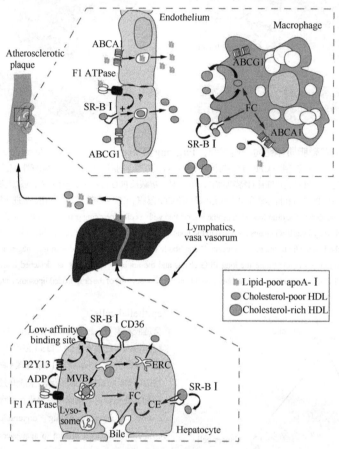

图 3-30　高密度脂蛋白的内吞作用；HDL endocytosis

FC：游离胆固醇；CE：酯化胆固醇；apoA-I：载脂蛋白 A-I；HDL：高密度脂蛋白；SR-B I：清道夫受体 B 类 I 型；ABCA1：ATP 结合盒转运体 A1；ABCG1：三磷酸腺苷结合盒转运 G₁；CD36 分化 36 簇；FC: free cholesterol；CE: esterified cholesterol；apoA-I, apolipoprotein A-I；HDL: high-density lipoprotein；SR-BI: scavenger receptor class B, type I；ABCA1：ATP-binding cassette transporter A1；ABCG1：ATP-binding cassette transporter G₁；CD36: cluster of differentiation 36

（2）Ephrin-B2 将细胞运动和侵袭的调控与血管内皮生长因子受体（VEGFR）的内吞作用和信号通路联系起来。Ephrin -B2 在血管出芽的尖细胞中的表达部分与在柄细胞（根基部分）Ephrin-B4 的表达重叠[44]。

挑战与展望

在过去数十年对内吞进行的研究中，已经明确了细胞内吞的主要过程，并发现了许多参与这一过程的分子，使我们对内吞的过程和机制都有了初步了解。细胞通过胞膜变形的内吞作用过程将胞外物质运输到细胞内。内吞作用一般分为两类：吞噬作用和胞饮作用。后者根据摄入物质的大小又分为四种：网格蛋白依赖的内吞作用（网格蛋白有被小泡的直径 100～150nm），小凹蛋白依赖的内吞作用（小凹蛋白包被的小泡直径 50～100nm），巨胞饮（胞饮颗粒直径 0.5～2μm，有时达 5μm），以及网格蛋白和小凹蛋白非依赖的内吞作用。已知细胞内吞并不是一连串蛋白依照严格的时间顺序按部就班进行的简单过程，而是一个有许多成员参加的、受到精密调控的复杂过程。许多蛋白（如 endophilin、dynamin、actin 和 Rab 家族系列等）在内吞的不同过程中发挥重要作用。内吞作用异常和许多疾病的发展有关。

虽然现在还不十分清楚生物体如何调控细胞内吞这个复杂的过程，但可以预期，随着越来越多新的研究手段在这一领域的应用，有助于进一步了解肿瘤细胞是否通过增加内吞比正常细胞获得更多的能量和营养物质，是否通过增加生长因子的内吞而增大自身体积，是否通过抑制细胞内吞来抑制肿瘤生长，是否通过诱导肿瘤细胞内吞特异性药物而达到治疗肿瘤的目的，肿瘤细胞中一些在细胞死亡信号通路中起重要作用的受体如磷酸-6-甘露糖受体的内吞是否受到抑制等一系列的问题，将使我们能更全面地认识细胞内吞机制。

思　考　题

1. 本章基本概念：胞饮作用，吞噬作用，网格蛋白依赖的内吞，小凹蛋白依赖的内吞，脂筏介导的内吞作用，巨胞饮，细胞膜微域。

2. 根据其产生的机制不同总结胞饮作用的类型。

3. 阐述下图内容。

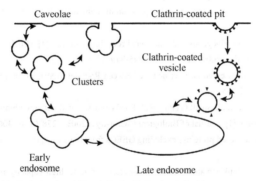

4. 比较小凹蛋白依赖的内吞和网格蛋白依赖的内吞作用。

5. 简述发动蛋白的特征及其在内吞中的作用。

6. 阐述肌动蛋白在内吞中的作用。

7. 阐述细胞分裂中有哪些内吞作用。

8. 阐述内吞作用对细胞极性的影响。

9. 阐述肿瘤发生中研究内吞的意义。

参 考 文 献

[1] Li Chen，Hui Li，Ren Zhao et al. Study progress of cell endocytosis [J].Chinese-German Journal of Clincal Oncology，2009，8（6）：360-365.

[2] Muñoz A，Costa M. Elucidating the mechanisms of nickel compound uptake：a review of particulate and nano-nickel endocytosis and toxicity[J]. Toxicology & Applied Pharmacology，2012，260（1）：1-16.

[3] Ewers H，Helenius A. Lipid-mediated endocytosis[J]. Cold Spring Harbor Perspectives in Biology，2011，3（8）：a004721.

[4] Sahay G，Alakhova D Y，Kabanov A V. Endocytosis of nanomedicines[J]. Journal of Controlled Release，2010，145（3）：182-195.

[5] Parkar N S，Akpa B S，Nitsche L C，et al. Vesicle formation and endocytosis：function，machinery，mechanisms，and modeling[J]. Antioxid Redox Signal，2009，11（6）：1301-1312.

[6] Fielding A B, Royle S J. Mitotic inhibition of clathrin-mediated endocytosis[J]. Cellular & Molecular Life Sciences, 2013, 70(18): 3423-3433.

[7] Kiss A L, Turi A, Müller N, et al. Caveolae and caveolin isoforms in rat peritoneal macrophages[J]. Micron, 2002, 33 (1): 75-93.

[8] Barrow E, Nicola A V, Jin L. Multiscale perspectives of virus entry via endocytosis[J]. Virology Journal, 2013, 10 (1): 1-11.

[9] Shivas J M, Morrison H A, Bilder D, et al. Polarity and endocytosis: reciprocal regulation[J]. Trends in Cell Biology, 2010, 20 (8): 445-452.

[10] Schwarz L A, Patrick G N.Ubiquitin-dependent endocytosis, trafficking and turnover of neuronal membrane proteins[J].Molecular and Cellular Neuroscience, 49 (2012) 387-393.

[11] Rajjayabun P H, Garg SDurkan G C, Charlton R, et al. Caveolin-1 expression is associated with high-grade bladder cancer[J]. Urology, 2001, 58 (5): 811-814.

[12] Frank P G, Woodman S E, Park D S, et al. Caveolin, caveolae and endothelial cell function [J]. Arterioscler Thromb Vasc Biol, 2003, 23 (7): 1161-1168.

[13] Krajewska W M, Maslowska I. Caveolins: structure and function in signal transduction[J]. Cellular & Molecular Biology letters, 2004, 9 (2): 195-220

[14] Fra A M, Pasqualetto E, Mancini M, et al. Genomic organization and transcriptional analysis of the human genes coding for caveolin-1 and caveolin-2[J]. Gene, 2000, 243 (1): 75-83.

[15] Cameron P L, Liu C, Smart D K, et al. Caveolin-1 expression is maintained in rat and human astroglioma cell lines[J]. Glia, 2002, 37 (3): 275-290.

[16] Williams T M, Cheung M W, Park D S, et al. Loss of Caveolin1 gene expression accelerates the development of dysp lastic mammary lesions in tumor prone transgenic mice [J]. Molecular Biology of the cell, 2003, 14 (3): 1027-1042.

[17] Pascariu M, Bendayan M, Ghitescu L. Correlated endothelial caveolin overexpression and increased transcytosis in experimental diabetes[J]. Journal of Histochemistry & Cytochemistry, 2004, 52 (1): 65-76.

[18] Gaudreault S B, Dea D, Poirier J. Increased caveolin-1 expression in Alzheimer's disease brain[J]. Neurobiology of Aging, 2004, 25 (6): 753-759.

[19] Donaldson J G. Phospholipase D in endocytosis and endosomal recycling pathways[J]. Biochimica et Biophysica Acta (BBA) - Molecular and Cell Biology of Lipids, 2009, 1791 (9): 845-849.

[20] Langley P A, Maly H. IRSp53 is an essential intermediate between Rac and WAVE in the regulation of membrane ruffling[J]. Nature, 2000, 408 (6813): 732-735.

[21] Sun P, Yamamoto H, Suetsugu S, et al. Small GTPase Rah/Rab34 is associated with membrane ruffles and macropinosomes and promotes macropinosome formation[J]. Journal of Biological Chemistry, 2003, 278 (6): 4063-4071.

[22] Nichols B. Endocytosis of lipid-anchored proteins: excluding GEECs from the crowd[J]. Journal of Cell Biology, 2009, 186(4): 457-459.

[23] Cousin M A. Activity-dependent bulk synaptic vesicle endocytosis—a fast, high capacity membrane retrieval mechanism[J]. Molecular Neurobiology, 2009, 39 (3): 185-189.

[24] Gad H, Ringstad N, Low P, et al. Fission and uncoating of synaptic clathrin-coated vesicles are perturbed by disruption of interactions with the SH3 domain of endophilin [J]. Neuron, 2000, 27: 301-312.

[25] Petrelli A, Gilestro G F, Lanzardo S, et al. The endophilin-CIN85-Cbl complex mediates ligand-dependent downregulation of c-Met[J]. Nature, 2002, 416 (6877): 187-190.

[26] Weinberg J, Drubin D G. Clathrin-mediated endocytosis in budding yeast[J]. Trends in Cell Biology, 2012, 22 (1): 1.

[27] Guichet A, Wucherpfennig T, Dudu V, et al. Essential role of endophilin A in synaptic vesicle budding at the Drosophila neuromuscular junction[J]. EMBO Journal, 2002, 21 (7): 1661-1672.

[28] Takei K, Mcpherson&Ast P S, Schmid S L, et al. Tubular membrane invaginations coated by dynamin rings are induced by GTP-[gamma]S in nerve terminals[J]. Nature, 1995, 374 (6518): 186-190.

[29] Wells W A. Twisting endocytosis[J]. The Journal of Cell Biology, 2006, 173 (4): 456.

[30] Damke H, Binns D D, Ueda H, et al. Dynamin GTPase domain mutants block endocytic vesicle formation at morphologically distinct stages[J]. Molecular Biology of the Cell, 2001, 12 (9): 2578-2589.

[31] Sun Y, Martin A C, Drubin D G. Endocytic Internalization in Budding Yeast Requires Coordinated Actin Nucleation and Myosin Motor Activity[J]. Developmental Cell, 2006, 11 (1): 33-46.

[32] Galletta B J, Mooren O L, Cooper J A. Actin dynamics and endocytosis in yeast and mammals[J]. Current Opinion in Biotechnology, 2010, 21 (5): 604-610.

[33] Voytek O, Drubin D G. Cofilin recruitment and function during actin-mediated endocytosis dictated by actin nucleotide state[J].

Journal of Cell Biology, 2007, 178（7）: 1251-1264.

[34] Kaksonen M, Toret C P, Drubin D G. A Modular Design for the Clathrin- and Actin-Mediated Endocytosis Machinery[J]. Cell, 2005, 123（2）: 305-320.

[35] Kazuya T, Shiro S, Nobunari S, et al. Coordination between the actin cytoskeleton and membrane deformation by a novel membrane tubulation domain of PCH proteins is involved in endocytosis[J].The Journal of Cell Biology, 2006, 172: 269-279.

[36] Sung J Y, Kim J, Paik S R, et al. Induction fo neuronal cell death by Rab5A-dependen endocytosis of alpha-synuclein. The Journal of Cell Biology, 2001, 276（29）: 27441-27448.

[37] Agola J O, Jim P A, Ward H H, et al. Rab GTPases as regulators of endocytosis, targets of disease and therapeutic opportunities[J]. Clinical Genetics, 2011, 80（4）: 305-318.

[38] Saito A, Sato H, Iino N, et al. Molecular mechanisms of receptor-mediated endocytosis in the renal proximal tubular epithelium[J]. Journal of Biomedicine & Biotechnology, 2010, 2010（1）: 403272.

[39] Musse A A, Melotykapella L, Weinmaster G. Notch ligand endocytosis: Mechanistic basis of signaling activity[J]. Seminars in Cell & Developmental Biology, 2012, 23（4）: 429-436.

[40] Sorkin A, Zastrow M V. Endocytosis and signalling: intertwining molecular networks[J]. Nature Reviews Molecular Cell Biology, 2009, 10（9）: 609-622.

[41] Fürthauer M, Gonzálezgaitán M. Endocytosis and mitosis: a two-way relationship[J]. Cell Cycle, 2009, 8（20）: 3311-3318.

[42] Vaccari T, Bilder D. At the crossroads of polarity, proliferation and apoptosis: the use of Drosophila to unravel the multifaceted role of endocytosis in tumor suppression[J]. Molecular Oncology, 2009, 3（4）: 354-365.

[43] Röhrl C, Stangl H. HDL endocytosis and resecretion[J]. Biochimica et Biophysica Acta-Moleular and Cell Biology of Lipids, 2013, 1831（11）: 1626-1633.

[44] Pitulescu M E, Adams R H. Eph/ephrin molecules--a hub for signaling and endocytosis[J]. Genes & Development, 2010, 24（22）: 2480-2492.

（王桂兰　刘　俊　陈　莉）

Chapter 3 Cell Endocytosis

In the process of cell metabolism, various kinds of materials including some ions, small molecules, macromolecular materials and some granular matters keep in and out of cells. The macromolecular substances and granular materials can not go through the membrane. They complete the transfer across the cell membrane in another way, that is, materials cross in and out of cell membrane in the form of vesicle which is fused with membrane and then sciss into the cell, which is currently recognized as the main pathway of intaking biological macromolecules – endocytosis. [1]

The recent study reported that the abnormal expression of endocytosis may be involved in the mechanism of certain diseases, such as diabetes and neurological diseases and also closely related to the malignant transformation of cells. The role of endocytosis was paid increasing attention. Further research in this area will help us understand these diseases, thereby found new treatments.

Randy Schekman, James Rothman and Thomas Südhof were awarded the Nobel Prize in Physiology and Medicine in October, 2013.The winning reason: "the main transport system is found in cells-vesicle transport regulation mechanism, extracellular or intracellular molecules are passed through the coating vesicles. Randy Schekman found a set of genes required for vesicle transport; James Rothman illustrated how did the vesicle fuse with the targeting proteins and pass its. Thomas Sudhof revealed that the signal is how to guide vesicles released by transport objects accurately.

Here we introduce about pathway of cell endocytosis, mechanisms of regulation, endocytotic proteins and the roles of endocytosis.

Section 1   Types and Mechanisms of Endocytosis

In general endocytic mechanisms can be roughly divided into two categories depending on whether the uptake substrate consists mainly of fluids and solutes (pinocytosis) or whether it is composed of large particles (phagocytosis). Within pinocytosis there is a further division depending on whether the mechanism is dynamin dependent (clathrin and caveolar) or dynamin independent (non clathrin/noncaveolar, lipid raft-mediated, micropinocytosis [2] (Fig. 3 -1).

The main organelles are EEs, LEs, REs, and lysosomes in trafficking in the endocytic pathway. EEs are complex organelles with tubular and vacuolar domains. The vacuolar domains dissociate with their contents and undergo microtubule-mediated, dynein-dependent movement to the perinuclear region. They mature to LEs, which can fuse with each other and eventually with lysosomes generating endolysosomes. At the level of EEs, LEs, and REs, the endocytic pathway is connected to the TGN and the Golgi complex by vesicle transport and possibly with the endocytic recycling compartment (ERC) at the level of endolysosomes[3] (Fig. 3-2).

There are multiple pathways for cellular entry of particles and solutes result to different types of endocytosis. So that Different mechanisms in the different types of endocytosis [4] (Fig. 3-3).

1. Phagocytosis

Phagocytosis refers to endocytosing large granular matters (> 250 nm), it provides the host a direct way digesting exogenous substances, which is one of the most important immune protecting mechanisms [1]. In mammalian, phagocytosis can only be completed by specific cells, such as macrophages and neutrophils which are called phagocytic cells. Phagocytic cells recognize and combine with IgFc and complement packing pathogens through IgFc receptor and complement receptor respectively. When the cell surface receptors combined with the corresponding ligands, downstream signal transduction was activated, which caused actin polymerization under plasma membrane of intaking site, actin contraction makes phagocytic cell membrane form pseudo-foot fusing into vesicle to pack pathogens. In cytoplasm, dynamin assembled into ring at the neck of vesicle, and hydrolysed the binding GTP, dynamin contraction forced vesicle to sciss from membrane at the neck and form phagosome which integrated with the lysosome, the acid hydrolysis enzyme of lysosomal digested pathogens. (Fig. 3-4). In addition to phagocytosing pathogens, macrophages of phagocytic cells can swallow foreign bodies through ligand - receptor binding pattern. Identify and kill tumor cells, identify and remove degenerative plasma protein, lipids, and other macromolecules. Remove aging and damaged cells and cell debris. (Fig. 3-5). The entry of a nanoparticles inside macrophages depends on the angle between the membrane normal at the point of initial contact and the line defining the particle curvature at this point (Ω). The internalization velocity is positive at $\Omega \leqslant 45°$, which indicates that the particle undergoes internalization [4].

2. Pinocytosis

Pinocytosis refers to the intake process that endocytoses extracellular liquid and the dissolving materials.

(1) Clathrin Mediated Endocytosis

Cathrin-mediated endocytosis (CME): Clathrin plays an important role in the regulation of compostion of plasma membrane proteins, research on clathrin can help us understand how cells interact with the surrounding environment, signal transduction of mitogenic, nutrition intake of the cell, establishment of extracellular environment, cell identity including the interaction with the immune system, keep a balance in the stability of the environment of cell. The process of CCV assembly. Once a cell-surface receptor is ligated by its specific ligand or cargo, intracellular adaptor protein and clathrin assemble on the membrane receptor, forming a clathrin-coated pit and, eventually, a clathrin-coated vesicle (CCV). Schematic diagram of clathrin-mediated endocytosis [5, 6] (Fig. 3-6)

Clathrin is the skeleton protein outside the vesicle, clathrin-coated vesicle is 100-150nm in diameter and exists in all eukaryotic cells and it mediates the way of transportation from the plasma membrane to intracellular of proteins, lipids, nutrients, antibodies and growth factors and also the vector through which proteins and lipids transport from trans Golgi net work (TGN) to endosome. Clathrin is spider-like and is polymerized by three chains at the top, which is known as triskelion [1].

Adaptor protein (AP) lies inside the clathrin-coated vesicle, which mediates membrane binding, localization, sorting signals, identification and inositol phosphate. It not only serves to combine cargo and clathrin, but also connect with polyphosphate dylinositol headgroup. It is now found four kinds of adapters (AP1-4), all of which comprise a pair of 100～130KD subunit. These subunits are able to identify 6-phosphate mannose receptor, transferrin, low-density lipoprotein and epidermal growth factor receptor, protease and de-sialic acid receptor [4].

Mechanism of CME

The process from recruitment to disassemble is very short. Comprise: ①recruitment of adapter and clathrin recruitment of AP2 complex to high activity, saturated, easy enzymolysis site, activate formation of clathrin-coated vesicle in the plasma membrane under the effect of sorting signal and docking protein [7]. ②Invagination, scission and budding of clathrin-coated vesicle the planar clathrin protein can be transformed into curved one without nucleic acid and cytoplasm in vitro; In vivo, clathrin-coated vesicle curves to some degree. Invagination may be due to structure changes or rearrangement of clathrin assembling in the crystal lattice or between clathrin. The budding of clathrin-coated vesicle is involved with GTPase dynamin, actin tubulizes or forms ring-shape in vitro, it is the trigger that vesicle dissociated from the membrane. ③Decapsulation of clathrin-coated vesicle. This is a wasting process that needs HSC70, auxilin and ATP. The large chain of Clathrin has two sites which interact with the adaptper and also with HSC 70.The interaction between clathrin and HSC70 destroyed the interaction between clathrin and adaptper. Over-expression of HSC70 mutant blocked the cycle of transferrin receptor so that the "assembly-dismantle"balance moved to the assembly direction. HSC70 dissociated clathrin from the vesicle in vitro, but could not dissociate adapter. Auxilin plays an important role in decapsulation. Auxilin can not only recruit HSC70 to clathrin-coated vesicle, but also stimulate activity of HSC70 ATP enzyme, such as the steps of virus entry via clathrin-mediated endocytosis [8, 9].

Endocytosis begins at the plasma membrane, where transmembrane proteins such as receptors and other membrane-associated proteins cluster into invaginating clathrin-coated pits (CCP). This clustering is dependent on recognition of appropriate cargo proteins by adaptor proteins such as the Adaptin complex (AP-2), which is also responsible for recruiting the clathrin coat subunits to the forming vesicle. Proteins such as the GTPase Dynamin (Dyn) are then recruited to the neck of the budded vesicle and promote membrane scission, freeing the vesicle from the plasma membrane. Once released, the clathrin coat disassembles from the vesicle, enabling interaction between the vesicle and the early endosome (EE) target membrane. The small GTPase Rab5 promotes cargo delivery into the early endosome through effector proteins that activate membrane fusion via a SNARE complex. From the early endosome, cargoes can be recycled back to the cell surface by a Rab4- or Rab11-mediated mechanism. Cargoes that are not recycled remain in the endosome, which acquires the marker Hrs. Proteins such as the ESCRT (endosomal sorting complex required for transport) complexes are recruited to the endosome and promote the budding and scission of intraluminal vesicles (ILVs), forming the late endosome/MVB compartment. Fusion between the MVB and the lysosome, which contains digestive enzymes such as proteases and lipases, ultimately leads to cargo degradation [9](Fig. 3-7).

(2) Caveolin Dependent Endocytosis

Caveolae / Caveolins mediate endocytosis of many substances and is the main form of clathrin-independent endocytosis. As early as 1950, Japanese scholar Yamada used transmission electron microscopy to observe some small caveolae which was about 50 ～ 100 nm in diameter for the first time. These vesicles appeared alone or string-like, in the form of invagination of the cytoplasmic membrane, it had typical lipid bilayer structure [7]. Caveolae is currently considered to be the signal transduction center, and many signal transduction receptors , protein kinase and binding proteins are highly enriched in Caveolae region. In the regulation of Caveolae endocytosis, activation of tyrosine kinase-dependent signal is an important step. After the treatment of phosphatase inhibitor, the endocytosis of the the cell by caveolae had increased notably. Caveolin dependent endocytic trafficking processes [5] (Fig. 3-8).

Degradation of ubiquitinated membrane proteins by the lysosome. Ubiquitination is a process whereby target proteins can be marked for degradation by the 26S proteasome. Ubiquitination, usually in the form of single (mono) or short-chain ubiquitin modifications (K63-linkages in many cases) can result in the endocytosis of membrane proteins. In early endosomes, non-ubiquitinated proteins can recycle back to the plasma membrane or be directed to other intracellular compartments. In contrast, ubiquitinated proteins are sorted into multivesicular bodies (MVB) and eventually targeted to the lysosome for degradation. De-ubiquitinating enzymes (DUBs) reverse the ubiquitination process. Deubiquitination of cargos plays a critical role in the regulation of intracellular trafficking through the endosomal sorting complexes required for transport (ESCRT) pathway and in some cases ensures recycling of internalized cargos to the plasma membrane [10] (Fig. 3-9) .

Biological Feature of Caveolin

Caveolin is the main surface marker of a caveolae, a kind of membrane integrin family modified in the inner surface of caveolae, 21～25kD. It consists of N-terminal region, transmembrane region and C-terminal region, N-terminal and C-terminal cytoplasmic moves inword into the cytoplasm fand its peptide chains like hairpin structure. Caveolin plays a critical role in the assembly process of Caveolae and cholesterol and is the signaling molecule of the scaffold proteins and negative regulatory proteins and belongs to a highly conserved integrity membrane protein family [11]. Frank, etc. [12] confirmed that Caveolin-1 was the key factor of Caveolae endocytosis. If Caveolin gene was knockout, Caveolae can not be formed. So far, four kinds of Caveolin isomers have been found in mammals: Caveolin-1α, 1β, 2 and 3, which are products of different genes, most cells expressed Caveolin-1 and Caveolin-2, the two form a stable heterologous oligomers complexes, particularly rich in terminal differentiated cells, such as fat cells, endothelial cells and fibroblasts, Caveolae as a signaling molecule plays a role as a platform in signal transduction. Caveolin-1 is in the center of signaling pathways at all these platforms. Caveolin, as a signaling molecule's scaffold protein and negative regulatory protein, inhibits kinase activitives of signaling molecules in the normal signal transduction pathways. Caveolin-2's skeleton region has no inhibitory activitives, other signaling molecules inhibitory regions may exit in it. Caveolin-1 has strong affinity to cholesterol, thus the cholesterol levels of Caveolae is far higher than other biofilm. The study showed that the absence of caveolae eventually resulted in formation of foam cells, suggesting that caveolae and caveolin-1 can maintain the cholesterol balance by removing the excessive lipoprotein cholesterol out of cells. Caveolin-3 mainly exists in various muscle cells (such as myocardial cells, rhabdomyosarcoma cells and skeletal muscle cells) and is closely related to the synthesis of muscle cells [13], and Caveolin-3 is involved in energy metabolismin in muscle cells. Neither Caveolin protein nor Caveolae structure appeared in peripheral blood cells and nerve cells.

The correlation between Caveolin and tumors have become one of the hot spots in tumor biology, among which, the relationship between Caveolin-1 and tumor occurrence and metastasis has been studied a lot. Gene coding for Caveolin-1 (CAV) locates in the suspicious tumor suppressive site (D7S522; 7q31.1).

This site depletes or fractures in a variety of tumors (such as liver cancer, ovarian cancer, breast cancer, uterine fibroids, gastric adenocarcinoma, etc.)[14]. The normal NIH3T3 cell which was introduced by antisense Caveolin-1 transplanted into nude mice to observe the formation of tumor, suggesting Caveolin-1has tumor suppressive function. In many tumors and activated oncogene transfected cells, the expression of mRNA and its protein of Caveolin-1 decreased or lost [15]. The experiments in vivo demonstrated mutation or deletion of Caveolin-1 could lead to the excessive proliferation of breast epithelial cells, and then increase the occurrence of breast cancers [16]. Besides, the expression of Caveolin uprehulated in diabetes [17] and hypercholesterolemia and play a significant role in Alzheimer's disease [18], degenerative muscle disease, heart and lung diseases.

Comparison of the structurein caveolae and CCVs shown in Fig. 3-10.

Clathrin-dependent and clathrin-independent endocytosis membrane systems [19](Fig. 3-11).

Macropinocytosis

Large and irregular original endocytosis vesicles are formed by folding membrane on the verge of extending cell under stimulation by certain factors, they are known as macrop inosome whose size varies with diameter generally 0.5~2 μm. Macrop inocytosis plays a major role in macrophages and dendritic cells, also in many tumor cells [18]. Macrop inosome has no clathrin or caveolins coating; it is closely related to actin at the early stages of formation, which provides an effective way for non-selective endocytosis of extracellular nutrients and liquid phase macromolecules. Macrop inocytosis and phagocytosis, regulated by a variety of proteins, such as actin, Scar protein, Ap21 complexes and RabB. Different membrane wrinkle results in different rates of developing macrop inocytosis. Such as particulate nickel uptake via macropinocytosis and/or clathrin mediated endocytosis, the dissolution of the crystalline Ni_3S_2 particle produces high concentrations of Ni^{2+} in the vesicle into the cytoplasm where they can interact with biomolecules or the vesicles will continue to travel towards the nucleus where they will aggregate at the nuclear membrane (Fig. 3-12). The presence of Ni^{2+} can lead to multiple effects including DNA condensation and the modification of epigenetic marks including increased DNA methylation and loss of histone acetylation in H2A, H2B, H3 and H4 as well as an increase in H3K9 dimethylation, H3K4 trimethylation and ubiquitylation of H2A and H2B [2].

Macrop Inosomes Mechanism

The formation of Macrop inosomes can be significantly inhibited by cytochalasin D and Colchicine, suggesting that microtubules and microfilaments play an important role in this process. The mechanism may be the stimulus by a variety of factors that activate corresponding receptor tyrosine kinase and then self-phosphorylate quickly. Phosphorylated residues recruit PI3 kinase and activate it, the activated PI3 kinase activates Rac1 which may cause microfilament reconstruction through two ways. Firstly, the activated Rac1 activates PAK1 which regulates phosphorylation of myosin light chain. The interaction between myosin and actin is regulated by the phosphorylated myosin light chain and the interaction promotes reconstructure of microfilaments, development of the cell membrane ruffles and formation of macrop inosomes; Secondly, the activated Rac1 binds with the amino-terminal of its target protein IRSp53, SH3 region at the carboxyl end of IRSp53 combines with WAVE to form three molecular complexes which could activate WAVE [20]. The latter further activates actin related protein Arp2/3 complexes which stimulate microfilament nucleation, promote microfilament reconstruction, development of cell membrane ruffles and formation of macrop inosomes [21]. Indepth regulation mechanism needs further study.

(3) Lipid Mediated Endocytosis

Such as individual SV40 virions recruits cholesterol to form a membrane microdomain or "lipid raft" and its bound to cells seem to imprint their shape onto the plasma membrane and are found its in small, tight-fitting invaginations [3] (Fig. 3-13).

(4) Microdomain

Microdomain has similar lipid composition with Caveolae but not function through caveolin. It functions through dynamin and RhoA-dependent mechanism, or through clathrin-independent, dynamin-2-independent, Cdc4 mediated pathway to endocytose glycosylated phosphatidylinositol-hexanol anchored proteins. The pathway plays a role in endocytosis of IL-2. The results of Bhagatji et al. (2009) suggest a model in which lipid-anchored proteins are excluded from clathrin-coated pits when they have a bulky ectodomain. In endocytosis via clathrin-independent carrier 1, lipid-anchored proteins are present at the same density in the rest of the plasma membrane. In the speculative clathrin-independent carrier 2, which is generated by oligomerization of a protein embedded in the cytosolic face of the plasma membrane (analogously to caveolins or flotillins), transmembrane domains are excluded. This could lead to selectivity for lipid-anchored proteins in the outer leaflet of the membrane without this latter class of protein being actively concentrated [23] (Fig. 3-14).

Comparison of the roles in caveolae (bulk) endocytosis with clathrin-dependent endocytosis [22](Fig. 3-15).

Utilize multiple pathways to entry cells.Such as nanoparticles gain cellular entry [4], including CME ①caveolae mediated endocytosis ②and macropinocytosis ③The shape of the particles appears to be important in regulating the rate of their cellular entry (not shown). Cube-shaped microparticles also utilize multiple routes of cellular entry but their macropinocytosis appears to be the most prominent (Fig. 3-16).

The Roles of Endocytosis in Different Conditions

Under the different conditions the foreign granular matters(such as Pluronic®) enter cell through caveolae-mediated endocytosis, caveolae-independent endocytosis and Clathrin dependent endocytosis, respectively [4] (Fig. 3-17).

Section 2   Features of Endophilin

The various steps of vesicle trafficking through the different endocytic pathways are each regulated by the activity of specific proteins.

1. Biological Features of Endophilin

The main function of Endophilin is related to the endocytosis of neurotransmitter. Endophilin has a common special structure, whose C-terminal has a unique SH3 domain with the unique binding ability [24], which can interact with a number of special proteins such as dynamin, thus affecting the functions of other proteins.While N-terminal participates in membrane invagination of vesicles. They were named endophilin A1, A2, A3 in 2002. Huntingtin belongs to binding protein of endophilin A1, the complex composed of it and the huntingtin binding protein 40 (HAP40) inhibited early microtubule-dependent endosome movement, increased connection between early endosome and actin [25]. Then a new family was discovered, which was named Endophilin B.

2. Endophilin and Its Roles in Signal Transduction

(1) Endophilin can interact with various proteins through which involved in different signal transduction pathway. Endophilins which interact with cell membrane receptors are mainly distributed in the cytoplasm and cell membrane, it can interact with cytoplasmic membrane receptor and conduct signals, such as beta 1-adrenergic receptor. Endophilin is also involved in phospholipid signal transduction. Many

endophilins contain the binding sites of inositol 4, 5 diphosphate (PIP2). The degradation of PIP2 is necessary for the completion of the endocytosis.Mark PIP2 connected domain by immunohistochemical fluorescent protein and track endocytosis movement of living cells, PIP2 was found present in the cell membrane surface in the form of many small plaques, these plaques entered gradually into the cell, which confirmed that the shift was the endocytosis.The disappearance of PIP2 matched the recruitment of phosphoinositide phosphatase enzyme, we can propose that the latter can degradate the former. When PIP2 degradation was blocked, abnormal invagination can be observed, shearing machine of endocytosis gathered around the plaque on the membrane and failed to complete endocytosis. Therefore, PIP2 degradation is the necessary step of vesicle scission. Timeline for endocytic vesicle formation and modular organization of proteins [26].

(2) Recycling of the neurotransmitter   Neurotransmitter recycle is essentially a process of cell endocytosis, clathrin interact with AP2 or AP180 (adapter protein) and membrane lipid to form clathrin-coated vesicles. The process of its formation is just that endophilin A1 drived the rupture of membrane vesicles from the donor membrane at the neck of vesicles, LPAAT at N-terminal of endophilin A1 can catalyze lysophosphatidic acid (LPA) and arachidonic ene-CoA to form phosphatidic acid (PA), LPA is a three-dimensional structure like inverted cone-type and PA is cone-type, the former structure is beneficial for positive membrane deformation, the later is conducive to negative membrane deformation.It is the transformation of lysophosphatidic acid that drive rupture between vesicle and the donor vesicle membrane. After endophilin mutation, it will severely affect recycle mechanism of synaptic particle [27].

(3) Function besides endocytosis   Endophilin A2 is actually involved in absorbing nutrients and growth factors and endocytosis of pathogens and receptors, participating in a variety of membrane transport mechanism. While endophilin B1 locates in the membrane of the cell and its main function is related to cell membrane dynamics. Apoptosis receptor Fas / CD95 can not correctly located in the membrane, leading to cell apoptosis mechanism is suppressed.

Section 3   Key Proteins in Endocytic Pathways

1. Dynamin

Dynamin is a 100 kD GTPase, and its GTPase region at N-terminal can bind and hydrolyse GTP, PH(pleckstrin homology) region can bind with membrane and mediate polymerization between dynamins, PRD (praline arginine rich) region at C-terminal mediate the interaction between other proteins. In addition, dynamin has a small GED (GTPase effector) region which is necessary in hydrolysis of GTP [28], and also plays an important role in some clathrin independent endocytosis. Dynamin is necessary in pinching and formation of vesicles. After its binding with ligand amphiphysin1, dynamin-1 plays a key role in dynamin dependent endocytosis under regulation of cycle-dependent kinase 5 (Cdk5). Dynamin-1-dependent endocytosis occurs quickly, usually only a few seconds, while dynamin-2 mediated endocytosis is slow, usually ten minutes.

Dynamin uses mechanochemical activity-specifically a twisting action-to pinch off endocytic vesicles[29]. Dynamin was, early on, localized to the collar around the neck of forming endocytic vesicles. This suggested that dynamin may use the energy of GTP hydrolysis to directly pinch a membranous neck. Indeed, dynamin could tubulate lipids and break apart the tubules in vitro. Meanwhile, Sandy Schmid had come up with a "regulatory GTPase" mode [30]: that dynamin was active not as it hydrolyzed GTP but in its GTP bound form, which recruited other proteins to do the pinching. Longitudinal tension was needed with constriction to achieve fission. In mammalian, the dynamin collars are relatively short, so cortical actin is the most likely source of tension that would help the dynamin to wrench an endocytic vesicle free.

Dynamin has intrinsic activity of GTP and is also the cerebellum Dyrk1A kinase substrate, with its own aggregation feature of the endometrium can help new processes from the cell membrane vesicles isolated. Dynamin is involved in tubulation by PH epsin and ENTH (epsin NH2-terminal homology).

Wild-type dynamin mutant block the tube, which can be restricted to speculate dynamin of these membrane protein of the ability to control grid protein coated vesicle endocytosis and other media invagination degree.

2. Actin

Actin is the main component of microfilament. Microfilament is involved in cell shape and polarity of the maintenance of endocytosis, intracellular transport, cell shrinkage and movement, cell division, and many other functions. Actin has two kinds: G-actin and F- actin. The importance of F-actin in endocytosis was clearly illustrated by the effect of addition of the actin-monomer sequestering drug latrunculin A. Within 5 minutes of its addition, actin patches were no longer visible and endocytosis was completely abrogated. This was the point at which the yeast WASP orthologue Las17p and the type I myosins (Myo3p and Myo5p) began to nucleate actin filaments through activation of the Arp2/3 complex.This group of proteins has been called the 'actin network growth machinery'. Some researchers combined epifluorescence with total internal reflection microscopy (TIRF) to follow the internalisation of individual coated pits in living cells expressing a fluorescently tagged form of clathrin light chain (DsRed clathrin). They showed that transient recruitment of actin coincides with the inward movement of vesicles, they also observed recruitment of the Arp2/3 complex to clathrin-coated pits. PH-sensitive probes have been developed that allow internalisation of cargo into individual clathrin-coated vesicles to be visualised, allowing us to follow the time course of invagination and identify the point of scission. The recruitment of actin during invagination is thought to provide the force that drives the invagination of the coated pit [31].

The initial curvature of the membrane is generated by clathrin and additional endocytic proteins, such as F-BAR containing Syp1. Syp1 can inhibit WASp/Las17-Arp2/3-mediated actin assembly and may serve to keep actin polymerization inhibited during early steps of CME. As invagination proceeds, the changing membrane curvature may be sensed by other BAR-domain containing proteins, for example, Bzz1, which is recruited along with other endocytic proteins and regulators of Arp2/3. Major models for actin assembly during endocytosis [32](Fig. 3-18).

Scission is accomplished by constriction of the bud neck, driven by BAR protein-driven membrane deformation, actin-generated force and the proposed Sjl2p-imposed line tension created by lipid phase separation. After scission, the Pan1 complex proteins Sla1p, Pan1p and End3p are phosphorylated by Ark1p/Prk1p, resulting in their dissociation. Ark1p/Prk1p are also responsible for turning off actin polymerization, allowing Cof1p/Aip1p/Crn1p to disassemble the actin filaments. Sjl2p is responsible for dephosphorylating PIP2, reducing the affinity of Sla2p and Ent1/2p for the vesicles. Arf3p, Gts1p and Lsb5p together are involved in the dissociation of the Pan1 complex [26] (Fig. 3-19).

It is currently identified that the vesicle scission module contains the two yeast amphiphysin proteins Rvs161p and Rvs167p. These proteins contain BAR (Bin-Amphiphysin-Rvs) domains that bind to and tabulate, actin and associated proteins recruit amphiphysins and thus mark the site at which membrane tubulation should occur. Tubulation is then suggested to facilitate the scission process. Following scission, the vesicle is uncoated and moves away from the membrane until it fuses with an endosome.There are two possible roles for actin at this final stage: vesicles could move along actin cables; alternatively actin could be nucleated at the vesicle surface to facilitate their movement within the cell. Then the actin depolymerized from the endocytosis site. The most representative depolymerizing factor is cofilin. Cofilin is necessary for endocytosis in mammals, but its mechanism is still unknown [33]. In the process of invagination, Sac 6p/ microfilament binding protein/fimbrin is also required, invagination induced by actin failed without Sac 6p [34]. Endocytic mutants affecting actin polymerization (Fig. 3-20).

3. HIP1

HIP1 (Huntingtin-The interacting protien 1) activates the Cdc4, accelerating the accumulation of actin through N-WASP and Arp2/3 complexes. CD2AP can also inhibit the activity of capping protein in vitro. In addition, HIP1-associated protein (HIP1R) also play an important role between the endocytic pathway and the actin cytoskeleton. More intetested is, in the case of missing HIP1R actin, dynein and cortical actin accumulation at sites of Endocytosis, show that HIP1R only regulate actin torsion in the endocytic sites.

4. PCH/F-BAR

PCH (Pombe Cdc15 homology) /F-BAR is another family of proteins which plays an important role in endocytosis. The BAR region of these proteins combine with phosphoinositide. FBP17 is a member of PCH family, containing PCH domain and extended FC domain. The EFC domains show weak homology to the Bin-amphiphysin-Rvs (BAR) domain. The EFC domains bound strongly to phosphatidylserine and phosphatidylinositol 4, 5-bisphosphate and deformed the plasma membrane and liposomes into narrow tubules. Most PCH proteins possess an SH3 domain that is known to bind to dynamin and that recruited and activated neural Wiskott-Aldrich syndrome protein (N-WASP) at the plasma membrane. FBP17 contributed to the formation of the protein complex, including N-WASP and Dynamin-2, in the early stage of endocytosis. Furthermore, knockdown of endogenous FBP17 impaired endocytosis, suggesting FBP17 is necessary for dynamin-dependent endocytosis [35].

5. Rab proteins

Rab protein which is a small GTP enzyme is an important regulator of endocytosis. Rab5 is involved in tubulization and its role in endocytosis has been clear. Rab 5 protein has three isomers, Rab5A, Rab5B and Rab 5C. Rab5 protein exists primarily on the plasma membrane, clathrin-coated vesicle and early endosome, regulates transport of endocytotic materials between membrane and early endosome, and help vesicle movement along microtubules, taking charge of vesicle fusion and recycling. Rab5 protein functions with ongoing GTP / GDP cycle. As molecular switch of vesicle transport, the activated state of combining with GTP is "open", the unactivated state of combining with GTP is called "close." HAP40 is an effective regulatory factor of Rab5, Rab5 increase connections of endosome with actin under exsitance of HAP40, Young etc. found Rab 5A protein was related to endocytosis of A-synuclein [36]. A-synuclein is the root of Parkinson's disease, Lewy body Dementia and Alzheimer's disease and other central nervous system diseases. Moreover, Young found the mutant can decrease endocytosis of A-synuclein according to Rab5A GTP mutant enzyme research while Lewy body-like decreased in cytoplasm, the cytotoxicity also decreased. Over-expression of Rab5A protein in immune system deficiency, which can slower macrophage phagocytosis of pathogens and decrease the rate of degradation of pathogens and IFN-C-mediated phagocytosis weakened.

Receptor mediated endocytosis occurs via clathrin-coated vesicles and is regulated by Rab5 and Rab21. Internalized cargo is delivered to early/sorting endosomes. From here molecules can return to the plasma membrane via fast or slow recycling routes through specialized recycling endosomes and the activities of distinct Rab GTPases. Newly synthesized plasma membrane proteins are delivered from the trans-Golgi network to recycling endosomes, while lysosomal hydrolases are delivered to early and late endosomes via two mannose 6-phosphate receptors. Recycling from early endosomes to the Golgi depends on Rab6, while Rab 9 controls transport from the late endosome to the trans-Golgi. Rab7 is a critical Rab GTPase on multiple degradative pathways; promoting late endosome, phagosome and autophagosome fusion with lysosomes in cooperation with specialized Rab GTPases on each of these pathways. In conjunction with Rac1, Rab7 is also pivotal in cadherin degradation by epithelia and neurons, as well as in bone resorption by osteoclasts. Rab GTPases in endocytosis, recycling, and degradative pathways [37].

6. Megalin and Its Associated Molecules

On the apical membrane of PTEC, various molecules are involved in the process of receptor-mediated endocytosis. Megalin, playing a central role in the process, cooperates with other membrane proteins such as the cubilin-amnionless complex (CUBAM), NHE3, and ClC5. Megalin and CUBAM directly bind a variety of ligands, whereas NHE3 and ClC5 are involved in endosomal acidification, which is important for further processing of endocytosed proteins. Megalin also interacts with intracellular adaptor proteins such as ARH, Dab2, and GIPC. Dab2 binds to motor proteins, myosin VI, and NMHCIIA, which may mediate endocytic trafficking of the molecular complexes through actin filaments. The cytoplasmic tail of megalin is released from the membrane by γ-secretase and is involved in intracellular signal transduction[38] (Fig. 3-21).

Section 4   Endocytosis Regulates Plasma Membrane Signalling

Endocytosis researches mainly fouces on the ligand-induced Notch signaling pathways [39].

1. Signal Attenuation after Endocytosis

Ligand-induced activation of receptor tyrosine kinases (RTKs) or G protein-coupled receptors (GPCRs) promotes signalling from the plasma membrane by the receptor-mediated recruitment of signalling effectors to phosphorylated RTKs, or the activation of G proteins associated with GPCRs when the Gα subunit is bound to GTP (Fig. 3-22, step 1). GPCRs signalling can be mediated both by the GTP-bound Gα subunit and by the Gβ–Gγ subcomplex. Receptor recruitment into coated pits (Fig. 3-22, step 2) and clathrin-dependent endocytosis (Fig.3-22, step3) attenuate signalling by separating the receptors from plasma membrane-delimited substrates and/or mediators. Some receptors traffic to lysosomes after endocytosis, which results in their downregulation by proteolysis and further attenuates signalling (Fig. 3-22, step 4). Schematic depicting signal attenuation [40].

2. Signal Pathway Switching during Endocytosis

The ability of some GPCRs to activate trimeric G proteins (Fig. 3-23, signal 1, step 1) is attenuated before endocytosis by receptor phosphorylation and β-arrestin binding (Fig. 3-23, step 2). Such desensitized receptor–β-arrestin complexes concentrate into clathrin-coated pits (Fig. 3-23, step 3) and are endocytosed into acidic (H⁺) endosomes (Fig. 3-23, step 4), which promotes various events that may include (depending on the receptor and cell type) ligand dissociation or destruction, dissociation of β-arrestin and phosphatase-catalysed dephosphorylation (Fig. 3-23, step 5). Recycling (Fig. 3-23, step 6) restores the receptors to the cell surface, re-sensitizing the cell for another round of signalling. In some cases GPCR recycling inserts receptors into a different G proteincontaining environment (Fig. 3-23, step 7), which produces a 'switch' in signalling specificity following subsequent receptor activation (Fig. 3-23, signal 2, step 8) [40].

Section 5   Significance in Endocytosis

1. Relationship between Mitosis and Endocytosis

(1) Inhibiting CME during Mitosis

Four mechanisms proposed to account for CME shutdown during mitosis. a: Mitotic phosphorylation. Important molecules in the basic layer or second layer of CME proteins are phosphorylated by mitotic kinases. This phosphorylation renders them unable to inter-act with their partners, thus stalling CME. b: Altered membrane tension. During endocytosis, the CME machinery (green arrow) must overcome three forces: the tension in the bilayer plane ™, interactions between the membrane and cytoskeleton (γ), and the stiffness of bending a membrane (B); B depends on the radius of the invaginated membrane. The CME machinery can overcome the sum of these forces easily during interphase, but cannot do so during mitosis. c: Mitotic moonlighting. This is a variation on the first mechanism where a key protein is involved in another function during mitosis and its unavailability for CME stalls the pathway. It may or may not involve mitotic phosphorylation. d: Mitotic spindle-dependent inhibition. The reorganization of the microtubule network and associated motors during mitosis could inhibit late stages of CME [6] (Fig. 3-24).

(2) Endocytic Trafficking Regulates the Surface Area of Dividing Cells.

In interphase cells, membranes undergo continuous internalization and recycling back to the cell surface as cells prepare for division, recycling is shut down and internalized material accumulates in endosomal compartments. As a consequence, cells decrease their surface area, retract their processes and round up. During cytokinesis, endocytosis occurs mainly close to the spindle poles. Recycling endosomes accumulate in the midzone region to rapidly deliver large amounts of membrane material to the ingressing cytokinesis furrow [41] (Fig. 3-25).

(3) Cell Cycle Dependent Localisation of the Endocytic Protein

In interphase, Numb and its binding partner Pon are detected throughout the cell cortex. Par 6 and aPKC form a trimeric complex with Lgl at the apical cell cortex. As the cell enters prophase, the mitotic kinases AuroraA (AurA) and Polo are activated. Par6 is localized at the posterior cell cortex and phosphorylated by AurA. As a consequence, Lgl is released from the membrane and Par6 and aPKC form a new complex with Par3. This enables aPKC to phosphorylate Numb, triggering its release from the posterior cell cortex. In addition, the phosphorylation of Pon by Polo promotes the localization of Pon and Numb at the anterior cell cortex [41] (Fig. 3-26).

2. Reciprocal Regulation between Polarity Proteins and Endocytic Regulators in Cells

Proteins are removed from the plasma membrane by endocytosis, trafficked through the endocytic pathwayand then either degraded in the lysosome or recycled back to the plasma membrane. Key polarity regulators (Cdc42 and the Par module) positively or negatively regulate traffic from the plasma membrane to endosomes, regulated by Dynamin and Rab5 to control the polarity of epithelial cells [9].

(1) Possible models for endocytosis in controlling polarity in epithelia. (a) Newly synthesized apical proteinscould first be delivered from the Golgi network to the basolateral membrane before being

endocytosed, sorted, and transported to the apical membrane in a process called transcytosis. The apical membrane is separated from the basolateral membrane by cell–cell junctions. When endocytosis is blocked, these apically-destined proteins may aberrantly accumulate on basolateral surfaces, disrupting apical–basal polarity. (b) Surface levels of hypothetical 'master polarity regulators might normally be kept in check by endocytosis. When endocytosis is blocked, these master regulators could accumulate on the cell surface, leading to mispolarization of the cell. (c) Intrinsic exocytosis error rates or lateral diffusion between membrane domains could occasionally lead to mislocalized basolateral polarity proteins on the apical surface, which are removed from the incorrect domain via endocytosis and degraded in the lysosome. Disruptions in endocytosis would lead to unmitigated delivery errors and subsequent polarity perturbation [9].

(2) Reciprocal regulation between polarity proteins and endocytic regulators in non-epithelial cells. In the C. elegans embryo, separate domains are marked by distinct, opposing PAR proteins, including PAR-6 and PAR-2. Dynamin promotes the anterior enrichment of endocytosis. PAR-6 maintains the anterior enrichment of dynamin and early endosomes. PAR-6/CDC-42 may be internalized and trafficked via association with the early endosomes. The polarizing cargo could be recycled rapidly from the early endosome, or associate with the recycling endosome and be recycled back to the anterior or posterior cortex. Speculatively, PAR-6/CDC-42 could associate with the Golgi apparatus, and dynamin could participate in vesicle scission here. Another putative function of dynamin-dependent endocytosis is preventing the expansion of PAR-2 into the anterior by promoting PAR-2 removal and recycling back to the posterior cortex [9].

3. Significance of Endocytosis in Tumorgenesis

Many tumors arise when multiple steps of endocytic trafficking are blocked. The genes that act as tumor suppressors at the step of internalization of cargoes, entry of cargoes into endosomes and ubiquitylation-dependent sorting of cargoes into MVBs were degragated to loss of epithelial architecture and growth control ,Disruption of major endocytic regulators in a number of the hallmarks of human cancer initiates a tumorigenic process. Speculative model of endocytic tumor suppression circuitry [42] (Fig. 3-27).

Using the cell's endocytosis mechanism facilitate to develop the transmission system of antioncology drugs, The cell-penetrating peptide(CPP) interacts with the cell membrane and facilitates endocytosis of the drug-loaded liposomes into tumor cells(Fig. 3-28) or targeting to tumors via crosslinked-micelles carrying a drug though cancer losting junctions [4] (Fig. 3-29).

4. Others

(1) HDL Endocytosis

ApoA-I is secreted by the liver and intestine and acquires phospholipids and cholesterol. To exert athero-protective effects, apoA-I and HDL have to be transported to macrophage foamcells through endothelial cells. ABCA1 is necessary for apoA-I transcytosis through endothelial cells, whereas SR-BI, ABCG1 and ecto-F1-ATPase facilitate HDL transport. Excess macrophage free cholesterol is transported to apoA-I by ABCA1 or to HDL by SR-BI. In addition, HDL retroendocytosis was shown to mediate cholesterol efflux. ABCG1 mainly seems to have a role in intracellular cholesterol trafficking. Cholesterol enriched HDL then leaves the plaque via the lymphatics and the vasa vasorum and is transported back to the liver. Here, SR-BI transfers cholesterol to hepatocytes by selective lipid uptake. After endocytosis, HDL is either rapidly recycled through the endosomal recycling compartment (ERC) and resecreted or transported to multivesicular bodies (MVBs). HDL degradation in lysosomes is limited and occurs rather slowly. During endocytosis, HDL exchanges cholesterol with hepatocytes. Cholesterol is then either used for the formation of newlipoproteins or secreted into the bile directly or indirectly after conversion to bile-acids [43] (Fig. 3-30).

(2) Ephrin-B2 links the regulation of cell motility and invasiveness to VEGF receptor (VEGFR) endocytosis and signaling. Expression of ephrin-B2 in the leading cells of the sprout (so-called tip cells) partially overlaps with EphB4 in stalk cells at the sprout base [44].

Challenges and Prospects

We have found many molecules involved in endocytosis in the past few decades, and had a preliminary understanding about its process and mechabism. Endocytosis is a process through which extracellular materials are transported into cell through membrane deformation. This process is not a simple step-by-step process in which a series of proteins function according to the chronological order, but rather a complex process comprising many members which are regulated precisely. The role of endocytosis is broadly divided into two categories, phagocytosis and pinocytosis, the latter is divided into four species in accordance with the size of endocytosis substances:clathrin dependent endocytosis, the diameter of clathrin-coated vesicle is 100~150 nm; caveolin dependent endocytosis, the diameter of caveolin protein-coated vesicle is 50~100 nm; macropinocytosis, the diameter of macropinocytosis is generally 0.5~2 μm, sometimes up to 5 μm; clathrin and caveolin independent endocytosis. We now know that the process of endocytosis is not a simple step-by-step process in which a series of proteins function according to the chronological order, but rather a complex process comprising many members which were regulated precisely.Many proteins including endophilin A1, A2, A3, and endocytotic protein B, B1a, as well as dynamin, actin and Rab protein family are involved in endocytosis and play an important role in different stages. The abnormal endocytosis may be involved in the development of certain diseases.

Although the mechanism of regulation of endocytosis is still unknown, it can be predicted that as more and more new research techniques applied in this area, we will be able to understand the mechanism of cell endocytosis more comprehensively. Whether tumor cells endocytose more nutrients than normal cells and whether tumor cells increase sizes through endocytosing more growth factors? Can we inhibit tumor growth through inhibiting cell endocytosis or can we cure tumor by inducing specific drug endocytosis of tumor cells? Whether the endocytosis of 6-phosphate mannose receptor (MPR) which plays a very important role in cell death signal transduction is restrained in tumor cells? The mechanism of cell endocytosis can be further elucidated by solving all of the above problems.

Consider/Questions

1. Basic concepts in this chapter

Pinocytosis, Phagocytosis, Clathrin dependent endocytosis, Caveolin dependent endocytosis, Lipid mediated endocytosis, Macropinocytosis, Microdomain.

2. Summary the types of pinocytosis depending different mechanisms?

3. Analyze the following figure 3-31.

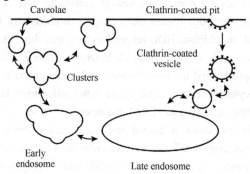

4. Comparison of the roles in caveolae (bulk) endocytosis with clathrin-dependent endocytosis.

5. Briefly descript the characteristics and roles of Dynamin in endocytosis.

6. Briefly descript the roles of Actin in endocytosis.

7.Which roles of endocytosis are in cells mitosis?

8. Briefly descript the endocytosis impact on cell plors.

9. Which significance of endocytosis research are in tumorgenesis?

第四章　细胞黏附分子

　　细胞-细胞，细胞-细胞外基质（extracellular matrix，ECM）的有序的结合是形成正常组织器官的必要条件，有赖于他们之间的识别、交换与黏附。细胞黏附分子（cell adhesion molecule，CAM）大多为糖蛋白，少数为糖脂，由细胞产生，存在于细胞表面或 ECM 中。多数 CAM 的作用依赖于二价阳离子（Ca^{2+}、Mg^{2+}等），介导细胞与细胞间、细胞与 ECM 间或同时介导两者间相互接触和结合（图 4-1）。通过配体-受体相互识别参与细胞的信号转导与活化、细胞的伸

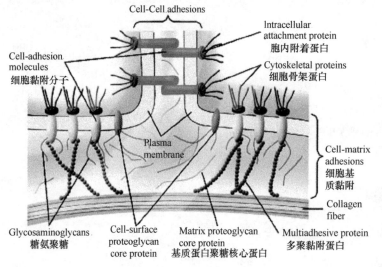

图 4-1　存在于细胞表面或 ECM 中的 CAM 介导细胞与细胞间或细胞与 ECM 间相互黏附；Cell adhesion molecules (CAMs), a class pf molecules that present on the cell surface mediated cells to cells or between cells and the extra-llular matrix (ECM) in contacting and being with each other

展和移动、细胞的生长及分化，以及炎症、血栓形成、肿瘤转移、创伤愈合等一系列重要生理和病理过程。CAM 是维持生物体正常发育、生长、形体及组织器官正常结构与生命活动的一类重要分子。

第一节　CAM 的概述

一、CAM 的主要功能

（1）介导配体和受体结合后的粘附反应（ECMs 间、细胞与细胞间、细胞与 ECMs 间）；

（2）通过增加细胞间的附着或传递信号来促进细胞功能（识别、激活、伸长、运动、生长、分化和信号转导等）；

（3）它参与了一系列重要的生理和病理过程：

1）维持正常细胞体在生理条件下的发育和生长，是正常器官结构和组织的一类重要分子。

2）在炎症、血栓、肿瘤转移、伤口愈合等病理过程中起着重要的作用。

二、CAM 的基本结构

CAM 的基本结构有胞浆区、穿膜功能区、胞膜外区三部分组成：①胞外区，肽链的 N 端部分，带有糖链，负责与配体的识别；②跨膜区，多为一次跨膜；③胞质区，肽链的 C 端部分，一般较小，与质膜下的骨架成分直接相连—迁移、变形，与胞内的化学信号分子相连—信号转导途径。

三、CAM 作用的三种模式

CAM 的作用模式（图 4-2）：①亲同性黏附：两相邻细胞表面的同种 CAM 分子间的相互识别与结合；②亲异性黏附：两相邻细胞表面的不同种 CAM 分子间的相互识别与结合；③中介性黏附：两相邻细胞表面的相同 CAM 分子借细胞外的连接分子相互识别与结合。

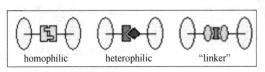

图 4-2　CAM 的作用机制有三种模式；Three patterns of CAM roles

四、CAM 的分类

目前按 CAM 的结构特点，可将其分为：整合素超家族（integrin superfamily）、免疫球蛋白超家族（immunoglobulin superfamily，Ig-SF）、选择素家族（selectin family）、钙离子依赖的 CAM 家族（Ca^{2+}-dependent cell adhesion molecule family）或称钙黏着蛋白（Cadherin），及其他未归类的 CAM。

五、肿瘤研究中 CAM 的意义

（1）诊断和评估

在肿瘤转移过程中伴随着一些 CAM 表达水平、表达类型的不同，因此，临床上通过对某些 CAM 表达水平和类型的检测，作为肿瘤诊断的一个有效的辅助手段，并且可以对肿瘤的分化程度、分期、转移潜能、复发及预后作出估计。

（2）确定肿瘤的起源

因某些 CAM（如整合素）在不同的组织、细胞有其特定的分布方式，而肿瘤组织在一定程度上保留了这种特定的分布方式，故可以通过对某些特定 CAM 的检测，来确定肿瘤的组织来源及其组织分型。

（3）作为治疗的靶点

1）CAM 可影响免疫细胞对肿瘤的杀伤作用，通过对某些 CAM 的研究，找出能增强细胞免疫作用的因子，并设想用合成的黏附多肽或细胞特异性 CAM 的单抗封闭肿瘤 CAM 或其配基上的识别位点，从而抑制肿瘤的浸润转移。通过抗血凝及抗血栓，阻止肿瘤细胞与血小板等的相互作用及瘤血栓的形成，抑制非特异性的肿瘤转移。

2）用肿瘤细胞特异性 CAM 的抗体与核素、化疗药物等结合进行导向治疗等。

CAM 不仅介导肿瘤与 ECM 的黏附，参与癌细胞之间、癌细胞与血管内皮细胞、淋巴细胞、实质器官细胞与其他细胞之间的相互作用，肿瘤细胞浸润转移过程中需要双向黏附[1-3]，一方面肿瘤细胞必须先从其原来黏附的原发灶脱离才能浸润；另一方面，肿瘤细胞又需借黏附才能移动。肿瘤细胞从连续的黏附接触和黏附解除中获得移动的迁移能力，故肿瘤浸润和转移的过程首先是黏附和去黏附的过程。

第二节　整合素超家族

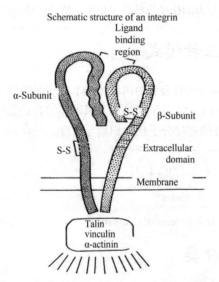

Schematic structure of an integrin
Ligand binding region
α-Subunit
β-Subunit
S-S
S-S
Extracellular domain
Membrane
Talin vinculin α-actinin

图 4-3　整合素的分子结构（示意图）；The molecular structure of the integrin（schematic）
图示 α 亚基位的二价阳离子（Mg^{2+}）结合区和 α、β 亚单位的重复序列；In the structure of the b integrin molecule show the two valence cation（Mg^{2+}）of the α subunit and the repeating sequence of α and β subunits.（diagram）

整合素（integrin）是一个跨膜蛋白大家族，作为一类细胞表面糖蛋白[1]，由 α、β 两条链通过非共价键连接组成异源二聚体。α、β 链均为 I 类跨膜蛋白，是介导细胞与 ECM 黏附作用的主要因子，参与细胞信号转导及细胞骨架改变。在细胞生长、分化、形成连接和维持极性等方面起重要作用。

一、整合素家族的分子结构

整合素中 α 链的分子量为 150～210kDa，β 链的分子量为 90～110kDa，个别 β 链（如 β4）分子量为 220kDa。两个亚基都有较长的细胞外片段、跨膜片段和较短的细胞内片段。各种 β 亚基中氨基酸序列具有 40%～48% 的同源性，β 亚基多肽链的羧基端位于胞质内。各种 α 亚基多肽链的氨基酸顺序更多地表现为相异性，它们的细胞外片段含有 Ca^{2+} 结合区。整合素细胞内片段通过纽带蛋白、辅肌动蛋白和尾蛋白与细胞骨架连接[2]（图 4-3）。

整合素的配体是 I 型、IV 型胶原，LN，FN，vitronectin，endotoxin，ICAM-1，VCAM-1。整合素与相邻细胞上或 ECM 中相应配体相结合发挥作用。在整合素配体中多含有 RGD（精氨酸-甘氨酸-天冬氨酸）序列，这一序列是整合素的结合位点。含有 RGD 序列的多肽具有抑制细胞-细胞外蛋白如纤维连接蛋白（FN）、层粘连蛋白（LN）的黏附反应，并具有抑制肿瘤细胞转移的作用[1]（图 4-4）。

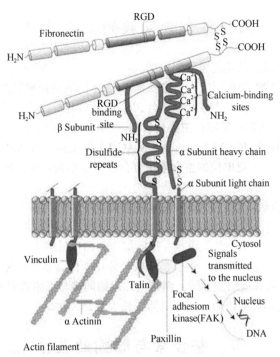

图 4-4　整合素引起细胞活化-细胞间质反应；Integrin causes cell activity and stroma reactions

黏着斑蛋白（vinculin）：又称纽带蛋白（linking protein），连接肌动蛋白（辅肌动蛋白）与质膜；踝蛋白（talin）：膜下的一种细胞骨架蛋白；聚焦黏附激酶（focal adhesion kinase，FAK）引起细胞膜磷脂酰肌醇代谢，将细胞外信号转导到胞质核糖体合成基因转录所需的蛋白质；vinculin(linking protein): connects with actin(actinin)and membrane; talin: a cytoskeletal protein under the membrane; focal adhesion kinase(FAK)causes cell membrane phosphatidylinositol metabolism, leading to the extracellular signal transducting to the cytoplasm ribosomal to synthesis requiring proteins for gene transcription

二、整合素家族的分类

目前已知至少有 18 种不同的 α 亚单位和 11 种 β 亚单位，多数 α 亚单位只能与一种 β 亚单位结合构成异源二聚体，但也有的 α 亚单位可与几种不同的 β 亚单位组合，而大部分 β 单位可以结合数种不同的 α 亚单位。至少有 24 种异源二聚体的整合素形式[3]。α/β 支链配对的形式决定了整合素主要与哪一个配体结合，同时受到整合素杂二聚体整体结构的限制[4]（图 4-5）。整合素分子表达于多种不同类型的细胞，或多种整合素表达于同一类型的细胞，但不同类型的细胞表达的整合素分子具有明显的组织细胞特异性（如 $\alpha_6\beta_4$ 特异性表达在上皮细胞），而且每一种细胞表达的整合素可随分化和生长状态而变化。

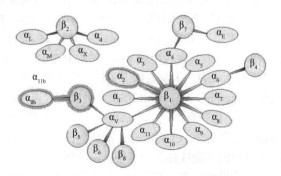

图 4-5　各整合素支链及配对形式图；Each integrin branched chain and pairing form diagram

三、整合素家族的主要功能

根据整合素作用方式，其功能可分为三类。

（1）介导细胞与 ECM 的黏附反应：主要是 β_1 亚单位的整合素包括 α_4/β_1、α_5/β_1、α_V/β_1 均可与 FN 相结合；α_V/β_3、α_V/β_5 可与 LN 相结合，α_V/β_3 还可与纤维蛋白原结合。

（2）介导细胞-细胞间黏附反应：主要是含 β_2 亚单位的整合素存在于各种白细胞表面，包括 α_L/β_2（LFA-1）的配体是 ICAM-1，α_M/β_2（MAC-1）的配体是 ICAM-1、C3bi、ENdotoxiN；α_4/β_1 的配体是 VCAM-1。β_3 亚单位的整合素主要存在于血小板表面，介导血小板的黏附，并参与血栓形成。

（3）既介导细胞-细胞，又介导细胞-ECM 的黏附反应：VLA-4 及 α_M/β_2。除 β_4 可与肌动蛋白及其相关蛋白质结合，$\alpha_6\beta_4$ 整合素以 LN 为配体，参与形成半桥粒。形成 ECM-整合素-细胞骨架跨膜复合体（既可诱导细胞骨架重排，加固细胞间的机械联系，又像座桥梁双向转导细胞内外的信号，广泛影响细胞的生存、生长、增殖、分化、侵袭和转移等生物学行为[3]。整合素细胞外片段可与 ECM 或邻近细胞黏附，细胞内片段则间接与细胞骨架连接，参与机体许多的生理过程，如免疫细胞间黏附作用，调节机体生长、发育，伤口修复及血栓形成等。

四、整合素与肿瘤的关系

整合素在肿瘤病理学上的研究，主要集中在两个方面，即整合素在肿瘤中的分布与表达及整合素对癌症发展的影响。许多恶性肿瘤的生长和转移均与整合素表达异常或分子结构改变相关。但由于整合素的多样性和复杂性，目前还不能总结出肿瘤转移过程中整合素改变的普遍规律。在一些肿瘤中其表达减少，肿瘤转移增强，而在另一些肿瘤中则相反。且同一整合素在不同的肿瘤发展阶段可呈现不同的表达，不同的肿瘤甚至同一种肿瘤可表达不同类型或不同水平的整合素[4]。

Matsuura 等[5]认为在肿瘤转移发生中整合素可能具有双重作用：整合素分子表达的减少使肿瘤细胞与基质间的黏附作用减弱，有利于肿瘤的浸润和转移，而某些整合素分子如层粘连蛋白受体表达的增加，可使肿瘤细胞得以与血管或淋巴管基底膜黏附，继而基底膜被肿瘤细胞分泌的或诱导宿主细胞产生的蛋白酶降解，肿瘤细胞通过管壁进入血管或淋巴管内。肿瘤细胞侵入血管或淋巴管后，首先导致局部栓塞，同时，整合素分子表达的增加，有利于肿瘤细胞黏附于血管内皮，然后通过前述机制，穿过管壁进入外周组织，并形成转移灶。

Wang 等研究发现，膨胀性生长的胃癌中 α_6 呈连续或断续状线形表达，而在浸润性生长的胃癌 α_6 表达减弱或消失。Su 等用免疫组化检测 FAK 和 $\alpha_2\beta_1$ 整合素亚基表达与肿瘤类型、分级及淋巴结转移的关系，发现 FAK 在癌组织中比非癌组织中高表达，在胃癌、直肠癌中与恶性程度、淋巴结转移、浸润深度呈正相关。Lindmark 等[6]研究 33 例直肠癌，发现 α_2、α_3 在正常上皮细胞和肿瘤细胞上都表达，但其表达模式不同，正常上皮细胞中 α_2、α_3 靠近基底侧表达，而肿瘤组织中 α_2、α_3 弥漫性表达或表达于基底侧但表达，失去连续性，与肿瘤分化、Dukes 分期及生存时间存在相关性。Zutter 等[7]发现，$\alpha_2\beta_1$ 在正常乳腺上皮表达正常，而在乳腺癌中表达降低，且与肿瘤分化有关。低分化肿瘤细胞中重新表达 $\alpha_2\beta_1$，表明肿瘤细胞有逆转倾向，$\alpha_2\beta_1$ 表达可上调 $\alpha_6\beta_4$。Yamanaka 等[8]发现，EGF 能与 $\alpha_2\beta_1$ 协同作用，上调 $\alpha_2\beta_1$ 表达，降低 FAK 磷酸化使 $\alpha_2\beta_1$ 表达增加，EGF 诱导的细胞迁移作用能被 $\alpha_2\beta_1$ 抗体抑制。宫颈癌中 α_6 表达增高，$\alpha_6\beta_4$、$\alpha_2\beta_1$、$\alpha_3\beta_1$ 在侵袭性宫颈癌中弥漫性分布，在良性组织中分布在基底侧，且 $\alpha_6\beta_4$ 的分布浓度与宫颈上皮内瘤变（CIN）的分级呈负相关。Wang 等[9]在研究原发性非小细胞肺癌中，发现 α_2、α_1 在肺鳞癌及腺癌中高表达，且 $\alpha_6\beta_4$、$\alpha_6\beta_1$ 表达增高，而在正常组织则表达水平比较低。Hangan[10]等[10]研究整合素 VLA-2（$\alpha_2\beta_1$）在人肝内横纹肌肉瘤上的作用，结果显示 VLA-2 整合素的高表达，使肿瘤转移力增强。Kawaguchi 等[11]研究整合素 VLA-4（$\alpha_4\beta_1$）在肿瘤转移中的作用，发现 VLA-4 分子在肿瘤细胞同血管内皮细胞 VCAM-1 分子开始黏附时，过度表达 α4 的细胞对 VCAM-1 的结合力增强，侵袭性亦增强。Demeure[12]的研究发现，β1 表达还与甲状腺癌侵袭基底膜并激活蛋白酶能力有关。

有关黑色素瘤的研究资料较多。原发性恶性黑色素瘤中 $\alpha_V\beta_3$ 高表达，与预后有关，特别与血行转移有关，$\alpha_V\beta_3$ 也能激活 MMP22，MT12MMP 促进细胞外基质降解和肿瘤的侵袭，抑制 $\alpha_V\beta_3$ 能减少血行转移，延长生存时间。有研究认为 β_3 只在恶性黑色素瘤细胞中表达，而 $\alpha_V\beta_1$ 的高表达与肿瘤转移呈正相关。以 α_VcDNA 转染低表达 $\alpha_V\beta_3$ 的黑色素瘤细胞可提高其转移力。以 $\alpha_V\beta_3$ 抗体、玻璃粘连蛋白抗体处理高转移黑色素瘤细胞，可降低其黏着性及转移力[13]。

Tennenbaum 发现，在鳞状细胞乳头状瘤发生癌变向内部浸润时，整合素 $\alpha_5\beta_4$ 的表达异常，是早期侵袭生长的标志，在咽部乳头状瘤也有 $\alpha_5\beta_4$、$\alpha_2\beta_1$、$\alpha_3\beta_1$ 三种整合素的表达。有研究证实 $\alpha_5\beta_4$ 整合素分子与鳞状细胞癌的复发密切相关，其表达较强者易发生早期复发，而表达较弱者则预后较好。

第三节 免疫球蛋白超家族

免疫球蛋白超家族（immunoglobulin superfamily，Ig-SF）是一类不依赖于 Ca^{2+}、与 Ig 结构相似的细胞表面跨膜蛋白质。Ig 样结构域系指借二硫键维系的两组反向平行 β 折叠结构（图 4-6）。

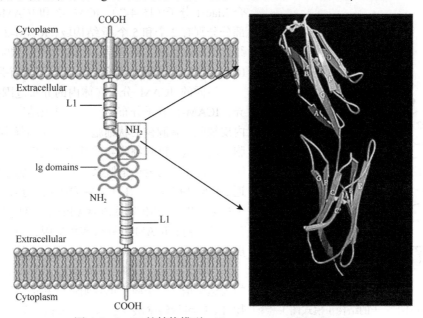

图 4-6 Ig-SF 的结构模型；The structure model of Ig-SF

一、Ig-SF 的分子结构

Ig-SF 包括分子结构中均含有 Ig 样结构域的所有分子，一般这些分子结构与 Ig 有很高的同源性，由 1 个或多个 Ig 同源单位组成，即与 Ig 的氨基酸序列中第 70～110 位氨基酸残基同源，中间由二硫键相连。二硫键的数目由肽链的长短决定。不同 Ig-SF 分子有着相同的 Ig 重复区，但 Ig 重复区数目各有不同。例如，细胞间黏附分子（intercellular adhesion molecule-1，ICAM-1）由 532 个氨基酸残基组成，含 5 个 Ig 样区域；血管细胞黏附分子-1（vascular cell adhesion molecule-1，VCAM-1）含 647 个氨基酸残基，含 6 个或 7 个 Ig 样区域，而血小板内皮细胞黏附分子（platelet endothelial cell adhesion molecule -1，PECAM-1）则有 6 个 Ig 样区域。

二、Ig-SF 分类

Ig-SF 是细胞表面分子数最丰富的家族，目前已发现 Ig-SF 包括 70 多种分子[8]，其主要成员：淋巴细胞功能相关抗原 2、3[lymphocyte function-associated antigen（LFA）-2, 3]，CD28，细胞毒性 T 淋巴细胞相关抗原 4（Cytotoxic T lymphocyte associated antigen 4，CTLA-4），B7-1，B7-2，ICAM-1、2、3，VCAM-1，神经细胞黏附分子（neural cell adhesion molecule，NCAM），PECAM-1，癌胚抗原（carcinoembryonic antigen，CEA），结肠癌缺失分子（deleted in colorectal carcinoma molecule，DCC）等。

（1）ICAM-1：它是最早发现的 Ig-SF 的 CAM 之一，以后又相继发现了 ICAM-2 和 ICAM-3，它们的 Ig 结构域氨基酸序列具有同源性，且都可以结合 LFA-1 分子。ICAM-1 分子为单链跨膜糖蛋白，核心多肽为 55kDa，由于不同种类细胞上 ICAM-1 分子所含寡糖分子数有所差别，ICAM-1 分子量可在 80～110kDa。ICAM-1 分子胞膜外部分具有 5 个 Ig 样结构域，第 2 和第 3 结构域之间有一段连接序列，富含脯氨酸，类似 Ig 的绞链区，可发生扭曲。以此连接区为界，氨基端的 D1 和 D2 结构域可结合 LFA-1 分子和鼻病毒，而羧基端的 D3 结构域可以结合 Mac-1 分子（图 4-7）。ICAM-2 和 ICAM-3 胞膜外部分分别有 2 个和 5 个 Ig 结构域，ICAM-2 分子 2 个结构域与 ICAM-1 氨基端 2 个结构域有 34% 同源性，ICAM-1 D1 结构域中结合 LFA-1 分子具有关键作用。

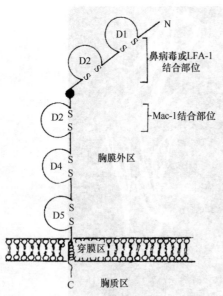

图 4-7　ICAM-1 分子的结构（模式图）；Molecular structure of ICAM-1

不同的 ICAM 分子在体内的分布范围有较大差异，ICAM-1 分子分布广泛，如淋巴结和扁桃体血管内皮细胞、胸腺树突状细胞、扁桃体和肾小球上皮细胞、白细胞、巨噬细胞和成纤维细胞等，在大多数组织，ICAM-1 的表达是低水平的，而在肺组织则高出近 30 倍。白介素-1（IL-1）、肿瘤坏死因子-α（TNF-α）、干扰素（INF）和植物血凝素（PHA）可促进 ICAM-1 分子的表达；ICAM-2 则分布较局限，主要在血管内皮细胞表达；而 ICAM-3 只在血细胞表达。

当使用 IL21、TNF2α 和 INF2γ 诱导时，ICAM-1 的表达会增加。来源于革兰阴性菌和革兰阳性菌的产物 LPS 和脂磷壁酸（LTA）对人微血管内皮细胞上 ICAM-1 的表达起重要的作用。氧化剂也能增加 ICAM-1 的表达[14, 15]。炎性细胞因子和细菌产物能诱导 ICAM-1 的表达，但是对 ICAM-2 基本无影响。ICAM-1 对于单核细胞、淋巴细胞、中性粒细胞黏附于内皮细胞是十分重要的，而 ICAM-2 在淋巴细胞聚集、ICAM-3 在调节 LFA/ICAM-1 途径的细胞间黏附中各自发挥作用。

（2）VCAM-1：又称诱导性细胞黏附分子（inducible cell adhesion molecule，INCAM），意指该类 CAM 在 IL-1、TNF-α 等细胞因子活化的血管内皮细胞上表达。VCAM-1 分子量为 100kDa 或 110kDa，最近命名为 CD106 的蛋白是 VCAM-1 的配体，分布在白细胞表面的 VLA-4 分子。VCAM-1 能在内皮细胞、巨噬细胞、成纤维细胞等表达，主要介导淋巴细胞、单核细胞、嗜酸性细胞和内皮细胞的黏附。虽然内皮细胞的 VCAM21 能够在皮肤和胸膜表达，但在 IL-4 介导的嗜酸性细胞聚集过程中，仅局限于在皮肤起作用[16]。

（3）PECAM 主要在内皮细胞表达，在淋巴细胞游走通过内皮时极为重要。

（4）CEA 是一种高度糖基化的细胞表面糖蛋白，分子量为 180kDa。近年来对 CEA 基因及蛋白结构分析表明，CEA 是 Ig-SF 的成员之一，是一种重要的细胞黏附分子，可能有细胞识别和相互作用的功能，作为黏附分子，CEA 可增强肿瘤细胞与正常细胞间的结合。

三、Ig-SF 的主要功能

Ig-SF 中的 CAM 主要介导非 Ca^{2+} 依赖性同种细胞和异种细胞之间的黏附反应。Ig-SF 大部分成员参与细胞间识别（包括那些免疫功能的分子，如 MHA、CD4、CD8 和 T 细胞受体），参与神经细胞发育（N-CAM，L1）、白细胞交流（ICAM-1、VCAM-1、PECAM-1）和信息传递[克隆刺激因子 1 受体（colony stimulating factor-1 receptor，CSF-1R）、血小板源性生长因子受体（PGFR）]等。

四、Ig-SF 与肿瘤的关系

（一）Ig-SF 杀伤肿瘤细胞的作用

ICAM-1 首先作为 LFA-1 的配体，在一些类型的鳞状细胞癌和黑色素瘤中表达，已被认为是皮肤癌发展的标志。研究发现，肿瘤组织内有淋巴细胞浸润时，肿瘤细胞多数表达 ICAM-1，而肿瘤患者血清中可溶性 ICAM-1 水平也高于正常人。因此推测，可溶性 ICAM-1 分子可能抑制 NK 细胞对肿瘤细胞的杀伤作用，而肿瘤细胞表达的 ICAM-1 分子可能与肿瘤浸润淋巴细胞（TIL）的杀伤作用有关。其他细胞因子如 IFN-γ、IFN-α、IL-4、TNF-α 可促进某些肿瘤细胞 ICAM-1 分子的表达[17]，增加其对杀伤细胞作用的敏感性。

（二）Ig-SF 与肿瘤发生、进展的关系

VCAM-1 是 VLA-4 的配体[18]，在骨髓基质细胞中持续表达，猜测它对骨髓中白细胞的滞留和骨髓淋巴瘤转移起一定作用。已发现在肿瘤患者的血液循环中 VCAM-1 的数量增加；在黑色素瘤转移实验模型和肺癌转移患者的血管壁上 VCAM-1 则表达缺失。

CEA 是富含多糖的蛋白复合物。胎儿早期的消化管及某些组织均含有合成 CEA 的能力，但孕六个月以后含量逐渐减少，出生后含量极低。CEA 含量无性别差异，但随年龄增高稍有上升。吸烟者有轻度增高。在结肠癌、胃癌、肺癌、胆管癌中 CEA 明显升高。CEA 也存在于肝癌、胰腺癌、肾癌、乳腺癌、食管癌、卵巢癌等肿瘤组织中。CEA 是目前研究得较多的肿瘤标志物之一，临床上用于肠道、乳腺及肺部恶性肿瘤的辅助诊断及预后判断。细胞分泌的 CEA 进入局部体液及血液中，在上述癌症的血清及胸腔积液、腹水、消化液内可出现 CEA 异常增高。肺癌胸腔积液中 CEA 高于血清。原发性结肠直肠癌在早期未转移时，CEA 阳性率为 45%～80%，血清 CEA 升高往往预示肿瘤的复发和转移。因此它对肿瘤的诊断、预后复发

判断有意义。

DCC 蛋白产物与 NCAM 同源，与细胞黏附有关。在大多数结肠癌、食管癌、胃癌中表达缺失，增生和分化中的细胞 DCC 蛋白表达增加。

（三）Ig-SF 对肿瘤血管生成的影响

Patey[19]研究发现，ICAM-3 在恶性淋巴瘤等恶性肿瘤血管内皮中呈高度阳性表达，在良性肿瘤的血管内皮细胞中呈低度阳性表达，在正常组织的内皮细胞缺乏表达，结果提示 ICAM-3 与肿瘤的血管形成及肿瘤的进展与转移有关。Penfold 等[20]在对口腔鳞状细胞癌行病理检查时，采用 JC70 抗体对 PE-CAM-1 作标志发现，随着肿瘤新生血管的增加及淋巴结转移，PE-CAM-1 的量明显增加。结果提示，研究开发某些 CAM 抑制剂将能阻止肿瘤血管生成。

第四节　选择素家族

选择素家族（selectin family）最初被称为外源凝集素 CAM 家族（lectin cell adhesion molecule family，LEC-CAM family）。选择素家族分子是一类以糖基为识别配体的 CAM，属 I 型跨膜糖蛋白。

一、选择素家族分子结构

其家族成员均由三部分构成。

（1）胞质区：选择素家族分子的胞质区与细胞内骨架相连，去除胞质部分的选择素分子虽仍可结合相应配体，但失去了其介导细胞间黏附的作用。

（2）一个跨膜功能区；各种选择素家族分子的跨膜区和胞质区没有同源性。

（3）胞膜外部分：该部分有较高的同源性，结构类似，均由三种结构域构成（图 4-8）：①钙离子依赖的 C 型外源凝集素结构域（calcium dependent ctypelectin domain）是选择素外侧氨基端（约 120 个氨基酸残基），可以结合碳水化合物基团，是选择素家族分子的配体结合部位；②表皮生长因子样结构域（epidermal growth factor-like domain），紧邻外源凝集素结构域，约含 35 个氨基酸残基，EGF 样结构域虽不直接参加配体的结合，但对维持选择素家族分子的构型是必需的；③补体调节蛋白（complement regulatory protein）样功能区近胞膜部分有 2～9 个补体调节蛋白样功能区，每个功能区包括 62～67 个氨基酸的同源性重复序列组成；补体调节蛋白样功能区的重复序列又称为补体结合蛋白（complement binding protein）重复序列，它们与补体受体（如 CR1、CR2 等）和 C4 结合蛋白（C4bp）等结构同源。

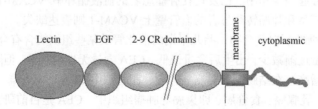

图 4-8　选择素分子的结构模式图；Molecular structure of selectin

虽然这些蛋白辖区在其他蛋白上也能发现，但只有在选择素上的这些蛋白辖区能产生对合作用，这对于受体功能是十分重要的[21]。

二、选择素家族的分类

目前已发现选择素家族中有三个成员：L-选择素、P-选择素和E-选择素[8]，L、P和E分别表示白细胞（leukocyte）、血小板（platelet）和内皮细胞（endothelium），是最初发现相应选择素家族分子的三种细胞，故得名（图4-9）。

（1）E选择素只在内皮细胞上表达，一般均是在内皮细胞受到IL-1、TNF-α或细菌脂多糖等炎性刺激后才表达。当内皮细胞受到内毒素及炎性细胞因子作用后 1小时内表达即开始增加，4～6小时达到高峰，24小时后下降，因此它在炎症部位的血管内皮细胞与中性粒细胞黏附中发挥重要作用，在体内炎性部位，E-选择素呈现慢性表达现象，很多能上调 ICAM-1 表达的刺激同时上调 E 选择素的表达。此外，在肿瘤的血道转移中介导肿瘤细胞与内皮细胞的黏附。转化生长因子β（TGF-β）能抑制 E-选择素的诱导和转录。在培养的人脐静脉内皮细胞（human umbilical vein endothelial cells，HUVEC），用TNF-α刺激后3～6小时 E-选择素表达即达高峰期，随

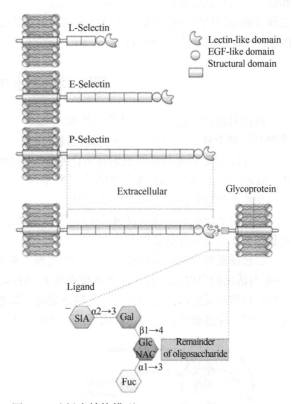

图4-9　选择素结构模型；The structure model of selectin

后，即使有细胞因子刺激，其表达亦会在 10～12 小时内回到基础水平。在培养的其他内皮细胞，一般不会超过24小时。

（2）P-选择素在内皮细胞和血小板上表达，且预先存储于血小板和内皮细胞的 α 颗粒及内皮细胞的 Weibel-Palade 小体内，所以其表达速度较快，在内皮细胞受到组胺、凝血酶、补体碎片和细胞因子激活以后，P-选择素能快速移向细胞表面，10 分钟内即可达到表达高峰，而在20 分钟后回到基线水平[22]。同时，经对 P 选择素 mRNA 表达的分析，其基因转录能被 LPS、TNF-α、IL-1 等诱导，导致其2～4 小时后再度表达，表明 P-选择素能对炎症做出早、晚两期反应。P-选择素有同源二聚体和异源二聚体等形式，不同的表达形式在结构和功能上略有差异[22]。

（3）L-选择素在淋巴细胞，单核细胞，大部分 T 细胞、B 细胞和 NK 细胞上表达，但不在内皮细胞上表达。L-选择素在早期炎症反应中起重要作用。新近的研究表明非类固醇类抗炎药能下调 L-选择素在中性粒细胞上的表达[23]。

三、选择素分子识别的配体

选择素中的凝集素样结构决定了其配体是糖类。与选择素结合的寡糖基团可存在于多种糖蛋白或糖脂分子上，并分布于多种细胞表面，因此选择素分子的配体在体内的分布较为广泛。已发现在白细胞、血管内皮细胞、某些肿瘤细胞表面及血清中某些糖蛋白分子上都存在有选择

素分子识别的碳水化合物基团。与选择素具有亲和力的结构有 3 类：①一些寡糖基团——唾液酸化的路易斯寡糖（寡糖 Lex）或类似结构的分子；②磷酸化的单糖和多糖；③硫酸化的多糖和糖脂。选择素的配体原型唾液酸 LewisX（slex），是一个含岩藻糖和唾液酸残留物的四糖。选择素的黏附依赖于唾液酸，而且 3 种选择素均需要岩藻糖。多数文献报道 3 种选择素都能和 P-选择素糖蛋白配体 1（PSG21）结合[24]。

四、选择素的功能

选择素是白细胞 CAM，其作用依赖于 Ca^{2+}，介导白细胞进入炎性损害区及与内皮细胞的黏附[17]，对于募集白细胞到达炎症部位具有重要作用。

E-选择素及 P-选择素所识别与结合的糖配体为唾液酸化及岩藻糖化的 N 乙酰氨基乳糖结构（sLeX 及 sLeA）。sLeA 结构存在于髓系白细胞表面（其中包括 L-选择素）分子中。多种肿瘤细胞表面也存在 sLeX 及 sLeA 结构。

炎症时活化的内皮细胞表面首先出现 P-选择素，随后出现 E-选择素。它们对于募集白细胞到达炎症部位具有重要作用。

L-选择素参与炎症部位血管内白细胞附壁、游出的过程。白细胞表面 L-选择素分子上的 sLeA 与活化的内皮细胞表面的 P-选择素及 E-选择素之间的识别与结合，可募集血液中快速流动的白细胞在炎症部位的脉管内皮上减速滚动（即通过黏附、分离、再黏附……，如此循环往复），最后穿过血管通过趋化作用进入炎症部位（图 4-10）。

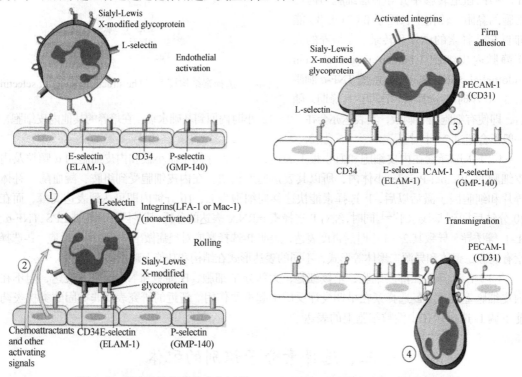

图 4-10　炎症中选择素的参与过程；The process of selectin in inflammation

①内皮细胞活化 L-选择素——EC-CD34，糖蛋白 sLeX——E-选择素；②白细胞在选择素介导下滚动；③与受体作用牢固黏附；④白细胞与 EC 表面的 CD31 相互作用介导细胞迁移；①endothelial cells（EC）activates L-selectin——EC-CD34, glycoprotein sLeX——E-selectin；②Leukocyte rolls through the interaction between selectins；③interaction between receptors firmed adhesion；④That the leukocyte interacting with shaped molecule（CD31）on EC surface mediates cells migration

五、选择素家族与肿瘤的关系

选择素参与肿瘤细胞-内皮细胞之间的黏附作用可作为血清肿瘤标志物来判断肿瘤进展、复发和转移，以及进行预后评估。Stone 等通过激活血小板、内皮细胞与癌细胞黏附的机制，发现两种肺癌细胞株和神经母细胞瘤细胞株均可与激活的血小板结合，这种结合是钙依赖性的且通过 P-选择素介导。人体黑色素瘤细胞的体外黏附和黏附抑制实验表明，血小板可增强肿瘤细胞与内皮细胞的黏附（2.2～2.5 倍）及与 ECM 的黏附。肿瘤细胞与内皮细胞-血小板的黏附主要由 GPⅡb-Ⅲa 所介导。Pice 等的研究表明，细胞分裂素激活内皮细胞后细胞膜上的 E-选择素能介导结肠癌细胞株 HT-29 与之结合。最近对成人 T 细胞白血病（ATL）易转移到肝、脾、肺和皮肤等器官的研究发现，ATL 细胞可黏附于 IL-1 激活的人脐静脉内皮细胞，E-选择素单抗能显著抑制 ATL 细胞的黏附。有实验表明，选择素与肿瘤转移的器官选择性有关。

在乳腺癌中，血清可溶性 E-选择素水平的升高表明肿瘤在进展或复发，进一步的升高常提示远处转移，转移的部位与血清可溶性 E-选择素的水平无关。血清可溶性 E-选择素的改变常在临床发现转移灶之前。血清中选择素水平有望成为继 CEA 和 CA 系列之后又一个重要的恶性肿瘤检测指标[25]。

Schadendorf 等研究恶性黑色素瘤组织中 E-选择素表达与患者临床的关系，结合长期随访资料发现，无转移者 E-选择素表达低，有转移者 E-选择素表达高，两者差异显著。肿瘤组织中 E-选择素表达少者 5 年生存率高。

另外，选择素的配体 sLeA、sLeX 在消化道肿瘤（如结肠癌、胰腺癌、胆管癌等）中常常高表达，且肿瘤复发时其含量再度升高，手术切除后其含量下降。因此，该指标对判断肿瘤复发有一定的参考价值。

第五节 钙黏着蛋白家族

Takeichi 最早发现一种在有 Ca^{2+} 存在时可以抵抗蛋白酶的水解作用，介导细胞间相互黏附的分子，遂将其命名为钙离子依赖性 CAM 家族（Ca^{2+}-dependent cell adhesion molecules family）简称钙黏着蛋白（cadherin）家族，是一组依赖细胞外 Ca^{2+} 的 CAM，介导 Ca^{2+} 依赖性细胞间黏附，对于生长发育过程中细胞的选择性聚集具有重要作用。

一、钙黏着蛋白分子的结构

钙黏着蛋白是钙依赖性跨膜单链糖蛋白，通过同类或同分子亲和反应相结合[1]。钙黏着蛋白参与建立和维持细胞间连接，可能是最重要的形成细胞间联系的 CAM 之一。已克隆了 4 种钙黏着蛋白，一级结构相似，由 723～748 个氨基酸组成，不同的钙黏着蛋白分子在氨基酸水平上有 43%～58%的同源性，其分子量约为 120kDa。钙黏着蛋白分子为 Ⅰ 型膜蛋白，分子结构包括细胞膜外区、跨膜区和胞质区三部分（图 4-11）。

（1）细胞外区：为 4 个由 110 个氨基酸组成的重复单位构成，并含有由 4～5 个氨基酸残基组成的重复序列，近膜部位另有 4 个保守的半胱氨酸残基，分子外侧 N 端的 113 个氨基酸残基构成钙黏着蛋白分子的配体结合部位。胞膜外部分这些重复的单位中每个单位均含有 Ca^{2+} 结合位点，这就是其依赖于 Ca^{2+} 存在的原因[26]。外区还含有由组氨酸-丙氨酸-缬氨酸（histidine-alanine-valine，HAV）序列组成的黏附识别位点（亲同性黏附，homophilic adhesion）。

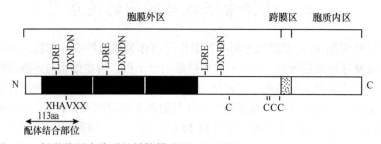

图 4-11 钙黏着蛋白分子的结构模式图；The molecular structure of the Cadherin

图中黑区部分显示钙黏着蛋白分子内重复结构域；LDRE 及 DXNDN 为重复序列

（2）跨膜区：由 4 个半胱氨酸组成，为跨膜锚定作用的高疏水区。

（3）细胞内胞质区：其氨基酸有高度的同源性，并通过与胞质联蛋白（catenin，Cat）形成复合物，从而与细胞内的微丝结合。钙黏着蛋白分子的胞质区高度保守，并与细胞内骨架相连，靠近 C 端的一半对于钙黏着蛋白分子介导的细胞黏附可能具有重要作用，去除此部分的钙黏着蛋白分子虽可与配体结合，但丧失介导细胞间黏附的作用。推测这是由于钙黏着蛋白分子与细胞内骨架相连，当钙黏着蛋白分子胞膜外区与相应配体结合后，向胞质内部分传递信号，导致胞质区与细胞骨架相接，稳定胞膜外区与配体的结合，发挥细胞黏附功能。

钙黏着蛋白选择性地与同种分子亲和性结合，这种黏附反应是利用其细胞外结构中 HAV 序列来识别和介导的，钙黏着蛋白的功能依赖于胞质内结构与细胞骨架元件之间的作用。但这种作用是间接地与三种胞质蛋白结合，这三种胞质蛋白为胞质联蛋白 α、β、γ，这些分子与钙黏着蛋白一起位于细胞的黏附小带（zonule adhesin）上，参与连接的形成与稳定。

二、钙黏着蛋白家族的组成和分布

根据钙黏着蛋白家族组织分布的不同分为 3 种亚型：E-钙黏素（首先在上皮中发现，E-Cad）、N-钙黏素（首先在神经中发现，N-Cad）和 P-钙黏素（首先在胎盘中发现，P-Cad）。E-Cad 也被称作 uvomorulin、L-CAM 或 cell-CAM120/80。后来又发现了一些新的成员，如 V-Cad、M-Cad、B-Cad、R-Cad 及 T-Cad。不同的钙黏着蛋白分子在体内有其独特的组织分布，它们的表达随细胞生长、发育状态不同而改变（表 4-1）。

E-Cad 基因定位于 16 号染色体 q22.1，cDNA 全长 4.8kb，于 1993 年被克隆；人类 E-Cad 基因组 DNA 全长 100kb，含 16 个外显子，于 1995 年由 Berx 首先克隆[27]。

表 4-1 钙黏着蛋白家族的组成、分布及其配体

cadherin 家族成员	分子量/kDa	主要分布组织	配体
E-cadherin	124	上皮组织	E-cadherin
N-cadherin	127	神经组织、横纹肌、心肌	N-cadherin
P-cadherin	118	胎盘、间皮组织、上皮细胞	P-cadherin

三、钙黏着蛋白的主要功能

钙黏着蛋白主要参与介导同型细胞间的黏附作用，在调节胚胎形态发生和维持成人组织结构完整性与细胞极性方面具有重要作用[21]。钙黏着蛋白的作用主要有以下几个方面。

（1）介导细胞连接，在成年脊椎动物，E-Cad 是保持上皮细胞相互黏合的主要 CAM，是黏合带的主要构成成分。桥粒中的钙黏着蛋白就是桥粒黏附蛋白（desmoglein/desmocollin）。钙黏素也是重要的形态分子，E-Cad 作用于形成完整的上皮层，P-Cad 则在基底层起作用，这些钙黏着蛋白的存在对于保持上皮和内皮结构很重要，其表达改变将导致细胞-细胞间正常连接完整性的丧失。

（2）参与细胞分化，钙黏着蛋白对于胚胎细胞的早期分化及成体组织（尤其是上皮及神经组织）的构筑有重要作用。在发育过程中通过调控钙黏着蛋白表达的种类与数量可决定胚胎细胞间的相互作用（黏合、分离、迁移、再黏合），从而通过影响细胞的微环境，参与细胞分化、器官形成的过程。

（3）抑制细胞迁移。

四、钙黏着蛋白与肿瘤的关系

恶性肿瘤中钙黏着蛋白系统失活或低表达的机制可能有 3 点[28]：①基因突变或丢失导致钙黏素表达下调或缺乏。例如，在肠癌基因研究中发现，50%细胞上钙黏着蛋白第 8（或 9）外显子缺失。②生物化学结构的改变，如钙黏素中的磷酸键结构改变。③胞质联蛋白（Cat）表达障碍。在某些钙黏素表达水平正常的癌组织中癌细胞仍有较强的侵袭能力。例如，人肺癌细胞系 PC9 细胞中钙黏素表达正常，但该肿瘤细胞系表现为侵袭性表型，研究发现是因为它不能合成 Cat 的缘故。

在钙黏着蛋白中 E-Cad 是近年来研究的热点。E-Cad 与肿瘤的侵袭转移密切相关，大量研究发现 E-Cad 分子在侵袭性肿瘤中表达下调（在中分化肿瘤中表现不一致，未分化癌中几乎没有表达），以致癌细胞易从瘤块脱落，成为侵袭与转移的前提。实验性上调或下调 E-Cad 可抑制或诱发肿瘤侵袭。因此，E-Cad 被认为是肿瘤侵袭抑制因子。虽然肿瘤钙黏着蛋白缺失与转移形成没有绝对的联系，但是，体积大、分化差、伴浸润和转移的肿瘤，其钙黏素表达水平多数降低，在食管癌、胃癌、乳腺癌、肺癌等中均体现出这种趋势[29]。因此，钙黏着蛋白表达的改变可能作为一种评价转移潜能的指标。研究发现，E-Cad 分子在正常的上皮组织及分化程度高的肿瘤细胞中分布于细胞的侧面，而在分化程度低的肿瘤细胞中分布于细胞的顶面或弥散分布。能表达一定水平 E-Cad 分子的肿瘤细胞，细胞间附着作用也有所减弱，可能与细胞表面的 E-Cad 异常分布有关。

第六节 其他未归类的黏附分子

除了上述四类 CAM 外，还有一些 CAM 目前尚未归类，包括一组作为选择素分子配体的寡糖决定簇或载有这类寡糖决定簇的糖蛋白，如 CD15、S-LewisX、S-LewisA；此外还有 CD44、MAd、MLA 等。本文在此主要介绍 CD44 分子。

一、CD44 分子结构

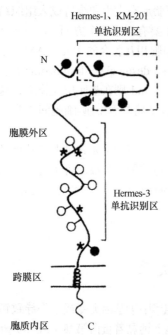

图 4-12　CD44 分子的结构；
Molecular structure of CD44
●：-N-连接的糖基化位点，○：C-连接的糖基化位点，★：硫酸软骨素连接位点

CD44 分子[也称为 Hermes 抗原，H-CAM、Pag-1 抗原，细胞外基质受体Ⅲ（ECM-Ⅲ）和淋巴细胞表面的归巢（homing）受体]是一种多功能的跨膜透明质酸受体，是由单一基因编码的具有高度异质性的单链膜表面糖蛋白家族，分子量为 85～250kDa，介导细胞与细胞间，细胞与 ECM 间的相互作用，可分为胞膜外区、跨膜区及胞质区三个部分：胞膜外区是 CD44 分子发挥生物学功能的重要结构，在此区域，CD44 分子信号肽的氨基端功能区（糖基化位点和硫酸软骨素连接位点）能够连接胞外基质及基底膜的透明质酸，从而调节细胞的运动及形态；跨膜区由 21 个疏水氨基酸组成；胞质区部分可作为 PKC 的底物被磷酸化，参与信号转导过程（图 4-12）。

二、CD44 的分类

人类 CD44 基因位于 11 号染色体短臂上[22]。其 cDNA 全长 50kb，有至少 20 个外显子。按其转录片段是否存在选择性拼接分为两种类型，一种是组成型外显子（constitutive exon，C-exon）；另一种是选择性拼接外显子，又称变异型外显子（variant exon，V-exon）。仅含 C-exon 的 CD44 转录子称作标准型 CD44（standard form CD44，CD44s），有 V-exon 插入的 CD44 转录子称为变异型 CD44（variant form CD44，CD44v）。V 区外显子有 10 种（CD44v1～10），分子量 85～160kDa，目前研究较多的是 CD44v6。

三、CD44 的功能

CD44 分子分布十分广泛，如 T 细胞、胸腺细胞、B 细胞、粒细胞、神经胶质细胞、成纤维细胞和上皮细胞等。作为细胞表面的 CAM，主要介导多种细胞与细胞、细胞与 ECM 之间的黏附作用。

（1）与透明质酸、纤黏连蛋白及胶原结合，介导细胞与细胞外基质之间的黏附。

（2）参与细胞对透明质酸的摄取及降解。

（3）介导淋巴细胞归巢。

（4）参与 T 细胞的活化。

（5）参与细胞伪足形成和促进细胞迁移。

（6）介导白细胞与活化的内皮细胞结合，参与炎症反应。

四、CD44 分子与肿瘤的关系

肿瘤细胞表达的 CD44 与宿主组织基质细胞及 ECM 作用可通过下列途径刺激肿瘤生长。

（1）固定肿瘤细胞，为肿瘤克隆形成提供病灶场所。

（2）肿瘤细胞与基质细胞相互作用产生生长因子及血管生成因子，此两种因子可促进肿瘤生长。

（3）肿瘤细胞通过 ECM 的蛋白聚糖获得隐蔽的生长因子，从而促进生长。

（4）CD44 还可识别宿主组织的额外配体，直接刺激肿瘤细胞增殖。

（5）CD44 的胞质内部分与细胞骨架蛋白作用，传导细胞分裂信号。

目前认为，不同的 CD44 分子在肿瘤浸润与转移过程中的作用不同。正常组织细胞或无转移能力的瘤细胞主要表达 CD44s，而具有转移能力的瘤细胞主要表达 CD44v。CD44 基因在许多肿瘤如胃癌、结肠癌、乳腺癌、宫颈癌、膀胱癌、肺癌及血液系统恶性肿瘤中均有异常表达[30]。研究发现，CEA 和 CD44s 在大肠癌原发灶中的表达呈显著正相关。由 CEA 介导的结肠细胞间的黏附可被 CD44 的单抗所阻断，表明 CEA 和 CD44 可能使用相同的抗原决定簇，在黏附过程中起协同作用，提示 CD44s 亦可作为一种新的肿瘤标志物，与 CEA 共同用于大肠癌患者的辅助诊断和无症状高危人群的筛选。

CD44 在很多种肿瘤细胞的表达比相应正常组织为高，并与肿瘤细胞的成瘤性、侵袭性及淋巴结转移性关。恶性肿瘤细胞表达 CD44 分子如同披上伪装的外衣，以逃避宿主免疫系统的识别而免于被杀伤，进而 CD44 分子与配体透明质酸等结合，使酪氨酸磷酸化激活信号转导系统，导致细胞形态、游走性的改变，促进了癌细胞的浸润和转移。Mayer 等认为 CD44v9 的表达与肿瘤的复发及生存率有关。CD44v9 在大肠癌组织中有明显的表达，这种表达与多种因素有关，如低分化者显著强于高分化者，Dukes C 期明显高于 Dukes A/B 期肿瘤，有淋巴结转移者明显强于不伴淋巴结转移者。结果提示 CD44v9 的表达与分化程度、Dukes 分期及转移密切相关，可以作为综合评价肿瘤生物学行为的指标。另外，CD44v6 可能通过促进癌细胞与血管内皮和 ECM 的黏附促进肿瘤向基质侵袭。

挑战与展望

近年来除了研究 CAM 在肿瘤细胞中表达，推测其在肿瘤生物学行为中的作用外，有学者开始研究 CAM 结构与配体、受体和反受体的相互作用，信号转导及调节机制的影响等。由于肿瘤及 CAM 本身的多样性和复杂性，肿瘤转移过程中许多现象还无法解释，CAM 的确切作用机制还没有完全清楚，相信随着分子生物学和分子病理学的发展，人们将会从本质上认识细胞黏附的机制和意义，认识 CAM 与疾病的内在联系，将为相关疾病的诊断和治疗提供更有效的途径。

思　考　题

1. 本章基本概念：细胞黏附分子（cell adhesion molecules，CAM），整合素（integrin），免疫球蛋白超家族（immunoglobulin superfamily，Ig-SF），癌胚抗原（carcinoembryonic antigen，CEA）、结肠癌缺失分子（deleted in colorectal carcinoma molecule，DCC），选择素家族（selectin family），钙黏着蛋白（cadherin），CD44。

2. 阐述 CAM 的基本结构和作用模式。

3. 简述细胞黏附分子在肿瘤研究中的意义。

4. 阐述 CEA 在肿瘤研究中的意义。

5. 为什么转移癌高表达 CD44?

参 考 文 献

[1] 陈莉，程纯. 现代病理学研究的基本问题[M]. 北京：科学出版社，2006.

[2] Bruijn J A，De H E. Adhesion molecules in renal diseases[J]. Laboratory investigation，1995，72（4）：387-394.

[3] Green L，Mould A，Humphries M. The integrin beta subunit[J]. International Journal of Biochemistry & Cell Biology，1998，30（2）：179-184.

[4] Sonnenberg A，Modderman P W，Hogervorst F. Laminin receptor on platelets is the integrin VLA-6[J]. Nature，1988，336（6198）：487-489.

[5] Ruoslahti E. Integrins[J]. Journal of Clinical Investigation，1991，87（1）：1-5.

[6] Lindmark G，Gerdin B，Påhlman L，et al. Interconnection of integrins alpha 2 and alpha 3 and structure of the basal membrane in colorectal cancer：relation to survival[J]. European Journal of Surgical Oncology，1993，19（1）：50-60.

[7] Zutter M M，Sun H，Santoro S A. Altered integrin expression and the malignant phenotype：the contribution of multiple integrated integrin receptors[J]. Journal of Mammary Gland Biology and Neoplasia，1998，3（2）：191-200.

[8] Wigle D A. Novel candidate tumor marker genes for lung adenocarcinoma[J]. Oncogene，2002，21（49）：7598-7604.

[9] Wang R N，Zhu Y B，Xue J Y. The relation between integrin，type IV collagenase and extracellular matrix in invasion and metastasis of gastric carcinoma[J]. Zhonghua Bing LI Xue Za Zhi，Chin J Pathol，1994，23（5）：278-281.

[10] Hangan D，Uniyal S，Morris C L，et al. Chau Integrin VLA-2（alpha2 betal）function in postectravasation movement of human rhabdomycsarcoma RD cells in the liver[J]. Cancer Research，1998，56（13）：3142-3149.

[11] Kageshita T，Hamby C V，Hirai S，et al. Alpha（v）beta3 expression on blood vessels and melanoma cells in primary lesions：differential association with tumor progression and clinical prognosis [J] .Cancer Immunol Immunother，2000，49（6）：314-318

[12] Demeure M J，Damsky C H，ELFMAN F，et al. Invasion by cultured human follicular thyroid cancer correlates with increased beta 1 integrins and production of proteases[J]. World J Surg. 1992，16（4）:770-776.

[13] Yamanaka I，Koizumi M，Baba T，et al. Epidermal growth factor increased the expression of alpha2beta 1-integrin and modulated integrin-mediated signaling in human cervical adenocarcinoma cells[J]. Experimental Cell Research，2003，286（2）：165-174.

[14] Panés J，Perry M，Granger D N，et al. Leukocyte-endothelial cell adhesion：avenues for therapeutic intervention [J]. British Journal of Pharmacology，1999，126（3）：537-550.

[15] True A L，Rahman A，Malik A B. Activation of NF-kappaB induced by H（2）O（2）and TNF-alpha and its effects on ICAM-1 expression in endothelial cells[J]. American Journal of Physiology Lung Cellular & Molecular Physiology，2000，279（2）：302-311.

[16] Larbi K Y，Allen A R，Tam F W，et al. VCAM-1 has a tissue-specific role in mediating interleukin-4-induced eosinophil accumulation in rat models：evidence for a dissociation between endothelial-cell VCAM-1 expression and a functional role in eosinophil migration[J]. Blood，2000，96（10）：3601-3609.

[17] Essani N A，Mcguire G M，Manning A M，et al. Differential induction of mRNA for ICAM-1 and selectins in hepatocytes，Kupffer cells and endothelial cells during endotoxemia[J]. Biochemical & Biophysical Research Communications，1995，211（1）：74-82.

[18] Nguyen K. VCAM-1 on activated endothelium interacts with the leukocyte integrin VLA-4 at a site distinct from the VLA-4/fibronectin binding site[J]. Cell，1990，60（4）：577-584.

[19] Polverini P J. Cellular adhesion molecules. Newly identified mediators of angiogenesis[J]. American Journal of Pathology，1996，148（4）：1023-1029.

[20] Penfold C N，Partridge M，Rojas R，et al. The role of angiogenesis in the spread of oral squamous cell carcinoma[J]. British Journal of Oral & Maxillofacial Surgery，1996，34（1）：37-41.

[21] Alahari S K，Reddig PJJuliano R L. Biological aspects of signal transduction by cell adhesion receptors[J]. International Review of Cytology-a Survey of Cell Biology，2002，220（220）：145-184.

[22] Wagner J G，Roth R A. Neutrophil migration mechanisms with an emphasis on the pulmonary vasculature[J]. Pharmacological Reviews，2000，52（3）：349-374.

[23] Barkalow F J，Barkalow K L，Mayadas T N. Dimerization of P-selectin in platelets and endothelial cells[J]. Blood，2000，96（9）：3070-3077.

[24] Norman K E，Katopodis A G，Thoma G，et al. P-selectin glycoprotein ligand-1 supports rolling on E- and P-selectin in vivo. [J]. Blood，2000，96（10）：3585-3591.

[25] Chen X L，Tummala P E，Olliff L，et al. E-selectin gene expression in vascular smooth muscle cells. Evidence for a tissue-specific repressor protein[J]. Circulation Research，1997，80（3）：305-311.

[26] Trikha M，De Clerck Y A，Markland F S. Contortrostatin，a snake venom disintegrin，inhibits beta 1 integrin-mediated human

metastatic melanoma cell adhesion and blocks experimental metastasis[J]. Cancer Research, 1994, 54 (18): 4993-4998.

[27] Bussemakers M J, Van B A, Mees S G, et al. Molecular cloning and characterization of the human E-cadherin cDNA[J]. Molecular Biology Reports, 1993, 17 (2): 123-128.

[28] Berx G, Staes K, Van H J, et al. Cloning and characterization of the human invasion suppressor gene E-cadherin (CDH1) [J]. Genomics, 1995, 26 (2): 281-289.

[29] Böhm M, Totzeck B, Birchmeier W, et al. Differences of E-cadherin expression levels and patterns in primary and metastatic human lung cancer[J]. Clinical & Experimental Metastasis, 1994, 12 (1): 55-62.

[30] Ahrens T, Sleeman J P, Schempp C M, et al. Soluble CD44 inhibits melanoma tumor growth by blocking cell surface CD44 binding to hyaluronic acid[J]. Oncogene, 2001, 20 (26): 3399-3408.

（顾婷婷　王建力　陈　莉）

Chapter 4 Cell Adhesion Molecules

Cell adhesion molecules (CAM), a class of molecules (glycoproteins or glycolipids) that presents on the cell surface mediated cell to cell or between cells and the extracellular matrix (ECM) in contacting and binding with each other (Fig. 4-1). Most CAM action depends on divalent divalent calcium (Ca^{2+} or Mg^{2+}).

Section 1   Outlines of Cell Adhesion Molecules

1. Main Functions of CAMs

(1) It mediates adhesion reaction with the interaction of ligand-receptors binding (between ECMs, or cells and cells, or to both cells and ECMs);

(2) It promotes cell function by increasing the intercellular adhesion or transmit signals (identification, activation, stretching, movement, growth, differentiation and signal transduction, etc.);

(3) It participates in a series of important physiological and pathological processes:

It maintains normal cell organism development, growth under physiological conditions. An important class of molecules of normal organ structure and tissue.

It plays important roles in pathological processes (inflammation, thrombosis, tumor metastasis, wound healing etc.).

2. Basic Structures of CAMs

CAMs are composed of three parts: cytoplasmic domain, transmembrane ribbon, extracellular domain:

(1) Extracellular domain, N-terminal portion of the peptide chain, having with a sugar chain, and it is responsible for ligand recognition;

(2) Transmembrane region, mostly for a transmembrane;

(3) Cytoplasmic region, C (carboxy)-terminal portion of the peptide chain, generally shorter, CAMs directly connected with under plasma membrane and cytoskeletal component -mediating cells migration, deformation. CAMs linked intracellular chemical signaling molecules ----mediating signal transduction pathways.

3. Three Patterns of CAM Roles (Fig. 4-2)

(1) Homophilic adhesion: Mutual recognition and binding between same types CAMs on two adjacent cell surface;

(2) Heterophilic adhesion: Mutual recognition and binding between two different types of CAMs on adjacent cell surface;

(3) Linker adhesion: Mutual recognition and binding between isotype CAMs on two adjacent cell surface through linked molecule outside the cells.

4. Classifications of CAMs

(1) Integrin superfamily

(2) Immunoglobulin superfamily

(3) Selectin family

(4) Ca^{2+}- dependent CAM family

(5) Unclassified CAMs

5. Significance of CAM in Cancer Research

(1) Diagnosis and Evaluation

Based on the locations and patterns of CAMs expressions in tumor tissues, may effectively assess the degree of tumor differentiation, stage, metastatic potential, recurrence and prognosis.

(2) Determining Tumor's Origin

Detecting the certain CAMs in different tissues, cells and its specific distributed manner may determine the source of the tumor tissue and its subtypes.

(3) Treating targets

Finding anti-factors for CAMs, or synthetic adhesion polypeptides or cell specific monoclonal antibody block tumor CAMs or recognize site on its ligands, may inhibit the invasion and metastasis of tumors. Now with antibodies combined with radionuclides or chemotherapy drugs targeting the cell-specific CAMs of tumor may carry on targeting therapy for patients.

Section 2   Integrin Superfamily

Integrin is a large family of transmembrane proteins, and it is major adhesion factors between cell and

ECM as a class of cell surface glycoproteins involving in cell signaling transduction and cytoskeletal changes. It plays an important role in cell growth, differentiation, forming connection and maintaining polarity and so on.

1. Molecular Structure of Integrin

Integrin is heterodimers of non-covalently linked which is composed by two strands α and β. Two subunits of α and β have a long extracellular fragment, the transmembrane segment and a shorter intracellular fragment. There are 40% -48% homology of amino acid sequence in various β subunits, the carboxyterminus of the β subunit polypeptide chain located in the cytoplasm. The polypeptide chain of amino acids sequences in various α subunit perform more heterophilic, its extracellular fragment contain divalent calcium (Ca^{2+} or Mg^{2+}) binding sites (Fig. 4-3).

Integrin causes cell activity and stroma reactions (Fig. 4-4)

2. Classification of Integrin Family

There are 18 kinds of α-subunit and 11 kinds of β subunit.α-subunit and β subunit binding to compose heterodimer integrin are at least 24 kinds (Fig. 4-5).

Different cells express different integrins. The same kind of cells express different integrins at different differentiation and growth stages. A cell can express many different integrins.

Integrin ligant：I type and IV type of collagen, LN, FN, Vitronectin, Endotoxin, ICAM-1, VCAM-1.There are RGD in integrin ligants, which sequence is the integrin binding motif.

Because polypeptides containing the RGD sequences can inhibit adhesion reactions between cell and extracellular proteins. So that synthetic peptides containing the RGD sequences can inhibit the binding of integrins and extracellular matrix, thus blocking platelet aggregation, infection, inflammation and tumor metastasis process that mediated by the integrin.

3. The main functions of the integrin family

There are three types according to patterns of integrin roles:

(1) Mediates the adhesion reaction between cells and ECM: mainly refers to the integrins containing beta 1 subunits, include α4/β1, α5/β1、αV/β1, which can be combined with FN；αV/β3、αV/β5 can be combined with LN, aαV/β3 can also be combined with fibrinogen.

(2) Mediates the adhesion reaction between cells-cells: mainly refers to the β2 subunits of integrin exists in various leukocytes, including the αL/β2 (LFA-1), its ligands is ICAM-1; αM/β2 (MAC-1) , ligands is ICAM-1, C3bi, ENdotoxiN; α4/β1, ligand is VCAM-1. The β3 subunit mainly exists in platelet surface, mediate platelet adhesion, and participate in thrombosis.

(3) Mediates the adhesion reaction of the cell - cell and the cell –ECM: mainly mediated by VlA-4 and αM/β2. In addition to β4, it can bind to actin and its related proteins, and α6β4 integrates is combined with LN to participate in the formation of half-bridge granule. Formation of ECM - integrin - cytoskeleton transmembrane complex, induce cytoskeleton rearrangement, reinforced mechanical connection between the cells; and   as a bridge, bi-directional transduce signal of intracellular and extracellular, widely affect biology behavior of cell, such as survival, growth, proliferation, differentiation, invasion and metastasis, etc. Extracellular fragment of integrin may adhere ECM or neighboring cells, and intracellular fragments indirectly connects to the cytoskeleton, then participate in many physiological processes, function of immune cell, regulate the organic occurrence, development, wound repair and thrombosis, etc.

4. Relationship between Integrins and Tumors

The expression of integrin molecule reduced in some tumors, weakened adhesion between tumor cells is in favor of tumor invasion and metastasis;

While in other tumors, integrin molecule expression increases, such as increasing in laminin receptor (LNR), are enable to promote tumor cells into the blood vessels or lymphatic vessels through degradating the basement membrane of vascular or lymphatic vessels.

And the same integrin at different stages of tumor development can present different levels of expressions and patterns.

Due to the diversity and complexity of the integrin, so now still have not been able to summarize the universal law of integrin in tumors.

Section 3　Immunoglobulin Superfamily (Ig-SF)

1. Molecular Structure of Ig-SF

The molecular structure of Ig-SF contains all molecules with Ig-like domains, and generally does not depend on Ca^{2+}. Ig-like domain means the β-sheet structure of two antiparallel by disulfide bonds. Molecular structure and Ig have high homology, which are composed by one or more Ig homology units, intermediate connecting by disulfide (Fig. 4-6). Different Ig-SF have same Ig repeats but the number of Ig repeats is different.

2. Classification of Ig-SF

Ig-SF is the most abundant family in cell surface molecules (more than 70 kinds of molecules), the main members are: Lymphocyte function-associated antigen (LFA) 2,3, CD28, Cytotoxic T lymphocyte associated antigen 4 (CTLA-4), B7-1, B7-2,Intercellular adhesion molecule (ICAM)1,2,3, Vascular cell adhesion molecule -1(VCAM-1), Neural cell adhesion molecule (NCAM), Platelet endothelial cell adhesion molecule-1 (PECAM-1), Carcinoembryonic antigen (CEA), deleted in colorectal carcinoma molecule (Colon deletion molecule, DCC), etc.

(1) ICAM-1 (80 kDa~110kDa)

The Ig's domain structure of the amino acid in ICAM-2 and ICAM-3have sequence homology, can be combined with LFA-1.ICAM-1 is a single-chain transmembrane glycoprotein (Fig. 4-7), core polypeptide is 55kDa. The ICAM-1 molecular weight can range from 80 to 110kDa because the ICAM-1molecule on different kinds of cells present the differences in the number of oligosaccharides.

Different ICAM are quite different in vivo distribution. ICAM-1 is distributed in lymph nodes and tonsils vascular endothelial cells, thymic dendritic cells, tonsil and glomerular epithelial cells, leukocytes, macrophages and fibroblasts and so on. In most tissues, the expressions of ICAM-1 are lower, while in the lung tissue is higher nearly 30-fold to other tissues. Inflammatory cytokines (IL-1, TNF-α, INF), phytohemagglutinin (PHA) and oxidants can promote the expression of ICAM-1 molecule. The bacteria products of G negative and G positive, LPS, and wall fatty acid (LTA) play an important role in the expression of ICAM-1 in human microvascular endothelial cells. ICAM-1 is also important to promote inflammatory cells (monocytes, lymphocytes and neutrophil's) adhesion to endothelial cells.

ICAM-2

There are two Ig domains presenting in outer membrane of ICAM-2 and have 34% homology with the two domains at ICAM-1 N-terminal. ICAM-2 distribution is more limit, and mainly expressed in vascular endothelial cells. ICAM-2 play a role in lymphocytes aggregation.

ICAM-3

There are five Ig domains present in outer membrane of ICAM-3, it only expressed in blood cells. ICAM-3 plays a role in regulation between the cell adhesion by LFA, CD11a / CD18) / ICAM-1 pathway.

(2) VCAM-1 or Inducible Cell Adhesion Molecule (INCAM)

VCAM-1 expressed in endothelial cells with activated IL-1, TNF-α and other cytokines, and also expressed in macrophages and fibroblasts, and mainly mediated adhesion of lymphocytes, monocytes, eosinophils and endothelial cells. Its molecular weight is 100kDa～110kDa.

(3) Platelet Endothelial Cell Adhesion Molecule (PECAM)

It is mainly expressed in endothelial cells, and it is extremely important in mediating the lymphocyte migrated through endothelial.

(4) CEA

It is a highly glycosylated cell surface glycoprotein. The molecular weight is 180KD.In recent years, analysis of CEA gene and protein structure have indicated that is a member of the Ig-SF, and is an important CAM, mediating adhesion reaction between non-calcium-dependent cancer cells or cells and extracellular collagen matrix. CEA can enhance tumor cells binding to normal cells. Early fetal digestive tract and some organizations have the ability to synthesize CEA, but gradually reduce the level after pregnancy of six months. After birth, it is very low. But slightly increased with age and slightly increased in smokers. CEA is carcinoembryonic antigen, a protein-rich polysaccharide complexes. In the serum of some cancer patients, it can be found that abnormally elevated the level of CEA. Based on the level of CEA may be judgment for prognosis and recurrence of tumor.

3. Main Functions of Ig-SF

It mainly mediates adhesion reaction of non-dependent Ca^{2+} cells with same cells or different cells. It participates in inter-cell recognition (including those with immune function of molecules, such as MHA, CD_4, CD_8 and T cell receptors).

(1) It participates in neural cell development (N-CAM, L1);

(2) It is involved in leukocyte cross-talks (ICAM-1, VCAM-1, PECAM-1);

(3) It is involved in the transmission of information, such as CSF-1R (colony stimulating factor-1 receptor), PGFR, and so on.

4. Relationship between Ig-SF and Tumors

(1) The role of Ig-SF killing tumor cells

Soluble ICAM-1 may inhibit NK cell killing effect on tumor cells, and tumor cells expressing ICAM-1 molecule may be associated with TIL (tumor-infiltration lymphocyte) killing effects.

(2) The relationship between the Ig-SF and tumor metastasis

There is a very close relationship between CEA and tumor metastasis.

CEA is significantly increased in colorectal cancer, stomach cancer, lung cancer and cholangiocarcinoma, liver cancer, pancreatic cancer, kidney cancer, breast cancer, esophageal cancer, ovarian cancer and other tumor tissues. Tumor cells secrete CEA into the local body fluids (chest fluids, ascites, digestive juices) and blood (serum) in above cancer. Lung cancer patients' CEA is higher in pleural effusion than that in serum. In early the primary colorectal cancer without metastasis, CEA positive rate is about 45% to 80%, and elevated serum CEA often indicates tumor recurrence and metastasis.

(3) The effect Ig-SF to tumor angiogenesis (ICAM-3, PE-CAM-1 promoting tumor angiogenesis)

Section 4   Selectin Family

Selectin, also known as lectin-like CAM, mainly involved in leukocyte and endothelial cell recognition and adhesion.

1. Molecular Structure of Selectin

A class of CAM which takes glycosylated as it's identify ligand, belongs to a transmembrane protein I. Its outer membrane portion has a high degree of homology, similar structure, constituting three domains:

(1) Calcium-Dependent Lectin Domains

The amino terminus outside selectin (about 120 amino acid residues) as the lectin-like domain (ligand binding and recognition) can bind to carbohydrate groups.

(2) Epidermal Growth Factor (EGF)-Like Domains

About 35 amino acid residues (synergy maintain selectin family molecule configuration).

(3) Complement Regulatory Protein-Like Ribbon

Near membrane area present $2\sim9$ complement regulatory protein functional areas, which includes homologous sequences repeats of $62\sim67$ amino acids, constituting different selectin (Fig.4-8).

2. Classfication of Selectin Family (Fig. 4-9)

(1) E (endothelium) Selectin

It only is expressed on endothelial cells. Generally the endothelial cells are inflammatory stimulated by IL-1, TNF-α or bacterial polysaccharidesit is expressed.

When endothelial cells was infected by endotoxin and inflammatory cytokines, it began to increase at less than 1h, peaked after 4-6h, and declined after 24h, so it plays an important role in vascular endothelial cells and neutrophil adhesion to sites of inflammation. In addition, it mediated tumor cell adhesion to endothelial cells in tumor blood metastasis. TGF-β can inhibit E selectin induction and transcription.

(2) P (platelet) Selectin

It is expressed on endothelial cells and platelets, and pre-stored in platelets α granules and Weibel-Palade small body of endothelial cells. It is expressed fast. When endothelial cells are activated by histamine, thrombin, complement and cytokine debris, P selectin can quickly move to the cell surface, and then it can be induced by LPS, TNF-α, IL-1, leading to its renewed expression, which suggesting that P selectin can make both early and late reactions to inflammation factors.

(3) L (leukocyte) Selectin

It is expressed on lymphocytes (mostly T, B cells and NK cells), monocytes, and not in endothelial cells. L selectin plays an important role in the early inflammatory response. Recent studies show that non-steroidal anti-inflammatory drugs can decrease the expression of L selectin on neutrophils.

3. Selectin Molecular Recognized Ligands

Lectin-like structure in selectin determines its ligand is sugar groups. There are three categories of structures having affinity to selectin:

(1) Some oligosaccharides --- sialylated Lewis oligosaccharides (FOS Lex) or similar structures

(2) Phosphorylated monosaccharides and polysaccharides

(3) Sulfated polysaccharides and glycolipids.

The oligosaccharide groups bind to selectin existed in a variety of glycoproteins or glycolipids, and distributed in a variety of cell surface, thus selectin molecule ligands distributed extensively in the body. It has been found selectin gene molecular recognised carbohydrate presented in the white cells, endothelial cells, the surface of some tumor cells and serum certain sugars protein molecules.

4. Selectin Functions

Selectin is leukocyte CAM, whose role is mediating leukocyte into the inflammatory damage zone and adhesion to endothelial cells depending on Ca^{2+}. Selectin plays an important role in the recruitment of leukocytes reaching the site of inflammation. L selectin on leukocyte surface recognized and binded to P selectin and E selectin on the surface of activated endothelial cells. Which can quickly raise the flowing leukocytes in blood and reduce rolling in inflammatory sites of vascular endothelium (i.e., by adhesion, separation, and then adhesion, so recycle), and finally into the site of inflammation through the blood vessels by chemotaxis (Fig.4-10).

5. Relationship between Selectin Family and Tumors

(1) Selectin as a serum tumor marker used to determine tumor progression, recurrence and metastasis, and assessment of prognosis.

(2) Selectin is related to tumor metastasis and organ selective.

(3) Soluble E- selectin often change in serum before clinical metastases, so serum selectin level is expected to become an important indicator of cancer detection.

(4) Selectin ligand sLeA, sLeX highly expressed in gastrointestinal tumors, and tumor recurrence when its content is increased again, the indicator for judgement of tumor recurrence has a certain value.

Section 5   Cadherin Family

Ca^{2+}-dependent cell adhesion molecules family (Cadherin) is a transmembrane glycoprotein with calcium-dependent single-chain, CAM of Cadherin family has a crucial role for the selective aggregation in process of growth and development of cells.

1. Moleculr Structure of Cadherin (I   Type Membrane Protein)

Extracellular domain: 110 amino acids repeating units with 4 to 5 repeats sequences. Each unit contains repetitive Ca^{2+} binding sites. Histidine-alanine-valine (HAV) sequence consist of the adhesion recognition site. (homophilic adhesion) (Fig. 4-11). Transmembrane region: By the four conserved cysteine residues, a transmembrane anchor role in a highly hydrophobic region. Intracellular domain aminoacids has a high degree of homology with the cytoplasmic-catenin (Cat) forms a complex binding to the intracellular action.

2. Composition and Distribution of Cadherin Family

Menbers and ligand	Molecule weight	Distribusion
E-Cadherin (E-Cad)	124kDa	epithelum

| N-Cadherin (N-Cad) | 127 kDa | nerve tissue, rhabdomyus, cardiomycyte |
| P-Cadherin (P-Cad) | 118KDa | placenta，mesothelnm,epithelum |

New discovered members: V-Cad, M-Cad, B-Cad, R-Cad and T-Cad. Different cadherin molecules have their own unique tissue distributions in the body, their expression are changed with cell growth, development and different states.

3. Main Functions of Cadherin

(1) It mediates cell connections, as the main component of the adhesive tape (desmosome). Cadherin is also an important form molecules and structure.

(2) It involves in cell differentiation and the process of organ formation. It plays an important role in early differentiation of embryonic cells and building of adult tissues (especially epithelial and nerve tissue). It decided interaction between embryonic cells in the development process through regulating the kinds and quantity of the Cadherin expression (adhesion, separation, migration, and then bonding).

(3) It inhibits cell migration. (E-Cad is as a metastasis suppressor molecule)

4. Relationship between Cadherin and Tumors

(1) E-Cad molecules locate in the side of the cell in epithelial tissue and high differentiated tumor cells. And they are distributed in the top surface or dispersed in poorly differentiated tumor cells. Abnormal distribution of E-Cad on cell surface decreased the adhesion between the tumor cells.

(2) The reduction of E-Cad is closely associated with tumor invasion and metastasis.

(3) E-Cad molecule downregulated in invasive tumors, and has no expression in most undifferentiated carcinoma.

Experimental up- or down-regulated E-Cad led to inhibitor induce tumor invasiveness. Therefore, E-Cad is considered as suppressor of tumor invasion.

Section 6   Unclassified CAM

In addition to the four categories of CAMs, which have not yet classified, including a group oligosaccharide determinant, as a selectin molecule ligand, or containing similar oligosaccharides determinants glycoproteins, such as CD15, S-Lewisx, S-Lewisa, CD44, MAd (mucosal addressin), MLA, etc.

1. Structure of CD44

CD44 molecules [also known as Hermes antigen, H-CAM, Pag-1 antigen, the extracellular matrix receptors III (ECM-III) and lymphocyte surface homingreceptor] is a multifunctional transmembrane hyaluronic acid receptors. It is a single chain membrane surface glycoprotein family with a high degree of heterogeneity encoded by a single gene (Fig. 4-12). A molecular weight is in the range of 85 KD-250KD.

(1) The outside of membrane area of CD44 molecules is an important structure that play its biological function where the nitrogen ribbon of CD44 signal peptide molecular can connect ECM with the hyaluronic acid of basement membrane to regulate cell motility and morphology;

(2) Transmembrane region consists of 21 hydrophobic amino acids;

(3) Cytoplasmic domain as a phosphorylated PKC substrate involved in signal transduction.

2. Classification of CD44

According to whether its transcription fragment has alternative splicing, it is classified into standard CD44s and variant CD44v.

(1) Standard CD44 (CD44s): containing only the constitutive exons (C-exon).

(2) Variant CD44 (CD44 v): There are variant exons (V-exon) inserted. CD44V1-10, molecular weight of about 85-160KD.

3. Functions of CD44

(1) Binding with hyaluronic acid, fibronectin and collagen, mediating adhesion between cells and ECM;

(2) Involving in cellular uptaking and degradating hyaluronic acid;

(3) Mediating lymphocyte homing;

(4) Involving in T cell activation;

(5) Involving in cell filopodia formation and promotes cell migration;

(6) Mediating the activation of leukocytes to bind endothelial cells, involving in inflammation

4. Relationship between CD44 Molecules and Tumors

(1) CD44 may fixe tumor cells and provide a forum for the tumor colony formation;

(2) CD44 mediated the interaction between tumor cells and stromal cell to produce the growth factors (GF) and tumor angiogenic factors (TAF), which may promote tumor growth;

(3) The tumor cells obtain hidden growth potency by CD44;

(4) CD44 may also identify additional host tissue ligands, directly stimulating the proliferation of tumor cells; especially the cytoplasmic portion of CD44v interact with cytoskeletal proteins to promote the transduction of cell division signals.

Malignant cells expressing CD44 molecule escape the host immune system recognition and avoid being killed. Subsequently, CD44 molecule bind ligands hyaluronic acid to activate tyrosine phosphorylation signal transduction system, which result in cell morphology changes, migration to promote cancer cell invasion and metastasis.

SLEX distributes in granulocytes, monocytes in normal adult, with containing four sugar fucose and sialic acid residues. It is also distributed in the epithelial tumor cell surface, such as lung cancer, stomach cancer, colon cancer and so on. Recent studies have pointed out that the sialylation SLEX on tumor cell surface acts as the ligands of E- selectin on endothelial cell, is the indicators for early diagnosis of colon cancer, cancer invasion, and poor prognosis.

Challenges and Prospects

The present study of CAMs is focus on the relationship between CAMs expression and location in tumor cells, and the tumor biological behavior to expose its roles and significance, and also begin to study the interaction between the ligand and structure of CAMs; the receptor and anti-CAM receptors; influence of regulatory and signaling mechanisms, etc.

Because of the diversity and complexity of tumor metastasis and CAM itself, now we still can 't explain many phenomena and exact mechanism of CAMs action.

With developing molecular biology and molecular pathology, we will understand the mechanisms of cell adhesion from nature and the intrinsic link between CAMs and cancer, providing more effective ways for tumor diagnosis and treatment.

Consider/Questions

1. Basic concepts in this chapter

Cell adhesion molecules(CAM), Integrin, Immunoglobulin superfamily (Ig-SF), Carcinoembryonic antigen(CEA), Selectin family, Cadherin,CD44.

2. Briefly describe the basic structures and roles patterns of CAMs.

3. Description of the significance of CAMs in cancer research.

4. Describe the function of CEA and its relationship with tumor.

5. Which significances are there tumor cells overexpressing CD44?

第五章 细胞周期的调控

  细胞周期的准确调控对生物的生存、繁殖、发育和遗传均是十分重要的。对简单生物而言，调控细胞周期主要是为了适应自然环境，以便根据环境状况调节繁殖速度，以保证物种的繁衍。复杂生物的细胞则需面对来自自然环境和其他细胞、组织的信号，做出正确的应答，以保证组织、器官和个体的形成、生长及创伤愈合等过程能正常进行，因此，需要更为精细的细胞周期调控机制。

第一节 细胞周期的基本概念

  自 1882 年发现细胞分裂以来，许多生物学家进行了大量的相关研究。直到 20 世纪 50 年代，随着 DNA 是遗传物质这一观念的形成及 DNA 双螺旋结构的确立，细胞周期的概念才逐渐成形。细胞从一次分裂结束起到完成另一次分裂结束止称为一个细胞周期（cell cycle）。细胞生长、分裂时，依次经过 G_1、S、G_2、M 期而一分为二，周而复始，因此又故称为细胞分裂周期（cell division cycle）。

  G_1 期：DNA 合成前期，其长短因细胞而异，主要为 S 期的 DNA 合成储备物质和能量。RNA 和蛋白质生物合成迅速进行，如合成各种与 DNA 复制有关的酶（数小时～数天～数月）。细胞体积明显增大，其中线粒体、核糖体增多，内质网更新扩大，来自内质网的高尔基体、溶酶体等也增加。动物细胞的两个中心粒彼此分离并开始复制。

  S 期：DNA 合成期，DNA 含量增加 1 倍（8～30 小时）是细胞周期的关键时期，使体细胞成为 4 倍体，每条染色质丝都转变为由着丝点相连接的两条染色质丝。与此同时，还合成组蛋白，进行中心粒复制。

  G_2 期：DNA 合成后期，DNA 合成终止（2～8.5 小时）为分裂期做最后准备。在 G_2 期中 RNA 和蛋白质的合成逐渐减少。其中微管蛋白的合成为分裂期（M 期）纺锤体微管的组装提供原料。中心粒完成复制而形成 2 对中心粒。

  M 期：细胞分裂期。细胞的有丝分裂（mitosis）需经前期、中期、后期、末期，是一个连续变化过程，由一个母细胞分裂成为两个子细胞。一般需 1～2 小时。

G_0 期：暂时离开细胞周期，停止细胞分裂，执行一定生物学功能的细胞所处的时期。处于此期的细胞接受刺激后可以进入细胞周期循环。

细胞在 G_1 期完成必要的生长和物质准备，在 S 期完成其遗传物质——染色体 DNA 的复制，在 G_2 期进行必要的检查及修复以保证 DNA 复制的准确性，然后在 M 期完成遗传物质到子细胞中的均等分配，并使细胞一分为二，循环周而复始。细胞周期的基本任务是保证 S 期的 DNA 复制和 M 期有同等的染色体分布到两个子细胞中去。

2001 年 10 月 8 日，美国人 Leland Hartwell、英国人 Paul Nurse、Timothy Hunt 因对细胞周期调控机制的研究而荣获诺贝尔生理学或医学奖。

第二节　细胞周期调控中的重要元素
一、细胞周期蛋白

1953 年霍华德等首先提出细胞分化是通过细胞周期完成的理论；1983 年，Evans 等首次在海洋无脊椎动物中发现一组蛋白质呈周期性出现，并调节细胞的生长，其被确定为细胞周期蛋白（cyclin）。1988 年科学家们发现细胞周期调节蛋白能与细胞分化周期编码蛋白结合并激活相应的蛋白激酶，从而促进细胞分裂。所以 cyclin 是一类合成和分解都与细胞周期同步、驱动细胞周期运转的特殊动力蛋白，能组成 cyclin 依赖性激酶的调节亚单位。迄今，至少发现有 11 种不同的 cyclin，分别为 cyclin A、cyclin B1、cyclin B2、cyclin C、cyclin D1、cyclin D2、cyclin D3、cyclin E、cyclin F、cyclin G 和 cyclin H。其中 8 种主要的 cyclin 已被分离。各类 cyclin 均含有一段约 100 个氨基酸的保守序列，称为周期蛋白框，介导 cyclin 与周期蛋白依赖性激酶（cyclin-dependent kinase，CDK）结合。不同的周期蛋白框识别不同的 CDK，组成不同的周期蛋白复合体，表现不同的 CDK 激酶活性。

根据 cyclin 调控细胞周期时相的不同，可分为 G_1 期和 M 期两大类。

（一）G_1 期 cyclin

G_1-cyclin（G_1 期周期蛋白）是指在 G_1 期或 G_1/S 交界期发挥作用，启动细胞周期和促进 DNA 合成的 cyclin，包括 cycln C、cyclin D、cyclin E。G_1 期是增殖细胞唯一能接受从外界传入的增殖或抑制增殖信号的时期。

1. cyclin D　其首先在酵母菌中被发现，它能激活 CDK4、CSK6，驱动细胞通过细胞周期限速点（START）。G_1 期 cyclin D 表达，并与 CDK4、CDK6 结合，使下游的蛋白质如 Rb 磷酸化，磷酸化的 Rb 释放出转录因子 E2F，促进许多基因的转录，如编码 cyclin E、cyclin A 和 CDK1

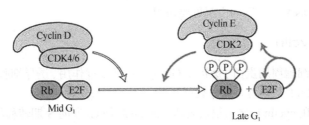

图 5-1　Cyclin D、Cyclin E、CDK4/6、CDK2，使 Rb 磷酸化促进细胞进入增殖周期；Cyclin D，Cyclin E and CDK4/6，CDK2 genes make phosphorylation of Rb to release E2F to promote cell cycle

的基因。E2F-1 介导 mRNA 转录使细胞进入增殖状态(图 5-1)。cyclin D 有 3 个亚型,包括 cyclin D1、cyclin D2、D3,具组织特异性。cyclin D1 与 cyclin D2 功能相似,都在酵母子细胞中起作用,cyclin D3 在酵母母细胞中起作用。许多研究表明在细胞周期的调节中 cyclin D 是一个比其他 cyclin 更加敏感的指标。

(1)cyclin D1 的编码基因位于 11q13 上,全长约 15kb,含有 5 个外显子,称为 PRAD1 或 CCND1,其编码蛋白含 295 个氨基酸,相对分子质量约 34000kDa,与其他 cyclin 相比最小,主要是因为其 N 端缺少一个"降解盒"片段,该蛋白半衰期很短,不足 25 分钟。它的 C 端有一个富含脯氨酸(P)、谷氨酸(E)、天冬氨酸(S)、丝氨酸和苏氨酸(T)残基的 PEST 序列,在蛋白质转化和降解中起作用。其 N 端有 LX-Cys-X-Glu 序列,是与 Rb 蛋白及 p107 蛋白结合所必需的位点。在有生长因子的情况下,cyclin D1 在细胞周期中首先被合成,并于 G_1 中期合成达到高峰,cyclin D1 的功能主要是促进细胞增殖,是 G_1 期细胞增殖信号的关键蛋白质,其过度表达可致细胞增殖失控而恶性化,因此被认为是癌基因。

(2)Cyclin D2 的编码基因位于 12p13,称为 CCND2,在正常的二倍体细胞及 Rb 阳性肿瘤细胞中 cyclin D2 的表达呈波动状态,其峰值在 G_1 晚期。给 G_1 期细胞微量注射 cyclin D2 抗体,可使表达 cyclin D2 的淋巴细胞停滞在 G_1 期,说明 cyclin D2 是细胞从 G_1 向 S 期转移所必需的。

(3)cyclin D3 的编码基因位于染色体 6p21,称为 CCND3。正常和恶性组织中未见 cyclin D3 基因异常及其蛋白的过度表达。目前认为 cyclin D3 似乎不直接反映恶性度,而是肿瘤发展到晚期的结果。

2. cyclin C 与所有 cyclin 的同源性最低,主要在果蝇及人类细胞中发现,它与其他 G_1-cyclin 不同的是其 mRNA 和蛋白质水平在 G_1 早期达最高,可能在 G_1 早期发挥作用。

3. cyclin E 是人类的 G_1-cyclin,在 cyclin D 之后出现,于 G_1/S 转化过程中表达,人类 cyclin E 基因定位于染色体 19q12-q13。由 4 个外显子和 3 个内含子组成,mRNA 长 2.2 kb。编码一个含 395 个氨基酸的多肽,分子量 50kDa。cyclin E 中 1/3 段有一大约含 87 个氨基酸的高度保守区为周期蛋白盒,此为 CDK 结合所必须。cyclin E 蛋白的 C 端存在 PEST 序列。此外,cyclin E 尚能被 SCF(SKP l-cullin-2-F-box protein)中的 S 期激酶相关蛋白-2(S-phase kinase-associated protein-2,SKP2)经泛素路径降解[1],缺乏 SKP2 的细胞表现 cyclin E 蛋白降解不足并不断积累。cyclin E 基因及其产物的表达在细胞周期的 G_1 中期上升,至 G_1 晚期或 S 早期达高峰,然后经与 PEST 序列有关的蛋白水解或泛素路径降解而迅速下降。cyclin E 在正常细胞和肿瘤细胞中主要在 G_1 晚期发挥正调控细胞周期的作用。

cyclin E 虽与 M-cyclin(M 期细胞周期素)的同源性很高,但它的 mRNA 及蛋白水平在 G_1/S 交界处急剧升高达峰值,因此它与 cyclin D 一样都是 G_1 期 cyclin,与相应的 CDK 形成复合物,从不同方面调节 G_1 期,促进细胞通过 G_1 期进入 S 期。cyclin E 对于 G_1/S 的转化更为重要,在人类细胞的 DNA 合成启动中起重要作用。

(二)M 期 cyclin

M-cyclin(M 期细胞周期蛋白)是指在 G_2/M 交界期发挥作用、诱导细胞分裂的一类 cyclin,包括 cyclin A 、cyclin B,均为有丝分裂所必需。

1. cyclin A 它在 cyclin E 之后很快表达。cyclin A 是 G_1 期向 S 期转移的限速因素,可促进细胞从 G_2 期向 M 期的转移。它由 CCNA 基因编码,与 CDK1 结合,CDK1 使底物蛋白磷酸化,发生染色体凝缩、核膜解体等下游细胞周期事件。

2. cyclin B 是有丝分裂蛋白激酶的一个亚单位,能促进 G_2 期向 M 期的过渡。哺乳动物

cyclin B 在 S 晚期合成。

3. cyclin A 与 cyclin B 之间存在多种差异

（1）周期积累方式不同，cyclin A 含量在 S 期及 G₂ 期初最高，cyclin B 在 G₂ 期末含量最高。

（2）结合的催化亚基不同，cyclin A 与 p33cdc2 结合，cyclin B 与 p34 cdc2 结合。

（3）功能不同，cyclin A 在 S 期发挥作用，与 DNA 的复制完成有关，cyclin B 在 G₂/M 交界处发挥作用，诱发细胞分裂。

（4）对细胞分裂的影响不同，cyclin B 持续升高可使细胞停滞于分裂期，而 cyclin A 的持续升高并不影响细胞分裂的完成。

（三）Cyclin 的降解

G₁ 期 Cyclin 其 N 端没有降解盒，C 端有一段 PEST 序列与其降解有关。G₁ 期 cyclin 经与 PEST 序列有关的蛋白水解或经 SKP2 泛素路径降解。M-cyclin 分子近 N 端含有一段 9 个氨基酸组成的破坏框，参与泛素介导的 cyclin A 和 cyclin B 的降解。分裂后期，cyclin 通过与泛素连接酶催化的泛素结合后被蛋白酶体（proteasome）水解。cyclin A、cyclin B 的降解是细胞脱离有丝分裂所必需。

综上所述，各种 cyclin 随特定细胞时相而出现（图 5-2）。

G₁ 早期：cyclin D-CDK2/CDK4（启动子）。

G₁ 晚-S 早期：cyclin E-CDK2（细胞进入 S 期）。

S 期：cyclinA- CDK2，cyclin D、cyclin E 降解。

S 晚-G₂ 早期：cyclin A- cdc2 、cyclin B-cdc2（细胞进入 G₂ 期）。

G₂/M 转化期：cyclin B-CDK1（细胞进入 M 期）。

cyclin H 与 cyclin C 有较高的同源序列，可以和 CDK7 装配成全酶对细胞周期各阶段行使调节作用。

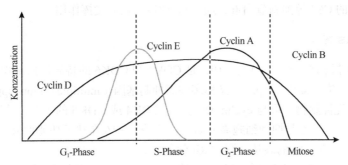

图 5-2　随特定细胞时相而出现的细胞周期蛋白；Various cyclins Appear with specificcquphases

二、周期蛋白依赖性激酶

周期蛋白依赖性激酶（CDK）是调节细胞周期的另一个重要蛋白，是一类重要的丝氨酸/苏氨酸蛋白激酶，包括 CDK1～CDK7。CDK 的主要生物学作用是启动 DNA 的复制和诱发细胞的有丝分裂，以复合物形式出现，该复合物分为催化亚基和调节亚基两部分，催化亚基为 CDK，调节亚基为 cyclin。CDK 有三个重要的功能区，第一功能区是 ATP 的结合部位，是该酶的活性部位；第二功能区是调节亚基的结合部位；第三功能区是 P13sucl 的结合部位（P13sucl 能抑制激酶的活性，阻止细胞进入或退出 M 期）。

　　G_0 期静止细胞可由丝裂原刺激而诱导 CDK4 的表达。CDK4 可能是 TGF-β 介导的生长抑制靶点，下调 CDK4 的表达可能在细胞分化过程中起重要作用。

　　在高等真核生物中，cyclin 主要有 cyclin A、cyclin B、cyclin C、cyclin D、cyclin E 五种，它们都能与 CDK 结合，相对应的 cyclin 与 CDK 装配成全酶，促进细胞分裂。不同 cyclin 在细胞周期不同时相表达量不同，并结合不同的 CDK。CDK 为调控中心，为催化亚单位；cyclin 是调节亚单元，起正调控作用；反应底物为 Rb 蛋白，通过 Rb 蛋白的磷酸化而实现细胞周期的转化（正调控）；真核细胞的细胞周期由 cyclin 依次激活相应的 CDK 所推动。

　　cyclin-CDK 协调周期中诸如 DNA 复制及分离，中心体的复制及分离，纺锤体的形成等重要事件。cyclin 必须与相应的 CDK 相结合，经磷酸化后方具活性，促使细胞周期有关蛋白表达。G_1 早期 cyclin D 表达并与 CDK2 或 CDK4 结合，成为始动细胞周期的启动子。

　　G_1 晚期、进入 S 早期后 cyclin E 表达，并与 CDK2 结合，推动细胞进入 S 期；进入 S 期后，cyclin A 表达，cyclin D、cyclin E 降解；S 晚期、G_2 早期，cyclin A、cyclin B 表达，并与 cdc2 结合，促进细胞进入 M 期。Cyclin A 和 CDK2 相结合可以调节 S 期进入 G_2 期；cyclin B_1、cyclin B2 可与 CDK1 结合并在 G_2/M 转化期间活性达到最高峰；与 cyclin C 匹配的 CDK 及其酶解底物目前尚不清楚；cyclin H 与 cyclin C 有较高的同源序列，可以和 CDK7 装配成全酶对细胞周期各个阶段行使调节作用。

三、周期蛋白依赖性激酶抑制剂

　　周期蛋白依赖性激酶抑制剂（CDK inhibitory protein，CKI）是 CDK 抑制蛋白，通过竞争性地抑制 cyclin 或 cyclin-CDK 复合物，导致 cyclin 生物学功能丧失；对细胞生长起负调控作用。

　　G_1 期 CDK 的负调节子有 2 个蛋白家族：INKs 和 CIP/KIPs。

　　CKI 为负调控因子，CKI 抑制 CDK 催化活性而发挥作用。癌基因和抑制基因产物及由抑癌基因诱导产生的 CKI 等抑制蛋白群，通过 G_1 期控制点而发挥作用。

（一）INKs 家族

　　INKs 家族包括 p15、p16、p18、p19，是 CDK4 和 CDK6 的特异性抑制物。

　　1. p16INK4 位于染色体 9p21，又称多肿瘤抑制基因（multiple tumor suppressor，MTS），是 CDK4 的特异性抑制物，可与 cyclin D 竞争与 CDK4 或 CDK6 的结合，抑制 CDK4 对细胞生长分裂的正向作用，参与抑制细胞周期 G_1/S 的转化。p16 在缺乏功能性 Rb 的细胞中水平上升，提示 Rb 可能抑制 p16 的表达，同时 Rb 刺激 cyclin D 的表达。

　　2. p15INKB 位于 9 号染色体紧邻 p16 的区域，它与 p16 在前 50 个氨基酸有 44% 相同，在其后 81 个氨基酸有 97% 相同。这两个蛋白质都有 4 个锚蛋白区，都只能结合并抑制 CDK4 或 CDK6。p15 与 p16 一样属于抑癌基因。

（二）KIPs 家族

　　KIPs 家族包括 p21、p27、p57 等，能抑制各种 cyclin-CDK 复合物，阻止 CDK 激酶的激活，或阻止活化的 CDK 激酶活性。

　　1. p27 目前被很多学者认为是有可能最直接地影响 G_1/S 期限制位点的调控。广泛抑制 cyclin-CDK 复合物。正常情况下 p27 在 G_0/G_1 时表达增高，进入 S 期后表达下降。p27 通过与 CDK 亚单位的结合，使 CAK（CDK 激活酶）不能诱导 CDK 磷酸化（CDK 活性状态是以磷酸化形式存在）。非活化的 CDK 不能使 Rb 蛋白磷酸化，使细胞停留在 G_1 期，对细胞周期进行负调控。

1994 年 Polyak 从用 TGF-β 处理抑制细胞生长和细胞间接触抑制生长的细胞系 MV1lu 中发现一个 27kDa 的热稳定蛋白，命名为 p27，并用亲和透析法分离出 p27，以自动 Edman 降解法获得了数个 p27 的肽链序列，据此设计出数个寡核苷酸探针，用 RT-PCR 法进行 cDNA 文库筛选，克隆出人（肾）、鼠（胚胎）、貂 p27 的 cDNA。其基因定位于染色体 12p13.1 及 12p13.2 处，至少包含 2 个外显子和 2 个内含子，人的 p27cDNA 全长 594bp，编码 198 个氨基酸，是高度保守的蛋白分子，在人、鼠、貂中 p27 的氨基酸主序列有 90% 的同源性，其 C 端均含有一个双支核定位信号。其 N 端介导抑制 CDK，12～87 氨基酸主序列与 p21 同源。当其丢失 N 端的 8 个氨基酸或 C 端的 15 个氨基酸，其抑制活性减弱。若再丢失 N 端 7 个氨基酸时其抑制活性完全丧失。p27 与 p21 在 N 端序列上有 42% 相同，且像 p21 一样能广泛抑制 cyclin-CDK 复合物，但是 p27 介导抑制 CDK 的区域与 p21 不尽相同。p27 还可阻止 Rb 蛋白磷酸化，其过度表达能抑制细胞进入 G_1 期。p27 在调节细胞进入和退出 M 期中也起重要作用，抗丝裂原环境中细胞生长停滞与 p27-CDK2 复合物的量相关。

p27 还参与对细胞分化的调控。同 p21 一样它可诱导未成熟细胞进行分化。有对少突神经胶质细胞分化进行研究发现，p27 在少突神经胶质前体细胞增殖时进行性地积聚，当其分化为少突神经胶质细胞时 p27 水平达最高峰，认为 p27 的积聚既部分地参与决定前体细胞何时停止增殖、启动分化的内在监控机制，又部分地参与在启动分化时使细胞周期停滞的效应机制。同时 p27 也可诱导肿瘤细胞分化，如外源性 p27 可诱导原巨核细胞白血病细胞分化，但 p27 不能诱导成熟正常细胞的衰老。

p27 表达水平受多种因素调控，如有丝分裂原、抗增殖信号因子、细胞因子、癌基因及接触抑制等。TGF-β 具有抑制细胞增殖、调节细胞分化、使细胞黏附亢进、调节血管生成和免疫抑制等多种功能。TGF-β 和接触抑制能共同调控转录 CKI p27 和 p15，通过靶因子 cAMP 介导 G_1 期停滞，其负调节信息的共同通路是抑制 CDK 和 cyclin G_1 功能，发挥 CKI 抑制作用。TGF-β 对 p27 表达的影响是双相的，在大多数细胞中，TGF-β 可诱导 p27 的表达，但是在正常垂体前部和垂体瘤细胞中，TGF-β 可下调 p27 mRNA 及蛋白的表达。PDGF、EGF 等也可下调 p27 的表达。p27 对细胞周期的调控主要依赖于其蛋白表达水平，而非基因突变。p27 的表达受多种因素调控，其表达下降或缺失会引起基因组不稳定，甚至导致肿瘤发生。p27 抑制 cyclin-CDK 复合物的负性调节作用。

2. p21　该基因位于染色体 6p21.2，第 17～71 氨基酸含有 cyclin 结合抑制区。p21 可能阻碍细胞进入 S 期；能抑制应激激活的蛋白激酶（stress-activated protein kinase，SAPK），参与细胞应激状态时的信号转导级联系统的调节。

p21 与 p27 的 N 端序列上有 44% 相同，都能广泛抑制 cyclin-CDK 复合物，但两者介导抑制 CDK 的区域不尽相同。

第三节　细胞周期调控中各元素间的相互作用

细胞周期的调控可分为外源性和内源性调控，外源性调控主要是由细胞因子及其他外界刺激引起；内源性调控主要是通过 cyclin-CDK-CKI 的网络调控来实现。细胞能否通过限制点从 G_1 期进入 S 期很大程度上取决于 G_1 期内 cyclin D1/cyclin E/cyclin A 的积累、CDK4/CDK6/CDK2 与细胞周期抑制蛋白的化学剂量关系及 INK4 的活性。

一、Rb 基因

细胞一旦从 G_0 期进入细胞周期，cyclin D（D1、D2、D3）开始表达，其作用是延迟对生长因子刺激的早期反应，其合成和与 CDK（如 CDK4、CDK6）的结合依赖于有丝分裂信号的刺激。探讨 G_1 调控机制可能为从细胞周期角度研究癌变机制和对癌症基因治疗提供重要依据。

Rb 基因位于 13q14.1，27 个外显子，编码 928 个氨基酸的 110kDa 蛋白质。30%的视网膜母细胞瘤中可见包括 Rb 基因在内的 DNA 缺失，甚至染色体片段的缺失。

Rb 基因转录产物 Rb 蛋白是主要的转录信号连接物，在细胞周期中起制动器功能。它能与转录因子 E2F 结合并阻止相应基因转录表达，从而抑制细胞生长。cyclin D 是 Rb 调节细胞周期的基础。cyclin D1-CDK4 复合物可看作 G_1 期 Rb 蛋白激酶，它能结合 Rb 的 N 端，磷酸化 Rb 蛋白，使转录因子释放，导致 G_1/S 转化。当细胞受到增殖刺激时 cyclin D1 与 CDK4、CDK6 结合形成二元复合物，使 Rb 磷酸化[2]，Rb 一旦被磷酸化，其结合 E2F-1 的作用丧失，E2F-1 介导的 mRNA 转录得以进行，细胞进入增殖状态（图 5-3）。

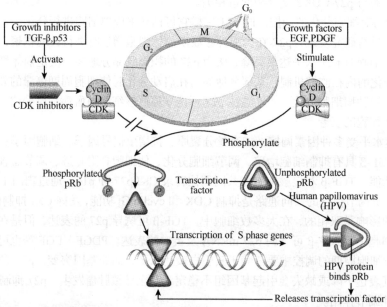

图 5-3　Cyclin D 介导的细胞周期中 *Rb* 基因的作用；Rb gene role in cell cycle mediated by Cyclin D

有报道认为 Rb 可抑制 DNA 聚合酶Ⅲ的功能，Rb 的磷酸化也可能负性调节该通路。低磷酸化的 Rb 蛋白能使细胞停滞于 G_1 期。简言之 cyclin D1 灭活 Rb 使细胞进入 S 期开始 DNA 复制。cyclin D1 与 Rb 的功能是相互依赖的，缺乏 Rb 功能的细胞显微注射 cyclin D1 抗体后，不能使细胞停滞于 S 期之前。低磷酸化的 Rb 还可刺激 cyclin D1 的转录，使其合成增加，并活化再导致 Rb 磷酸化，这样形成负反馈环以调节 cyclin D1 的表达。

二、细胞转录因子

在许多 DNA 合成基因和细胞生长调控基因的启动子中（如 C-myc、N-myc、C-myb、DNA 聚合酶等）均含有 E2F 的位点，E2F 可以直接活化这些基因启动 DNA 合成，使细胞进入 S 期。在 E2F 基因活化转录的功能区内有一段 18 个氨基酸的残基序列可与 Rb 结合，Rb 通过与 E2F

功能区的结合遮盖其功能区，而抑制其活性转录功能，使 E2F 介导的二氢叶酸还原酶基因、CDK 基因及 E2F 自身基因不能转录，抑制 DNA 合成。其中二氢叶酸还原酶是体内四氢叶酸库稳定的关键酶，该酶不能转录时，与一碳单位转移有关的生化反应及 DNA 合成受阻（图 5-4）。

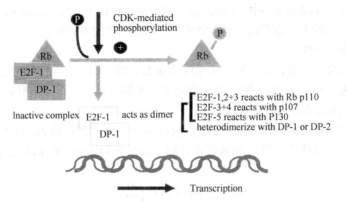

图 5-4　CDK 介导 E2F 活化；CDK mediated E2F activation

三、S 期激酶相关蛋白-2

SKP2 是一种肿瘤标志物，SKP2 在正常组织中只表达于扁桃体和胎盘组织中，但在肿瘤组织中 SKP2 表达广泛，包括部分结肠癌、前列腺癌、胰腺癌和皮肤癌，尤其在肺癌、乳腺癌、卵巢癌和子宫内膜癌高表达，并在淋巴瘤和乳腺癌肿瘤发生中起重要作用。在结肠癌和肝癌中 SKP2 的表达与 p27 表达水平下降有一定的相关性[21]。SKP2 还能使 E2F 通过泛素路径降解。

四、cyclin E，cyclin A 和 cyclin B

cyclin E 和磷酸化的 CDK2 结合成复合物。cyclin E-CDK2 的作用是通过正反馈以促进 Rb 磷酸化和 E2F 的释放[1, 2]。另外，E2F-1 刺激其自身转录，E2F 和 cyclin E 在细胞进入 G_1/S 转换时，其活性快速升高。与不可逆性进入 S 期一致的是由 cyclin D 操纵的有丝分裂原依赖性 Rb 的失活转变为 cyclin E 操纵的有丝分裂原非依赖性 Rb 的失活。通过 Rb 磷酸化或直接损害 Rb 基因而使 cyclin E 失活缩短 G_1 期，使细胞变小，但不能消除细胞对分裂原和黏附信号的要求，因为 Rb 阴性细胞保留了一些对生长因子的需求。cyclin E 也能干扰 p107 和 E2F 的功能。cyclinE-CDK2 复合物受相应的 CKI 如 P21WAFl 和 p27kipl 的抑制而失去活性。

CKI 与 cyclin E 竞争 CDK 配体，阻止底物磷酸化，将细胞阻滞于 G_1 期，抑制细胞增殖。当抑制物的活性丢失或水平下降后，细胞可以通过 G_1 期进入 S 期。另外 cyclin D1 的过度表达可以诱导 cyclin E 的表达及 CDK2 的磷酸化，从而在静止的细胞中激活 cyclin E-CDK2 复合物的活性，因此 cyclin D 和 cyclin E 共同高水平表达是使 G_1 期缩短的主要原因。此外，当外来信号如生长因子（growth factor）的刺激使 cyclin D1、cyclin D3 大量合成并与 CDK4 和（或）CDK6 结合成复合物，调节 G_1 和 S 期的转化。

cyclin A 在 S 期与 CDK2 结合，在 M 期与 cdc2 结合。cyclin B 与 Cdc2 结合，结合后的复合物立即由于 Cdc2 的 14、15 位酪氨酸磷酸化而被灭活。S 期及 G_2 期灭活的复合物在胞质内积累，直到 G_2 晚期由 Cdc25 介导 Cdc2 的 14、15 位酪氨酸去磷酸化而激活。正常细胞 DNA 损伤后会阻止 Cdc2 的 14、15 位酪氨酸去磷酸化，使细胞停滞于 G_2 期。此时细胞体积较大，核深染，不能进行核分裂。有实验发现，在细胞质中存在一种因子叫 M 期促发因子（促成熟因子）（Maturation promoting factor，MPF）是一种由 Cdc2 蛋白激酶和 cyclin 蛋白构成的复合物，当 cyclin 蛋白与 Cdc2 激酶结合形成一个有活性的 MPF 时，与转录有关的因子即被磷酸化，DNA 合成有关基因活化。当细胞分裂完成后，cyclin 蛋白自行降解，而 Cdc2 蛋白继续参与下一个细胞循环。在细胞周期中，Cdc2 蛋白的含量是稳定的，而 cyclin 的含量和种类则是处于一种动态变化过程中，在不同的生物中或一个细胞周期的不同时期，cyclin 都不尽相同，有丰富的多样性或变化性。

细胞周期进行时，可使 cyclin A-CDK 和 cyclin B-CDK 保留高度的磷酸化状态，直到完成有丝分裂和重新进入 G_1（或 G_0）期。许多细胞进入 S 期对生长因子和黏附信号有双重要求，既要有 cyclin A 基因表达，也要有 Rb 磷酸化。

在 S 晚期 cyclin A-CDK2 激活后，嵌合的 cyclin A 可以干扰正常的 cyclin A 与 Rb 相关蛋白 p107 和转录因子 E2F 的相互作用，导致转录抑制。刺激 S 期必需依赖 E2F 的基因转录。

五、p21 和 p27

（1）p21 结合并抑制多种 cyclin-CDK 复合物，包括 cyclin A-CDK2、cyclin D-CDK4、cyclin E-CDK2，负性调节 CDK 功能，并结合及灭活 DNA 复制机制中的成分（如 PCNA 和 DNA 聚合酶Ⅵ等）。实验证明，正常细胞多数 cyclin-CDK 复合物都与 p21 结合，而多数转化细胞中则不结合。p21 是 p53 作用的靶点，p21 启动子含有 p53 结合位点，野生型 p53 可激活 p21 转录。p21 在 p53 介导的 DNA 损伤所致的 G_1 期停滞中起重要作用：G_1 期 DNA 损伤可激活 p53，诱导 p21 转录，导致 cyclin D-CDK4 和 cyclin E-CDK2 抑制，从而阻止细胞进入 S 期。而缺乏 p53 的细胞，DNA 损伤后不能诱导 p21 转录合成，从而不能使损伤 DNA 得到修复，导致染色体异常和基因不稳定。在 G_1 期细胞对 DNA 损伤的反应中，p53 和 Rb 起关键作用。较低水平的 DNA 损伤即可诱导 p53 依赖的 G_1 期停滞的延长，并长时间诱导 p21，提示 p53 的关键作用是阻止损伤的 DNA 复制，其在 DNA 损伤诱导的凋亡中起重要作用。通过凋亡可剔除 DNA 损伤的细胞以抑制肿瘤发生的重要作用已被人们所接受。p21 基因多态性在增强某些肿瘤的易感性中起重要作用。

（2）p27 主要通过与 CDK 或 cyclin-CDK 复合物结合，实现对 CDK 活性的抑制。CDK 活性状态是以磷酸化形式存在的。CAK 可诱导 CDK 磷酸化，而 p27 通过与 CDK 亚单位的结合，使 CAK 不能与 CDK 直接发生作用，从而阻断了 CAK 诱导 CDK4 Thr172 和 CDK2 Thr160 的磷酸化过程，使 CDK 处于非活性状态。非活化的 CDK 不能使 Rb 蛋白磷酸化，对细胞周期进行负调控。p27 还可阻止 Rb 蛋白磷酸化，其过度表达能抑制细胞进入 G_1 期。同时，CDK 在 S 期是必需的，该基因不能表达，细胞则不能实现从 G_1 到 S 期的转换。Rivard 等发现在体外 p27 能与 cyclin E-CDK2、cyclin D-CDK4、cyclin D-CDK6、cyclin A-CDK2 等具有活性的复合物结合，且能抑制其活性，使细胞停留在 G_1 期。

p27 在调节细胞进入和退出 M 期中起重要作用，抗丝裂原环境中细胞生长停滞与 p27-CDK2 复合物的量相关。p27 的功能可能建立了一个 G_0 期 CDK 激活和进入 S 期前必须超越的抑制性门槛。

G_1-S 期调控中各元素间的相互作用见图 5-5。

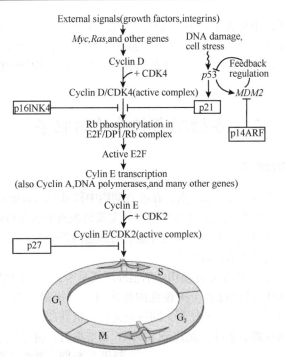

图 5-5　G₁-S 期调控中各元素间的相互作用；The interaction between various elements in G₁-S phase regulation

第四节　细胞周期检测点

细胞在长期的进化过程中发展出了一套保证细胞周期中 DNA 复制和染色体分配质量的检查机制，通常被称为细胞周期检测点（check point），又称为限制点（restriction point）。这是一类细胞周期的负反馈调节机制。

一、细胞周期检测点功能

当细胞周期进程中出现异常事件，如 DNA 损伤或 DNA 复制受阻，这类调节机制就被激活，即对 DNA 损伤检查（确定有无损伤、合成、复制错误，细胞周期时相检查）以确保细胞周期时相的严格秩序和不重复性，保证了在细胞周期中上一期事件完成以后才开始下一期的事件。细胞周期检测点构成了 DNA 修复的完整元件。在应激和损伤的情况下阻止细胞周期循环；在修复过程中，限制点对保持基因组的稳定性特别重要。检测点通过延缓细胞周期的进展，为 DNA 复制前的修复、基因组的复制、有丝分裂及基因组的分离提供更多的时间。待细胞修复或排除了故障后，细胞周期才能恢复运转。

根据细胞周期的时相，细胞周期检测点主要有 G₁-S 期检测点、S 期检测点、G₂ 期检测点和 M 期检测点（图 5-6）。作为一种保护

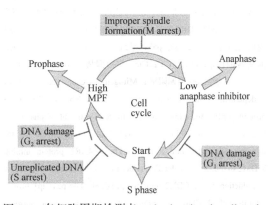

图 5-6　各细胞周期检测点；check points in cell cycle

机制在真核生物生命活动中起着十分重要的作用。每一完整的检测点应由四个步骤组成，即发现或传感（detect or sensor）、制动或扣留（stop or arrest）、修复（repair）和继续分裂或死亡（division or death）。检测点功能缺陷可能会导致遗传基因突变和染色体结构异常的细胞获得增殖，从而导致肿瘤发生[3]。

二、各检测点相关的细胞事件

（一）G_1-S 期检测点

G_1-S 期检测点在酵母中称 START 点，在哺乳动物中称 R 点（restriction point），控制细胞由静止状态的 G_1 进入 DNA 合成期，这是细胞顺利完成细胞周期最关键的检测点。细胞在该检测点对各类生长因子、分裂原及 DNA 损伤等复杂的细胞内外信号进行整合和传递，决定细胞发展方向（分裂、凋亡或进入 G_0 期）[4]。

该检测点相关的事件：DNA 是否损伤？细胞外环境是否适宜？细胞体积是否足够大？

细胞顺利完成其周期需经过若干关键性的检测点，其中最重要的控制点是 G_1 晚期的 START，此时细胞开始又一轮 DNA 复制，同时也是正、负外部信号整合入细胞周期的部位。肿瘤发生时，这些控制点调节紊乱，尤其是 START 调节失灵，将导致细胞越过正常的程序限制进入 S 期，并允许细胞复制未修复的突变 DNA，从而积累形成肿瘤表现型的基因改变。而 START 的异常可能由正调节子（如 cyclin）的过度表达所致，也可能由负调节子（如 CKI）的减少所致。哺乳动物细胞中 START 的调节主要靠 cyclin D 及其相应的 CDKs（图 5-7）。许多肿瘤的发生都与 G_1-S 期检测点缺陷有关[5-7]。G_1-S 期检测点缺陷导致肿瘤的原因主要是 p53 缺失和 cyclin D1 上调。当细胞出现 DNA 损伤时，p53 诱导细胞周期阻滞在 G_1 期，并试图在 DNA 复制之前修复损伤的 DNA 或者诱导细胞凋亡。cyclin D1 上调可加速细胞周期，或使细胞逃避检测点，进而使肿瘤发生的风险增加。

一旦发生癌变，失控的癌细胞倾向于保留在细胞周期中持续循环；一旦细胞通过 G_1 晚期限制点，将对胞外生长调控信号产生不应期而代之以自律性程序，并带着这些信息进入有丝分裂。对限制点调控的研究是搞清癌细胞是怎样和如何持续进入细胞周期的关键所在。

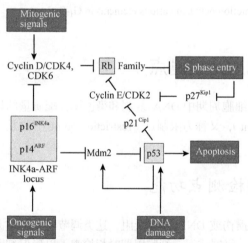

图 5-7　细胞周期检测点；Cell cycle check points
有丝分裂信号激活磷酸化 Rb 和 Rb 家族蛋白质（p107 和 p130）细胞周期素 D 依赖性激酶，促进细胞进入 S 期。p16INK4a 蛋白质抑制 cyclin D/CDK4,6 活化 Rb 以抑制细胞进入 S 期。p14ARF 蛋白质抑制 MDM2 诱导 p53，导致 p53 依赖性凋亡或对 CDK2 抑制剂 p21Cip1 的诱导。p21Cip1 蛋白抑制 cyclin E/CDK2 而诱导 Rb 依赖性细胞周期阻滞；Mitogenic signals activate cyclin D-dependent kinases，which phosphorylate Rb and Rb family proteins（p107 and p130）to facilitate cells entry into S phase. The p16INK4a protein inhibits cyclin D/CDK4, 6 to activate Rb and prevent cells entry into S phase. The p14ARF protein inhibits MDM2 to induce p53，leading either to p53-dependent apoptosis or to induction of the CDK2 inhibitor p21Cip1. The p21Cip1 protein inhibits cyclin E/CDK2 and induces Rb-dependent cell cycle arrest

（二）S 期检测点

S 期检测点的主要任务是解决 DNA 复制是否完成，包括损伤检测和复制检测两方面。损伤检测点与复制检测点的关系密切，损伤检测点的作用因子正是复制检测点的上游调控因子。S 期检测点允许细胞通过阻滞复制叉的组装来使复制暂停，以修复损伤或复制异常，同时稳定已组装的复制叉，防止损伤的 DNA 结构和复制过程中的异常导致基因组不稳定性和肿瘤发生。关于如何稳定复制叉的机制还不是很清楚，但 S 期检测点缺陷的细胞在复制暂停时会在染色体脆性部位发生染色体重排，形成非整倍体细胞。复制重新开始时，DNA 会复制有损伤的 DNA 模板，在这种情况下，可产生 DNA 继发性损伤或双链缺口，形成双链断裂，导致细胞表型改变或形成肿瘤。S 期 DNA 复制检测点的功能常常是通过参与 DNA 复制的蛋白质来进行，如 DNA 聚合酶（pol）α、β 和 ε。Waga 等[8]在非洲爪蟾（Xeropus）卵提取物中证实了 polε 在 DNA 复制中起重要作用。polε 和复制因子（RFC）的亚基 RFC5 能够结合在 DNA 复制起始区，并探测 DNA 复制异常从而阻滞复制，另外 polε 还参与初生态 DNA 复制叉处复制蛋白的合适组装。Bergoglio 等[9]研究认为 polβ 表达的改变会导致肿瘤细胞恶性表型的增加。

（三）G_2/M 期检测点

G_2/M 期检验点：是决定细胞一分为二的控制点，可防止受损的 DNA 和未完成复制的 DNA 进入有丝分裂。DNA 损伤诱导的 G_2 期检测点途径主要是抑制 Cdc2 活性。细胞损伤后，磷脂酰肌醇-3 激酶（PI-3K）家族成员（DNA-PK、ATM 和 ATR）被激活，并开始转录与 DNA 损伤修复和细胞周期转换相关的基因。PI-3K 家族的成员可直接磷酸化 p53，导致 Chk1 和 Chk2 激酶的激活[10]。Chk1 和 Chk2 磷酸化 Cdc25C 的 Ser-216，从而在 Cdc25C 上生成一个结合位点。14-3-3σ 蛋白可以结合在该结合位点，使 Cdc25C 从核中运出，抑制细胞质中的磷酸化，从而抑制 Cdc2 活性，使细胞阻滞在 G_2 期[11]。同 G_1-S 期检测点一样，p53 是 DNA 损伤诱导 G_2 期阻滞的关键机制，因此 p53 缺失导致的 G_2 期检测点缺陷与许多肿瘤的发生有关。另外 14-3-3σ 蛋白缺失引起的 G_2 期检测点缺陷会使细胞过早进入有丝分裂而导致肿瘤发生。在乳腺癌中发现有 14-3-3σ 的高频缺失[12]。而 Osada 等[13]亦发现在 13 种小细胞肺癌细胞系中有很高比例（69%）的 14-3-3σ 甲基化所导致的基因沉默。在 7 种大细胞肺癌细胞系中 14-3-3σ 基因沉默的比例是 57%。成纤维细胞中 cyclin B1 或 Cdc25C 过表达使 GADD45 诱导的 G_2 期阻滞失败，从而使细胞异常扩增形成肿瘤[14]。

（四）M 期检测点

M 期检测点又叫纺锤体组装检测点，主要是阻止细胞分裂，阻止细胞两极形成纺锤体，阻止染色体附着到纺锤体上。任何一个着丝点没有正确连接到纺锤体上，都会抑制相关激酶的活性，引起细胞周期中断。参与该检测点最重要的两类基因是 Mad2 和 Bub。Mad2 和 Bub1 存在于尚未结合微管的着丝点上，这两种蛋白在着丝点上可以探测着丝点与微管的结合，并诱导检测点信号途径。对酵母的研究显示 Mps 和 Cdc20 在有丝分裂检测点中也起作用，Cdc20 在人类的同源基因是 p55 Cdc 或 Cdc20。已证实是哺乳动物细胞中有丝分裂检测点的调节因子[15]。在有丝分裂后期 APC 会降解 M 期的 cyclin，从而推动细胞从 M 期又进入 G_1 期。纺锤体装配检查点可诱导 Mad2 与 Cdc20 的结合，使 Cdc20 无法激活 APC，导致细胞周期停止在 M 期[16]。染色体与纺锤体如果不能正常结合，姐妹染色体就不能有效分离，从而导致染色体的缺失或倍增。如果在检测点有缺陷的情况下，细胞仍然分裂，则会产生带有不稳定性染色体的细胞增殖，从而导致肿瘤发生。有丝分裂检测点缺陷与具有染色体不稳定表型的癌症密切相关，如研究发现有丝分裂检测点中起重要作用的蛋白 Mad2 表达下降会导致乳腺癌的发生[17]。在白血病和淋巴瘤中都有 Bub1 基因的缺陷[15]。MAD1L1 基因是 HILV21 反转录病毒素 Tax 蛋白的靶点，它能够使感染的 T 细胞中的 M 期检测点失活，从而导致肿瘤发生[18]。目前检测点基因如 Bub1 已被作为肿瘤治疗中引人注意的候选基因[20]。正常细胞一旦进入 M 期，在 M 中期末有一控制点，若有染色体错排或有丝分裂装制错误，则会导致停滞；肿瘤细胞 M 中晚期控制点调节失控可能破坏 cyclin B 的机制。

理论上说，检测点的任何一部分出了问题，如发现不了 DNA 损伤（如 ATM 突变）、不能使细胞周期停下来（如 p53 突变）、DNA 修复错误（如 MLH1/PSM 突变）、决定错误（如 Bcl-2 突变）等都会导致遗传的不稳定性、（基因）受损细胞的存活和复制或细胞遗传物质的改变。这样突变基因累积而促使的细胞多步骤进化将最终导致肿瘤。

细胞周期检测点功能的减弱，会导致突变基因的累积和遗传的不稳定性，但只有当累积的突变基因破坏了细胞周期驱动机制时，细胞才能进入失控性生长。有人将细胞周期驱动机制比作一辆汽车，驱使其运行的因素（positive agents）好似"油门"，制动其运行的因素（negative agents）犹如"刹车"；持续踏住"油门"或"刹车"失灵都将导致失控。

检测点功能的丢失或减弱可能通过降低 DNA 复制效率来增加和诱导基因突变和染色体畸变。在某些遗传性癌症和细胞转化早期中，已经能观察到检测点调控的缺失，后者可能导致遗传失稳态，促使向肿瘤的转化。

第五节　细胞周期的调控与肿瘤

细胞周期紊乱与多种人类疾病相关，其中最重要的莫过于与肿瘤的关系。正常组织中细胞数增加与丢失保持动态平衡。肿瘤发生的机制之一是细胞周期调控机制的破坏，使细胞增殖大于细胞丢失，并呈相对无限制生长。

一、在肿瘤中细胞周期调控的异常

从分子水平上分析，是由于基因突变致使细胞周期的促进因子异常活化和（或）抑制因子失活，造成细胞周期调节失控。其中，破坏检测点的正常控制、由癌蛋白"谎报军情"使细胞周期调控系统总得到"增殖"的指令，如多数肿瘤中 cyclin A、cyclin D1 过表达，p15、p16 失表达，并可导致肿瘤的发生和进展[19]。

（一）cyclin D 与原癌基因

很多原癌基因与细胞周期的调控有关。与 G_0/G_1 期转化有关的原癌基因有 myc、Ras 等，它们在转化细胞中与 cyclin D 共同作用。静止的成纤维细胞中 myc 可诱导 cyclin D1 的表达，这提供了丝裂原通路与 G_1 期过程的联系。但持续过度表达 myc 会抑制 cyclin D1 的表达。这说明 myc 对 cyclin D1 的调节是复杂的。cyclin-CDK 复合物介导的 Rb 磷酸化使 Rb 释放转录因子 E2F，E2F 刺激 c-myc 和 cyclin A 的表达。E2F 释放可以进一步增加 c-myc 的表达，诱导 cyclin E 和 cyclin A。Ras 活性的抑制，E2F 靶基因的活化，导致细胞停滞于 G_1 期。Ras 激活是 G_1 期 CDK 活性的产生所必需的，而 cyclin E-CDK 的激活则依赖于 Ras 和 myc 的共同作用。

正常情况下，cyclin D1 在 G_1 期恒定的保持极低水平，在正常组织中除了扁桃体（检测 cyclin D1 最理想的组织）、血管内皮细胞、一些组织细胞和鳞状上皮的基底细胞表达 cyclin D1 外，其他组织均不表达 cyclin D1。cyclin D1 过度表达导致 G_1 期缩短。cyclin D_1 的表达在许多人类原发肿瘤和细胞系中被检出。cyclin D_1 由于基因的扩增或重排，在多种肿瘤中有过度表达，但在有些肿瘤中，如乳腺癌、肝癌、食管癌及胰腺癌中，cyclin D_1 RNA 和（或）蛋白出现了过

第五章　细胞周期的调控　·161·

度表达，但相应的基因却没有出现扩增，表现出扩增与表达不一致的现象。在肿瘤中 cyclin D1 基因扩增 11%～20%，cyclin D_1 蛋白过度表达率约为 50%或更高，这可能是基因启动子区域的改变或调节转录因子如 c-Jun 的异常表达所致，或是由于 cyclin D_1 mRNA 3'非翻译区的截短导致其稳定性增加引起，或 mRNA 半衰期延长也可能导致这种结果。

在肿瘤中 cyclin D1 过表达的意义：cyclin D1 过表达与某些肿瘤的组织类型相关，在不同肿瘤中阳性检出率不同；与组织分化程度相关，在分化差的肿瘤中表达增强；与预后相关，在多种肿瘤中是独立的预后差的指标。

cyclin D1 在正常和反应性淋巴细胞中总是阴性；但套细胞淋巴瘤（mantle cell lymphoma，MCL）中 cyclin D1 阳性。仅约 7%的 MCL 是阴性。MCL 遗传学的主要特征是 t（11，14）（q13，q32），该区正好是 Bcl-1 基因编码细胞周期蛋白 cyclin D1。该基因的易位就造成 cyclin D1 mRNA 的过度表达，因此大多数 MCL 中均有 cyclin D_1 蛋白的过表达。国际淋巴瘤协会认为 MCL 中染色体 11q13 的易位和 cyclin D1 的过表达是很重要的特征。在 MCL 中，由于 cyclin D1 具有高度的敏感性和相对的特异性，成为区别 MCL 与其他淋巴瘤的特异性标志。

尽管 cyclin D1 与肿瘤的关系最为密切。但单独的 cyclin D1 过度表达不足以使原代细胞发生转化，不足以造成细胞的恶性转化，还必须与其他能使细胞退出 G_0 期的原癌基因共同作用，如与 Ras 共同导致幼鼠肾细胞转化，与 myc 共同诱导转基因小鼠 B 细胞淋巴瘤等。

（二）Cyclin A 在人类恶性肿瘤中研究的意义

最早使人们将肿瘤与细胞周期机制联系在一起的是 cyclin A，当时有两条线索提示 cyclin A 的改变可能与细胞转化(癌变)有关。在肝细胞癌的细胞中，乙肝病毒的 DNA 片段整合到 cyclin A 的基因中；这是克隆肝细胞中 HBV 的唯一插入点。病毒插入后整合入宿主 DNA 形成嵌合体，cyclin A 的 N 端直至 cyclin 盒（cyclin box）的区域被病毒的基因序列取代，所形成的蛋白质缺乏 cyclin 降解盒（cyclin destruction box）不能在正常的有丝分裂期被降解。同样从腺病毒转化细胞中可以看到 cyclin A 与腺病毒转化蛋白 ElA 结合在一起。ElA 能促进释放出更多的游离 E2F，影响一些与转化表型有关的特定基因表达在正常细胞的 S 期，而 cyclin A 蛋白与 ElA 结合形成的复合物使具有高活性的游离 E2F 减少，因此 cyclin A 可以对基因转录起到一定的限制作用。

（三）P27 在人类恶性肿瘤中研究的意义

p27 作为一种抑癌基因，其蛋白表达水平与肿瘤的形成有关。p27 的表达与 ki-67 呈显著负相关。p27 的表达增加还可抑制脑肿瘤的生长和异倍体细胞的积聚，而敲除了 p27 基因的小鼠则出现多种组织器官增生综合征，表现为体态肥胖，细胞生长加速，多器官肥大，组织增生，视网膜变性，雌性不育。多种肿瘤中 p27 的蛋白表达水平、恶性肿瘤的恶性程度、侵袭性的强弱及预后明显有关，低 p27 表达与预后不良显著相关，高 p27 表达与良好预后相关。翻译后期调节可能是影响癌组织中 P27 蛋白水平的关键。

某些癌基因对 p27 有调节作用[20]。Valch 等报道：c-myc 表达增加可防止 cyclin E-CDK2 灭活，允许细胞在 p27 存在的情况下继续增殖。c-myc 在此过程中，既没有改变 cyclin E-CDK2 对 p27 抑制作用的易感性，也没有改变 p27 原有的抑制作用，只是诱导 p27 以一种不能与 cyclin E-CDK2 结合的形式存在。表面免疫球蛋白交联激活脾脏 B 细胞过程中，c-Fos 高表达可下调 p27 水平而使 cylcin E-CDK2 复合物活性增强，促使细胞增殖。c-myc 与 Ras 在细胞内共表达时可使细胞内 p27 消失。

二、细胞周期的调控与肿瘤治疗

实际上多数肿瘤化疗药物均是细胞周期的抑制剂，但缺点是它们"良莠不分"，也抑制正常细胞。对细胞周期分子机制的研究，不仅使我们能深刻认识这一重要生命活动的本质，还可能通过针对性的设计和筛选，开发出更专一、更有效的治疗药物及治疗方法，使相关疾病病因的基因诊断和针对性基因治疗成为可能。

（一）不同细胞对肿瘤治疗敏感性

处于细胞周期的细胞对抗肿瘤药物或放射治疗较为敏感。暂不增殖处于休止状态的 G_0 期细胞对抗肿瘤药物、放射治疗不敏感，可成为肿瘤复发的根源。

（二）针对肿瘤细胞周期各时相的药物

有些药物是周期非特异性药物，可作用于细胞周期各个时相，包括 G_0 期细胞。有些药物是周期特异性药物，仅对增殖周期中处于某些时相的细胞敏感、对 G_0 期细胞不敏感。

（三）细胞周期调控与肿瘤治疗的策略

限制 CDK 活性抑制瘤细胞过度生长。抑制 cyclin 表达阻止瘤细胞异常增殖。提高 CKI 水平减轻肿瘤细胞增殖失控。利用细胞周期检测点的缺陷，或将其作为靶点，加快肿瘤细胞死亡。

挑战与展望

细胞周期通常受到信号转导途径和反馈环路的精确调控，其正常与否和细胞及个体的生长、分化、衰老和癌变密切相关。经过一个完整的细胞周期后，有的细胞继续增殖，有的细胞可能暂不增殖或永不增殖。决定细胞周期后各类细胞命运的关键则是细胞周期的调控。目前对细胞周期的调控研究已作为生命科学研究的热点，随着研究的深入将进一步揭示细胞周期调控的分子机制及其与疾病的相关性，并对认识细胞生长的动力学、有目的地调控细胞周期，对肿瘤的防治干预具有重要的指导意义。

思 考 题

1. 本章基本概念：细胞分裂周期（cell division cycle）、细胞周期素（cyclin）、周期蛋白依赖性激酶（cyclin-dependent kinase, CDK），周期蛋白依赖性激酶抑制剂（CDK inhibitory proteins, CKIs），细胞周期检测点（check point）Rb，E2F，p27。
2. 简述细胞周期调控中 cyclin D1 的作用和病理学意义
3. 简述 *Rb* 基因在细胞周期调控中的作用。
4. 简述随特定细胞时相而出现的 cyclin 和 CDK。
5. 简述细胞周期检测点的功能。
6. 阐述细胞周期 G_1 期的调控因子和肿瘤形成的相关性。

参 考 文 献

[1] Nakayama K，Nagahama H，Minamishima Y A，et al. Targeted disruption of Skp2 results in accumulation of cyclin E and p27

（Kip1），polyploidy and centrosome over duplication[J]. EMBO Journal，2000，19（9）: 2069-2081.

[2] Chen J，Peters R，Saha P，et al. A 39 amino acid fragment of the cell cycle regulator p21 is sufficient to bind PCNA and partially inhibit DNA replication in vivo[J]. Nucleic Acids Research，1996，24（9）: 1727-1733.

[3] Pietenpol J A，Stewart Z A. Cell cycle checkpoint signaling: cell cycle arrest versus apoptosis[J]. Toxicology，2002，s181–182（1-3）: 475-481.

[4] artek J，Lukas J. Mammalian G_1-and S-phase checkpoints in response to DNA damage[J]. Gurrent Opinion in Cell Biology，2001，13（6）: 738-747.

[5] Zhou J X，Niehans G A，Shar A，et al. Mechanisms of G_1 checkpoint loss in resected early stage non-small cell lung cancer[J]. Lung Cancer，2001，32（1）: 27-38.

[6] Feakins R M，Nickols C D，Bidd H，et al. Abnormal expression of pRb, p16, and cyclin D1 in gastric adenocarcinoma and its lymph node metastases: relationship with pathological features and survival[J]. Human Pathology，2003，34（12）: 1276-1282.

[7] Rose S L，Buller R E. The role of p53 mutation in BRCA1-associated ovarian cancer[J]. Minerva Ginecologica，2002，54（3）: 201-209.

[8] Waga S，Masuda T，Takisawa H，et al. DNA polymerase epsilon is required for coordinated and efficient chromosomal DNA replication in Xenopus egg extracts[J]. Proceedings of the National Academy of Sciences of the United States of America，2001，98（9）: 4978-4983.

[9] Bergoglio V，Pillaire M J，Lacroix Triki M，et al. Deregulated DNA polymerase beta induces chromosome instability and tumorigenesis[J]. Cancer Res earch，2002，62（12）: 3511-3514.

[10] Yang J，Yu Y，Hamrick H E，et al. ATM, ATR and DNA-PK: initiators of the cellular genotoxic stress responses[J]. Carcinogenesis，2003，24（10）: 1571-1580.

[11] Duckworth B C，Weaver J S，Ruderman JV. G_2 arrest in Xenopus oocytes depends on phosphorylation of cdc25 by protein kinase A[J]. Proceedings of the National Academy of Sciences of the United States of America，2002，99（26）: 16794-16799.

[12] Umbricht C B，Evron E，Gabrielson E，et al. Hypermethylation of 14-3-3 sigma（stratifin）is an early event in breast cancer[J]. Oncogene，2001，20（26）: 3348-3353.

[13] Osada H，Tatematsu Y Y，Nakagawa T，et al. Frequent and histological type-specific inactivation of 14-3-3sigma in human lung cancers[J]. Oncogene，2002，21（15）: 2418-2424.

[14] Han C，Demetris A J，Michalopoulos G K，et al. PPARgamma ligands inhibit cholangiocarcinoma cell growth through p53-dependent GADD45 and p21 pathway[J]. Hepatology，2003，38（1）: 167-177.

[15] Ru H Y，Chen R W, Chen J H. hBUB1 defects in leukemia and lymphoma cells[J]. Oncogene, 2002, 21（30）: 4673.

[16] Lew D J，Burke D J. The spindle assembly and spindle position checkpoints[J]. Annual Review of Genetics，2003，37（1）: 251-282.

[17] Kraft C，Herzog F，Gieffers C，et al. Mitotic regulation of the human anaphase‐promoting complex by phosphorylation[J]. EMBO Journal，2003，22（24）: 6598-6609.

[18] Percy M J，Myrie K A，Neeley C K，et al. Expression and mutational analyses of the human MAD2L1 gene in breast cancer cells[J]. Genes Chromosomes & Cancer，2000，29（4）: 356-362.

[19] 陈莉，王桂兰，曹晓蕾. 鼻咽癌中 cyclin D1、p16、Rb 蛋白表达及意义[J]. 临床与实验病理学杂志，1999，15（4）: 362-362.

[20] Chen L，Lu P，Song HJ，et al. The relationship between the expression of p27Kip1, p53 and the infiltration, metastasis and prognosis in gastric carcinoma[J]. The Chinese-German Journal of Clinical Oncology，2005，4（3）: 155-160.

（薛玉文 陈 莉）

Chapter 5 Cell Cycle Regulation

The regulation of simple organism cell cycle mainly is in order to adapt to the natural environment, so that it regulates reproduction rate based on environmental conditions.

Complex organism needs to make the right response to natural environment and signals of the other cells and tissues to ensure that the formation, growth and wound healing process can work on tissues, organs and individual. It needs more elaborate cell cycle control mechanism.

Section 1　Conception of Cell Cycle

Cell cycle is the process of cells from the first divided end to finish next divided end.Cell cycle contain four phases, G_1, S, G_2, M.When cells enter cell cycle and pass the G_1, S, G_2, M phase to divide two daughter cells, so it is also called the cell division cycle. The basic tasks of cell cycle are to ensure that the DNA replication of S phase and has the same chromosome distribution into two daughter cells in M phase.

G_1 phase: Early DNA synthesis phase, its length (hours $\sim$ days $\sim$ months)depends on the cells, mainly reserves material and energy for DNA synthesis of S -phase.Rapid RNA and protein biosynthesis, such as the synthesis of various enzymes associated with DNA replication.Cell volume increases significantly involve in mitochondria and ribosomes increase, the endoplasmic reticulum update to expand, the Golgi apparatus from the endoplasmic reticulum and lysosomes also increased.

S phase: DNA synthesis phase. DNA content increases 1 time (8~30h).It isa critical moment in the cell cycle. Somatic cells become tetraploid, each piece of filament in chromatin is connected with two chromatinfilaments by a centromere.Meanwhile, also histones are synthesized and centrioles replication.

G_2 phase: Later phase of DNA synthesis. Termination of DNA synthesis (2~8.5h) and prepares for the final mitotic.RNA and protein synthesis during the G_2 period are gradually reduced. Microtubulin apparatus supplies raw material to spindle microtubule assembly in mitotic phase.The centriole replication completesand two pairs of centrioles are formed.

M phase: Cell mitosis phase. Cells mitosis needs to go through the early, middle, late and final phases. It is a continuous process of change, in which a mother cell divides into two daughter cells. It normally takes 1~2 h.

G_0 Quiescent phase:Cells leave the cell cycle and stop division, to carry out certain biological functions.

On October 8, 2001, American Leland Hartwell and English Paul Nurse, Timothy Hunt due to the research of cell cycle control mechanism, so they won the Nobel Prize in Physiology or medicine.

Section 2   Important Factors in Cell Cycle Regulation

The important regulating factors in cell cycle include cyclin-dependent kinase (CDK), cell cycle protein (Cyclin) and CDK inhibitory protein (CKIs).

1. Cyclin

In1953 Howard and others, first proposed the theory that cellular differentiation is done through the cell cycle.In 1983, Evans and others first found a group of proteins that appear periodically in marine invertebrates, and regulate cell growth. It is identified as "cyclin". In 1988, scientists found that cell cycle regulatory proteins can bind to cell division cycle encoding proteins and activate the corresponding protein kinases to promote cell division.

Definition:It is a kind of synthesis and decomposition that is synchronized with the cell cycle, a specific dynamic protein to drive cell cycle works and Cyclin - dependent kinase (CDK) regulatory subunit is composed.

At least there are 11 kinds Cyclins, namely, A, B1, B2, C, D1, D2, D3, E, F, G, and H. Among them, 8 kinds Cyclins have been separated. According to Cyclins regulating different phases in cell cycle, Cyclins can be divided into two major categories of G_1 and M phases.All types of Cyclins contain a conserved sequence of about 100 amino acids, called cyclin box, it mediates the combination of Cyclin and CDK. Different cyclin box identify the different CDK to compose of different Cyclin complexes, express the different CDK kinase activity.

(1) G_1 Phase Cyclins

G_1 phase is a period in which proliferating cells only accept the signals to promote or inhibit cells proliferation. Mainly: Cyclin D (D1, D2, D3),Cyclin C and Cyclin E (Cyclin E 1,Cyclin E 2).

1) Cyclin D

Cyclin D was first discovered in yeast, it can activate the CDK6, drive the cell through the START. It has three subtypes, D1, D2, D3, all with tissue specificity.The functions of cyclin D1 and cyclin D2 are similar, both work in yeast daughter cells. Cyclin D3 works in yeast mother cells. In regulating cell cycle, Cyclin Dl is a more sensitive index than other Cyclin D. Coding Cyclin D1 gene is located on 11q13, is about 15kb length.Compared with other Cyclins, it is the smallest Cyclin mainly because its N-terminus lacks a "degradation box" segment, the protein half-life is very short, less than 25mins.

In the case of growth factors, Cyclin D1 was first synthesized in the cell cycle and synthesis peak is in the mid-G_1. It is a key protein in G_1 phase of the cell proliferation signals. Expression of cyclin D in the G= phase and its combination with CDK4, CDK6, makes the downstream proteins phosphorylate, such as Rb. The phosphorylating Rb releases E2F of transcription factors to promote transcription of many genes, such as coding Cyclin E, A and CDK1 genes. E2F-1-mediated mRNA transcription make cells enter the proliferation state (Fig. 5-1). The major function of Cyclin D1 is to promote the cell proliferation, its over-expression can cause uncontrolled cell proliferation causing malignant. It is considered a cancer gene.

Cyclin D2: Coding cyclin D2 gene is located on 12p13, called CCND2. In normal diploid cells and Rb-positive tumor cells, the expression of Cyclin D2 with fluctuation, the peak is in late stage of G_1phase. Microinjection of Cyclin D2 antibodyin cell with G_1 phase can lead the Cyclin D2 expressing lymphocytes to arrest in G_1 phase. It is description that Cyclin D2 is required to the cell transfer from G_1 to S phase.

Cyclin D3: Coding Cyclin D3 gene located on chromosome 6p21, called CCND3. Having not reportedCyclin D3 gene abnormal and its protein overexpression in normal and malignant tissues. Now that the Cyclin D3 does not seem to directly reflect the degree of malignancy, but yet the result of tumor development late.

2) Cyclin C

Cyclin C is the lowest homology with all other Cyclins, mainly found in drosophila and human cells. Because its mRNA and protein levels peaked in the early stage of G_1, may play a role in early stage of G_1, so it different with the other G_1-Cyclins.

3) Cyclin E

Cyclin E appears and expression in G_1/S conversion process after the expression of Cyclin D. The expression of cyclin E gene and its products rises in the middle stage of G_1 phase, reached its peak until late G_1 phase or early S phase.

Cyclin E binds with CDK2, which promotes cell through G_1/S restriction point then enters to S phase.

(2) M Phase cyclins

M phase cyclins - at the junction of G_2/M induce cell division.

1) Cyclin A

Cyclin A expresses after following cyclin E. It is the rate -limiting factor of G_1 phase transfer to S phase, but can also promote cells from G_2 phase to M phase. It is encoded by CCNA gene and combined with the CDK1. CDK1 makes substrate protein phosphorylate, leading to chromosome condensation, the disintegration of the nuclear membrane, etc., a sires of downstream cell cycle events.

2) Cyclin B

Cyclin B is a subunit of mitotic protein kinase, which can facilitate the cells transiting from G_2 phase to M phase. The synthesis of mammals Cyclin B is in the late S phase.

(3) Every Phase cyclin——Cyclin H

Cyclin H and Cyclin C have high homology sequence and can assemble to holoenzyme with CDK7 to have a regulating effect on every stage of the cell cycle.

(4) Degradation of Cyclins——Destruction Box

There is no destruction box in N-terminal of G_1 Cyclins, but C-terminal has a sequence of PEST which is related to its degradation. Cyclins of G_1 phase are hydrolyzed by the "PEST" sequences related protein or degraded by ubiquitin pathway of S-phase kinase-associated protein 2 (SKP2).

N-terminal of M phase Cyclin molecules contains a destroy box of 9 amino acids, involving ubiquitin-mediated degradation of Cyclin A and B. In anaphase, ubiquitin is catalyzed by ubiquitin ligase combines with cyclins, which is then hydrolyzed by proteasome.Cyclin A and Cyclin B in M phase are degraded by the ubiquitin pathway, which is necessary for cell getting out of mitosis.

Various Cyclins Appear with Specific Cell Phases (Fig. 5-2).

The early G_1 phase: Cyclin D-CDK2/CDK4 (promoter)

The late G_1 phase——the early S phase: Cyclin E-CDK2 (Cells into S phase)

S phase: Degradation of CDK2, Cyclin D, Cyclin E

The late S phase——the early G_2 phase: CDK2, Cyclin D, Cyclin E (Cells into G_2 phase)

DuringG_2 / M phase: Cyclin B-CDK1 (cells into M phase).

Every Phase Cyclin:Cyclin H

2. Cyclin-Dependent Kinase (CDK)

CDK is an important complex of serine / threonine protein kinases, including CDK1-7. The main biological effect of CDKs is to initiate DNA replication and induce cell mitosis.

3. CDK Inhibitory Proteins (CKIs)

CKIs is the inhibition protein of CDK. It competitively inhibitingCyclin or Cyclin-CDK complexes, resulting in loss of biological function of Cyclin. It plays a negative role in cell growth.

(1) There are 2 protein families in the G_1 phase of CKIs

1) INKs: p15、p16、p18、p19 are specific inhibitors of CDK4 or CDK6.

2) CIP / KIPs: p21、P27、p57 etc, are the inhibitors of various Cyclin-CDK complexes. They block the activation of CDK kinase, or prevent the active roles of CDK kinase.

(2) The roles of major CKIS molecules

1) P16: P16INK4 is located on chromosome 9p21, and is also known as MTSI (multiple tumor suppressor gene). It is CDK4's specific inhibitor, that can inhibitCyclin D to combine with CDK4 or CDK6, inhibiting the positive effect of CDK4 in cell growth and division. It is involved in inhibition of cell cycle G_1/S transformation. The level of P16 rises in cells lacking functional Rb, suggesting that Rb may inhibit the expression of P16 and at the same time stimulates the expression of Cyclin D.

2) p15INKB: P15INKB is located on a region of 9th chromosome near by the P16. Like P16, it is a tumor suppressor gene.

3) P27: P27 has probably the most direct impact on G_1/S regulation of restriction sites by widely inhibiting the functions of Cyclin-CDK complexes. It increases the P27 expression in G_0/G_1 under normal circumstances. After entering S phaseP27 expression is decreased.Regulation of p27 expression level is affected by many factors, such as mitogens, anti-proliferative signals, cytokines, cancer genes and contact inhibition, etc. The effects of TGF-β on the expression of p27 are biphasic. In most cells, TGF-β's induces the expression of p27, but in front of the normal pituitary and pituitary adenoma cells, TGF-β can down-regulate the expression of p27 mRNA and proteins.The expression of p27 also can be down-regulated by PDGF, EGF.P27 regulates cell cycle depending on its protein level, rather than its gene mutation. If expression of p27 decreased or its deficiency can lead to genomic instability, and even cancer genesis.P27 has negative regulatory effect on inhibiting Cyclin-CDK complexes. By combining with CDK subunit, p27 makes CAK (CDK active enzymes) which do not induce CDK phosphorylation (CDK activity state). Non-activation of CDK cannot stimulate the Rb protein phosphorylation, so the cells remain in the G_1 phase and have negative regulation to cell cycle. P27 may also prevent Rb protein phosphorylation and its overexpression to inhibit cells entering the G_1= phase.P27 plays an important role in regulating cell entry and exit to M phase.In anti-mitogen environment, the cells growth is arrested, related to the amount of p27-CDK2 complex.P27 is also involved in regulation of cell differentiation: As p21, it can induce the differentiation of immature cells;P27 can induce tumor cell differentiation (such as exogenous p27 can induce the original megakaryocytic leukemia cell differentiation); P27 does not induce normal cells aging.

4) p21: It is located on chromosome 6p21.2. The 17th to 71st amino acids contain the Cyclin binding inhibitor regions. P21 may hinder cells into S phase; can inhibit the SAPK (stress-activated protein kinase), involving the regulation of signal transduction cascade system in cellular stress states.

44% are the same N-terminal sequence of P21 and p27. All can widely inhibit Cyclin-CDK complexes, but both mediate the inhibition of CDK in the different regions.

Section 3　Interaction of Various Elements in Cell Cycle

Exogenous regulation is primarily caused by cytokines and other external stimuli; Endogenous regulation is mainly realized by Cyclin-CDK-CKIs network regulation.

1. Rb Gene

Rb gene is located in 13q14.1. It has 27 exons, encoding 110kD protein with 928 amino acids.The deletion of Rb gene can be seen in 30% retinoblastomas, including the deletions of DNA or even chromosome fragments.

Rb protein, as a major transcript, has a brake function in the cell cycle. It can combine with transcription factor E2F and stop the corresponding gene transcription and expression, thereby it can inhibit cell growth.

Cyclin D is the foundation of Rb regulating the cell cycle. Cyclin D1-CDK4 complex can be seen as Rb protein kinase in G_1 phase. It can combine with N-terminal of Rb, phosphorylating Rb protein, releasing transcription factors, resulting in G_1/S transformation (Fig.5-3).

Functions of Cyclin D1 and Rb are interdependent.

Low phosphorylating Rb can also stimulate the transcription of Cyclin D1, which increases Cyclin D1 synthesis and activation , again leads to the phosphorylation of Rb, the latter forms a negative feedback loop to regulate the expression of Cyclin D1.The role of Cyclin E-CDK2 is through positive feedback in order to promote phosphorylation of Rb and release E2F.

2. Cell Transcription Factor (E2F)

Many DNA synthesizing genes and promoters of cell growth regulation genes contain E2F sites. E2F can directly activate these genes, initiate DNA synthesis to make cells enter S phase.

There is an 18 amino acid sequence that can be combined with Rb in E2F gene transcription activating functional area. Rb covers its functional area by binding with the E2F functional area to inhibit the function of active transcription and DNA synthesis.Release of more E2F, when the E1A intervene, will affect some specific gene expressions associated with the transformed phenotypes (Fig. 5-4).

3. SKP2 (S phase kinase associated protein 2)

SKP2 is a tumor marker. In normal tissue, it only expresses in placenta tissue and tonsils, but in tumor tissue, SKP2 has wide expression. In oral epithelial carcinoma and colon cancer, expression of SKP2 has a certain correlation with p27 lower level expression. SKP2 make E2F degraded by ubiquitin pathway.

4. P21

There are negative regulatory effects of P21 inhibiting cyclin-CDK complexes.

P21 binding and inhibiting various cyclin-CDK complexes, negatively regulate the function of CDK. The experimental results show that Cyclin-CDK complexes are combined with p21 in most normal cells, but are not combined in most transformed cells. P21 is the target of P53. P21 promoter contains P53 binding site. Damage to the DNA in G_1 phase can activate p53, induce P21 transcription, leading to Cyclin D-CDK4 and Cyclin E-CDK2 inhibition that prevents cells from entering S phase. Therefore, damaged DNA is repaired. P21 plays an important role in the stagnation of G_1 phase which induces the repair of damaged DNA mediated by p53.

Summary in the interaction of various elements in cell cycle regulation (Fig. 5-5)

Section 4   Cell Cycle Checkpoints

During the long period of evolution, cells developed a set inspection mechanism that ensure the cell cycle DNA replication and quality distribution in chromosomes. It is known as the cell cycle check-point, or restriction point. This is a negative feedback mechanism.

Function of cell cycle check-point: To check the damaged DNA——Checking with or without injury, synthesis and replication errors of cell cycle phase——Ensure the strict sequence and no repetition of cell cycle phase. Guaranteeing the cell cycle. The event of next phase starts after finished the last event. Cell cycle checkpoints constitute a full component of DNA repair.

1. Major Checkpoints in Cell Cycle

G_1-S phase check-point, S-G_2 phase check-point, G_2-M phase check-point. Composition of the check point decided to detect or sense, stop or arrest, repair, continue to divide or death of cells (Fig. 5-6).

2. Relevant Cells Events of Cell Cycle CheckPoints

G_1-S phase check-point: In yeast it is called start point. In mammals it is called the restriction point, and control cells enter DNA synthesis phase from resting G_1 phase. This is the most important checkpoint that means the cells has successfully completed its cycle. Cells in this check-point integrate and deliver all kinds of growth factors, mitogens, as well as DNA damage and other complex internal and external signals to determine the direction of cell development (division, apoptosis or entering the G_0 phase).

Related events include: Whether does the DNA damage? Whether there is suitability of the extracellular environment? Whether the cell size is big enough?

(1) The primary cause of G_1-S phase check-point defection leading to tumorigenesis is the deletion of p53 and upregulation of cyclinD1.

START regulating failure in the late G_1 phase will make the cell to cross the normal checking procedures into S phase, and allow cell to replicate the unrepaired mutated DNA, which is not repaired, and then accumulate the genetic changes of tumor phenotype (Fig. 5-7).

The uncontrollable proliferating cancer cells tend to remain in a continuous cell cycle.Once the cells cross G_1 terminal limit point, they will have a refractory period on extracellular growth regulating signals to be replaced with a self-regulatory program, and take this information into mitosis. Study of limit point adjustment isa key to find out how and why cancer cells continue to enter cycle.

(2) S phase check-point

G_2/M check-point: It is the control point which determines the cell into two, and prevents DNA which is damaged or unfinished to enter mitosis. P53 is the key mechanism that DNA damage repair- induces G_2 phase arrest. The defection of G_2 check-point caused by p53 deficiency is related to the occurrence and developments of many tumors.

(3) M phase check-point (spindle assembly checkpoint)

It mainly prevents cell division. Cell surface forms the spindle and chromosomes attach from spindle. If any of the centromeres is not properly connected to the spindle, it will inhibit the activity of related kinases causing the cell cycle to stop.

The functional defect of check-point will cause gene mutations, chromosome aberrations, genetic instability. Only when the accumulated mutations gene destruct the driven mechanism of cell cycle, cells can enter the uncontrolled growth.

Someone takes driving mechanism of cell cycle as a car that factors drive to run like the throttle, break its running mechanism like the brakes, and take hold of the accelerator or the brake fail will both cause out of control.

Section 5　Cell Cycle Regulation in Human Cancer Research and Treatment

Normal tissue maintain homeostasis between increase and decrease of the number of cells.

Tumor cell cycle control mechanism damage makes cell proliferation more than cell loss, presents relatively unlimited growth. Analysis on the molecular level shows that cell cycle regulation disorders is due to gene mutation caused by abnormal activation of promotor factors and (or) inhibitor inactivation in cell cycle. For example, over-expressionsof Cyclin A and Cyclin D1, loss of p15 and P16 expression in tumor that can leadto the development and progression of tumors.

1. Cyclins and Proto-oncogenes

Proto-oncogenes Myc and Ras have an interaction with Cyclin D in transformed cells.

E2F stimulates the co-expression of Cyclin A and c-myc.

Activation of Cyclin E-CDK is dependent on the interaction of Ras and Myc.

Increased c-myc expression can induce p27 exisence, which cannot be combined with cyclin E-CDK2, preventing CyclinE-CDK2 inactivating, and allowing cells to continue to proliferate.

Overexpression of C-fos can reduce the level of p27, enhance Cylcin E-CDK2 complexes activity, and promote cell proliferation.

When intracellular C-myc and Ras co-expression, they can make intracellular p27 disappear.

2. CyclinD1

In normal tissue besides the tonsils (detection of Cyclin D1 the ideal organization), vascular endothelial cells, some histocytes and basal cells of squamous epithelium may express Cyclin D1. Other organizations are not expressed.

Cyclin Dl, due to gene amplification or rearrangement, is over-expressed in a variety of tumors. Cyclin Dl gene amplification is in about 11%~20% tumors, over-expression rate of Cyclin D1 protein is about 50% or higher in tumors.

Significance of Cyclin D1 over-expression in tumors includes:

1) Associated with some tissue types of tumor, different positive rate in different tumors and different cell states;

2) Associated with tissue differentiation degree, increased expression in poorly differentiated tumor;

3) Associated with prognosis, in a variety of tumors, over-expression of Cyclin D1 is an independent prognostic indicator;

Although there is a close relationship between Cyclin D1 and tumor, Cyclin D1 overexpression alone is insufficient to cause malignant transformation of cells, there must be an interaction effect with other cells which can exit the G_0 phase oncogenes, such as the interactionwith Ras and Myc.

Chen Li's study showed that over-expression of Cyclin D1 in nasopharyngeal carcinoma (56%),in the nest and expanding growth patterns, positive rate of Cyclin D1 significantly higher than other growth patterns.In nasopharyngeal carcinoma, Cyclin D1, P16 and Rb co-exceptions may exist simultaneously. Cyclin D1, P16 and Rb abnormal expression are common molecular events in nasopharyngeal carcinoma growth, differentiation and metastasis.LMP1 (EBV) infection was positively correlated with Cyclin D1 overexpression, and negatively correlated with expression of P16 and Rb.

The combined effects of p16 deletion and Cyclin D1 overexpression can make tumor cells obtain more growth trend.

P16 has rearrangement, deletion or mutation in many tumors, suggesting that p16 inactivation is related to many tumors. P16 methylation may be the genetic basis of familial melanoma.

Mantle cell lymphoma (MCL):

In addition to the characteristic T (11, 14) (q13, q32) of MCL, where are Bcl_2 lode for Cycling, which makes Cyclin Dl protein over-expression. Therefore, International Lymphoma Society believes that chromosome 11q13 translocation of MCL and over-expression of Cyclin D1 are both very important characteristics. In MCL, because the Cyclin D1 has high sensitivity and relative specificity, it can be a specific marker to distinguish other lymphomas.

3. Cyclin A

The earliest tumor linked with mechanisms of cell cycle is Cyclin A. There are two clue hints of Cyclin A changes, that may be associated with cell transformation (cancerous).

(1) In hepatocellular carcinoma(HCC) cells, HBV DNA fragments integrate into Cyclin A gene; This is only insertion point for clone of HBV liver cells. The virus insert then integrate into host DNA and form chimeras. The regions between the N-terminal Cyclin A and cyclin box is replaced by gene sequences of the virus, which forms proteins that are not degraded in the normal mitosis phase.

(2) As can be seen from the adenovirus-transformed cells, Cyclin A binds with ElA—the adenovirus transforming protein.

4. P27

Study shows that expression levels of p27 protein is clearly relevant with the degree of malignant tumor, invasion and prognosis, which can be used as indicators of prognosis in some malignant tumors.

Chen Li's study in 100 cases of gastric cancer pointed that the significantly relationship between p27Kip1 expression and gastric carcinoma invasion, metastasis and prognosis. The positive rate of p27Kip1 protein expression in gastric cancer tissue was 44%. The expression of p27Kip1 was significantly lower in the group of deep infiltration of gastric cancer, death within 5 years and lymph node metastasis, respectively.The 5-year survival rate in group of p27Kip1 higher expression was 70.59%, significantly higher than that in lower expression (54.55%) and negative (26%). p27Kip1 is a good independent prognostic indicator.

5. Cancer treatments

(1) The sensitivity of tumor therapy in different cells is different

1) Cells in cell cycle are more sensitive to antitumor drugs or radiation therapy.

2) G_0 cells without proliferating temporarily in the resting state; Not sensitive to antitumor drug and radiation therapy that can be a source of tumor recurrence.

(2) Medicine against tumor cells in each phase

1) CCNSA (cell cycle non-specific agents): Effect in various phases, including G_0 phase cells

2) CCSA (cell cycle specific agents): The drugs that are only sensitive to certain phases of the cell cycle and insensitive to cells in G_0 phase.

(3) The strategies of cancer treatment targeting cell cycle

Limit the activity of CDKs to inhibit the excessive growth of tumor cells

Inhibit the expression of Cyclins to block tumor cell proliferation.

Raise the level of CKIs, ease out the control of tumor cells proliferation.

Use of the check point defects of cell cycle, as it a target to accelerating tumor cell death.

Challenges and Prospects

Cell cycle is usually precisely regulated by signal transduction pathways and feedback loops whether. It is normal or not, it is closely related to cell as well as individual growth, differentiation, aging and cancer.After going through a complete cycle, some cells continue to proliferate. Some cells may be temporary or never proliferate. The key to decide the fate of various cells cycle is the regulation of cell cycle. Current research on cell cycle regulation is a hot-spot in life science. The development of research will further reveal the molecular mechanism of cell cycle regulation. It will have an important guiding significance to understand the kinetics of cell growth, the regulation of the cell cycle, cancer prevention and treatments interventions.

Consider/Questions

1. Basic concepts in this chapter

Cell division cycle, Cyclin, Cyclin-dependent kinase (CDK), CDK inhibitory proteins (CKIs), cell cycle checkpoint, Rb gene, E2F.

2. Summarize the roles of Cyclin D1 in cell cycle regulation, and its pathological significance.

3. Summarize the roles of Rb gene in cell cycle regulation.

4. Summarize the Cyclins and CDKs appearance within specific cell phases.

5. Summarize the functions of cell cycle checkpoints.

6. Summarize the regulators in G_1 phase relateol to tumorgenesis.

第六章 端粒与端粒酶

　　细胞学家 Hayflick（海弗利克）在五十年前发现培养的人体成纤维细胞在营养充分供给的情况下，细胞分裂到 50 代左右就停止活动，真正地进入衰老期。随着对端粒、端粒酶结构和端粒酶激活及调节机制的深入研究，阐明了端粒酶可有效地调控端粒的长度，而端粒的长度直接影响细胞的增殖或凋亡，从而决定人体寿命的长短。进一步揭示了端粒酶与人类衰老和肿瘤发生、发展的关系，端粒、端粒酶的功能失调将影响细胞的生物学行为，包括细胞周期的稳定性、细胞增殖、癌变、凋亡和衰老。

第一节　端粒与端粒酶的发现

一、端粒的发现

　　端粒（telomere）一词最早由果蝇遗传学家 Hermann J. Muller（赫尔曼·约瑟夫·穆勒，1946 因辐射遗传学研究获诺贝尔奖）命名。其含义为末端的部分，由两个希腊词根 "telos"（末端）和 "meros"（部分）合并而成。这一命名方式是按照 "centromere"（着丝粒）和 "chromomere"（染色粒）这类构词方式组成，此类构词在二十世纪三四十年代带有明显的细胞学和遗传学含义。

　　Muller 通过 X 射线对果蝇进行人工诱变，导致果蝇染色体断裂和重排，对染色体断端进行了早期研究。1938 年 9 月，Muller 在一次精彩演讲中对端粒（图 6-1）做出了完整阐述[1]，"末端基因一定具有某种特殊功能，即可对染色体的末端起到封闭的作用"，"为区别于其他基因，采用端粒命名""端粒具有单极性，只与一个（而不是两个）基因连接"。

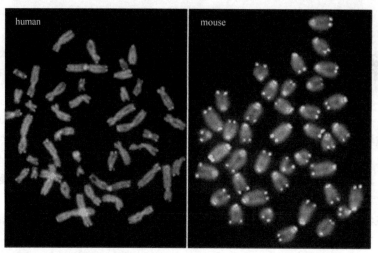

图 6-1　通过原位杂交技术可见位于染色体末端的端粒结构；Telomere structure at the ends of chromosomes is visible by in situ hybridization

　　几乎同一时期，Barbara McClintock（巴巴拉·麦克林托克，1983 年因玉米转座子研究获诺贝尔奖）在进行玉米减数分裂实验中发现[2]，减数分裂后期偶然产生的染色体断端极易重新融合形成"桥"，并出现染色体"断裂—融合—桥—断裂"的重复循环。新形成的染色体断端比较黏，易于与其他片段结合，若"断裂的末端愈合，整个循环完全终止"，而正常的染色体末端则非常稳定，不易发生相互融合。

　　两名遗传学家在不同实验室用不同物种进行的实验中，都发现了染色体末端结构对保持染色体功能的稳定性十分重要，明确了端粒是真核生物染色体末端的特殊结构，由端粒 DNA 和端粒结合蛋白组成，其功能在于维持染色体的稳定性和完整性。通过原位杂交技术可见位于染色体末端的端粒结构（图 6-1）。

　　随着研究手段的进步，1978 年 Elizabeth 实验室成功用化学方法测定出了四膜虫（*Tetrahymena*）的端粒序列。四膜虫被誉为研究端粒和端粒酶的最佳生物模型，四膜虫属于原生动物门，纤毛虫纲，进化地位处于原核生物和高等真核生物之间。四膜虫有两个细胞核[3]。小核很稳定，含 5 对染色体，用于生殖传代。大核在接合细胞的发育过程中，rDNA（核糖体 DNA）从染色体上断裂后通过复制可形成高达 10 000 多个小染色体，能够提供非常丰富的端粒资源，因此四膜虫是研究端粒得天独厚的材料（图 6-2）。Elizabeth 实验室利用这种特殊的模式生物进行化学实验，证实四膜虫端粒具有六聚体重复序列，同时还证明该序列具有极性，即从 5′→3′方向由 TTGGGG 序列构成[4]。随后的大量实验表明，大多数生物中端粒的序列和结构具有保守性，基本都以富含 G 碱基的重复序列为特征，几乎所有生物的端粒重复序列都可以写成：G_n（A/T）$_m$ 的形式。

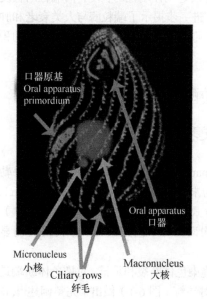

口器原基
Oral apparatus
primordium

Oral apparatus
口器

Micronucleus
小核

Ciliary rows
纤毛

Macronucleus
大核

图 6-2　四膜虫结构示意图；The structure of Tetrahymena

二、端粒酶的发现

对端粒酶（telomerase）结构的关注大概源自如何解决"末端隐缩问题"的一些猜想。20世纪70年代初，对 DNA 聚合酶特性的深入了解引申出了一个染色体的复制问题。DNA 聚合酶在复制 DNA 的时候必须要有 RNA 引物来起始，但线性染色体最末端的 RNA 引物因为没有办法被 DNA 取代，所以每复制一轮，RNA 引物降解后末端都将缩短一个 RNA 引物的长度。James Watson[5]（詹姆斯·沃森，DNA 分子双螺旋模型的发现者之一，1962 年获诺贝尔奖）最早明确指出此"末端隐缩问题"，并猜想染色体也许可以通过复制前联体（染色体末端与末端连起来）的方式来解决末端复制的问题。1980 年 Elizabeth 实验室报告了四膜虫的端粒发现，立即引起了 Jack Szostak（杰克·绍斯塔克）的兴趣。当时他正在世界范围内率先开展酵母菌中合成人造染色体的研究，希望人造染色体能够在细胞中像自然染色体一样复制，但是当线性染色体转入酵母细胞后往往很快被降解。线性染色体的降解是否因其末端没有端粒保护？端粒序列的发现让 Jack Szostak 有机会把线性染色体末端连接四膜虫的端粒 DNA，然后再导入酵母细胞。奇迹发生了，线性染色体不再降解，它可以在细胞内复制，合成人工染色体的想法实现了！人工染色体的实现当初也许仅仅是满足人们的异想天开，但它实际上使 DNA 的大片段克隆成为可能，为后来人类基因组测序的工作立下了汗马功劳。这也是 Jack Szostak 共同获得诺贝尔奖的重要原因。随后 Elizabeth 实验室发现了一个有趣的现象：带着四膜虫端粒 DNA 的人工染色体导入到酵母后，被加上了酵母的端粒而不是四膜虫的端粒序列。由于端粒是由重复序列组成的，当时人们普遍猜想同源重组是延伸端粒补偿染色体末端隐缩的机制。但是同源重组只能复制出更多本身的序列，而四膜虫端粒上被加上酵母的端粒序列，而不是四膜虫端粒本身序列，这个现象用同源重组理论无法解释，科学家拟推断酵母中可能存在专门的"酶"来复制端粒 DNA。经过多次优化条件后，1984 年圣诞节，该酶在 Elizabeth Blackburn（伊丽莎白·布莱克本）和其博士生 Carol Greider（卡罗尔·格雷德）的共同努力下被发现和确认，这种酶活性不依赖于 DNA 模板和 DNA 聚合酶，只对端粒 DNA 进行延伸，而对随机序列的 DNA 底物不延伸[6]。后来证实，这确实是一种 RNA 依赖的 DNA 聚合酶（RNA dependent DNA polymerase），并被命名为"端粒酶"。端粒酶是在染色体末端不断合成端粒序列的酶，是一种核酸核蛋白酶，即 RNA 依赖的 DNA 聚合酶。能以自身的 RNA 为模板合成端粒 DNA 的重复序列，具有逆转录酶活性，它的活性不依赖于 DNA 聚合酶，对 RNA 酶、蛋白酶和高温均敏感。

1989 年 Carol Greider 通过跟踪端粒酶活性，纯化并克隆了四膜虫的端粒酶 RNA 亚基。1996 年 Tom Cech（汤姆·切赫，1989 年因发现核酶而获诺贝尔奖）实验室纯化端粒的催化亚基，并确认其含有逆转录酶的结构域。

2009 年瑞典卡罗林斯卡医学院宣布，将该年度诺贝尔生理学与医学奖授予美国加利福尼亚旧金山大学的 Elizabeth Blackburn、美国巴尔的摩约翰·霍普金斯医学院的 Carol Greider、美国哈佛医学院的 Jack Szostak 及霍华德休斯医学研究所，以表彰他们对揭示"染色体是如何被端粒和端粒酶保护的"这一古老课题作出的巨大贡献。这三人"解决了生物学上的一个重大问题"，即在细胞分裂时染色体如何进行完整复制，如何免于退化。其中奥秘全部蕴藏在端粒和端粒酶上。

三、端粒和端粒酶发现大事记

1938 年，端粒一词命名。

1939 年，发现玉米细胞的染色体断裂末端容易融合。

1972 年，提出染色体复制的末端隐缩问题。

1978 年，报道四膜虫的端粒序列。

1982 年，端粒的发现导致人工染色体的发明。

1984 年，报道酵母的端粒序列。

1985 年，报道四膜虫的端粒酶活性。

1989 年，报道四膜虫端粒酶的 RNA 亚基。

1994 年，报道酵母端粒酶的 RNA 亚基。

1995 年，报道酵母端粒酶活性。

1996 年，纯化了四膜虫端粒酶的催化亚基，遗传筛选到酵母端粒酶的催化亚基。

1997 年，证明了四膜虫和酵母端粒酶的催化亚基。

2009 年，诺贝尔生理学或医学奖授予发现了端粒和端粒酶保护染色体的机制。

第二节　端粒与端粒酶的特征

一、端粒的结构与功能

端粒是真核生物染色体末端的特殊结构，由端粒 DNA 和端粒结合蛋白组成，其功能在于维持染色体的稳定性和完整性。

（一）端粒的结构

端粒 DNA 为不含功能基因的简单、高度重复序列，在生物进化过程中具有高度保守性。不同物种的端粒 DNA 序列存在差异（表 6-1），但都以富含 G 碱基的重复序列为特征。例如，四膜虫端粒重复序列为 TTGGGG，酿酒酵母端粒重复序列为 $T(G)_{2\sim3}(TG)_{1\sim6}$，脊椎动物人和鼠的端粒重复序列均为 TTAGGG。

端粒结合蛋白是与端粒 DNA 特异序列相结合的蛋白质。人端粒结合蛋白称为端粒重复序列结合因子（telomeric repeat factor，TRF），包括 TRF1 和 TRF2。TRF1 大小约 60kDa，可与同源二聚体双链 TTAGGG 重复序列结合，包含一个 C 端螺旋-转折-螺旋区和一个 DNA 结合折叠同源区，其 N 端是酸性区。通过负反馈调节机制抑制端粒增长，起到稳定端粒长度的作用。研究发现其抑制端粒酶在端粒末端的行为，但不抑制端粒酶活性。TRF2 与 TRF1 相似，但 N 端碱性强，可以防止染色体末端相互融合。

表 6-1　经典生物端粒重复序列

生物	序列	报道者	报道时间
四膜虫	TTGGGG	Blackburn、Gall [4]	1978
尖毛虫	TTTTGGGG	Klobutcher et al.[7]	1991
锥虫	TTAGGG	Blackburn、Challoner [8]	1984
酿酒酵母	$T(G)_{2\sim3}(TG)_{1\sim6}$	Shampay, et al.[9]	1984
番茄	TT（T/A）GGG	Ganal, et al. [10]	1991
人	TTAGGG	Moyzis et al.[11]	1988
鼠	TTAGGG	Kipling、Cooke, et al.[12]	1990

端粒结构较为稳定，以人端粒为例，端粒 DNA 由两条互相配对的 DNA 单链组成，其中一条稍长于另一条，其双链部分通过与端粒结合蛋白 TRF1（依赖于端粒酶）和 TRF2（不依赖于端粒酶）结合使端粒的 3′单链端（G 尾）重复取代了双链 DNA 中的同源重复序列以形成一个 t 环（t loop）[13]（图 6-3）。t 环的这种特殊结构可维持染色体末端的稳定，保持染色体及其内部基因的完整性，从而使遗传物质得以完整复制。

（二）端粒的功能

端粒的基本功能之一是对染色体的保护作用。缺少端粒的染色体不能稳定存在，这是因为端粒 DNA 与结构蛋白形成的复合物如同染色体的一顶"帽子"，它既可保护染色体不被降解，又避免了端粒对端融合（end-end fusion）。同时端粒能帮助识别细胞中完整染色体和受损染色体。

端粒的另一重要意义体现在细胞有丝分裂过程中。细胞学家 Hayflick 发现，体外培养人成纤

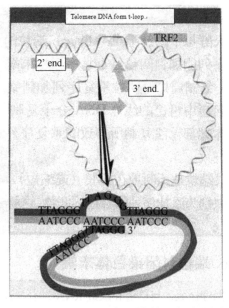

图 6-3　端粒 DNA 形成 t 环结构示意图（人）；Telomere DNA at the end of chromosomes form a special DNA t loop

维细胞，即使在营养充分供给的情况下，细胞分裂到 50 代左右也将停止复制，进入衰老期。而端粒长度的丢失在这一过程中扮演重要的角色，至少可以成为有丝分裂能力的一种标记。由于每次 DNA 复制中，每条染色体的 3′端均有一段 DNA 无法得到复制，随着细胞每次分裂，染色体 3′端将持续丧失 50～200bp 的 DNA，因而细胞分裂具有一定的限度，即分裂寿命[14]。所以端粒的长度可作为细胞的"分裂时钟"（division clock），反映细胞分裂能力。随着每次细胞分裂，染色体末端逐渐缩短，当端粒缩短到一定关键性长度时，染色体的稳定性受到破坏，细胞将停止分裂，出现衰老迹象。目前的研究发现，生殖细胞中可稳定维持较长的端粒，其他组织细胞如皮肤、肺和血管中，端粒往往随年龄增长而逐渐缩短。许多证据都表明端粒长度的丢失对于人类细胞的衰老具有重要的生物学意义，因此端粒也被称为"生命时钟"（life clock）。

二、端粒酶的结构和功能

（一）端粒酶的结构

端粒酶实质上是一种特殊的逆转录酶，能通过明显的模板依赖方式每次添加一个核苷酸，它由三个主要亚单位构成：端粒酶 RNA（TR）、端粒酶逆转录酶（TERT）和端粒酶相关蛋白（TEP）。

1. 端粒酶 RNA（telomerase RNA，TR）　是第一个被克隆的端粒酶成分。端粒酶 RNA 富含 C_yA_x 序列，可与富含 T_xG_y 的端粒 DNA 序列形成互补将端粒序列添加到染色体末端（图 6-4）。端粒酶 RNA 转录模板内的远端区参与和底物的结合。近端区能添加特定的核苷酸，对底物识别并不重要。模板边界区（端粒酶 RNA 内最后复制入 DNA 的位置）可与 TERT 和 TEP（Est1p）等结合[15]。端粒酶 RNA 是端粒酶执行功能的关键成分，体外实验中使用 RNA 酶 H 切割端粒酶 RNA，能消除端粒酶延长端粒的功能。

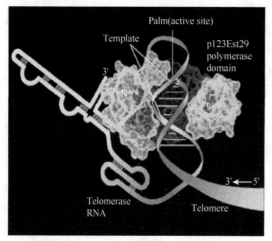

图 6-4　端粒酶, RNA 依赖的 DNA 聚合酶; Telomerase, RNA dependent DNA polymerase

2. 端粒酶逆转录酶　几乎所有存在端粒酶的细胞均含有单独的端粒酶逆转录酶 (telomerase reverse transcriptase, TERT) 基因, 哺乳动物 TERT 的转录由许多转录因子、激素和细胞外信号严格控制。不同的转录因子调节 TERT 在不同的细胞内的表达。TERT 能够催化端粒 DNA 转录合成, 破坏 TERT 将消除端粒酶活性并致端粒缩短。

TERT 晶体结构由三部分组成: RNA 结合区 (TRBD)、逆转录区 (reverse transcriptase domain) 和 C 端延伸区 (carboxy-terminal extension, CTE)。TRBD 主要由螺旋组成, 含有 CP 和 T 两个保守区域, 与单链和双链 RNA 结合。逆转录区由 α 螺旋和 β 折叠组成, 呈现像手指 (figer) 和手掌 (palm) 形状的结构。CTE 区由延长的螺旋组成, 其表面有长的 loop 结构。

TERT 内的 N-残基的功能包括与端粒酶 RNA 结合、装配和催化作用, 与 p53 的相互作用和细胞永生化。TERT 的 C-残基也在人类原始成纤维细胞的永生化、端粒组装的竞争、核仁内定位、引物结合和渐进性延长等方面起重要作用[16]。

人类 TERT (hTERT) 基因为一单拷贝基因, 定位于 5p15. 33, 具有 7 个保守序列结构域单元和端粒酶特异性结构域单元 T。有报道认为癌基因 c-myc 为一重要的端粒酶激活剂, 存在于 hTERT 核心启动子中有两个重要的 c-myc 结合位点 (CACGTG, 亦被称为 E 盒)。 c-myc 是一个受特殊信号调节的可诱导癌基因, 并可与 H-Ras、N-Ras、多瘤病毒 MTLT 等癌基因协同作用, 促进细胞无限增殖, 获得永生化并发生癌变。Fujimoto 等[10]用 c-myc 反义寡核苷酸转染白血病细胞 HL260、U73 和 K562, 这些细胞端粒酶活性均下调, 而 c-myc 正义寡核苷酸无此作用。Wang 等[17]研究发现 c-myc 在正常人乳腺上皮细胞 (HMECS) 和双倍体成纤维细胞中可诱导端粒酶活性, 并能延长 HMECS 的寿命。c-myc 诱导的 hTERT 表达起始速度快, 不受细胞增殖或额外的蛋白合成的影响, 与 c-myc 引起直接的转录激活一致。但癌基因 c-myc 不是唯一与 hTERT 基因调节有关的转录因子。近期研究表明, Sp1 协同 c-myc 激活 hTERT 的转录。可能还有其他因子, 如 Bcl-2 抗凋亡基因、E6 人乳头状瘤病毒 16 型蛋白等均可使 hTERT 上调。但在诸多不同类型的瘤细胞中, 致 hTERT 上调的基本激活剂是 c-myc[18]。

3. 端粒酶相关蛋白(telomerase associated protein, TEP)

(1) TEP1 是一多功能的 RNA 结合蛋白, TEP1 缺失导致 rRNA 水平的显著降低, 但不导致端粒酶活性或端粒长度的紊乱[19]。

(2) 运动神经元存活基因 (SMN) 产物, 即一种被喻为 RNP 生物源的蛋白, 已被证实为另一种人端粒酶相关蛋白。热休克蛋白 (HSP) 90 可能是芽殖酵母端粒酶活性和端粒长度维持的调节剂。其他涉及 TERT 转录后修饰的蛋白包括磷酸酶-A、Akt、cAbl、P53 和 PARP 等。

(3) 芽殖酵母蛋白 Est1p 和 Est3p 与体内端粒酶的功能有关。Est1p 使端粒延长。但无 Est1p 的情况下, Est2p-Cdc13pDBD 融合也可以维持端粒长度[20]。

（二）端粒酶的功能

在端粒酶被发现以前，人们就推测生殖细胞之所以能世代相传，其中可能存在一种维持端粒长度的特殊机制，体细胞可能正是由于缺乏这种机制，它的染色体末端才面临着致死性缺失（deletion）的危险。因此在正常人体细胞向永生化细胞（immortalized cells）及肿瘤细胞的转化过程中可能也存在着与生殖细胞类似的机制。这些细胞怎样保持细胞具有继续分裂或长期分裂的能力呢？科学家们发现端粒确实随着每次分裂而缩短，但细胞可通过端粒酶使已缩短的端粒延长，从而维持端粒长度，保持细胞增殖潜能，抑制细胞的衰老。在生殖细胞和干细胞中可检测到高水平的端粒酶活性。

在端粒的复制中，端粒酶的催化亚基利用端粒酶 RNA 亚基作为模板，通过转位不断重复复制出端粒 DNA，从而补偿在染色体复制过程中的末端隐缩，保证染色体的完全复制。没有端粒酶的细胞中，端粒会逐渐缩短至损害基因。有端粒酶存在的细胞，则端粒长度得到补充更新，使端粒处于一种动态平衡状态。

端粒酶的另一功能是修复断裂的染色体末端。当断裂的染色体末端有丰富的 G、T 碱基存在时，即使没有完整的端粒重复序列存在，端粒酶也能以此为引物延伸该染色体端粒序列，从而使末端免遭外切酶的破坏。此外，端粒合成过程中，端粒酶还具有纠错作用，可去除错配碱基。

第三节　端粒与端粒酶的作用机制

一、DNA 的半保留复制

真核生物的染色体主要由 DNA 和组蛋白构成。DNA 是遗传信息的载体，生物体以 DNA 为模板合成 RNA 的过程称为转录，即将储存于 DNA 中的遗传信息通过转录和翻译得到表达。逆转录过程是指以 RNA 为模板，由脱氧核苷三磷酸（deoxy-ribonucleoside triphosphate，dNTP）聚合形成 DNA 分子，此过程中，核酸合成与转录的过程与遗传信息流动的过程相反，故称为逆转录。逆转录酶是依赖 RNA 的 DNA 聚合酶。一般认为，端粒酶是一种特殊的逆转录酶，能以自身的 RNA 为模板合成端粒的重复序列，以维持端粒长度的稳定性。

核酸的基本组成单位是核苷酸，由碱基、戊糖和磷酸三种成分连接而成。DNA 分子中的碱基成分是 A（腺嘌呤，adenine）、T（胸腺嘧啶，thymine）、G（鸟嘌呤，guanine）和 C（胞嘧啶，cytosine），碱基之间具有严格的互补配对关系，A-T、G-C 配对，彼此之间以氢键连接。RNA 分子中的碱基成分是 A-U（尿嘧啶，uracil）和 G-C 配对。

DNA 复制最重要的特征是半保留复制。复制时，亲代的 DNA 双链解开螺旋，形成两条单链，各自作为模板指导子代合成新的互补链。子代细胞的 DNA 双链，其中一条是从亲代完整接受过来，另一条则是由底物完全重新合成。由于碱基互补，两个子细胞的 DNA 双链都和亲代 DNA 碱基序列一致。DNA 复制是在多种酶催化下进行的核苷酸聚合过程，相邻核苷酸之间以磷酸二酯键聚合形成 DNA 长链，由底物的 5′-P 加合到原有的游离 3′-OH 上形成，新链合成只能从 5′→3′方向进行，此即为复制的方向性。

二、冈崎片段和染色体末端隐缩问题

（一）冈崎片段

子代 DNA 复制过程中，顺着解链方向由 5′→3′复制的新链，复制是连续进行的，称为前导链。另一条新链的复制方向与解链方向相反，复制时必须等待模板解开足够的长度，才能从 5′→3′复制，顺着解链方向，等到下一段又暴露出足够长度的模板，再进行另一段从 5′→3′的复制。这种复制称为半不连续复制，这条不连续复制的 DNA 链被称为后随链，其中不连续的 DNA 片段即冈崎片段（Okazaki fragment）。因日本学者冈崎令治在研究大肠杆菌中的噬菌体 DNA 复制时发现此现象而得名。1968 年冈崎用含有 3H-dTTP（脱氧胸苷三磷酸，deoxy-thymidine triphosphate）的培养液短时间标记大肠杆菌，分离纯化 DNA，变性后用超离心方法得到许多 3H-dTTP 标记的短片段，长度约为 1000～2000bp。延长标记时间后，这些片段可转变为成熟的 DNA 链，因此这些片段是复制过程中的中间产物，这些小分子片段就被称为冈崎片段。

（二）末端隐缩问题

DNA 的复制需要 RNA 引物，这是由 DNA 聚合酶和 RNA 聚合酶的特性决定的。在复制时，已知的 DNA 聚合酶都不能直接启动复制，必须在 RNA 聚合酶作用下，以 DNA 为模板合成一小段 RNA 作为引物提供一个 3′-OH，这样 DNA 聚合酶才能在此基础上按照 5′→3′的方向聚合脱氧核糖核苷三磷酸来延伸 DNA 新链。当复制延伸反应启动之后，5′-端的 RNA 引物便被降解掉，这样母链的 5′-端将会有一小段无法拷贝到子链当中去，造成 DNA 信息的丢失。DNA 复制结束时，前导链 5′端会留有引物消除后的空缺，而在后随链中，由于 DNA 合成是不连续进行，上一次引物消除所留下的空缺将被下一次复制补完整，因此当最后一次不连续复制的引物被消除后无法得到弥补。

所以线性染色体 DNA 每复制一轮，RNA 引物降解后末端都将缩短一个 RNA 引物的长度。尽管这个引物不长，但是细胞持续不断复制，如果不进行补偿，染色体不断缩短，最终就会消失。此即"末端隐缩问题"，最早由 James Watson 明确提出，当时人们猜想染色体也许可以通过在复制前联体（染色体末端与末端连起来）的方式来解决末端复制的问题（图 6-5）。

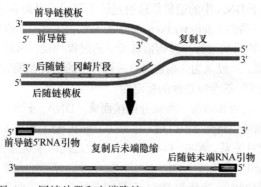

图 6-5 冈崎片段和末端隐缩；Okazaki fragment and at the end of hidden problems

（三）端粒酶使端粒延长的作用机制

人类对端粒-端粒酶结构和功能的探索是一个漫长而严谨的过程。真核生物的端粒具有特殊的复制难题，如前文所说，由于 DNA 聚合酶不能完整地复制后随链，通常 DNA 复制中染色体末端会发生序列丢失。20 世纪 80 年代，对于端粒复制特点有两个重要发现：①锥虫在宿主体内连续传代时端粒长度增加[21]，在类似的四膜虫实验中，维持在对照生长期的细胞内端粒长度也增加[22]；②把四膜虫端粒转入亲缘关系较远的酿酒酵母中也可以起到端粒的作用，并且酵母特有的端粒重复序列可以添加在其线性质粒的末端[23]。人们提出两种模型解释端粒序列是如何添加的，第一种模型认为 DNA 重组或聚合酶在重复序列上的滑动可延伸端粒序列，即可能通过基因重组机制来获得端粒结构[23]。第二类模型认为端粒序列是由目前尚未知的聚合酶添加上的，此酶可以在没有模板条件下将序列添加到染色体末端[9]。后一种模型显然可以更好地解释酵母特异重复序列在四膜虫端粒上的添加。1985 年 Greider [24]在四膜虫中鉴定出这一"目前尚未知的聚合酶"。该酶可通过对端粒不依赖模板的复制，补偿由于去除引物而可能造成的 DNA 线性末端缩短，此即端粒酶。1989 年 Elizabeth 实验室在反复多次试验的基础上[25]，以四膜虫为例，提出了端粒酶合成端粒重复序列的模型，尽管此模型的细节还需要完善，但总的来说，该模型经受住了时间的考验。其延伸机制：①端粒酶与染色体末端结合，端粒酶 RNA 模板区 5'-CAACCCCAA-3'序列与端粒 TTGGGG 重复序列形成碱基配对；②端粒 DNA 通过在 3'端添加 TTG 而延伸；③端粒酶 RAN 移位，使末端新形成的 TTGGGG 序列重新和暴露的模板序列配对；④另一轮模板复制产生新的 TTGGGG 重复序列（图 6-6）。体内端粒酶的延长功能是一复杂的动态过程：受双链端粒结合蛋白包括 RAP1（芽殖酵母）、存在于 t 环的 TRF1 和 TRF2 的负调控。

第四节 疾病中端粒与端粒酶研究的意义

"端粒-端粒酶假说"认为端粒酶的激活与细胞永生化和恶性肿瘤的发生、发展密切相关。

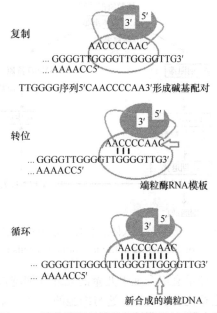

图 6-6 端粒酶延长端粒机制模型（四膜虫）；The mechanism of telomerase prolonging telomeres

一、细胞衰老及永生化中端粒-端粒酶假说

染色体末端的端粒 DNA 进行性缩短是限制人细胞寿命的先决条件。目前的资料证实，端粒酶对长期成活的组织和长期进行有丝分裂的细胞是必需的[26]。

细胞的死亡过程分为两个阶段，即第一致死期（mortality stage1，M_1）和第二致死期（mortality stage 2，M_2）。当端粒缩短至一关键性长度 2~4kb 时，染色体的稳定性就会遭到破坏，细胞开始衰老进入 M_1 期。在 M_1 期细胞对生长因子等失去反应，产生 DNA 合成蛋白抑制因子，细胞周期检查点（cell cycle checkpoint）发送细胞周期停止信号，DNA 合成即告停止，DNA 断裂，活化 p53 依赖（或非 p53 依赖）的 DNA 损伤修复途径。并诱导 CDK 抑制物如 P21、P27 产生，导致细胞 G_1 期生长停滞，最终走向死亡。如果这一过程中一些癌基因的激活和 Rb、p53 和 p16 等抑癌基因失活或功能丧失，均能使 M_1 期的机制被抑制使细胞逃逸 M_1 期，继续生长获得额外的增殖能力，此时端粒酶仍为阴性，端粒继续缩短，经过 20~30 次分裂后，最终到达 M_2 期。虽然上述情况可使细胞生命周期延长，但仍不能使其永生化，处于 M_2 期的细胞由于端粒过短，基因不稳定，绝大多数细胞将在这一时期死亡，只有极少数细胞由于端粒酶活性的上调或重新激活，端粒的功能得到恢复，使细胞超越 M_2 期，成为永生化细胞[27]（图 6-7）。

研究发现，不但在正常组织的永生化细胞（如造血干细胞、精子），而且在非永生的、正常生理状态下增殖活跃的细胞（如受抗原刺激的 T 淋巴细胞及 B 淋巴细胞、口腔和食管黏膜上皮、皮肤基底层角质形成细胞、宫颈上皮、小肠上皮）也可检出端粒酶活性。一般情况下，在生殖组织中极易检测到端粒酶的活性，并且在生殖细胞中可稳定维持较长的端粒；而大多数出生后的稳定的组织和细胞很难检测到端粒酶活性，且端粒长度随年龄逐渐缩短。端粒-端粒酶

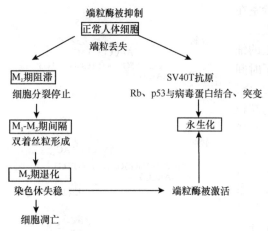

图 6-7　端粒酶在人体细胞永生化中的作用特点；The roles of telomerase in the immortalized cells of the human

假说将端粒的丢失同细胞衰老联系起来，另一方面，也将端粒酶再激活同肿瘤联系起来。许多证据都表明，对于衰老的人类细胞，端粒的丢失具有重要的生物学意义，如在多种类型的衰老体细胞中，都呈现出共同的端粒平均长度缩短，在体外衰老细胞及体内淋巴细胞中有与端粒丢失有关的染色体畸变的聚积。

端粒的缩短引起衰老。在早老患者中表现出端粒过度的缩短，进而缩短的端粒允许染色体融合，这些现象与年老患者的细胞中或培养的老化细胞中染色体组型衰老异常的高发生率密切相关。对患有郝-吉二氏病（Hutchinson-Gilford progeria，

一种早衰综合征）儿童的成纤维细胞进行体外培养后发现[28]，其端粒长度与同龄人正常细胞相比明显变短，这与细胞的复制力降低相一致。另外，端粒的丢失可以用来衡量培养基中再生细胞的衰老程度，也可根据它来判断细胞供体的年龄。对唐氏（Down）综合征患者外周血淋巴细胞端粒进行检测发现其细胞内端粒丢失程度是同龄人的三倍之多[29]。TERT 在神经退行性病变实验模型中展现出神经保护性功能，提示在神经细胞中若能提高端粒酶的活性可能会抑制与衰老相关的神经退行性病变，如 AD 和脑老化的发生等[30-32]。

端粒酶延长端粒长度以减慢细胞衰老最早的证据来自 Bodnar 等的研究，1998 年其在 Science 上刊文报道：在培养细胞中将人的端粒酶基因导入端粒酶阴性的正常人体细胞中激活其表达，与未导入该基因的细胞比较，发现前者端粒明显增长，细胞分裂旺盛，细胞寿命比后者大大延长，更令人关注的是细胞并无肿瘤样改变。例如，在神经细胞中激活端粒酶与 TERT 功能，能较好地避免神经细胞死亡，还可以促进神经细胞在各种神经元退行性病变条件下的恢复。端粒酶活性和细胞凋亡可作为伴有（或不伴有）子宫内发育延迟的胎盘衰老的标志。端粒缩短加快还可在许多病变中观察到，如 Werner 综合征、共济失调毛细血管扩张症、先天性角化不良等，虽然有些遗传异常和端粒缺陷的关系还不清楚，但可能的原因有①端粒核酸外切酶活性和（或）有效利用的增加。②端粒过度丢失。③在发育或出生后端粒补偿机制的不足。端粒缩短加速可由于环境应激介导的 DNA 损害或对这些损害敏感度增加所致。不管何种原因，端粒缩短速率增加可致增殖组织的早衰。

尽管端粒酶能使端粒长度延伸，但生物整体的老化是一个非常复杂的问题。即使仅在早老性疾病中，端粒缩短过快发生的原因和调控因素，端粒长度延伸后染色体是否能够稳定存在，端粒酶活化是否导致细胞肿瘤化，这些问题都有待于进一步深入研究予以解决。能否通过对端粒-端粒酶的研究，使细胞年轻化，进而延长人类生命，仍是一个漫长的课题。

二、端粒、端粒酶与肿瘤

自从 1994 年 Kim 等[33]创立 TRAP 法（端粒重复序列扩增法，telomeric repeat amplification protocol，TRAP）检测端粒酶活性以来，越来越多的文献报告了在大多数人类原发性肿瘤标本及肿瘤衍生细胞系中可检测到较高的端粒酶活性。证明肿瘤细胞持续增殖是端粒酶激活或端粒维持机制改变的结果，这是恶性肿瘤细胞显著的生物学特征之一，是癌变机制中一个十分重要的环节。

美国学者检测 400 多例来源于 12 种不同组织的原发肿瘤病例发现，肿瘤组织的端粒酶阳性率高达 84.8%，而肿瘤周围组织或良性病变中阳性率仅为 4.4%。Shay 等[34]总结了肿瘤端粒酶的检测结果，在正常组织（196 例）、原位癌（410 例）、恶性肿瘤（2031 例）和癌旁组织（690 例）中端粒酶的阳性率分别是 0.5%、30%、85%和 11%。在前列腺癌，乳腺、胰腺、肺、肝的早期癌中端粒酶的阳性率为 85.0%～95.0%，而对应的癌旁组织或良性病变组织中，端粒酶基本上不能检出或活性极微弱（表 6-2）。

表 6-2 人类肿瘤和非瘤组织中端粒酶活性的比较

肿瘤部位/类型	瘤旁正常组织/良性病变	肿瘤组织（%）
肺	3/68（4.4%）	108/136（80.1%）
乳腺	2/28（7.1%）	19/24（79.6%）
前列腺	1/18（5.6%）	23/27（85.1%）
结肠	0/45（0）	22/23（95.6%）
肝	—	1/1（100%）
卵巢	0/8（0）	7/7（100%）
肾	0/55（0）	40/55（72.7%）
成神经细胞	0/17（0）	94/100（94%）
血（淋巴瘤，CLL，ALL）	—	21/23（91.3%）
脑	—	6/8（75%）
其他（颅顶，Wilms 瘤）	8/93（8.6%）	24/26（92.3%）
总计	14/332（4.2%）	365/430（84.8%）

CLL：慢性淋巴细胞性白血病（chronic lymphocytic leukemia, CLL）；ALL：急性淋巴细胞性白血病（acute lymphocytic leukemia, ALL）

在慢性髓细胞白血病（chronic myelocytic leukemia，CML）和急性髓细胞白血病（acute myelocytic leukemia，AML）的端粒动力学研究中，用 Southern 印迹法测量端粒长度，用 stretch-PCR 法测出端粒酶活性，在 CML 白细胞中，端粒酶活性非常低，与正常组织相似。但若 CML 急性发作时，肿瘤细胞中端粒酶活性显著升高，表明 CML 由慢性到急性过程高度激活了端粒酶。端粒酶水平与某些肿瘤恶性程度相关。TRAP 法检测膀胱癌患者尿液中端粒酶的活性，Ⅰ期肿瘤患者端粒酶阳性率为 79%，Ⅱ期和Ⅲ期肿瘤患者端粒酶阳性率分别为 84%及 87.5%；66 %的膀胱炎患者端粒酶阴性；而健康者均为阴性[35]。在区分良性与恶性甲状腺瘤中，hTERT 是敏感的标志物[36]，从 24 例患者的甲状腺结节穿刺物中提取 RNA，进行 RT-PCR，扩增 hTERT 基因，与细胞学和组织学检查结果比较，hTERT 阳性与甲状腺癌的符合率为 93%，hTERT 阴性与良性甲状腺瘤的符合率为 90%。因此，随着研究的不断深入，端粒酶和 hTERT 有望成为肿瘤诊断及恶性程度分类的标志物[37, 38]。这些研究结果表明，端粒酶的激活，合成端粒的 DNA 被认为是细胞永生化和癌症发展的重要步骤。但端粒酶的激活常是恶性肿瘤发生过程中的一个后期事件。

在一些肿瘤存在端粒危机（telomere crisis），即端粒酶激活和端粒缩短的现象同时存在，特别见于造血系统的恶性肿瘤。由于这些瘤细胞的增殖和循环往往都是单细胞的，因此每一个肿瘤细胞都将竞争更有效的增殖，使突变细胞在短期内形成群落。肿瘤细胞中虽有端粒酶激活，但肿瘤细胞分裂次数大大增加仍使端粒缩短，即发生端粒危机。与此相反，实体肿瘤细胞常固定在局部，因此子代细胞对于不同突变的竞争被其紧邻细胞所限制。实体肿瘤细胞的克隆将比白血病细胞有更稳定的遗传特性。因为位于特殊环境中的特殊表型必须保持相当长的时间才能克隆形成群落，所以实体肿瘤只有具备较长的端粒，才能有较稳定的遗传特性，具备"最好"的表型从而被选择、生长和增殖。其次端粒危机的发生也可能由于异常修复事件使染色体发生端端融合。端端融合的后果是在随后的细胞分裂过程中发生染色体断裂，进而导致遗传不稳定和肿瘤易感性。

三、端粒酶活性与细胞周期的相关性研究

端粒酶活性与细胞周期密切相关。细胞周期所处阶段不同，端粒酶活性亦不同。紫外线照射四周后裸鼠（SKH-1）的表皮细胞端粒酶活性开始上升，Cyclin D1 和 Cyclin E 及其催化亚单位 CDK4 和 CDK2 的表达均上调，说明端粒酶活性与细胞周期 CDK-CKI 网络调控系统有关[39]。具有正常周期的永生化细胞株 HT-1080 和 HL-60 细胞在各个时相都有端粒酶活性，而静止期细胞中活性降低，随着肿瘤细胞进入 G_1/S 期，端粒酶活性逐渐升高，在 DNA 复制 S 期端粒酶活性最高，而在 G_2/M 期端粒酶活性逐渐下降，当培养细胞处于无血清条件而进入 G_0 期时，端粒酶活性不受影响。在人乳腺癌中，端粒酶的高活性水平伴有周期蛋白 Cylin D 或 Cyclin E 的高表达，某些周期蛋白可能参与酶活性的调控[40]。

四、端粒酶活性与细胞凋亡的相关性研究

启动凋亡的某些基因位于端粒结构附近，完整的端粒结构可以抑制这些基因的表达，而维持端粒长度主要依赖于端粒酶。Holt 等[41]在血清饥饿和基质非依赖性生存实验中发现，通过异位表达端粒酶而使端粒长度保持稳定的某些正常细胞对凋亡的抵抗力增强；用实验方法使端粒酶阳性细胞 IDH4 和 DU145 端粒延长，子代细胞生存和抗凋亡能力将增强；端粒酶阳性永生化细胞 SW39 要比端粒酶阴性永生化细胞 SW13 和 SW26 有更强的抗凋亡的生存能力。深入研究发现，这种抵抗性的增强与两个主要的凋亡途径——核内钙依赖核酸内切酶诱导途径和半胱氨酸蛋白酶家族中 IL-1β 转换酶活化途径存在缺陷有关。此外，Zhang 等[42]发现，诱导人端粒酶催化亚单位 hTERT 显性突变，降低肿瘤细胞内源性端粒酶活性，肿瘤细胞端粒将持续缩短，继之异常有丝分裂增多，并最终出现大量凋亡细胞。

Mattson 等[30]亦认为在研究神经细胞分化和存活中激活端粒酶与 TERT 功能，能较好地避免神经细胞死亡，还可以促进神经细胞在各种神经元退行性病变条件下的恢复。AD 患者的脑血管壁中可分离出致神经元退行性病变的 β-淀粉样蛋白。Zhu 等[31]利用反义技术和端粒酶抑制剂引发胎鼠海马区神经细胞中 TERT 的功能抑制，发现显著增加了由 β-淀粉样蛋白引起的细胞凋亡；而嗜铬细胞瘤细胞中 TERT 的过量表达会降低此种细胞凋亡，其原因是 TERT 功能降低的神经细胞在暴露于 β-淀粉样蛋白中能增强其氧化性，并使线粒体功能发生障碍，因而引起细胞凋亡。

五、不依赖端粒-端粒酶的细胞增殖

一些端粒酶阴性的肿瘤通过一种或几种端粒延长替代（altematire lengthening of telomere，ALT）机制（添加端粒重复序列）维持端粒的长度。例如，少数永生化的肿瘤细胞株和一些软组织肿瘤虽然没有端粒酶活性，但仍有较长端粒，提示还存在不依赖端粒酶的端粒延长机制[43]。此外用识别 hTR 3′端不同序列的三种核酶作用于肿瘤细胞，4 周内端粒酶活性降低，端粒缩短，增殖速度没有改变。其他研究如黑色素瘤细胞 8 周内端粒酶活性降低，但是传代超过 20 代后，端粒长度不缩短，细胞持续增殖[44]，说明除了端粒、端粒酶引起细胞增殖外，还有其他引起细胞增殖的机制。

细胞穿过亿万年的时光，在漫长的进化中"尝试"了各种可能性。端粒酶复制只是其中一种最为普遍的解决染色体末端隐缩问题的方式。细胞也可以通过同源重组的方式延伸端粒。裂殖酵母通过染色体头尾相连环化的方式来避开染色体末端隐缩的问题，在缺乏端粒酶和端粒的情况下生存传代。果蝇能通过转座子的不断复制延伸端粒。病毒能够利用蛋白或 tRNA 作为引物启始基因组 DNA 的合成，使染色体本身解决复制隐缩问题。

第五节　以端粒酶为靶标的抗癌药物研究

端粒酶对维持肿瘤细胞的无限增殖具有重要作用，在 85%以上的肿瘤细胞和组织中高度表达，因此端粒酶是一个较理想的抗癌药物的靶标。但仍有几个问题：①使用端粒酶抑制剂后，肿瘤细胞端粒缩短直至足以对增殖产生负面效应，这种时间上的滞后与起始端粒的长度有关。②至少在理论上肿瘤细胞存在抗端粒酶抑制剂或不依赖端粒酶的端粒延长替代机制（ALT）的可能。③端粒酶抑制剂对人表达端粒酶的体细胞可能有作用，如造血干细胞、生殖细胞、表皮基层细胞和肠腺管细胞，但这种作用可能很小，因为新生组织的干细胞比肿瘤细胞的端粒要长得多。④在细胞静止期，端粒不缩短，端粒酶活性很低。端粒酶抑制剂对肿瘤细胞和端粒酶阳性的正常细胞的作用是不同的；肿瘤细胞对端粒酶抑制剂很敏感，作用一定时间后细胞出现生长抑制或凋亡；生殖细胞在端粒酶抑制剂的作用下，端粒长度稍有缩短，然后继续生长，端粒不再缩短；干细胞与端粒酶阴性的细胞相比，其端粒缩短的速度慢得多，经端粒酶抑制剂作用后，干细胞中端粒缩短的速度有所加快，一旦去除抑制剂，端粒缩短的速度又降低。当然部分肿瘤细胞有较长的端粒（>10kb），随细胞有丝分裂，端粒缩短是个缓慢的过程，这种情况下端粒酶抑制剂是否有效尚待进一步证实。

近年来，端粒酶抑制剂的研究取得了很大进展，具体包括以下几个方面。

一、以端粒酶 RNA 为靶标

（1）通过反义寡核苷酸（antisense oligodeoxynucleotides，ASODN）技术阻断端粒酶 RNA 的模板作用对端粒酶活性的抑制。被动抑制基于 ASODN 与 RNA 的简单竞争结合，而主动抑制机制涉及 RNA-ASODN 杂合体激活 RNA 酶 H，从而降解 mRNA。

Zhang 等[45]将 hTR 的反义 cDNA 通过腺病毒载体整合到乳腺癌细胞 MCF-7 中，结果发现端粒酶活性受到抑制，端粒长度从 9.25 kb 缩短至 7.28 kb，细胞凋亡增强。在宫颈癌细胞中同样观察到端粒酶活性被抑制导致细胞凋亡，而端粒不缩短[46]。

（2）核酶对端粒酶活性的抑制：核酶是具有特殊核酸内切酶活性的小分子 RNA，通过催化中心的反义序列识别靶位。Kanazawa 等[47]设计了一种锤形的核酶（Telo-R2），具有特异性的切割 hTR 模板区的功能。核酶有望成为广谱、低毒、高效的抗癌新药。

二、抑制端粒酶逆转录酶活性

（一）hTERT 突变

hTERT 突变表现为丧失催化活性，能结合 hTR。在体内和体外实验中，hTERT 突变后端粒酶活性均明显被抑制。Zhang 等[42]在人表皮肿瘤细胞系和永生化胚肾细胞系中通过含点突变的 cDNA 介导 hTERT 突变，结果端粒酶活性被抑制，端粒缩短，其中表皮肿瘤细胞的端粒变得非常短（1～4 kb），早期表现出形态学改变和生长抑制，32 天后细胞成片死亡；相反，胚肾细胞表现为端粒长度在不同的克隆之间有明显差异（3～12 kb），端粒长的克隆（10～12kb）继续以一定速度增殖，直至端粒长度缩短到约 4 kb，此时，端粒酶蛋白为阴性。另外的研究表明，端粒酶抑制剂诱导端粒进行性缩短，当细胞端粒缩短到临界点时细胞进入凋亡期。

（二）逆转录酶抑制剂

逆转录酶抑制剂（reverse transcriptase inhibitor，RTI）在 HIV 治疗中广泛使用，它能结合到病毒 DNA 上阻断逆转录酶的链延伸。由于端粒酶是 RNA 依赖的 DNA 聚合酶，所以 RTI 可以成为肿瘤治疗药物。其中对于齐多夫定的研究最多，体外研究的剂量为 IC_{50} 为 0.10～1.75 $mmol \cdot L^{-1}$ 时端粒酶活性被抑制，细胞生长变缓，但延长用药时间并没有观察到端粒变短或最终细胞生长抑制[48]。这一现象可能是因为该药抑制线粒体 DNA 复制，导致剂量依赖的端粒酶活性下降，从而产生细胞毒性作用。

（三）靶向 hTERT mRNA 的 ASODN

针对 hTERT mRNA 设计的 ASODN 能选择性地与靶基因杂交，阻断靶基因的表达。1997 年 Webb 等[49]首次使用针对 hTERT mRNA 的 ASODN，成功地选择性阻断了端粒酶的表达。在以端粒酶 hTERT 基因为靶标的 ASODN 体外抗肿瘤活性评价中，发现 ASODN 对肝癌、肺癌、胃癌、乳腺癌、脑胶质瘤等细胞均有不同程度的抑制作用，其作用有明显的序列依赖性，其中对胃癌抑制作用最强，IC_{50} 仅为 0.25$\mu mol \cdot L^{-1}$[50]。hTERT mRNA 的 ASODN 作用于 AML、CML 细胞 24 小时后再加入顺铂，可促进顺铂诱导的细胞凋亡[51]。

三、G 四联体的稳定

端粒 3′端突出链富含鸟苷，在体外可形成四链 DNA 结构，称为 G 四联体。形成 G 四联体后端粒酶活性受到抑制。因此，能稳定 G 四联体的药物就可能是有效的端粒酶抑制剂。已发现很多此类化合物，这些药物可以抑制端粒酶，但尚无缩短端粒的报道[52]。

四、小分子抑制剂

通过分子结构模拟软件（NCI-COMPARE）进行拟合分析或通过其他高通量模式快速筛选端粒酶的小分子抑制剂是近年来发展较快的一个领域，此方法是基于化学结构的生物信息学策略去搜寻先导化合物。用这一策略已发现了几个端粒酶抑制剂（如 FJ5002），但其作用机制有待进一步研究[53]。

第六节 检测端粒酶的方法

鉴于端粒酶在肿瘤组织、非肿瘤组织或正常组织中阳性率的差异，1996 年美国召开的国际肿瘤会议上，有专家讨论认为端粒酶可以作为肿瘤特异性标志物，并认为利用端粒酶作为肿瘤基因治疗的靶点具有很大的潜在应用价值[54]。近几十年来，端粒酶的检测方法陆续取得了较大进展，方法的稳定性和可操作性逐渐提高。

一、端粒重复序列延伸方法

端粒重复序列延伸方法（telomere extension assay）是根据端粒酶具有逆转录酶的功能，可以自身 RNA 模板，合成、延伸端粒而设计。主要方法是从组织中制备端粒酶提取液，加入 TTAGGG 重复引物，合成延伸 TTAGGG 重组序列。反应液中，含 ^{32}P 标记的脱氧鸟苷三磷酸（deoxyguanosine triphosphate，dGTP），使同位素掺入。反应以 0.1mg/ml RNA 酶终止。反应产物进行聚丙烯酰胺（PAGE）凝胶电泳，放射自显影，阳性标本可见梯形条带。因端粒含 RNA 成分，在提取和检测过程中要求无 RNA 操作，防止模板 RNA 降解。此方法是最早建立的方法，稳定性好，特异性高。缺点是所需样本量较大，无放大作用，不适合临床标本的大量检测，且试验中使用同位素用量较大，不利于实验人员的身体健康和大规模推广。

二、TRAP 检测法

1994 年 Kim 等创立的 TRAP 法（telomerase report amplification protocol，TRAP）被誉为端粒酶活性检测首选方法，该方法为设计引物，在体外通过 PCR 方法扩增端粒酶反应的产物，再通过 PAGE 凝胶电泳显示碱基梯带。

TRAP 检测法与传统方法相比敏感性增加了一万倍。该技术标本获得来源广泛，可包括术中获取组织，针吸活检组织，脱落细胞和体外细胞株等，组织于冰上裂解获得端粒酶提取物。将获得的端粒酶提取液通过 PCR 反应体系扩增[55]，反应体系中包括 dNTP 和 TS（5'-AAT CCG TCG AGC AGA GGT-3'）引物。TS 是一段长度为 18bp 的寡核苷酸，端粒酶可与 TS 结合，以其本身的 RNA 组分作为模板，在 TS 的 3'端合成延伸 TTAGGG 重复序列。将此延伸反应合成的产物作为模板，加入另一条引物 CX（5'-CCCTTACCCTTACCCTTACCCTAA-3'）和 Tag 酶，以 TS 引物为上游引物，CX 为下游引物，通过 PCR 方法扩增。反应的产物观察，经典方法是在 PCR 反应中加入 ^{32}P 标记的核苷酸，并将扩增产物通过放射自显影分析结果，大约需在 PAGE 凝胶电泳后−80℃经 24~48 小时自显影。鉴于此观察方法耗时长且同位素放射污染，有学者提出将反应产物通过银染法进行分析。该方法将反应产物通过凝胶电泳 50 分钟后经硝酸银染色分析端粒酶活性，明显缩短了检测时间。TRAP 法是检测端粒酶的经典方法，所需标本少，敏感性高。此后在该方法的基础上出现了 PCR-ELIA、PCR-荧光、PCR-银染等多种改良。该方法的缺点一方面是实验步骤仍较为复杂，结果定量困难，另一方面由于某些组织中含有 Tag 酶抑制剂，可能导致假阴性结果出现。

三、酶联免疫吸附法（ELISA 方法）与 TRAP 法相结合

20 世纪 90 年代后期采用酶联免疫吸附法（ELISA 方法）与 TRAP 法相结合，将 TRAP 法进一步改良，缩短实验时间，简化实验步骤。该方法的基本原理是以生物素标记 TS 引物，然后将延伸的 TS 与第二引物 CX 一起进行 PCR 扩增，扩增产物与地高辛标记的端粒特异寡核苷酸探针杂交，最后经过氧化物酶分解底物 TMD 形成有色反应物，酶标仪测定实验数据。实验周期一般为 6~8h。已有商品化的试剂盒，实验步骤较为简化，有较广阔的临床使用前景。缺点是定量困难，一般为半定量检测端粒酶活性[56, 57]。

四、实时荧光定量 PCR 技术

近年来，实时荧光定量 PCR（RT-QPCR）技术被引入端粒酶活性测定。有端粒酶活性的肿瘤细胞中几乎均存在 hTERT 表达，而正常细胞中却无 hTERT 表达，说明端粒酶活性主要由 hTERT 表达水平的高低决定[58]。Kyo 等[59]观察多例卵巢癌患者及卵巢良性病变患者，发现 hTERT 仅表达于卵巢癌，而 hTR 和 TP1 在癌性和非癌性组织中均有表达，提示 hTERT 是端粒酶活性的敏感指标。使用一步法 RT-QPCR，通过将 hTERT 的 mRNA 逆转录，扩增出互补脱氧核糖核酸（complementary DNA，cDNA），利用特异杂交探针，对扩增子进行荧光检测，利用荧光共振能量转移（fluorescence resonance energy transfer，FRET）定量检测 hTERT mRNA 含量。此方法重复性好、稳定可靠，除去样品处理时间，一般在 1 小时内可得到实验结果。

端粒酶检测方法由早期的粗略定性正朝着准确定量的方向发展。如何增强其实验的重复性、稳定性，增强临床操作的简便性和推广性，并将其在不同细胞的表达形成量化乃至标准化判断，仍是端粒酶能否从实验研究到实际应用于临床需要攻克的难题。

挑战与展望

人类对端粒-端粒酶的认识始于 20 世纪 30 年代乃至更早，从 1938 年端粒一词命名，到 1985 年端粒酶被发现，在漫长的时间里，人们经历了无数个提出假设—验证假说—否定假说—重新提出假说的过程。遗传学家们最初在不同的生物中均发现了染色体末端结构对于维护染色体功能稳定的重要性，科技手段的进步使 DNA 序列可以被成功检测，对端粒的认识由最初的形态学逐渐过渡到分子生物学。随着对 DNA 聚合酶特性的深入研究，人们提出了染色体末端隐缩问题并思考生物如何解决这一复制难题。在当时提出的同源重组和新的未知的酶之间，实验数据更支持后者，这种酶后来被成功发现，即以自身为模板，逆向合成端粒的端粒酶。在整个端粒-端粒酶的研究过程中，科学家从现象观察中提出问题，并通过严谨合理的实验分析问题、解决问题，端粒和端粒酶的发现过程充分体现了科学思想的智慧之光和大自然造物的神奇。

随着对端粒和端粒酶的结构、功能及作用机制的深入研究，使端粒-端粒酶因其与人类衰老和肿瘤的密切关系而越来越受到人们重视。目前的研究热点多集中在端粒酶与人类早老性疾病及以端粒酶作为肿瘤患者诊断、预后及抗癌药物靶标等方向。体内端粒酶的延长功能是一复杂的动态过程，端粒酶的持续合成能力到底是如何实现的？在端粒长度调节过程中，端粒相关蛋白的亲和力发挥何种作用？如何将端粒酶作为肿瘤诊断和分型标志物？以及在体内每一次细胞分裂有多少端粒 DNA 合成？……这些问题的解决依赖于临床上检测方法的可操作性和稳定性的进一步提高；依赖于开发更灵敏和特异性的定量准确的评价体系；依赖于对端粒和端粒

酶新组分的克隆和鉴定。同时，对端粒-端粒酶的精细结构及激活调控机制，端粒-端粒酶与衰老、长寿因素之间的关系，以及是否存在不依赖端粒-端粒酶模式的染色体修复机制等问题的研究和探索仍在继续。但现阶段的研究多局限在理论阶段，真正将端粒酶应用于临床还有很多工作要做。

思 考 题

1. 本章基本概念：端粒（telomere），端粒酶（telomerase），DNA 的半保留复制，冈崎片段（Okazaki fragment），端粒危机（Telomere crisis）。

2. 为什么选用四膜虫作为研究端粒的材料？

3. 阐述端粒的结构特点和主要功能。

4. 阐述端粒酶的基本结构和主要功能。

5. 简述端粒酶延伸端粒的机制。

6. 概述端粒酶作为抗癌药物靶标的主要研究进展。

7. 阐述常见端粒酶的检测方法。

8. 尝试以端粒、端粒酶的发现过程归纳科学研究的过程。

参 考 文 献

[1] Muller H J. The remaking of chromosomes[J]. Collecting Net：Woods Hole，1938，8：181-198.

[2] McClintock B. The stability of broken ends of chromosomes in Zea mays[J]. Geneitics，1941，26：234-282.

[3] Ruehle M D，Orias E，Pearson C G. Tetrahymena as a Unicellular Model Eukaryote：Genetic and Genomic Tools[J]. Genetics，2016，203（2）：649-665.

[4] Blackburn E H，Gall J G. A tandemly repeated sequence at the termini of the extrachromosomal ribosomal RNA genes in Tetrahymena[J]. Journal of Molecular Biology，1978，120（1）：33-53.

[5] Watson J D. Origin of concatemeric DNA[J]. Nature：New Biology，1972，239（94）：197-201.

[6] Carol W. Greider，Elizabeth H.Blackburn. Identification of a specific Telomere Terminal Transferase Activity in Tetrahymena Extracts[J]. Cell，1985，43：405-413.

[7] Klobutcher L A，Swanton M T，Donini P，et al. All gene-sized DNA molecules in four species of hypotrichs have the same terminal sequence and an unusual 3′ terminus[J]. Proceedings of the National Academy of Sciences of the United States of America，1981，78（5）：3015-3019.

[8] Blackburn E H，Challoner P B. Identification of a telomeric DNA sequence in Trypanosoma brucei[J]. Cell，1984，36(2)：447-457.

[9] Shampay J，Szostak J W，Blackburn E H. DNA sequences of telomeres maintained in yeast[J]. Nature，1984，310(5973)：154-157.

[10] Ganal M W，Lapitan N L，Tanksley S D. Macrostructure of the tomato telomeres[J]. Plant Cell，1991，3（1）：87-94.

[11] Moyzis R K，Buckingham J M，Cram L S，et al. A highly conserved repetitive DNA sequence，（TTAGGG）n，present at the telomeres of human chromosomes[J]. Proceedings of the National Academy of Sciences of the United States of America，1988，85（18）：6622-6626.

[12] Kipling D，Cooke H J. Hypervariable ultra-long telomeres in mice[J]. Nature，1990，347（6291）：400-402.

[13] Griffith J D，Comeau L，Rosenfield S，et al. Mammalian telomeres end in a large duplex loop[J]. Cell，1999，97（4）：503-514.

[14] Levy M Z，Allsopp R C，Futcher A B，et al. Telomere end-replication problem and cell aging[J]. Journal of Molecular Biology，1992，225（4）：951-960.

[15] Livengood A J，Zaug A J，Cech T R. Essential Regions of Saccharomyces cerevisiae Telomerase RNA：Separate Elements for Est1p and Est2p Interaction[J]. Molecular & Cellular Biology，2002，22（7）：2366-2374.

[16] Lai C K，Miller M C，Collins K. Template boundary definition in Tetrahymena telomerase[J]. Genes & Development，2002，16（16）：415-420.

[17] Wang J，Xie L Y，Allan S，et al. Myc activates telomerase[J]. Genes & Development，1998，12（12）：1769-1774.

[18] Gunes C, Lichtsteiner S, Vasserot AP, et al. Expression of the hTERT gene is regulated at the level of transcriptional initiation and

repressed by Mad1[J]. Cancer Res earch, 2000, 60（8）: 2116-2121.

[19] Kickhoefer V A, Liu Y, Kong L B, et al. The Telomerase/Vault-Associated Protein Tep1 Is Required for Vault RNA Stability and Its Association with the Vault Particle[J]. Journal of Cell Biology, 2001, 152（1）: 157-164.

[20] Teng S C, Zakian V A. Est1p as a cell cycle-regulated activator of telomere-bound telomerase[J]. Science, 2002, 297（5583）: 1023-1026.

[21] Bernards A, Michels P A, Lincke C R, et al. Growth of chromosomal ends in multiplying trypanosomes[J]. Nature, 1983, 303: 592-597.

[22] Larson D D, Spangler E A, Blackburn E H. Dynamics of telomere length variation in Tetrahymena thermophila[J]. Cell, 1987, 50（3）: 477-483.

[23] Walmsley R W, Chan C S, Tye B K, et al. Unusual DNA sequences associated with the ends of yeast chromosomes[J]. Nature, 1984, 310: 157-160.

[24] Greider C W, Blackburn E H. Identification of a specific telomere terminal transferase activity in Tetrahymena extracts[J]. Cel, 1985, 43: 405-413.

[25] Greider C W, Blackburn E H. A telomeric sequence in the RNA of Tetrahymena telomerase required for telomere repeat synthesis[J]. Nature, 1989, 337（6205）: 331-337.

[26] Meyerson M. Role of telomerase in normal and cancer cells[J]. Journal of Clinical Oncology, 2000, 18（13）: 2626-2634.

[27] 邵晋晨. 端粒酶与细胞周期及细胞凋亡关系的研究进展[J]. 临床与病理杂志, 2002, 22（1）: 36-39.

[28] Allsopp RC, Vaziri H, Patterson C, et al. Telomere length predicts replicative capacity of human fibroblasts[J]. Proceedings of the National Academy of Sciences of the United States of America, 1992, 89（21）: 10114-10118.

[29] Vaziri H, Schächter F, Uchida I, et al. Loss of telomeric DNA during aging of normal and trisomy 21 human lymphocytes[J]. American Journal of Human Genetics, 1993, 52（4）: 661-667.

[30] Mattson, Klapper.Emerging roles for telomerase in neuronal development and apoptosis[J]. Journal of Neuroscience research, 2001, 63（1）: 1-9

[31] Zhu H, Fu W, Mattson M P. The catalytic subunit of telomerase protects neurons against amyloid beta-peptide-induced apoptosis[J]. Journal of Neurochemistry, 2000, 75（1）: 117-124.

[32] Mattson M P. Emerging neuroprotective strategies for Alzheimer's disease: dietary restriction, telomerase activation, and stem cell therapy[J]. Experimental Gerontology, 2000, 35（4）: 489-502.

[33] Kim N W, Piatyszek M A, Prowse K R, et al. Specific association of human telomerase activity with immortal cells and cancer[J].Science, 1994, 266: 2011-2014.

[34] Shay J W, Bacchetti S. A survey of telomerase activity in human cancer[J]. European Journal of Cancer, 1997, 33（5）: 787-791.

[35] Wei S, Wei S, Sedivy J M. Expression of catalytically active telomerase does not prevent premature senescence caused by overexpression of oncogenic Ha-Ras in normal human fibroblasts[J]. Cancer Research, 1999, 59（7）: 1539-1543.

[36] Zeiger M A, Smallridge R C, Clark D P, et al. Human telomerase reverse transcriptase（hTERT）gene expression in FNA samples from thyroid neoplasms[J]. Surgery, 1999, 126（6）: 1198-1199.

[37] Kirkpatrick K L, Mokbel K. The significance of human telomerase reverse transcriptase（hTERT）in cancer[J]. European Journal of Surgical Oncology the Journal of the European Society of Surgical Oncology & the British Association of Surgical Oncology, 2001, 27（8）: 754-760.

[38] Matthews P, Jones C J. Clinical implications of telomerase detection[J]. Histopathology, 2001, 38（6）: 485-498.

[39] 陈泉，杨德同. 影响端粒酶活性的相关因素[J]. 现代医学, 2002, 30（2）: 137-138.

[40] 王韫芳. 肿瘤细胞端粒、端粒酶调节机制研究进展与临床意义[J]. 国际检验医学杂志, 2002, 23（2）: 102-104.

[41] Holt S E, Glinsky V V, Ivanova A B, et al. Resistance to apoptosis in human cells conferred by telomerase function and telomere stability[J]. Molecular Carcinogenesis, 1999, 25（4）: 241-248.

[42] Zhang X, Mar V, Zhou W, et al. Telomere shortening and apoptosis in telomerase-inhibited human tumor cells[J]. Genes & Development, 1999, 13（18）: 2388-2399.

[43] Reddel R R. Alternative lengthening of telomeres, telomerase, and cancer[J]. Cancer Letters, 2003, 194（2）: 155-162.

[44] Folini M, Colella G, Villa R, et al. Inhibition of telomerase activity by a hammer head ribozyme targeting the RNA component of telomerase in human melanoma cells[J]. Journal of Investigative Dermatology, 2000, 114（2）: 259-267.

[45] Zhang X, Chen Y, Tong T. Effect of antisense telomerase RNA on apoptosis of breast cancer cells[J]. Chinese Journal of Biochemistry & Molecular Biology, 2001, 17（4）: 447-452

[46] Kondo Y, Koga S, Komata T, et al. Treatment of prostate cancer in vitro and in vivo with 2-5A-anti-telomerase RNA component[J]. Oncogene, 2000, 19（18）: 2205-2211.

[47] Yatabe N, Kyo S S, Kanaya T, et al. 2-5A antisense therapy directed against human telomerase RNA inhibits telomerase activity

and induces apoptosis without telomere impairment in cervical cancer cells[J]. Cancer Gene Therapy，2002，9（7）：624-630.

[48] 陈莉. 病理临床与进展[M]. 上海：第二军医大学出版社，2000.

[49] Webb A，Cunningham D，Cotter F，et al. BCL-2 antisense therapy in patients with non-Hodgkin lymphoma [J].Lancet，1997，349（9059）：1137-1141.

[50] 王升启，林莉，陈忠斌，等. 端粒酶 hEST2 基因为靶的反义寡核苷酸体外抗肿瘤活性评价[J]. 科学通报，2002，47（5）：378-381.

[51] Yuan Z，Mei H D. Inhibition of telomerase activity with hTERT antisense increases the effect of CDDP-induced apoptosis in myeloid leukemia[J]. The Hematology Journal，2002，3（4）：201-205.

[52] Harrison R J，Gowan S M，Kelland L R，et al. Human telomerase inhibition by substituted acridine derivatives[J]. Bioorganic & Medicinal Chemistry Letters，1999，9（17）：2463-2468.

[53] Naasani I，Seimiya H T，Tsuruo T. FJ5002：a potent telomerase inhibitor identified by exploiting the disease-oriented screening program with COMPARE analysis[J]. Cancer Research，1999，59（16）：4004-4011.

[54] Lundblad V，Wright W E. Telomeres and telomerase：a simple picture becomes complex[J]. Cell，1996，87（3）：369-375.

[55] 张传宝，郭健，张克坚. 端粒酶检测方法研究进展[J]. 中国实验诊断学，2005，9（3）：477-480.

[56] 张友忠，江森，刘文君. 卵巢肿瘤组织中端粒酶活性测定及其临床意义的研究[J]. 现代妇产科进展，1999（2）：115-118.

[57] 蔡春友，张维铭，刘霜，等. PCR-ELISA 检测端粒酶活性的方法及其在人体肿瘤中的应用[J]. 中国肿瘤临床，2000，27（1）：14-16.

[58] 朱晓应，符伟军，洪宝发. 端粒酶与肿瘤靶向治疗[J]. 国际遗传学杂志，2005，28（6）：366-368.

[59] Kyo S，Kanaya T，Takakura M，et al. Expression of human telomerase subunits in ovarian malignant，borderline and benign tumors[J]. International Journal of Cancer，1999，80（6）：804-809.

（周家名　陈　莉）

Chapter 6　Telomere and Telomerase

Forty years ago ctologist Hayflick found that cultured human fibroblasts division about 50 generations would stop in the case of nutritionally adequate supply, and then relay into the aging period.

Experiments show that telomerase can effectively regulate the length of telomere, furthermore the length of telomeres directly worked on the cell proliferation or apoptosis, thus to determine the survival of human cells. With the further study on the structures of telomeres and telomerase, telomerase activation and regulatory mechanisms, the relationship among telomerase, aging, cancer occurrence and development will be further defined.

Section 1　Discovery of Telomere and Telomerase

1. Telomere Discovery

Early in the 1930s, two geneticists Ms. Muller and Barbara McClintock (because of their discovery in maize transposons, won the Nobel Prize) at different laboratories to experimented with different organisms found on the ends of chromosomes, this structure was very important to maintain chromosome stability, Muller named the structure telomeres (Fig.6-1).As early as 1939, Barbara McClintock who concentrated to studying of heredity in maize, noted that occasionally production of chromosomal breaks easily re-integrate form a "bridge" in meiosis anaphase.

In the subsequent mitosis, this chromosome "break-fusion-bridge-break" cycle continues this process,it shows they is easily undergo mutual fusion of broken ends of chromosomes.

Question one: why do the natural ends of chromosomes not easily undergo mutual fusion?Reasonable speculation is that the natural ends of chromosomes should have a special structure to avoid the mutual fusion of chromosomes.

End of telomeres in eukaryotic chromosomes shorten after the cell division, after the shortening of telomeres are passed on to daughter cells, cells mitosis again is further reduced. With each time cell of division, chromosome ends gradually reduced until the cell aging. Human somatic cells follow this rule from birth to aging, single-celled organisms also follow this rule and maintains its passage survival after division involving some other mechanisms, the same as germ cells.

Tetrahymena has two nucleus [3]. Micronucleus is very stable, and it has 5 pairs of chromosomes for reproductive passage. The big nucleus in the process of engaging the cell development caused the chromosome to break into 200—300 microchromosomes, further copying up to 10,000 microchromosomes (Fig. 6-2). So Tetrahymena is a good material for studying telomeres. In 1978, Ms ELiz found tetrahymena telomerase was made up of many repeating sequence of six base 5'-CCCCAA-3'. she reported her findings in 1980. Almost all telomeres repeat sequences of living organisms and can be written as: the form Gn (A/ T)$_m$. Yeast telomere sequence is TG1-3/C1-3A without rule.

2. Telomerase Discovery

Cell division has certain limits that is divided life. Telomere restriction fragments (TRFs) of somatic cells are more significantly shorter than the germ cells. TRFs in youth are significantly longer than that in older people, suggesting TRFs constantly shorter with cell division or aging, mainly due to DNA polymerase which cannot replicate telomere of linear DNA ends.

In 1972, James Watson, won the Nobel Prize due to the discovery of double helix of the DNA, clearly pointing out the hidden shrinking at the chromosome ends.

Question two: How to identify hidden shrink at the end of chromosome when replicating?

In 1980, Ms ELiz reported her findings of tetrahymena telomerase that immediately aroused the interest of Jack Szostak. He was trying to construct artificial linear chromosome in yeast, and hoped that it replicated in cells like a natural chromosome did. But after the artificial linear chromosomes transfected into yeast cells and it was degraded soon.

Question three: Whether is the degradation of linear chromosomes due to its end without telomeres protection?

The finding of telomere sequence let Jack Szostak have a chance to make the end of linear chromosome connect to the telomeres DNA of tetrahymena, then introduce it into the yeast cells. The miracle happened. The chromosome was no longer degraded, it replicated in the cells and ideas synthesizing artificial chromosome come true!

The realization of artificial chromosome originally may just satisfy people's wishful thinking, but it actually makes it possible for large segments of DNA cloning, and later contribute to the sequencing of the human genome. This is also an important reason for Jack Szostak to share the Nobel Prize in 2009.

In 1984 in the same article reported the yeast telomeric sequence, ELiz laboratory found an interesting phenomenon: With artificial chromosome of tetrahymena telomeric DNA into yeast, was given the telomeres of yeast instead of the tetrahymena telomeric sequence. Because telomerase is made up of repeated sequences, it was generally thought that homologous recombination is to extend telomeres to compensate the ends of chromosomes hidden shrink mechanism. But homologous recombination only can copy more sequences itself, why add in the tetrahymena telomere is yeast telomeric sequence instead of the tetrahymena telomeric sequence itself? This phenomenon cannot be explained by homologous recombination. Thus only one possible answer: the presence of a special "enzyme" in yeast can copy yeast telomeric DNA.

As mentioned earlier, during the development of macronuclear of Tetrahymena junction cells, produced very rich microchromosomes, the head of each microchromosome has a telomere. Presumably, if the "enzyme" hypothesis was established, the "enzyme" activity in cells should be very high at this time.

In 1984, Ms. Carol as a doctoral student joined ELiz laboratory. They both use Tetrahymena nuclear extracts (enzyme) respectively incubated telomere DNA and the DNA with random sequence, they hope to see the extension of the telomere to detect this "enzyme" activity in vitro.

Through continuous optimizing conditions, especially after the substrate was changed for in vitro synthesis telomeric DNA with high concentrations, on the Christmas of the same year, diligent Ms. Carol, opening cassette exposure X-ray, finally clearly saw the "enzyme" activity. On the isotopes-exposure of the sequencing gel, telomere substrates obviously were added by new DNA bases, and each of the six bases that form a dark zone, and coincide with six bases of the Tetrahymena telomeric repeats. This enzyme activity did not depend on DNA templates, only extended the telomeric DNA of Tetrahymena, while the substrates of DNA with random sequence did not extend; So that the activity did not depend on DNA polymerase. At this point, they proved an "enzyme" that can extend Telomere DNA, which was later named "telomerase".

(1) Revealed RNA Subunit

ELiz laboratory further to determined the nature of telomerase activity. At that time Tom Cech won the Nobel Prize for the finding of catalytic activity of RNA and just visited ELiz laboratory, she / they together made a simple experiment, using RNA enzyme treated sample to degrade the RNA, then check if telomerase activity is affected. The result is the activity of enzyme even disappeared, indicating that telomerase activity is dependent on RNA.

Is the telomerase a special RNA catalytic enzyme?

Tom Cech was attracted by telomerase, and intervened in this area. Of course, at that time, telomerase is known to be dependent on the protein: After protease digestion samples telomerase activity also was disappear.

In 1989, by tracking the activity of telomerase, Carol purified and cloned tetrahymena telomerase RNA subunit. She found that RNA subunit had a RNA sequences which was complementary to telomere DNA sequence of tetrahymena. Telomerase is used in this sequence of RNA subunit as a template to repeat replicate the telomere DNA. ELiz's laboratory reported the yeast telomerase activity in 1995.

(2) Revealed Protein Subunits of Telomerase

Since telomerase can use the RNA template subunits to copy DNA, it's easy to speculate that the subunits of protein might have the activity of RNA depending DNA polymerase, is the activity of reverse transcriptase. Its protein sequence should contain specific domains of reverse transcriptase. Although there is no experimental evidence, this mystery through the logical reasoning has actually guessed half. To reveal this mystery, different laboratories were competing fiercely.

In 1989 another heroine in this area—Vicki Lundblad who worked in Jack Szostak's lab, using ingenious genetic screening methods screened the genes of EST1 from the yeast. Knock down the EST1 genes, telomere shortened following yeast genera, in the last telomeres shortened to a critical length causing aging and death.

(3) Revealed Catalytic Subunit of Telomerase

In 1996, Tom Cech's laboratory by means of biochemical methods to purify the telomerase complex of Tetrahymena, which according to the molecular weight of a protein named p123. The same period, Vicki

Lundblad's lab has screened several genes closely related to yeast telomeres copy, named it EST2, EST3, and EST4 (also called CDC13). Later, the p123protein of tetrahymena which purified by biochemical method and the Est2 protein of yeast which screened by genetics method are both proved to be human telomerase catalytic subunits by Tom Cech lab, which contain the reverse transcriptase domain. If mutating that domain's key amino acid, telomerase activity is disappearing.

Since then, people in vitro transcription and translation system expressed telomerase catalytic subunits and RNA subunits to reconstruct the telomerase activity in vitro, that proved the existence of these two core subunits is a sufficiency condition of telomerase activity.

3. Summary Important Events in Telomeres and Telomerase Discovery

In 1939, Barbara McClintock found maize chromosomes ends easily undergo fusion

In 1972, James Watson raised an issue about hidden contraction at the replicating chromosome end.

In 1978, telomeric sequence of tetrahymena had been reported.

In 1982, telomere discovered led to the invention of artificial chromosomes.

In 1984, yeast telomeric sequence had been reported.

In 1985, telomerase activity of tetrahymena had been reported.

In 1989, telomerase RNA subunit of tetrahymena had been reported.

In 1994, the report of RNA subunit of yeast telomerase.

In 1995, the report of yeast Telomerase activity.

In 1996, catalytic subunit of Tetrahymena telomerase had been purified and get yeast telomerase catalytic subunit by genetic screened methods.

In 1997, catalytic subunit of Telomerase in tetrahymena and yeast had been proved.

In 2009, Nobel Prize in Physiology or medicine awarded to which found the mechanism of telomere and telomerase protecting chromosomes.

Karolinska Institute in Sweden announced that the 2009 Nobel Prize in Physiology and Medicine awarded to United States Elizabeth Blackburn who at the San Francisco University in California, Carol Greider who at the school of John Hopkins medicine at Baltimore, and Jack Szostak of Harvard Medical School and the Howard Hughes Medical Institute for their discovery for the mechanism of protecting chromosomes by telomeres and telomerase. Karolinska Institute said the three persons " solved a major problem in biology", that is how toper form a fullreplication of chromosomes when cells divide and how to avoid degradation. All the secrets are hidden in the telomere and telomerase.

Section 2   Structure and Functions of Telomere and Telomerase

Telomere: The special structure of linear chromosome ends in eukaryotic cells.Composed of telomere DNA and telomere-associated protein.

Telomerase is the enzyme which continues to synthesize the telomeres sequence at the ends of chromosomes. It is a nucleic acid proteinase, that is, RNA is dependent on DNA polymerase. With its own RNA template synthesis of telomeric DNA repeat sequences, it has reverse transcriptase activity, but the activity does not depend on DNA polymerase and is sensitive to RNA enzymes, protease and heat.

1. Structure of Telomere

Telomere structure at the ends of chromosomes is visible by in situ hybridization.

Telomere DNA: is simple and highly repetitive sequences without functional genes, which has highly conserved in biological evolution. There are differences of telomere DNA sequences among different species (Table 6-1).In 1978, Ms ELiz found tetrahymena telomerase was made up of many repeating sequence of six base 5'-CCCCAA-3'. She reported her findings in 1980. Almost all telomere repeats sequences of living organisms can be written as: the form Gn $(A/T)_m$. Yeast telomere sequence is TG1-3/C1-3A without rule.

Table 6-1   The repeat sequences classical biological telomere

biological	Sequence	reporter	reports on time
Tetrahymena	TTGGGG	Blackburn、Gall	1978
Peak caterpillars	TTTTGGGG	Klobutcher et al.	1991
trypan	TTAGGG	Blackburn、Challoner	1984
saccharomyces cerevisiae	$T(G)_{2\sim3}(TG)_{1\sim6}$	Shampay et al.	1984
tomatoes	TT(T/A)GGG	Ganal et al.	1991
human	TTAGGG	Moyzis et al.	1988
rat	TTAGGG	Kipling、Cooke et al.	1990

Telomere with GT enrichment extends in CA enrichment chain. Due to CA enrichment chain is limitedly degradated G tail is to produced.

Without free ends it is a critical of chromosome ends to bestable. The telomere at the end of chromosomes forms a special DNA loop resultingin telomere structure to be relatively stable.Human telomeres, for example, telomere DNA is formed by two mutually matched DNA single strand, one of them slightly longer than the other, the double chain part with telomere binding protein TRF1 (depend on) telomerase and TRF2 (does not depend on telomerase) combined with the telomere 3'single end tail (G) repeat the homologous double-stranded DNA are replaced in order to form a t ring loops (t).T-loop, this special structure, may maintain the stability of the chromosome ends and maintain the integrity of chromosomes interior genes, so that the genetic material are reproduced in full (Fig. 6-3).

2. Functions and Significances of Telomerese

(1) The complexes formed by telomere DNA and structural proteins like a "hat" of chromosome, can protect the chromosomes from degradation, and avoid end-end fusion as well as chromosome loss, and maintain the integrity and stability of the chromosome. Chromosome lacking telomere cannot present stabilitily.

(2) Telomere help to identify the intact and damaged chromosomes.

(3) In physiological conditions, telomeres act as cells "division clock" which can be shortened, eventually leading to cell from the cell cycle.

Telomere length could be used as cell's "division clock," reflecting the capacity of cell division. Telomerase is what scientists call "life clock".

3. Structure of Telomerase

Telomerase is a special reverse transciptase, includes three important components Telomerase RNA

(TR). Telomerase Reverse Transciptase (TERT) and Telomerase associated protein (TEP) (Fig.6-4).

(1) Telomerase RNA (TR)

Telomerase RNA (hTR)——Telomerase RNA was the first cloned human telomerase components. Telomerase RNA has a complementary sequence with homologous Telomeres DNA TTAGGG sequence. DNA enzyme H cuts this template region and can eliminate telomerase activity and extend telomeres in vitro.

Mammalian telomerase RNAs are widely expressed in different developmental stages in many organizations, even those that don't have telomerase activity of the organization.

The existence of telomerase RNA in vivo is essential for telomerase function, it affects telomerase stability and mutations, and also can change telomere length in vivo, and through the change of telomere integrity or telomereend-binding sites to make anaphase cell death.

(2) Telomerase Reverse Transcriptase (TERT)

Almost all cells with telomerase have a separate TERT gene. TERT transcription in mammals is controled by many transcription factors, hormone and extracellular signals. Different transcription factors regulate hTERT (Human Telomerase reverse transcriptase) expression in different cells.

The function of N-residues in TERT includes that it combines with telomerase RNA, assembles and catalysis, interaction with p53 and cell immortalization.

C-residues in TERT played an important role in raw human fibroblasts immortalized, the competition of telomerase assembly, positioning within the nucleolus, primer binding and the progressive extension.

hTERT gene is a single copy gene, located at 5p15. 33, it has 7 conservative sequence of domain element and telomerase-specific domain element T. Damage TERT will eliminate telomerase activity and Telomere shortening.

Oncogene C-Myc is an important telomerase activator. There are two important C-Myc binding site exist in the hTERT core promoter (CACGTG, also known as the E-box).c-Myc could induce with H-Ras, N-Ras, polyoma virus MT, LT and other oncogenes synergies roles to promote cell proliferation then getimmortalized and become cancerous. In many types of tumor cells, the basic activator inducing hTERT is c-myc. c-myc induce the expression of hTERT starting speed, and it isn't affected by cell proliferation or extra protein synthesis, and consistent with c-myc causing direct transcriptional activation. With c-myc antisense nucleotide transfected to leukemia cells, telomerase activity in these cells can be reduced. C-myc in normal human mammary epithelial cells and in diploid fibroblasts induce telomerase activity, and can extend to the life of the cells. But c-myc gene is not the only factor which relates to the hTERT gene regulation. Sp1 synergistic c-my cactivate the transcription of hTERT. Anti-apoptosis gene Bcl-2, E6HPV16-protein can raise hTERT. In many types of tumor cells, the basic activator inducing hTERT is c-myc.

(3) Telomerase-associated Protein (TEP)

1) TEP1 is a polyfunctional RNA-binding protein. Absence TEP1 can lead to rRNA levels significant reduction, but does not cause the disorder of telomerase activity and telomere length.

2) Survival dynamic neurocyte gene (SMN) product. HSP90, other concerns TERT post-translational protein including phosphatase-A, Akt, cAbl, p53, and PARP. PinX1 and TERT co-expressioninvitro can inhibit telomerase activity

3) Budding yeast proteins Est1p and Est3p These two proteins are associated with the function of telomerase in the body. Est1p extends telomere. But without the Est1p, Est2p-Cdc13pDBD fusion can also maintain telomere length.

4. Functions of Telomerase

Germ cells can be passed down through generations, there may be a special mechanism maintaining telomere length, somatic cells may precisely lack such mechanism, the ends of its chromosomes face lethal deletion risks.So in the process that normal human cells and tumor cells transform to immortalized cells may also exist such mechanism which are similar to the germ cells.

How do these cells maintain the ability to continue to divide or survive for a long time? Scientists found that telomerase would extend by the new synthetic fragments of telomere.

Normal conditions the telomeres are in a state of dynamic balance.In cells without telomerase, the telomeres length gradually reduced to damage cells. In cells with telomerase, the telomere length get updates, cells are survival.

(1) Expression of telomerase activity can stabilize the length of telomeres and maintain cellular proliferative potential, inhibition of cell sequence. In the germ cells and stem cells high levels of telomerase activity can be detected.

(2) Telomerase is responsible for replication of telomeres. Telomerase RNA subunit as a template for telomerase catalytic subunit toreplicate the telomere DNA by transposition of repeated copying to compensate for the chromosome end hidden in replication process, and guarantee full replication of a chromosome. In the cells without telomerase, the telomeres length gradually is reduced to damage genes. In the cells with telomerase, the telomeres length get updates, the telomerase are in a state of dynamic balance.

(3) The other function of telomerase is to repair the end of broken chromosomes. When the end of chromosomes fracture off chromosomes rich in G, T base exist, even if there is no complete telomere repeat sequences, telomerase can also extend the telomere sequence so that the end of chromosome is saved from the destruction of the enzyme.

(4) During the synthesis process of telomeres, telomerase has a function of correction, removes mismatches bases.

Section 3   Role Mechanism of Telomere and Telomerase

1. Half Reserved Copy of DNA

The eukaryotic chromosomes are mainly made up of DNA and histones. DNA is the carrier of genetic information, biological DNA as template RNA synthesis process is called transcription, genetic information stored in the DNA is expression by transcription and translation. Reverse transcription process refers to as a template of RNA, is formed of DNA molecules by deoxy-ribonucleoside triphosphate (dNTP) aggregation. The process of nucleic acid synthesis and transcription are in contrast to the process of genetic information flow, it is called the reverse transcription. Reverse transcriptase is, DNA polymerase relying on RNA. It is generally believed that telomerase is a special kind of reverse transcriptase, it can synthesize the telomere repeat sequence with itself with RNA as a template, in order to maintain the stability of the telomere length.

The basic unit of nucleic acid is nucleotides, which is connected with the three components, composed of base, pentose sugar and phosphoric acid. The basic components of DNA molecules are A (adenine) and T (thymine), G (guanine) and C (cytosine), has the strict complementarity relationship between bases, pairing A-T, G-C, with hydrogen bonds between each other. The basic components of RNA molecules are A-U (uracil) and G-C matches.

The most important characteristics of DNA replication is half reserved copy. During replication, parental double-stranded DNA unlock spirally, forming two single, each as a template to guide the child synthesize a new complementary strand. In new double-stranded DNA, the one completely accept from parental, another one is completely renew synthesized from substrate. Due to the base complementation, the double-stranded DNA in two daughter cells is completely consistent to parental DNA base sequence. DNA replication was nucleotide polymerization process conducted under a variety of enzyme catalytic, dihydrogen phosphate ester bond polymerization long chain between the adjacent nucleotides, consistng of substrate 5'-p adduct formed on the original free 3'- OH, new synthetic chain only from 5' to 3', this is the direction of the copy.

2. Okazaki Fragment Chromosomes and End-Hidden Problems

(1) Okazaki Fragment

DNA replication direction copy new chains along the 5'-3' solution chain, replication is continuous, known as the leading chain. Another copy direction of the new chain opposite the solution chain direction. replication have to wait for a template loose enough length to copy from 5'-3', along the direction of the unlock chain, wait until the next, and then exposed the enough length of the template, then another section from 5'-3' replication. This copy is called a half discontinuous replication, the discontinuous replication of DNA called the back following chain, the discontinuous DNA fragments namely Okazaki fragments. Because of the Japanese scholar okazaki to cure phage DNA replication in the research of e. coli found this phenomenon thus the name.

(2) End of Hidden Problems

The replication of DNA needs RNA primer, which is decision made by the nature of DNA polymerase and RNA polymerase. When copying, DNA polymerase can't directly start the replication, must in the function of RNA polymerase, a piece of RNA template synthesized by DNA as a primer provides a 3'- OH, the DNA polymerase on the basis of the according to the direction of 5'-3' can aggregate triphosphate DNA nucleotides to extend new DNA chain. When copying the extension reaction, 5' - RNA primer breaks down, so a short of the 5' parent chain cannot copy it into sub chain, causing the loss of DNA information. At the end of the DNA replication, a leading chain end will leave vacant by eliminating the primer, in the back following chain, because the DNA synthesis is discontinuous, the primer vacancy preceding left will be fill fulled by the next copy, so it couldn't supply primer vacancy, after the primers of discontinuous replication that was eliminated in the last time.

So linear chromosome DNA replicate in every round, the end of chromosome will shorten the length of a RNA primer. Although the primer is not long, but cells continue to copy, without compensating, chromosome is continuously shortened and will eventually disappear. This was known as "the end of the hidden problem". That is first presentation by James Watson. (Fig. 6-5).

3. Mechanism of Telomerase Extending Telomere

Human explore the structure and function of the telomeres - telomerase is a long and rigorous process. Eukaryotes telomeres have a special replication problem, as previously mentioned, due to the DNA polymerase it can't completely replicate the back following chain, usually the chromosomes sequence loss will happen in DNA replication. In the eighty, there were two important findings in the telomere replication features: (1) the trypanosome in the host telomere length increase when the successive batches. In similar Tetrahymena experiment, maintaining cell in growth period the telomere length in cell also increased; (2) transform the Tetrahymena telomeres to distant relatives saccharomyces cerevisiae can also play the role of telomeres in latter, and the telomere repeat sequence can be added at the end of the line plasmid.

People put forward two kinds of models to explain how telomere sequence is added, the first model thinks that DNA recombinant or polymerase sliding on repetitive sequence to extension telomere sequence, which telomere structure may be through genetic recombination mechanisms. The second model think that telomere sequence is added by the not yet known polymerase, this enzyme can be added sequence to the end of chromosomes in the condition of no template. Clearly, the latter model can better explain the yeast specific repeat sequences add the telomere of Tetrahymena. In 1985, Greider in Tetrahymena identified this "has not been known polymerase" enzyme independ on the template to telomere replication, which is compensation to the shorten end of the linear DNA due to the removal of primers, that is telomerase.

In 1989, on the basis of many experiments in Elizabeth laboratory, Tetrahymena, for example, puts forward the telomerase synthesis telomere repeat sequence model, although the details of this model is also need to perfect, in general, this model has stood with the test of time. This extension mechanism(Fig. 6-6):

(1) Telomerase combine with the end of chromosomes, telomerase RNA template area 5′-CAACC CAa-3′ sequence form base pairs with telomere TTGGGG repeat sequences;

(2) The telomere DNA extension by adding in the 3′TTG;

(3) Telomerase RAN shift, exposed to the end of the newly formed TTGGGGTTG sequence and the template sequence is paired;

(4) Another template copy produce new TTGGGG repetitive sequence.

The extended function of telomerase in the body is a complex dynamic process: which is negatively control by the double chain telomere binding protein, including RAP1 (budding yeast), TRF1 exists in T ring (depend on telomerase) and TRF2 (independ of telomerase).

Section 4　Studies of Telomere-telomerase in Diseases

The dysfunction of telomere and telomerase will affect the biological behavior of cells, including the stability of the cell cycle, apoptosis, proliferation, carcinogenesis, aging, etc.

1. Telomere-telomerase Effect on Cell Aging and Immortalization

"Telomere-telomerase hypothesis" deem that telomerase activation with the occurrence and development of immortalization and malignant transformation are closely related. The telomere DNA of chromosome ends with progressive shortening is a prerequisite to limit human cell lifespan. In contrast, activation of telomerase can synthesize telomere DNA as it is considered to be a necessary step on cell immortalization and cancer development. The current data confirms that telomerase is required for the long-term survival of the organization and long-term mitotic cells.

Cell death process is divided into two phases. When telomeres shorten to a critical length of $2 \sim 4kb$, the stability of the chromosome will be destroyed, the cells begin to age into the M_1 period (mortality stage1). In M_1, cell is unresponsive to growth factors and produce DNA synthesis protein inhibitor. Cell cycle checkpoints sends the signal to stop cycles, stop DNA synthesis, DNA breakage, and activation of DNA damage pathway with p53-dependent or non-p53-dependent. And inducting CDK inhibitors such as P21, P27, lead to cell G_1 phase arrest and ultimately to death. In this process a number of oncogenes undergo activation, like SV40T antigen, PRB, p53, p16 and other tumor suppressor gene inactivation, takeplace, both inhibit the M_1 mechanism and lead to the cells to escape M_1. They continue to grow with additional proliferative potential however in this stage telomere is still negative, telomeres continue to shorten, after mitosis $20 \sim 30$ times, and finally reach to the M_2 period. Cells due to telomere being too short, genetic instability, result the vast majority of cell death, but only a very few cells up-regulating telomerase are activated or reactivated, the function of telomere is restored and make the cell to go beyond

M_2 period to become immortalized cells (Fig. 6-7).

Telomerase activity can be detected not only in the immortalized cells of normal tissue (such as blood-forming stem cells, sperm), but also in proliferative activity non-immortalized cells under the normal physiological condition (such as the antigen stimulated T and B lymphocytes, epithelium   in mouth and esophagus mucous membrane, keratinocytes in basal layer of the skin, cervical epithelium, intestinal epithelium).

Because telomere shortening causes aging, early old patient have a premature shortening of telomeres, thus shortened telomeres allow chromosome fusion. These phenomena are related with the high incidence of abnormal aging karyotype which are seen in cells of elderly patients or in incubatory aging cells.

The study of telomerase prolonging and telomere length to slow down the cell aging was early evidenced by Bodnar and others. Who in 1998 published an article in Science reporting: The human telomerase gene import telomerase-negative normal human cells to activate its expression and cultivate these cells. And then compared with the cells without imported telomerase gene, found the former significantly length telomere, stronger cell division, longer cell life span than the latter. Of greater concern was not the tumor-like change.Kudo, at al. reported that telomerase activity and cells apoptosis can both be a sign of aging of placenta, that it with or without intrauterine growth slowly.

TERT in experimental models of neurodegenerative lesions demonstrated neuroprotective function. Suggesting that in nerve cells, it can increase telomerase activity and may inhibit neurodegenerative disorders related with aging, such as the AD, brain aging and so on.

Telomere's accelerating shortening can be observed in many diseases: such as Down syndrome, Werner syndrome, capillary expansion disorders, congenital dyskeratosis and so on. Although the relationship between some genetic abnormal and telomere defects remains unclear, but possible causes include: ①Increase the exonuclease activity of telomere and /or the effective use.②Over-loss of telomeres; ③Lack of the compensation mechanism of telomer during development or after the birth.

Telomere accelerated shortening may be caused by environmental emergencies - mediated DNA damage or the sensitivity increases to these damages. No matter what the cause, increased telomere shortening rate can improve the premature senility characteristic of proliferative organization. The discovery of telomerase function opens up a new road to anti-aging for us.

Since the expression of telomerase activity is to stabilize the length of telomeres, the telomere is not lost in cellular replication process, the cell aging process can also be blocked, so as to live longer. Whether extending the telomere length of the old person can achieve the purpose of youth—is a research hot topic about the relationship between telomerase and aging which is under research.

2. Activation of Telomerase in Tumors

Since 1994, Kim found telomeric repeat amplification Protocol (TRAP) to detect telomerase activity. More and more literature show that telomerase activity can be detected in most human primary tumor specimens and tumor-derived cell lines.

Increasing telomerase activation makes telomeres of cancer cells to no longer progress shortening so as to maintain and avoid the restricting mechanism of copy-death in normal cells to obtain immortality. This is one significant biological characteristics of malignant cells, which is a very important part in cancerous mechanism.United States scholars reveal in more than 400 cases from 12 different organizations a primary tumor. The positive rate of telomerase in tumor tissue was as high as 84.8%, but in tumor surrounding tissue and benign lesions the positive rate was only 4.4%. Shay et.al summed up the telomerase-positive rate respectively as 0.5%, 30%, 85% and 11% in normal tissue (196), carcinoma in situ (410), malignant neoplasms (2031) and adjacent tissue (690). Among prostate cancer, breast cancer, pancreatic cancer, lung cancer, liver cancer, thyroid cancer and urinary system cancer (kidney, bladder), all showed a good correlation of the positive rate of telomerase and tumorgenesis. (Table 6-2).

Table 6-2　Comparison the telomerase activity in human tumor and non-tumor tissues

Tumor location/type	normal tissue near the tumor/benign lesions(%)	tumor tissur(%)
Lungs	3/68(4.4%)	108/136(80.1%)
Mammary gland	2/28(7.1%)	19/24(79.6%)
prostate	1/18(5.6%)	23/27(85.1%)
colon	0/45(0)	22/23(95.6%)
liver	—	1/1(100%)
ovary	0/8()	7/7(100%)
kidney	0/55(0)	40/55(72.7%)
neuroblast	0/17(0)	94/100(94%)
blood(lymphoma, CLL ALL)	—	21/23(91.3%)
brain	—	6/8(75%)
other(parietal region, Wilms tumor)	8/93(8.6%)	24/26(92.3%)
Total	14/332(4.2%)	365/430(84.8%)

In the study of telomere dynamics in AML and CML, the measurement of telomere length by Southern blotting and detection of telomerase activity is by stretch-PCR method. In CML, telomerase activity was very low and similar to normal tissue. However, when CML appear on acute onset, the telomerase activity in tumor cells will increase significantly. Showing that the telomerase is highly activated by the process of CML from chronic to acute. Increased telomerase activation is a late event in malignant development process.

In a variety of gene toxicity or environmental stress-induced cellular DNA Double-strand break can make wild-type p53 to activate, thereby causing cell cycle arrest or induce cell apoptosis, allowing cells to avoid malignant transformation of phenotype.Whether double-stranded DNA damage of telomeres can activate p53-dependent signaling pathway?

Kusumoto and others, constructing either telomerase or p53 single deficient or double-deficient mice in vivo studies, confirmed that loss of telomere DNA could induce activation of p53 and p21WAF1 and leads cell cycle arrest, and the loss of p53 may promote the loss of telomere sequence, increasing the frequency of chromosome fusion. Lack of telomere function and following gene instability coordinated with p53 defects result to activate the process of cells malignant transformation.

Telomere Crisis

The phenomenon that telomerase is activated in some tumor cells, but telomere still shorten is known as the telomere crisis.

The hypothesis of the telomere crisis may be interpreted as: in the many malignant tumors of hematopoietic system, the tumor cells of proliferation and circulation are unicellular. Therefore every tumor cell will compete for more effective proliferation, so that mutant cells form cloning communities in the short term. Activation of telomerase in tumor cells, when compared with the corresponding normal cells, the shortening of telomeres still happens resulting the telomere crisis. This may be due to tumor cell divisions are so much more than the number of normal cells.

On the contrary, solid tumor cells do not move in the local, so that daughter cells compete different mutations is limited by the close cells. Cloning of solid tumor cells have more stable genetic characteristics than leukemic cells. The specific phenotype in special circumstances needs to be maintained for a long time to clone form community. So the solid tumors only with longer telomeres can have more stable genetic traits, and have the "best" phenotype in order to be selected, growth and proliferation.Due to increase cell division causes telomere shortening, resulting in abnormal repair events that end to end fusion of chromosome. The consequence of end to end fusion is chromosome breakage occurring in the subsequent process of cell division, which lead to genetic instability and cancer susceptibility.

3. Effects of Telomerase on Cell Cycle

Telomerase activity is closely related to the network control systems of cell cycle CDK-CKIs. There will be different telomerase activity in different stages of the cell cycle. It was found that immortalized cell lines in each cell cycle phase also have telomerase activity, whereas in resting cells havea decreased activity. As the tumor cells go into the G_1 / S phase, the activity of telomerase is gradually increased and reach the highest levels in S phase, but in G_2 / M phase is gradually lost. In human breast cancer, telomerase high activity levels are associated with high expression of Cyclin E or Cylin D, some Cyclins may be involved in the regulation of telomerase activity.

Lehner and others used quantitative RT-PCR method and detected hTERT mRNA expression values. They found that there were significantly different among endometrial cancer, proliferative phase endometrium, secretory endometrium and atrophic endometrium. Obviously, different degrees of endometrial proliferation express telomerase activity, but at different levels.Therefore, the significance in judging benign and malignant proliferation by telomerase qualitative detection was not as good quantitatively.

4. Effects of Telomerase on Cell Apoptosis

Starting apoptosis genes located near the telomeres and full telomeres structure can inhibit the expression of these genes, but cells go into apoptosis when the telomere shortening over the edge.Increasing the expression of telomerase in cells can enhance and resistance to apoptosis in cells with a stable telomere length. Using experimental methods to extend telomeres of telomerase positive cells (IDH4 and DU145), descendant cell survival and anti-apoptotic capacity will be enhanced. The anti-apoptotic capacity in telomerase-positive immortalized cells (SW39) is stronger than that in telomerase- negative immortalized cells (SW13 and SW26). Inducing hTERT dominant mutations, reducing the activity of endogenous telomerase in cancer cells, telomeres of tumor cells will continue to shorten, finally emerging a number of apoptotic cells. The over-expression of TERT in pheochromocytoma can reduce tumor cells apoptosis.

Mattson and others activated research in the aspect of activation telomerase and TERT function in nerve cells, can better prevent nerve cell death, but also promote the recovery of nerve cells in a variety of neuronal degenerative disease conditions.

AD (Alzheimer's disease) is a common degenerative disease of the nervous system in the elderly. In cerebral blood vessel wall of their patients they could separate β-amyloid protein which could lead to AD neuron degeneration. Zhu and others used the antisense technology and telomerase inhibitors leading to inhibit TERT function of fetal rat hippocampus neurons and found a significant increase in cells apoptosis by the β- amyloid peptide-induced. The reason is that reduce TERT function of the neurons can enhance the oxidative and lead to barrier of mitochondrial function through exposed β-amylase protein, thus causing apoptosis.

5. Cell Proliferation Independing Telomere Extension Mechanism

Some telomerase-negative tumors through one or more alternate lengthening of telomere (ALT) mechanism (add telomere repeat sequences) to maintain telomere length. A few immortalized tumor cell lines and some soft tissue tumors, although there is no telomerase activity, there still has long telomeres, suggesting that there is a telomere extension mechanism independing on telomerase.Also using three ribozyme which identify the different sequences of hTR 3′ end effect on tumor cells, telomerase activity was reduced within 4 weeks, the telomeres shorten, but the growth rate was not changed, suggesting that there was a proliferation mechanism without depending on telomerase.

Other studies, such as in melanoma cells, the telomerase activity was reduced within 8 weeks, but after the passage of more than 20 generations, telomere length is not shorten, and cells continued to proliferation. Showing that besides telomerase maintain telomere length to cause cell proliferation, there are other mechanisms maintaining telomeres length and cell proliferation.

Section 5　Telomerase as A Target for Anti-cancers

More than 85% cancer cells and tissues show high expression of telomerase, so telomerase is a better anti-cancer drug targets—Use telomerase inhibitor-induced telomere can cause progressive shortening. But it is necessary to consider the following factors: ①After using telomerase inhibitors, telomere of tumor cells continue shortening until proliferation is inhibited. This time lag is associated with the initial length of the telomeres in cells. ②At least in theory, there is a possibility that anti-telomerase inhibitor as or do not rely on telomere maintenance mechanisms of telomerase (ALT) in tumor cells. ③ Telomerase inhibitor may have a role of somatic cells of the human telomerase expression. For example, hematopoietic stem cells, germ cells, epidermis cells of basal layer and intestinal gland cells. ④In cell resting phase, telomeres do not shorten, telomerase in almost no activity.

The telomerase inhibitors effects are different on tumor cells and telomerase-positive of normal cells: tumor cells are sensitive to telomerase inhibitors, the cells may arise growth inhibition or apoptosis after treated with telomerase inhibitors .Under the action of telomerase inhibitors, the telomere length of germ cells shortened slightly, and then the cells continued to grow, but the telomeres no longer shortened. As compared with telomerase-negative cells, the rate of telomere shortening are much slower in stem cells. After treating telomerase inhibitors, accelerated telomere shortening in stem cells, once removing inhibitor, the speed of telomere shortening got slow again. Some cancer cells have longer telomeres (>10kb), telomere shortening is a slow process following mitosis. In this case, whether telomerase inhibitor is effective need to be further confirmed.

1. Targeting Telomerase RNA

Inhibiting telomerase activity by blocking the effect of telomerase RNA template.

(1) Anti-sense oligonucleotides are hot spots in the studying area of telomerase inhibitors. It is a short chain of DNA which is paired with target RNA. According to the principle of base pairing formed hybrid with target RNA, it then passively or actively inhibits RNA transcription.

(2) Ribozyme is a small molecule RNA which owns specific endonuclease activity, identifying targeting sites through the antisense sequence of enzyme catalytic center. That Ribozyme inhibits the telomerase activity may will become a new anticancer drug that has broad spectrum, low toxicity and is highly effective.

2. Inhibiting Telomerase Reverse Transcriptase (TERT)Activity

(1) Mutation of hTERT

In vitro and in vivo experiments, after mutation of hTERT, the telomerase activity was inhibited significantly.

(2) Reverse transcriptase inhibitors (RTI)

Because telomerase is RNA which is dependent DNA polymerase, so RTI (such as zidovudine) may become a treatment drug for cancer.

(3) ASODN which targets hTERT mRNA can hybridize selectively with target genes and block the expression of target genes.

3. Stabilization of G-quadruplex

The 3′ end of telomere prominent chain is rich in guanine. In vitro it can form four chains of DNA structures, it named as the G-quadruplex. The telomerase activity was inhibited after forming the G-quadruplex. Therefore, the drugs which can make G - quadruplex get stable might be the effective telomerase inhibitors. Many of these compounds have been found and these drugs can inhibit telomerase, but there is no report about telomeres shortening in this area.

4. Small Molecule Inhibitors

With fitting analysis by the simulation software of molecular structure or by other high-through mode for rapid screening small molecule inhibitors of telomerase, this is a fast developing area in recent years. This method is based on bioinformatics strategy of chemical structures to search for the leading compounds. Using this strategy a few of telomerase inhibitors (such as FJ5002) have been found, but its mechanism is unclear.

Section 6   Detection Methods for Telomerase

Given the differences in the positive rate of telomerase in tumor tissue and normal tissue, at the international conference in 1996, the United States, some experts presented telomerase as a tumor specific mark, and using telomerase as a target of tumor gene therapy has great potential application value. In recent decades, telomerase detection methods have made great progress, its stability and vulnerability gradually improve.

1. Telomere Extension Assay

Its main principle is based on the function of reverse transcriptase telomerase. They themselves make a RNA template to be synthesized and undergo extension. Main methods is to prepare telomerase extract from organization, add the repeated TTAGGG primers, synthesize and extend the restructuring TTAGGG sequences. In the reaction liquid, including 32 p labeled dGTP (dexoyguanosine triphosphate), the isotope incorporation. Response to 0.1 mg/ml RNA enzymes to terminate. Reaction products are detected by polyacrylic amide gel electrophoresis and radiation developing, positive specimen visible trapezoidal bands. Because telomerase contains RNA components, in the process of extraction and detection for no RNA operation, prevents the template of RNA degradation. This method is the earliest set up, with good stability and high specificity. The disadvantage is that they required more sample, no amplification, is not suitable for clinical specimens of a large number of samples tests, and tests with large dosage of isotope, against the experimenter health and mass promotion.

2. Telomerase Report Amplification Protocol Assay

Telomerase Report Amplification Protocol (TRAP) method was founded by Kim et al. in 1994 known as the preferred method of telomerase activity detection, the reaction product of telomerase is amplified by design guide objects polymerase chain reaction (PCR), and showed the bases of ladder by polyacrylamide gel electrophoresis (PAGE).

Test cells at least up to 1×10, compared with the traditional method sensitivity increased 10000 times. Specimen sources of the technology, can be obtained from organization, including intraoperative needle aspiration biopsy samples, exfoliated cells and in vitro cell lines. The telomerase extract in cracking tissues must be on the ice. PCR amplification the extract of telomerase PCR reaction system includes dNTP and TS (5'-the AAT CCG TCG AGC AGA GGT-3') primers. TS is a length of 18 bp oligonucleotides, telomerase can be combined with TS, on its own RNA component as template, in TS 3'extension synthesis the repeated TTAGGG sequences. Which extend product as a template, add another pair of primers CX (5' CCCTTACCCTTACCCTTACCCTAA-3') and the Tag enzyme, with TS as upstream primer, CX as downstream primers, by PCR amplification. Reaction products are observation with the classical approach adding 32 p labeled nucleotides and PCR amplification product, radiation imaging analysis results, about - 80 ℃ after 24 ~ 48 h after the enhancement. In view of this observation method it is time-consuming and isotope radioactive pollution, some scholars proposed to reaction products by silver staining. The TRAP is a classic method of detection of telomerase, only need less samples, high sensitivity. The many kinds of modified methods such as PCR - ELLSA, fluorescent PCR-, silver stain and so on. Defects on the one hand is the experimental steps is more complex, and the results of quantitative difficulties, on the other hand, due to the Tag enzyme inhibitors is contained in some organizations, may lead to false negative results.

3. Enzyme-linked Immunosorbent Method

In the late 90s by using binding Enzyme-linked Immunosorbent method (ELLSA) method and the TRAP method, further improved the TRAP method, shortened the experiment time, simplified the experimental steps. The basic principle of this method is with biotin labeling TS primer, and then extended TS and CX with PCR, and the amplification products are hybridization with digoxin labeled telomerase specific oligonucleotide probe, finally forms color reactants through oxide substrate enzyme decomposition TMD substrate. The data used in the determination of the instrument. Experiment cycle is 6~8 h, commonly used kits, experimental steps are simplified, has a wide prospect of clinical use. The disadvantage is that the quantitative difficulties, generally for the semi-quantitative detection of telomerase activity.

4. Real-time Fluorescent Quantitative PCR Technique

In recent years, the real time fluorescence quantitative PCR (RT - QPCR) technology was introduced into telomerase activity test. Due to human telomerase including telomerase RNA (hTR), telomerase related protein (TP1) and telomerase catalytic subunit (hTERT) three main components. Telomerase activity, hTERT is almost expressed in the all tumor cells, but no expression of hTERT in normal cells, which suggests that telomerase activity is mainly determined by the level of hTERT expression. hTERT is a sensitive indicator of telomerase activity. The method repeatability, stable and reliable, the sample processing time generally is within 1h, and the results can be obtained.

The methods of telomerase detection are developing in the direction of the accurate quantitative from early rough qualitative. How to enhance its experimental repeatability, stability, ease of clinical operation and popularization, and its expression in different cells form a quantitative and standardization, is still the problem of telomerase practical application from experimental study to clinical.

Challenges and Prospects

Human understanding telomeres - telomerase began in the 1930 s and even earlier, from 1938 naming telomeres, to the telomerase was found in 1985, in a long time, people have been processing to experience countless hypothesized - to verify these hypothesis - negative hypothesis- put forward the hypothesis. Geneticists have found the importance of chromosome end structure for maintaining chromosome stability in different biologicals. The progress of the technology to make DNA sequences can be successful in testing, understanding of telomeres by initial morphology and gradually transit to the molecular biology. With the further study of the characteristics of the DNA polymerase, people put forward the chromosomes end hidden problems and think about how to solve this copy problem. At the time put forward between the homologous recombination and new unknown enzyme, the experimental data more supported for the latter. This enzyme was later found telomeres that gave success to reverse synthesis telomeres in itself as a template. In the process of research the telomeres - telomerase, scientist questions from the phenomena were observed, analyzed and solved through rigorous reasonable experiments. In the process of the telomere and telomerase discovery, fully embodies the wisdom in light of the scientific thought and magical nature of creation.

1. Discover Process is the General Programs of Research in Life Sciences

(1) Presentating questions in the observation.

(2) Conducting a preliminary interpretation and investigation of the mentioned questions, thenput forward the hypothesis that make scientific predictions

(3) Establishment of experimental model to test the prediction.

(4) Statistical analysis of experimental data, and draw conclusions

(5) Revising a hypothesis and further observation and experimentation to the next known cycle.

The whole process is like a relay race, filled with brilliance of scientific ideas, inspiring future generations. A series of discoveries of telomere and telomerase is indeed a very perfect found journey. However, not only in showing the inherent simplicity of living organisms, but also will demonstrate its diversity and complexity of the internal. In fact, cell through millions years of time and "tries" a variety of possibilities in the long process of evolution.

Cells through one hundred million years, in the long evolution "try" to find different possibilities. Telomerase replication is one of the most common ways to solve the chromosomes hidden problem. Back to the initial speculation that homologous recombination extending telomere hypothesis is not wrong, cellscan actually also be extended with telomeres through homologous recombination. Fission yeast chromosome end connecting cyclization ways to avoid the chromosomes hidden problems, extend the survival in the absence of telomerase and telomere. Flies can pass the transposon copied extension of telomeres. Virus is able to use proteins or tRNA as primer starting genomic DNA synthesis, the chromosome solve itself a copy hidden problem. The result of evolution, different (individual, organs, tissue, cells, molecules) levels are natural selection's magic so that human are extremely skillful.

2. Unsolved Mysteries and Research Prospect

As the further study of mechanism of the structure and function of telomere and telomerase, make the telomeres - telomerase is more attention by people because of its close relationship with human aging and cancer. Current researches focus more on telomerase and alzheimer disease, telomerase as a diagnosis, prognosis and anti-cancer drug targets. The extended function of telomerase in the body is a complex dynamic process. How exactly the continuous synthesis ability of telomerase is real? Which roles do the affinity of telomere related proteins play in the process of telomere length regulation? How is the telomerase a tumor marker in diagnosis and classification of tumor? And it is not clear in the body how many telomere DNA synthesis in every cell division? The solution of these problems depends on the clinical detection methods to further improve the maneuverability and stability; Depends on the development of evaluation system with more sensitivity and specificity of accurate quantitative; Relies on the cloning and identification of new components of the telomere and telomerase. Now, research and exploration continues in the fine structure and the regulatory mechanism of the telomeres - telomerase, the relationship between the aging and longevity factors, and whether there is no dependence on telomeres - telomerase mode of chromosome repair mechanisms. How to make telomerase detection as the marker in tumor diagnosis is still the future research direction. At the same time, it is very important to further explore the relationship among telomeres, telomerase and aging, longevity factors, and to carry out research projects of the cloning human telomerase genes for human aging and anti-aging research. But at this stage of the study are limited in theoretical, detecting telomerase was applied to real clinical still has a lot of work to do.

Consider/Questions

1. Basic concepts in this chapter

Telomere, telomerase, half reserved copy of DNA, half discontinuous replication, Okazaki fragment, the end of the hidden problem, Telomere crisis, Alternative Lengthening of telomere (ALT).

2. Why choose Tetrahymena as the study material of telomere?

3. Brief introduction of the structure characteristics and main function of telomere.

4. Brief introduction of the basic structure and main function of telomerase.

5. How to explain the mechanism of telomere extension induced by telomerase?

6. An overview of research progress of telomerase as the main anti-cancer drug targets.

7. Summarizes the common methods in detection of telomerase (5 kinds).

8. In order to the discovery process of telomere and telomerase, summarizes the general process of scientific research.

第七章 肿瘤干细胞

关于干细胞的研究是现代生物医学研究中最吸引人的课题之一，其代表性的新领域的核心为再生医学。目前基本对干细胞使用持有相对开放的观点，认为干细胞可能是继药物，手术和物理治疗之后的第四大治疗手段，对其寄予厚望。前期一系列临床研究的结果也令人兴奋，如在抗器官移植后免疫排斥、自身免疫性疾病治疗、糖尿病治疗、肿瘤治疗等方面都取得了较好的结果，无疑给未来的临床应用领域提供巨大想象空间，在损伤性疾病、遗传性疾病、退行性疾病及再生医学中都可能将得到广泛应用。干细胞研究不仅具有不可估量的医学价值，而且也将加速科学家对细胞生长分化、生物发育机制等基本生命规律的重新认识。

但关于干细胞的研究也面临两方面的挑战：①建立生物概念；②将干细胞作为细胞疗法用于疾病（如癌症和神经变性）和人体组织损伤修复（包括心、脑和骨骼肌）的治疗。

第一节 干 细 胞

细胞是机体组成的基本单位，在其分化过程中，细胞往往由于高度分化而完全失去再分裂的能力，最终衰老死亡。机体在发展、适应过程中为了弥补这一不足，保留了一部分未分化的原始细胞，即为干细胞（stem cell）。

一、干细胞定义

干细胞（stem cell）是一类未分化的原始细胞，在体内能发展为具有特定功能的特殊细胞类型。干细胞可通过有丝分裂保持自我长期更新的状态。因此干细胞的两大生物学特性为多潜能分化能力和自我更新增殖能力。

干细胞存在于人和动物发育的各阶段（包括早期胚胎和成熟组织），一方面进行自我更新（self-renew），产生与亲本完全相同的子代细胞，以保持干细胞数量的恒定；另一方面在一定条件下可以进入分化程序，通过不对称分裂产生分化的子代细胞，最终形成功能特异的细胞类型。现在已经明确干细胞存在于成年动物的许多组织中，并有助于维持组织平衡。体内细胞数可以通过干细胞输入的增加或减少而改变。损伤或衰老引起的细胞丧失可通过不稳定细胞群和稳定细胞群中的干细胞池的新细胞来取代。永久型细胞也可由干细胞来源的新细胞取代。

界定干细胞有 4 条标准：①干细胞可进行多次的、连续的、自我更新式的细胞分裂，这是维持群体稳定的首要条件；②起源于单一干细胞的子细胞可分化出 1 种以上的细胞类型，如造血干细胞可分化为所有的血细胞；有些成熟干细胞只能分化成单一的细胞类型，如角膜干细胞；③当干细胞被移植入损伤部位时，它有重建原来组织的功能，这一点已被造血干细胞的功能所证实，最近发现肝脏干细胞和神经干细胞也有此特点；④不易确定的标准：即使无组织损伤，干细胞也能在体内扩增和分化。

近年来，许多努力已经致力于干细胞的分离和研究其表型特征。虽然产生识别干细胞的特殊标志物仍是一个持续的挑战，但一系列新的观察和研究手段使干细胞的研究充满活力，列举如下。

（1）鉴定干细胞及其在各种组织中的生态位，包括脑，曾被认为是一种永久性的静止器官。

（2）识别源自各种组织的干细胞，特别是骨髓中的干细胞可能具有广泛的发育可塑性。

（3）认识到在人类和小鼠组织中有些干细胞可能与胚胎干细胞相似。

二、干细胞的特征

（1）生化特征上具有较高的端粒酶活性。

（2）干细胞能无限增殖分裂，具有缓慢性、自稳性（区别与肿瘤细胞的特征）。

（3）干细胞本身不处于分化途径的终端。

（4）干细胞既可连续分裂几代，也可在较长时间内处于静止状态。

（5）干细胞具有两种方式生长，一种是对称分裂，即形成两个相同的干细胞，保持亲代的特征，仍作为干细胞保留下来。另一种是非对称分裂，即由于细胞质中的调节分化蛋白的不均匀分配，使得一个子细胞不可逆地走向分化的终端，成为功能特异的分化细胞；分化细胞的数目受分化前干细胞的数目和分裂次数控制（图 7-1）。

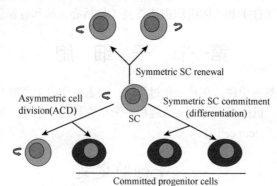

图 7-1　干细胞自我更新和分化之间的关系；Relationship between stem cell self-renewal and differen- tiation
干细胞自我更新是由弯曲的箭头表示。只有单向干细胞用直箭头描述；The stem cell（SC）self-renewal is indicated by curved arrows. Only a unipotent progenitor cell is depicted

三、干细胞在正常生理条件下的发展状态和在受损及应激刺激时的可塑性

干细胞多向分化的潜能称为发育可塑性。祖细胞一旦分化为不同的细胞时，即失去了自我更新的能力（图 7-2）。

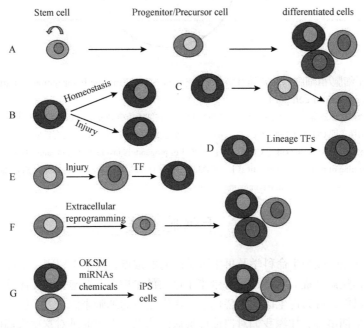

图 7-2 干细胞在正常生理条件下的发展状态和在受损及应激刺激时的可塑性；Stem cell development under normal（physiological）conditions and different forms of plasticity of the stem cell progeng during injury and upon induction

干细胞在正常生理条件下的发展状态，处于自我更新而相对静止的干细胞形成增殖性干细胞（通常称为前体细胞），然后形成非增殖性的终末分化细胞（A）；一个分化细胞可以直接产生另一个同类型的分化细胞（B）；可塑性是指一种分化细胞转化为祖细胞后转化为另一种类型的分化细胞（C）或一种分化细胞直接转化为另一种类型的分化细胞（D）；祖细胞因受损形成一种特殊的细胞类型，然后通过谱系特异转化因子（TF）转分化形成另一种特殊的细胞类型（E）；可塑性指祖细胞（或分化细胞）重新编程形成一种更原始的细胞，然后形成不同类型的分化细胞（F-G）；stem cell development under normal（physiological）conditions, a self-renewing, relatively quiescent stem cell gives rises to a proliferative progenitor cell（sometimes called a precursor cell），which then develops into non-proliferative terminally differentiated cells（A）；A differentiated cell directly generates another differentiated cell of the same type. The best example is mouse pancreatic β-cells（B）；Plasticity by which one differentiated cell type is converted（C）or directly converts（D）to another differentiated cell type（C, D）；A progenitor cell gives rise to a specialized cell type upon injury, which is then transdifferentiats into another specialized cell type by a lineage-specific TF（E）；Plasticity by which progenitor（or differentiated）cells are reprogrammed to a more primitive cell, which then develops into various specialized cells（F, G）

四、干细胞的标记

干细胞的常见标记有：SSEA-3、SSEA-4、TRA-1-60、 TRA-1-81、OCT-4 蛋白、CD133、CD44、CD34，干细胞和祖细胞在分子表达中具有异质性，如人造血干细胞/祖细胞（图 7-3）。

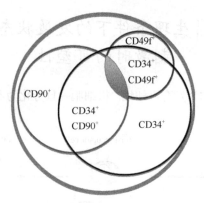

图 7-3　人类造血干细胞/祖细胞池的异质性特征；A cartoon depicting the heterogeneous nature of human hematopoietic stem/progenitor cell pool

三个圆圈分别代表三个祖细胞亚群（即 CD90$^+$，CD34$^+$和 CD49f$^+$），在圆圈重叠处分别是 CD34$^+$和 CD90$^+$，CD34$^+$和 CD49f$^+$ 细胞，合并三重标记阳性（即 CD34$^+$CD90$^+$CD49f$^+$；阴影）。在骨髓或脐带血细胞中富含具有长期重新增殖活性的造血干细胞；Illustrated are three subsets（i.e., CD34$^+$, CD90$^+$ and CD49f$^+$）of progenitors inside the CD34$^+$ and CD90$^+$, CD34$^+$and CD49f$^+$ population. Combined sorting of triple marker-positive（i.e., CD34$^+$CD90$^+$CD49f$^+$; shaded）blood cells（in either bone marrow or cord blood）greatly enriches HSCs with long-term repopulating activity

五、干细胞分类

近年来，干细胞已成为生命科学及再生医学研究的重点，其根本原因是干细胞和干细胞技术为人类战胜难治疾病和提高生活质量等带来了巨大的希望。干细胞具有在体外大量增殖和分化为多种细胞的潜能，可为再生医学的替代治疗提供充足的细胞来源。人胚胎干细胞还可以用于研究人类发育早期事件，加深我们对遗传性疾病的认识，进而促进对这些疾病的治疗。近年来诱导多能干细胞（iPSC）的获得绕开了胚胎干细胞研究一直面临的伦理和法律等诸多障碍，在医疗领域的应用前景非常广阔。

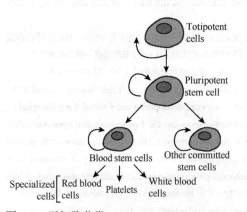

图 7-4　干细胞分类；Classifications of stem cells

（1）根据个体发育过程中出现的先后次序不同，干细胞可分为胚胎干细胞（embryonic stem cell，ESC）和成体干细胞（adult-derived stem cell，ASC），后者包括造血干细胞、表皮干细胞等（图 7-4）。

（2）按分化潜能的大小，干细胞还可分为三种类型。

1）全能干细胞（tyotipotent stem cell）：它具有形成完整个体的分化潜能。例如，ESC 具有与早期胚胎细胞相似的形态特征和很强的分化能力，可以无限增殖并分化成为全身 200 多种细胞类型，进一步形成机体的所有组织、器官。人类的全能干细胞可以分化成人体的各种细胞，这些分化出的细胞构成人体的各种组织和器官，最终发育成一个完整的人。人类的精子和卵子结合后形成受精卵，这个受精卵就是一个最初始的全能干细胞。受精卵继续分化，在前几次分化过程中，可以分化出许多全能干细胞，提取出这些细胞中的任意一个放置到妇女子宫中都可以发育成完整的个体。

2）多能干细胞（pluripotent stem cell）：这种干细胞具有分化出多种细胞组织的潜能，但不具备发育成完整个体的能力，发育潜能受到一定的限制。例如，骨髓多能造血干细胞，它可分化出至少十二种血细胞，但不能分化出造血系统以外的其他细胞。

3）专能干细胞（multipotent stem cell）：也称单能、偏能干细胞。这类干细胞只能向一种类型或密切相关的细胞类型分化，如上皮组织基底层的干细胞、肌肉中的成肌细胞或肌卫星细胞。

传统观点认为：ESC 是全能的，具有分化为几乎全部组织和器官的能力。而成年组织或器官内的干细胞一般认为具有组织特异性，只能分化成特定的细胞或组织。目前这个观点受到了挑战。最新的研究表明，组织特异性干细胞同样具有分化成其他细胞或组织的潜能，也就是说干细胞具有横向分化的能力。这为干细胞的应用开创了更广泛的空间。

（3）根据干细胞组织发生的名称，干细胞又可分为胚胎干细胞、造血干细胞、骨髓间充质干细胞、肌肉干细胞、成骨干细胞、内胚层干细胞、视网膜干细胞和胰腺干细胞等。

第二节　胚胎干细胞

胚胎干细胞（ESC）是在人胚胎发育早期——囊胚（受精后 5～7 天）中未分化的细胞。囊胚含有约 140 个细胞，外表是一层扁平细胞，称滋养层，可发育成胚胎的支持组织如胎盘等。中心的腔称为囊胚腔，腔内一侧的细胞群，称内细胞群。这些未分化的细胞可进一步分裂、分化、发育成个体（图 7-5）。由于这些细胞是首先从胚胎中鉴定的多能干细胞，能产生人体的所有组织，故称为 ESC。

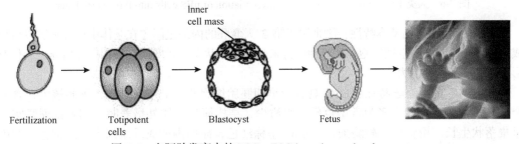

图 7-5　在胚胎发育中的 ESC；ESC in embryos development

ESC 是一种高度未分化的细胞，包括生殖细胞（胚胎性生殖细胞，embryonic germ cell，EGC），它可来源于畸胎瘤细胞（EC）、桑葚球细胞（MS）、囊胚内细胞团（BS）、拟胚体细胞（ES）、生殖原基细胞（EG）等。它具有发育的全能性，能分化出成体动物的所有组织和器官。

一、ESC 的特征

（1）ESC 可以从正常囊胚中分离（图 7-5），在胚胎发育过程中约有 32 期细胞的结构。

（2）ESC 在细胞培养中可以保持未分化状态，也可诱导分化成许多不同的细胞系，以及产生人体的所有组织的细胞，内细胞群在形成内、中、外三个胚层时开始分化。每个胚层将分别分化形成人体的各种组织和器官。例如，外胚层将分化为皮肤、眼睛和神经系统等，中胚层将形成骨骼、血液和肌肉等，内胚层将分化为肝、肺和肠等。由于内细胞群可以发育成完整的个体，这些细胞被认为具有全能性，故又称为全能干细胞（图 7-6）。

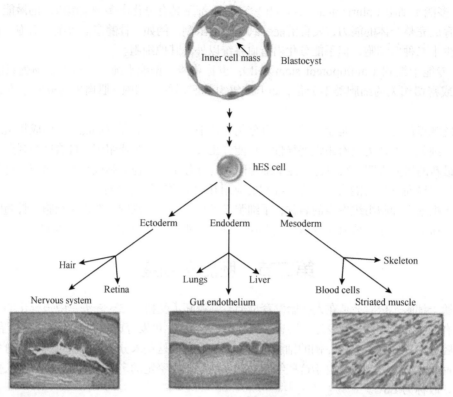

图 7-6　人类 ESC 分化为三个胚层；Differentiation of hES cells into three germ layers

　　脊椎动物 ESC 的基本特性：①来源于第 3 天囊胚的内细胞团（在孕体中这种细胞以后形成胚胎本身）或原始生殖细胞；②长期保持未分化增殖状态；③即使在长期体外培养之后仍有形成三胚层细胞的能力。

　　（3）ESC 的形态学特征：ESC 具有与早期胚胎细胞相似的形态结构，细胞核大，含一个或几个核仁，胞核中多为常染色质，胞质少，结构简单。体外培养时，细胞排列紧密，呈集落状生长。用碱性磷酸酶染色，ESC 呈棕红色，而周围的成纤维细胞呈淡黄色。细胞克隆和周围存在明显界线，形成的细胞克隆中细胞彼此界线不清，细胞表面有折光较强的脂状小滴。细胞克隆形态多样，多数呈岛状或巢状（图 7-7）。

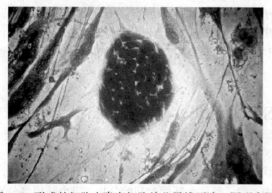

图 7-7　形成的细胞克隆中细胞彼此界线不清，圆形卵圆形，呈岛状或巢状；Morphological features of ESC clones pack closely round or oval without clear boundaries and it looks like a bird nest

　　（4）ESC 表面标志：由于不同种系胚胎在发育早期的基因表达、调控和细胞分化有差异，因此人和动物 ESC 表面标志物有差别。在分析鉴定 ESC 表面标志物的研究中，发现未分化的人 ESC 表面表达与未分化状态相关的表面抗原，包括特异性的胚胎抗原（SSEA-3、SSEA-4）和肿瘤抑制抗原（TRA-1-60、TRA-1-81）及其碱性磷酸酶。其中，SSEA-4 呈强阳性，SSEA-3 呈弱阳性。分化的人 ESC 表现出 SSEA-1 强阳性。这些表达的抗原与其他灵长类

ESC 一致。而小鼠 ESC 的表面抗原表达为 SSEA-1 阳性，SSEA-3、SSEA-4 阴性。ESC 表面表达的转录因子 Oct4，是 ESC 多能性的标志，其随着 ESC 的分化表达下降。

（5）细胞核型：ESC 应具有正常的、完整（双倍）、稳定的染色体核型。Thomson 等分离的人 ESC 系 H1、H13 和 H14 具有正常的 XY 核型，H7 和 H9 具有正常的 XX 核型。其中 H9 经长期培养后核型没有改变。Inzunza 等分离的人 ESC 系 HS181、HS235 和 HS237 经 30～42 周连续培养后，比较基因组杂交（CGH）检测均为正常核型（46，XX）。

二、ESC 的来源

ESC 可来源于早期体外受精形成的胚胎、早期胚胎细胞核置换（图 7-8）、脐带血液或胎儿组织，以及成人组织中的相应细胞。

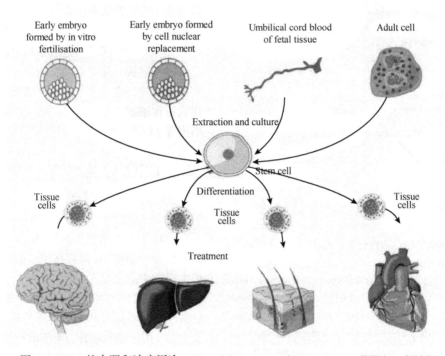

图 7-8 ESC 的来源和治疗用途；Potential sources and treatment possibilities of ESC

建立稳定的永生化的 ESC 细胞系更为实用和可行的方案有三个：①应用克隆技术，用人成熟细胞核置换人卵细胞的遗传物质，然后在体外将其培养至胚泡期，分离 ESC，用于研究和治疗（图 7-9）。此时胚胎尚未开始分化，各系统也未开始发育，故不能称之为 "人"，因此这一技术与 "克隆人" 有明显区别。这一策略具有很大的诱惑力，如将正常细胞核植入受体无核卵细胞中，培养和分离 ESC，再将其体外定向诱导分化为各种特定的功能细胞，用于治疗因这些细胞损伤而引起的多种严重疾病。例如，诱导 ESC 分化为多巴胺神经元治疗帕金森病，分化为胰岛细胞治疗糖尿病，分化为肝细胞和肌细胞治疗肝纤维化和肌萎缩，甚至还可以分化为 CD4⁺细胞治疗艾滋病。目前利用核移植技术获取 ESC 已在羊和小鼠实验中得到验证，但距其应用于人类疾病的治疗还需较长时间。②将人类的细胞核置入到其他哺乳动物的无核卵细胞以获取 ESC。通过对牛、羊、鼠的研究已经证实，克隆的后代看起来都与提供起源细胞核的供核动物的后代相像，而不像供卵者的后代。因此，这一策略可以用来获取 ESC，并已开始在牛和鼠中进行实验。如果可行，那么便可以避免应用人的卵细胞。目前异种核移植尚未得到令人鼓

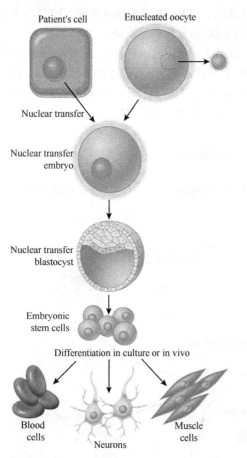

图 7-9　早期胚胎细胞核置换；Early embryo formed by cell nuclear replacement

将患者成熟细胞的二倍体细胞核植入到去核卵母细胞中。卵母细胞被激活，并在受精卵分裂成为含有供体 DNA 的胚泡。分离胚泡以获得 ESC。无论是在培养或移植到供体之后这些细胞能够分化成各种组织；The diploid nucleus of an adult cell from a patient is introduced into an enucleated oocyte. The oocyte is activated, and the zygote divides and becomes a blastocyst that contains the donor DNA. The blastocyst is dissociated to obtain ES cells. These cells are capable of differentiating into various tissues, either in culture or after transplantation into the donor

舞的结果。此外在伦理学上，这种通过其他动物的卵细胞获得的胚胎能否被称为人的胚胎也将成为一个新的课题。③将成人的细胞核植入 ESC 的胞质内，通过 ESC 的胞质与供体细胞核的作用，诱导表达 ESC 特异性的基因。已有研究发现，将成纤维细胞核植入肝细胞的胞质中，结果可以表达一个肝细胞特异性的基因，但这一技术目前还不成熟。

在体外 ESC 的培养：培养胚泡，分离内细胞团，在衬有小鼠成纤维细胞（作为营养细胞）的培养基中培养内细胞团，形成第一次接种平板，9～15 天后分离培养的内细胞团，移入新的营养细胞培养基中，形成第二次接种平板。建立克隆，7～10 天后，分离培养克隆，建立未分化的干细胞，最后分化成特种细胞（血液细胞，神经细胞或肌肉细胞等）（图 7-10）。

三、ESC 对生物学和医学的影响

ESC 又称为永生干细胞，作为组织工程的新型种子细胞，在器官移植和组织修复的再生医学中意义重大。

（1）ESC 已被用于研究许多组织发育中所需的特异性信号和分化步骤及基因调控。

（2）用于细胞治疗：细胞治疗是指用遗传工程改造过的人体细胞直接移植或输入患者体内，达到治愈和控制疾病的目的。ESC 经遗传操作后仍能稳定地在体外增殖传代。以 ES 细胞为载体，经体外定向改造，使基因的整合数目、位点、表达程度和插入基因的稳定性及筛选工作等都在细胞水平上进行，克服目前基因治疗中导入基因的整合和表达难以控制，以及用作基因操作的细胞在体外不易稳定转染和增殖传代的主要问题开辟了新的途径。

（3）进行新药开发、筛选及毒性试验等：ESC 作为新药的药理、药效、毒理及药代等研究的材料，大大减少了药物实验所需动物的数量。目前上述实验使用的细胞系或来自其他种属的细胞系，很多时候并不能真正代表正常人体细胞对药物的反应。ESC 还可用来研究人类疾病的发生机制和发展过程，以便找到有效和持久的治疗方法。

干细胞培养过程

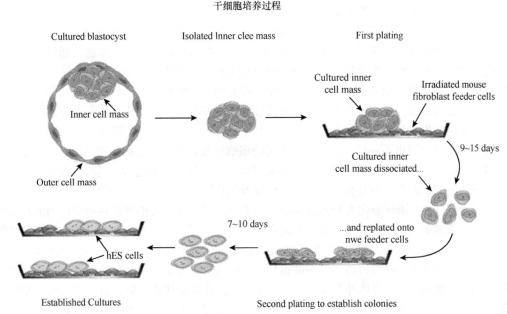

图 7-10　ESC 的培养；Human ESCs cultivation in vitro

（4）在将来 ESC 可以用于重塑受损器官，如肝细胞坏死后肝脏、梗死后心肌。从培养的 ESC 中已经获得了一些特定的细胞类型。培养出产生胰岛素的胰腺细胞和神经细胞分别植入糖尿病动物和神经缺陷的小鼠，尝试治疗。用 ESC 的治疗性克隆还可对神经退行性病变、肝硬化、重度烧伤、心肌梗死等疾病进行治疗。

（5）生产克隆动物和转基因动物：ESC 从理论上讲可以无限传代和增殖而不失去其正常的二倍体基因型和表现型。以其作为核供体进行核移植后，在短期内可获得大量基因型和表现型完全相同的个体。ESC 与胚胎进行嵌合克隆动物，可解决哺乳动物远缘杂交的困难，生产珍贵的动物新种。亦可使用该项技术进行异种动物克隆，对于保护珍稀野生动物有着重要意义。

用 ESC 生产转基因动物，可打破物种的界限，突破亲缘关系的限制，加快动物群体遗传变异程度，可以进行定向变异和育种。利用同源重组技术对 ESC 进行遗传操作，通过细胞核移植生产遗传修饰性动物，有可能创造新的物种；利用 ESC 技术，可在细胞水平上对胚胎进行早期选择，这样可以提高选样的准确性，缩短育种时间。

四、ESC 研究的技术和伦理问题

干细胞治疗是指人自体或异体来源的干细胞及其诱导分化的功能细胞经体外操作后输入（或植入）人体，用于疾病的预防和治疗的过程。用于干细胞治疗的干细胞主要来源于自体或同种异体不同组织的 ESC（系），以及具有发育全能性的 ESC 和细胞重编程获得的诱导多能干细胞（ipsc）细胞及谱系干（祖）细胞。用于干细胞治疗的细胞制备技术和治疗方案，具有多样性、复杂性和特殊性。然而，作为一种新型的生物治疗产品，所有干细胞制剂，都可遵循一个共同的研发过程，即从干细胞制剂的制备、体外实验和体内动物实验（即临床前研究），到植入人体的临床治疗研究全过程。

（一）ESC 研究中的技术难题

ESC 的研究还需要解决很多技术难题。这些问题包括：①ESC 极易分化为其他细胞，如何维持体外扩增时不分化？虽然在防止体外培养时干细胞分化方面已取得了很大成绩，如在培养基中加入白血病抑制因子等可抑制干细胞分化，但仍需进一步研究干细胞的培养条件。②如何定向诱导干细胞分化？细胞分化（cell differentiation）指的是同一来源的细胞，通过细胞分裂在细胞间产生形态结构、生化特征和生理功能有稳定性差异的细胞类群的过程。这个过程是个体发育中组织器官形成的基础，是发育生物学的中心问题。细胞分化包括时间上的分化和空间上的分化；前者是指一个细胞在不同的发育阶段有不同的形态结构、生化特征和生理功能，如骨髓内血细胞的发生过程；后者是指同一种细胞的子代细胞所处的环境位置不同，其形态结构、生化特征和生理功能也不一样，如外胚层来源的细胞可发育成表皮细胞、神经细胞等。细胞分化是多种细胞因子相互作用引起细胞一系列复杂的生理生化反应的过程，因而要诱导产生某种特异类型的组织，需要了解各种因子在何时何地开始作用，以及何时何地停止作用。科学家们认为，只要将 ESC 诱导分化为所需组织细胞的前体即祖细胞，将祖细胞移植到适当的环境中就能够产生所需的组织，因为机体能够分泌所有指导细胞正确分化的因子。并且，不必在体外形成结构精确得多细胞组织后再移植，只需要将已诱导的分散的胚胎细胞或细胞悬液注射到发病部位就可发挥作用，因为这些移植的细胞与周围细胞及胞外基质相互作用便可有机地整合到受体组织中。③由 ESC 在体外发育成一完整的器官，尤其是像心、肝、肾、肺等大型精细复杂器官这一目标还需要技术上的突破。因为器官的形成是一个非常复杂的三维过程。很多器官是两个不同胚层的组织相互作用而形成的。例如，肺中的肌组织、血管和结缔组织来源于中胚层，而上皮组织源自内胚层。每个细胞要获得营养和排泄代谢废物，分化的组织中就需要产生血管，而组织血管化目前还处于研究的起步阶段。退一步而言，即便是一来自自然机体的发育完整的器官，要离体培养并维持其正常的生理功能目前还无法做到，器官的体外保存和维持仍是器官移植中的难题。一种可能的方法是将干细胞注射到重度免疫缺陷动物的脏器中，让移植的人干细胞逐步替代动物细胞，使其脏器人源化，成为可供移植的器官。④如何克服移植排斥反应？创造一种"万能供者"细胞，需要破坏或改变细胞中的许多基因，其可行性尚不清楚；核移植后的卵细胞能否激活沉默基因，启动 DNA 的合成，是否会改变染色体的结构等问题，还有待进一步研究。⑤ESC 的安全性问题：ESC 有形成畸胎瘤的倾向，必须对 ESC 及其衍生细胞的移植安全性做全面、客观、深入的评价。

（二）围绕该研究的伦理道德问题

尽管人 ESC 有着巨大的医学应用潜力，但围绕该研究的伦理道德问题也随之出现。这些问题主要包括人 ESC 的来源是否合乎法律及道德，应用潜力是否会引起伦理及法律问题。从体外受精人胚中获得的 ES 细胞在适当条件下能否发育成人？干细胞要是来自自愿终止妊娠的孕妇该如何处理？为获得 ESC 而摧毁人胚是否道德？是不是良好的愿望为邪恶的手段提供了正当理由？使用来自自发或事故流产胚胎的细胞是否恰当？

毫无疑问，ESC 研究仍面临着一些难题和障碍，但其孕育的巨大价值是有目共睹的。随着人 ESC 基础研究的不断深入，必将在再生医学、人早期胚胎发育、治疗性药物筛选基因治疗中有着广泛的应用前景。

第三节　成体干细胞

成体干细胞（ASC）存在于成年动物许多组织和器官，如表皮和造血系统。在特定条件下，ASC 或者产生新的干细胞，或者按一定的程序分化，形成具有新功能的细胞，从而使组织和器官保持生长和衰退的动态平衡。ASC 主要包括神经干细胞（neural stem cell，NSC）、造血干细胞（hematopoietic stem cell，HSC）、骨髓间充质干细胞（mesenchymal stem cell，MSC）、表皮干细胞（epidermis stem cell）等。

相比于 ESC 的多分化潜能特点，ASC 有一个严格的分化方向，通常是谱系特异性的。作为具有广泛分化潜能的干细胞存在于成人骨髓和其他组织中（可塑性）。位于骨髓外的干细胞是组织干细胞。

ASC 常位于特定的微环境中。微环境中的间质细胞能够产生一系列生长因子或配体，与干细胞相互作用，控制干细胞的更新和分化。干细胞位于的部位称为生态位，在不同的组织中不同。干细胞分化程序并不固定，干细胞分化从一种类型变为另一种类型称为横向分化。

由于对干细胞的横向分化的研究，发现人体各个系统内的干细胞都可以通过诱导而相互转化。机体多种成熟分化的组织中普遍存在 ASC。大部分 ASC 都可以"横向分化"为至少 2～3 种以上其他组织的细胞。ASC 横向分化不仅具有相当的普遍性，而且具有多能性。这种"横向分化"的分子机制一旦被研究清楚，就有望利用患者自身健康组织的干细胞，诱导分化成可替代病变组织的功能细胞来治疗各种疾病。这样既克服了由于异体细胞移植而应起的免疫排斥，又避免了 ESC 来源不足及其他社会伦理问题。人们可望从自体中分离出 ASC，在体外定向诱导分化为靶组织细胞并保持增殖能力，将这些细胞回输入体内，从而达到长期治疗的目的。因此横向分化的发现在干细胞研究中具有革命性意义，它为干细胞生物工程在临床治疗中的广泛应用奠定了基础。探讨 ASC "横向分化"的机制已成为干细胞研究的另一个热点。

ASC 可以由下列几个方面获得：① 胚胎细胞，由 ESC 定向分化或移植分化而成。②胚胎组织，由分离胚胎组织、细胞分离或培养而成。③成体组织，由脐血、骨髓、外周血、骨髓间质、脂肪细胞等得到。利用从成年患者获得的自体细胞或异源性细胞进行再生性细胞治疗将是一种更易行的方法。

限制 ASC 利用的因素如下。

（1）有多少种 ASC，他们存在于何处？人们尚未从体内的全部组织中分离出 ASC。尽管多种不同类型的专能干细胞已得到确定，但所有类型细胞和组织的 ASC 尚未在成人体内发现。例如，人们尚未发现人类的成体心脏干细胞或成熟胰岛干细胞。

（2）在体内 ASC 是残留的 ESC 还是另有来源？为什么包绕其周围的细胞均分化而它可保持不分化？

（3）是否可通过控制 ASC 生长条件来提高增生能力，从而产生足够的组织细胞用于移植。因为 ASC 含量极微，很难分离和纯化，且数量随年龄增长而降低。有证据表明，成人身上获得的干细胞，其增殖能力可能不如年轻人的干细胞。如果尝试使用患者自身的干细胞进行治疗，那么首先必须从患者体内分离干细胞，并进行体外培养，直至有足够数量的细胞才可用于治疗。对于某些急性病症，恐怕没有足够的时间进行培养。

（4）存在于骨髓或外周血中的单个干细胞是否可分化为组织或器官的细胞？

（5）在一些遗传缺陷疾病中，遗传错误很可能也会出现于患者的干细胞中，这样的干细胞不适于移植。

（6）由于日常生活的暴露，包括日光、毒素及在一生中 DNA 复制过程中的某些错误，ASC 可能包含更多的 DNA 异常。

（7）干细胞有规律地分化和增生的信号是什么？刺激干细胞在受损伤或病变的部位出现的条件或因子是什么？

（8）在实验性操纵下 ASC 是否能正常地展现其可塑性或仅仅是横向分化？

这些问题限制了 ASC 的使用。

一、造血干细胞

造血干细胞（hematopoietic stem cells，HSC）又称多能干细胞，是存在于造血组织中的一群原始造血细胞。可以说它是一切血细胞（其中大多数是免疫细胞）的原始细胞，是体内各种血细胞的唯一来源，主要存在于骨髓、外周血、脐带血中。HSC 定向分化、增殖为不同的血细胞系，并进一步生成血细胞。人类 HSC 首先出现于胚龄第 2～3 周的卵黄囊，在胚胎早期（第 2～3 月）迁至肝、脾，第 5 个月又从肝、脾迁至骨髓。在胚胎末期一直到出生后，骨髓成为 HSC 的主要来源。HSC 具有多潜能性，即具有自身复制和分化两种功能。在胚胎和迅速再生的骨髓中，HSC 多处于增殖周期之中；而在正常骨髓中，则多数处于静止期（G_0 期），当机体需要时，其中一部分分化成熟，另一部分进行增殖，以维持 HSC 的数量相对稳定。HSC 进一步分化发育成不同血细胞系的定向干细胞。定向干细胞多数处于增殖周期之中，并进一步分化为各系统的血细胞系，如红细胞系、粒细胞系、单核-吞噬细胞系、巨核细胞系及淋巴细胞系。由 HSC 分化出来的淋巴细胞有两个发育途径，一个受胸腺的作用，在胸腺素的催化下分化成熟为胸腺依赖性淋巴细胞，即 T 细胞；另一个不受胸腺作用，而受腔上囊（鸟类）或类囊器官（哺乳动物）的影响，分化成熟为囊依赖性淋巴细胞或骨髓依赖性淋巴细胞，即 B 细胞。并分别由 T 细胞、B 细胞引起细胞免疫及体液免疫。如机体内 HSC 缺陷，则可引起严重的免疫缺陷病。

骨髓中有 HSC 和间质细胞能分化成各种细胞系。HSC 产生所有的血细胞，可以在疾病或辐射导致耗尽后重建骨髓（图 7-11）。

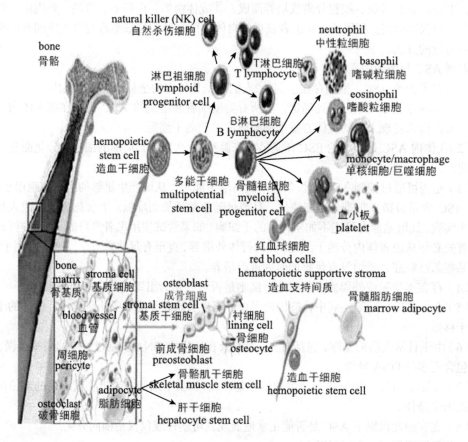

图 7-11　HSC 能分化成各种间质细胞系；HSCs are capable of differentiation into various lineages

HSC 可以直接来源于骨髓、脐血中。在人循环血中接受细胞因子，如粒细胞-巨噬细胞集落刺激因子可动员 HSC 产生。

由 HSC 到祖细胞再到外周血细胞的这种分化调节过程相当复杂，依赖于各种造血生长因子、造血基质细胞、细胞外基质等多种因素的相互作用与平衡，并涉及细胞的增殖分化、发育成熟、迁移定居、衰老凋亡和癌变等生命科学中的许多基本问题，这也是基础研究的主要热点。

（1）HSC 不同于其他多能干细胞：①在个体发育过程中，HSC 历经多次迁移，先由卵黄囊转移到胎肝，最后到达骨髓，而其后的某些条件下又可出现髓外造血的情况；而其他多能干细胞多在固定的场所发育成特定的组织。②由于生理需要，HSC 始终处于较为活跃的增殖与分化状态，能从骨髓源源不断地进入外周血而到达全身各处，而成熟个体中的多能干细胞多局限于相应的组织器官中，一般情况下处于类似休眠的状态。③HSC 具有可塑性，可以分化为肝脏、肌肉及神经等组织的细胞，一定条件下又可来源于肌肉干细胞、神经干细胞等，而这种分化大多在相应组织病变的情况下完成。

（2）HSC 的临床应用：在临床治疗中，HSC 应用较早。

1）HSC 移植就是应用超大剂量化疗和放疗以最大限度杀灭患者体内的白血病细胞，同时全面摧毁其免疫和造血功能，然后将正常人 HSC 输入患者体内，重建造血和免疫功能，达到治疗疾病的目的。但是，HSC 并不能在人群中随意移植，正如输血需要配 ABO 血型一样，HSC 移植需先进行人白细胞抗原（HLA）配型。HLA 是人体细胞表面的"主要组织相容性复合物"（MHC），只有两个个体 HLA 配型相同，才能进行 HSC 移植，否则会发生移植物抗宿主反应（GVHR）或移植排斥反应，严重者可危及患者生命。HLA 由遗传决定，理论上说，每五个同胞兄弟姐妹中可能有两人的 HLA 抗原完全相合，而在无血缘关系的人群中，约 10 万人以上才可能有两个 HLA 完全相同的个体。鉴于我国国情，在年轻患者的同胞中寻找 HLA 相合供体的可能性极小。由于 HSC 具有自我复制功能，因此捐赠骨髓一般不影响健康。而且由于科技进步，现在可通过 HSC "动员"技术，采集分离约 200ml 外周血就可得到足够数量的 HSC，称为外周血干细胞移植。所谓骨髓库，是抽取自愿者数毫升血用于 HLA 定型，并将资料储存于电脑。有患者需要供体时，将其 HLA 资料经电脑检索配型，由配型相合者捐献骨髓或外周血用于移植。发达国家现已建立了多达数百万人的骨髓库网络，多达 70% 需要移植的患者可获捐赠 HSC 而得以挽救生命。此外，科学研究证明，脐带血中含有丰富的 HSC，可用于 HSC 移植，如能建立脐血干细胞库，将会使大批患者受益。目前全球已有数百例患者接受了脐血移植。脐血干细胞移植的优点在于无来源的限制，对 HLA 配型要求不高，不易受病毒或肿瘤的污染。HSC 疗法除了可以治疗急、慢性白血病外，HSC 移植也可用于治疗重型再生障碍性贫血、地中海贫血、恶性淋巴瘤、多发性骨髓瘤等血液系统疾病，以及小细胞肺癌、乳腺癌、睾丸癌、卵巢癌、神经母细胞瘤等多种实体肿瘤。对急性白血病无供体者，也可在治疗完全缓解后采取其自身 HSC 用于移植，称为自体 HSC 移植。

2）在损伤修复中，HSC 的主要贡献不在于生成这些组织的细胞，而是干细胞可以产生生长因子和细胞因子，作用于组织细胞迁移，促进损伤修复和细胞复制。

虽然 HSC 能够取代受损组织中的细胞，但这些组织在生理（稳态）条件下 HSC 并不发挥作用。也许 HSC 来源的组织细胞的产生只发生在损伤部位，在损伤反应中从骨髓招募干细胞为局部组织的再生。

二、骨髓间质细胞/间充质干细胞

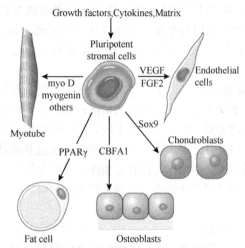

图 7-12　MSC 有不同的分化途径；Differentiation pathways for MSCs

骨髓间质细胞/间充质干细胞（bone marrow stromal cells /mesenchymal stem cells，MSCs），是属于中胚层的一类多能干细胞，主要存在于结缔组织和器官间质中，以骨髓组织中含量最为丰富，由于骨髓是其主要来源，因此统称为骨髓间充质干细胞（bone marrow mesenchymal stem cells，BMMSCs）。

（1）根据不同的组织环境，MSC 有不同的分化途径（图 7-12）。

该细胞可以分化成软骨细胞、成骨细胞、脂肪细胞、成肌细胞、内皮细胞的前体等。

生长因子，细胞因子或基质成分均可引起关键性调控蛋白的活化导致干细胞定向分化成特定的细胞系。特殊细胞的分化需要不同的因子。

（2）MSCs 具有以下特性

1）MSCs 具有强大的增殖能力和多向分化潜能，在适宜的体内或体外环境下不仅可分化为造血细胞，还具有分化为肌细胞、肝细胞、成骨细胞、软骨细胞、基质细胞等多种细胞的能力（图 7-13）。

2）MSC 具有免疫调节功能，通过细胞间的相互作用及产生细胞因子抑制 T 细胞的增殖及其免疫反应，从而发挥免疫重建的功能。

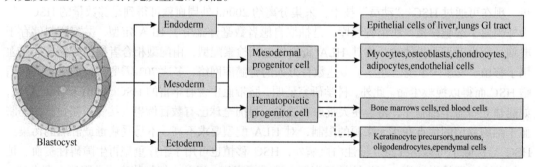

图 7-13　胚胎细胞分化和骨髓前体细胞引起的组织细胞产生；Differentiation of embryonic cells and generation of tissue cells by bone marrow precursors

通过胚胎发育的三个胚层内胚层、中胚层和外胚层的形成产生人体的所有组织。成体干细胞定位于这三层细胞形成的器官中。然而，一些成人骨髓干细胞，除了生产血细胞系（中胚层来源）外，也可以产生起源于内胚层和外胚层细胞组织（用虚线箭头表示）；During embryonic development of the three germ layers-endoderm，mesoderm，and ectoderm are formed，generating all tissues of the body. Adult stem cells localized in organs derived from these layers produce cells. However，some adult bone marrow stem cells，in addition to producing the blood lineages(mesodermal derived)，can also generate cells for tissues that originated from the endoderm and ectoderm（indicated by the dashed arrow）

3）MSC 具有来源方便，易于分离、培养、扩增和纯化，多次传代扩增后仍具有干细胞特性，不存在免疫排斥的特性。正是由于 MSCs 所具备的这些免疫学特性，使其在自身免疫性疾病及各种替代治疗等方面具有广阔的临床应用前景。通过自体移植可以重建组织器官的结构和功能，并且可避免免疫排斥反应。

　　MSCs 是组织修复与再生过程中重要的细胞来源之一。当组织损伤发生时，受损部位往往释放大量的"创伤信号"并伴有多种炎症性细胞浸润和炎症因子分泌。在"创伤信号"的作用下，MSCs 会被募集或动员至受损部位，发挥调控炎症反应和促进组织修复的作用。研究发现，MSCs 的免疫抑制作用不是与生俱来的，它需要炎症因子（IFN、TNF 或 IL-1 等）的"授权"。这一过程主要依赖于炎症因子刺激 MSCs 分泌大量的趋化因子和免疫抑制因子，前者能把淋巴细胞招募至 MSCs 周围，后者则在短距离内能发挥其对淋巴细胞的抑制作用。进一步的研究发现，介导 MSCs 免疫抑制作用的核心分子具有物种差异性，即鼠源 MSCs 主要通过分泌高水平的一氧化氮来执行对淋巴细胞的抑制作用，而人源 MSCs 主要通过表达高水平的吲哚胺-2, 3-双加氧酶，促进色氨酸消耗，发挥抑制淋巴细胞的作用。基于此，在移植物抗宿主的动物模型中，阻断 IFN-γ 在体内的表达或 IFN-γ 受体在 MSCs 上的表达可以消除 MSCs 对移植物抗宿主反应的治疗作用，进一步明确了炎症因子对 MSCs 免疫抑制功能的调控作用。更有意思的是，炎症因子对 MSCs 免疫抑制能力的可塑性调节，即当炎症因子浓度高时，MSCs 发挥免疫抑制作用；当炎症因子浓度不足时，MSCs 则发挥免疫促进作用。因此，这些研究不仅揭示了炎症对 MSCs 发挥免疫调节作用的重要性，而且为以免疫与 MSCs 之间作用为基础探寻炎症性疾病的有效治疗手段提供了新方向。

　　以年龄相关性黄斑变性（age-related macular degeneration，AMD）和视网膜色素变性为代表的视网膜变性疾病是全球性重要的致盲眼病。临床上，AMD 分为渗出性（湿性）和萎缩性（干性）两大类。尽管眼内注射抗 VEGF（vascular endothelial growth factor）药物治疗对干性 AMD 与湿性 AMD 有一定效果，但对更为常见的干性 AMD 目前尚缺乏有效治疗办法，加之眼部的特性，使之成为世界性干细胞应用研究热点。与美国以 ESC 进行视网膜前体细胞和视网膜细胞分化获得的供体细胞、日本以诱导多能干细胞来源的视网膜色素上皮细胞（RPE）为主要供体细胞开展视网膜下腔移植不同，我国研究团队以 MSC 和脂肪来源干细胞（ADSC）为供体细胞，并利用大鼠遗传性视网膜变性模型（RCS 大鼠）为工具，进行视网膜下腔移植的研究取得了进展，特别是 MSC 和 ADSC 在 RCS 大鼠的移植后能存活、迁移、整合、分化，并且这些干预治疗具有安全性。

三、多能成体祖细胞

　　成人骨髓中还有一个异质种群的干细胞，该细胞有非常广泛的分化潜能。他们在培养中增殖而不衰老，并能分化为内胚层、中胚层和神经外胚层的细胞类型。这些细胞称为多能成体祖细胞（multipotent adult progenitor cells，MAPCs）。

　　MAPCs 也不局限于骨髓，可在肌肉、脑、皮肤中孤立存在，类似于骨髓 MSC，可分化为内皮细胞、神经细胞、肝细胞和其他细胞类型。

　　从骨髓、肌肉、脑组织分离获得的 MAPCs 具有相似的基因表达谱，提示他们可能有共同的起源。MAPCs 的干细胞群可能来源于 ESC（如 MAPCs 中有些可能是成熟的 ESC 成分）。如果这一观点成立，那么在成熟组织中干细胞的转向分化和可塑性可能代表了多潜能胚胎样干细胞分化为特殊细胞系的过程。研究证实注射鼠骨髓 MAPCs 到囊胚中可得到体细胞系，证明了MAPCs 的多能性。

四、神经干细胞

1992 年，Reynodls 等从成年小鼠脑纹状体中分离出能在体外不断分裂增殖，且具有多种分化潜能的细胞群，并正式提出了神经干细胞（neural stem cells，NSC）的概念，从而打破了认为神经细胞不能再生的传统理论。Mckay 于 1997 年在 Science 上总结 NSC 的概念：NSC 是一类具有分裂潜能和自我更新能力的母细胞，它可以通过不对称的分裂方式产生神经组织的各类细胞，如分化为神经元、星形胶质细胞及少突胶质细胞，因此能自我更新并足以提供大量脑组织中的细胞。需要强调的是，在脑脊髓等所有神经组织中，不同的 NSC 类型产生的子代细胞种类不同，分布也不同。

（1）根据分化潜能及产生子细胞种类不同分类如下

1）神经管上皮细胞：分裂能力最强，只存在胚胎时期，可以产生放射状胶质神经元和成神经细胞。

2）放射状胶质神经元：可以分裂产生本身并同时产生神经元前体细胞或是胶质细胞，主要作用是幼年时期神经发育过程中产生投射神经元完成大脑皮质及神经核等的基本神经组织细胞。

3）神经细胞（neuroblast）：成年人体中主要存在的 NSC，具有分裂能力可以产生神经前体细胞、神经元和各类神经胶质细胞。

4）神经前体细胞（neural precursor cells）：各类神经细胞的前体细胞，如小胶质细胞是由神经胶质细胞前体产生的。

（2）根据部位分类主要有两类。

1）神经嵴干细胞（neural crest stem cell，NC-SC）和中枢神经干细胞（CNS-SC），一般是指存在于脑部的中枢神经干细胞（CNS-SC），其子代细胞能分化成为神经系统的大部分细胞。

2）外周神经干细胞（PNS-SC），既可发育为外周神经细胞、神经内分泌细胞和施万细胞，也能分化为色素细胞（pigmented cell）和平滑肌细胞等。

以往认为，中枢神经系统的神经元在出生前或出生后不久就失去再生能力。但近来的一些研究表明，成年哺乳动物的脑组织仍可不断产生新的神经元，成人脑组织中同样存在 NSC，主要是在侧脑室下层（嗅球）和海马齿状回两处。

（3）NSC 具有以下特点。

1）自我更新：NSC 具有对称分裂及不对称分裂两种分裂方式，以保持干细胞库稳定。

2）多向分化潜能：NSC 可以向神经元、星形胶质细胞和少突胶质细胞分化。

NSC 的分化能力不仅限于神经系统，在适当的微环境中 NSC 还具有向其他组织细胞多向分化的能力，如 NSC 植入肌肉分化成肌细胞，植入骨髓能分化成血细胞。

3）低免疫源性：NSC 是未分化的原始细胞，不表达成熟的细胞抗原，不被免疫系统识别。

4）组织融合性好：可以与宿主的神经组织良好融合，并在宿主体内能长期存活。

NSC 定向诱导分化调控是目前神经干细胞研究的重大课题。大脑的功能主要依赖于神经元并通过神经信息的传递方式来实现。脑内神经元种类繁多且功能极为复杂，如胆碱能神经元、儿茶酚胺能神经元、5-羟色胺能神经元及肽能神经元等。不同功能的神经元分布在脑内不同的部位，通过合成及释放相应的神经递质发挥各自独特的功能。

NSC 的分化受基因调控。基因表达的时空方式受到其自身固有的分子程序的调控和周围环境的影响。ESC 向 NSC 的分化需要基因调控，特别是不同发育分化阶段决定 NSC 向所需功能神经细胞定向分化的主要调控基因。目前，虽然基因组测序已完成草图，但基因组序列分析仅仅反映遗传信息复杂性的一面，而有关遗传信息有序地、时相性地表达等复杂性的另一面尚未完善。生物的类型变化主要是其内在的，所表达的基因是确定的，如分化细胞与祖细胞，肿瘤细胞与正常细胞等都存在着基因表达差别。若能在这些关系密切的细胞群之间发现那些有表达差异的基因，则可为这些相关细胞群所发生的复杂代谢和功能变化提供有意义的信息。Pevny 等将神经元特异性的 Sox 2 基因转染 ESC，再经维 A 酸诱导，可获得 90%以上的神经细胞。Giebel 等表达 Nurrl 基因对于中脑神经前体细胞分化为多巴胺能神经元起决定作用。这些研究表明基因调控与 NSC 的定向分化密切相关。

细胞因子与 NSC 的增殖、分化密切相关。不同的细胞因子在 NSC 的诱导分化中起重要作用，但尚没有一种细胞因子能在体外将 NSC 全部诱导分化为所需的功能性神经细胞，参与 NSC 诱导分化的细胞因子有白细胞介素类，如 IL-1、IL-7、IL-9 及 IL-11 等；生长因子类，如上皮生长因子（EGF）、神经生长因子（NGF）及碱性成纤维细胞生长因子（bFGF）等也影响 NSC 的分化。神经营养因子对 NSC 分化到终末细胞的整个过程均有影响，如果将培养的 NSC 置于脑源性神经营养因子作用下，大量的 NSC 可以表现出分化神经元的特性。NSC 对不同种类、不同浓度，以及多种因子联合应用的效应各不相同，在 NSC 发育分化的不同阶段，相同因子的作用也不同。例如，在 EGF 及 bFGF 存在的条件下，胚胎 NSC 主要向神经元、星形胶质细胞和少突胶质细胞分化，而出生后及成年的脑 NSC，则无论是否有 EGF 及 bFGF，都主要分化为星形胶质细胞。这些研究提示，EGF 及 bFGF 对 NSC 向功能细胞的诱导分化是复杂的。

NSC 研究起步较晚，由于分离 NSC 所需的胎儿脑组织较难取材，加之胚胎细胞研究的争议尚未平息，NSC 的研究仍处于初级阶段。理论上讲，任何一种中枢神经系统疾病都可归结为 NSC 功能的紊乱。由于血脑屏障的存在使脑和脊髓在干细胞移植到中枢神经系统后不会产生免疫排斥反应，如给帕金森病患者的脑内移植含有多巴胺生成细胞的 NSC，可治愈部分患者症状。除此之外，NSC 的功能还可延伸到药物检测方面，对判断药物有效性、毒性有一定的作用。

目前的研究主要集中于 NSC 在脑中的起源、分布及在治疗中的应用等方面。在发育和成熟的中枢神经系统中均存在着 NSC。近来研究者已从人胎儿大脑皮质中分离出中枢 NSC。同时使用 EGF、NGF-2 等扩增出细胞群。脑内的 NSC 是多能干细胞，它可以分化为脑内三种神经细胞。目前尚不清楚干细胞是否还能分化为它们所在部位的其他细胞类型，是否具有向其他胚层细胞转化的能力。最新研究发现，小鼠 NSC 被移植到辐射后的小鼠体内，可产生各系血细胞。提示起源于外胚层的神经细胞可向中胚层细胞转化，同时也表明 NSC 有更广泛的分化潜能和应用前景。

（4）NSC 治疗优点：中枢神经系统疾病中有很多是因为某种特定的脑细胞发生退行性死亡，导致一些重要的神经递质、蛋白质因子或某些重要结构的匮乏所致。因此，在成功培养了 NSC 之后，人们很自然地想到利用它直接进行移植治疗，或利用病毒载体，携带目的基因，导入 NSC，将筛选得到的体外高效表达目的基因的克隆进行移植。这种细胞治疗方法具有以下优点。

1）NSC 在脑中能根据其周围微环境的诱导而分裂，分化成为相应的细胞类型，其形态和功能与附近的宿主细胞非常类似。即使是将因转入原癌基因而永生化的 NSC 植入脑后也未长出肿瘤。

2）中枢神经系统特殊的血脑屏障结构使淋巴细胞很难进入。因此不同个体之间，甚至是不同物种之间的 NSC 移植，都几乎没有排斥反应，大大提高了 NSC 的用途。

3）NSC 可以在体外根据不同的需要导入相应的外源基因，成为一种广谱的细胞载体。根据 NSC 的这些特性，从不同角度加以应用，已在神经系统疾病的治疗上取得了很大进展。

对大脑和神经修复的再生医学研究显示：干细胞研究提供了对脑损伤、视神经损伤和长期神经修复后功能恢复的创新疗法。干细胞不仅存在于发育中的大脑和视神经系统，而且也存在成人神经系统。在开放性脑损伤常引起大脑和视神经损害中，如果大脑的神经组织脱出颅外它通常被丢弃。但现在研究人员已经能将这些组织作为 NSC 的来源，即从开放性脑外伤患者的脑组织分离和传代 NSC，然后在 MRI 引导下立体定向将 NSC 植入患者，治疗神经缺损造成的创伤。研究显示移植的 NSC 显著改善了患者的神经功能。干细胞疗法的研究中需要分析移植 NSC 的存活率和迁移。研究人员通过纳米颗粒标记人类 NSC 和视网膜干细胞，跟踪猴子和人类中枢神经系统证明了人类 NSC 疗法在中枢神经系统的可行性。

总之，NSC 是一种具有广泛应用前景的干细胞，随着其研究的不断深入，人类的 NSC 将有望作为脑移植的供体细胞及基因治疗的载体用于临床。而其增殖和定向诱导分化机制的最终阐明将有赖于分子生物学、发育生物学等生物学科的相互协作和研究方法的进一步完善。

五、其他组织干细胞

除了骨髓中的干细胞在组织损伤时能迁移到不同组织外，还有永久定居在组织中的干细胞称为组织干细胞，这些细胞可以产生该器官的成熟组织。

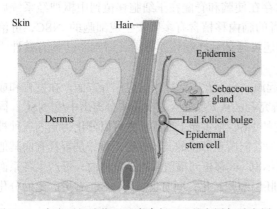

图 7-14　表皮干细胞位于毛囊隆起区，基底层与基底层相邻，作为毛囊和表皮的干细胞；Epidermal stem cells locate in the bulge area of the hair follicle，in the basal layer adjacent to the basement membrane serve as stem cells for the hair follicle and the epidermis

（一）表皮干细胞

表皮干细胞（epidermal stem cells），是皮肤发生、修复、改建的重要源泉。

表皮干细胞在胎儿期主要集中于初级表皮嵴，成人时则呈片状分布于表皮基底层。皮肤皮脂腺开口处与立毛肌毛囊附着处之间的毛囊外根鞘处含有丰富的干细胞（图 7-14），而在没有毛发的部位如手掌、脚掌，表皮干细胞位于与真皮乳头顶部相连的基底层。表皮干细胞可用于自体和异体移植治疗重度烧伤、慢性溃疡等，也可转向分化成神经元、胶质细胞、平滑肌细胞和脂肪细胞。

损伤后，自我更新的上皮以三个非相互排斥的策略进行重组：①增加活跃分裂的干细胞数量；②再扩增细胞成分增加细胞复制次数；③为细胞复制减少细胞周期时间。

（二）肠道干细胞

肠道干细胞（intestinal stem cells）位于结肠隐窝的基底，又称为隐窝细胞，其上为帕内特细胞（图 7-15）。

（三）肝干细胞

　　肝干细胞（liver stem cells），通常称为卵圆细胞（oval cells）是具有双向分化潜能的祖细胞，能够分化为肝细胞和胆管细胞。肝干细胞位于黑林管上，在肝细胞和毛细胆管最小分支连接处（图 7-16）。目前对于肝干细胞的存在，以及其分化产生肝细胞和胆管上皮细胞，进而参与肝脏结构和功能动态平衡维持的基本生物学特性，已进行了越来越多的研究。当肝细胞增殖受阻时，肝干细胞作为一个继发或储备成分被激活。在肝细胞生长过程中，如部分肝切除后肝再生、大多数类型的急性坏死性损

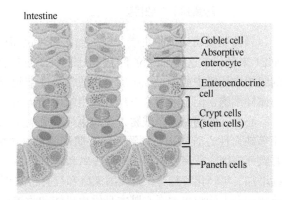

图 7-15　肠道干细胞位于结肠隐窝的基底，又称为隐窝细胞，其上为帕内特细胞；Intestinal stem cells are located at the base of a colon crypt（known as crypt cells），above Paneth cells

伤等，肝细胞本身很容易复制而不需激活干细胞。另一方面，在肝细胞增殖缓慢或受阻时卵圆细胞的增殖和分化是明显的，如重症肝衰竭、肝癌、慢性肝炎和肝硬化时，可见此种细胞明显增生，参与损伤肝脏的修复过程。虽然干细胞在肝切除术后代偿性增生中并没有发挥重要作用，但在某些形式的毒性肝损伤后会引起卵圆细胞的增生，从而诱导肿瘤性转化。

（四）角膜干细胞

　　角膜缘干细胞（corneal stem cells）位于角膜缘，即结膜和角膜之间（图 7-17），是角膜上皮细胞再生的来源，终生不断分化，并向角膜中心移行，以补充损伤及凋亡的上皮细胞，在保持角膜的生理生化环境、完整性，在维持局部免疫反应中占有重要地位。此外，角膜缘干细胞还能阻止结膜上皮细胞移行至角膜表面，对保持角膜的透明与正常生理功能有重要意义。

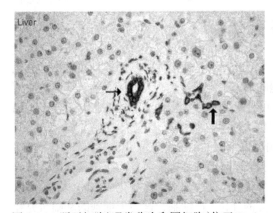

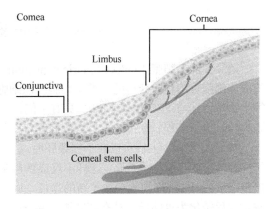

图 7-16　肝干细胞(通常称为卵圆细胞)位于 Hering 管上，在肝细胞和毛细胆管最小分支连接处（胆管和 Hering 管角蛋白染色阳性）；Liver stem cells（commonly known as oval cells）are located in the canals of Hering，in the junction between hepatocytes and the smallest segments of the biliary tree（bile duct and Hering canals are stained for cytokeratin）

图 7-17　眼角膜干细胞位于角膜缘，即结膜和角膜之间；Eye corneal stem cells are located in the limbus region，between the conjunctiva and the cornea

（五）骨骼肌干细胞

骨骼肌损伤后细胞不能分裂，损伤后骨骼肌的生长和再生由肌卫星细胞（muscle satellite cell）来替代。这些细胞位于骨骼肌膜下，即在损伤后能产生肌细胞的干细胞储存库。在不同的组织微环境中肌卫星细胞能分化成骨源性细胞或脂肪源性细胞。尽管已经有报道心肌中含有前体样细胞，但至今尚未发现心肌组织中的干细胞。

心血管疾病是当今威胁人类健康最严重的疾病之一，其中由于冠状动脉病变引发的心肌梗死等缺血性心脏病和心梗致死的心肌细胞被纤维瘢痕代替发生的心力衰竭是心血管疾病的主要致死病因。其高发病率、高致残率和高死亡率已成为我国重大健康问题，并且呈现发病率持续增加、年轻化等趋势，给我国家庭和社会带来更加沉重的负担。缺血性心脏病和心力衰竭的药物和介入治疗可增强心脏本身供血机能和收缩功能，但由于无法修复坏死的心肌细胞和逆转纤维瘢痕，只能延缓而不能阻止心力衰竭的发生；心脏移植可根治末期心力衰竭患者，然而受限于心脏供体缺乏。因此，寻找更有效、可广泛应用于治疗心力衰竭尤其是使纤维瘢痕转变为健康的心肌细胞的治疗手段是这一领域的前沿热点和探索目标。干细胞生物学为心肌再生医学开辟了广阔天地，也为解决心力衰竭治疗这一难题提供了希望。近年干细胞生物学和医学研究的进展显示如下三类可形成新生心肌细胞的起始细胞具有临床应用的前景，即人多能干细胞（包括人 ESC 和 iPSC），成体心脏来源的心脏前体细胞和重编程的成纤维细胞。

干细胞治疗心肌梗死成为近年的研究热点和未来的发展方向。目前全球已有上百个干细胞治疗心肌梗死的临床试验，这些结果虽然证明干细胞移植有一定疗效，但其效果并不理想。其中一个重要原因是干细胞在缺血、缺氧、超氧应激的移植微环境下的存活率及功能低下，这也是本领域亟待解决的难题。

总之，干细胞在促进组织修复和细胞再生中具有重要作用。利用干细胞修复或替代因疾病、意外事故或遗传因素所造成的组织、器官残缺已成为可能。干细胞及其衍生组织器官的应用在生命科学和医学中前景广阔，必将给人类带来全新的医疗理念和医疗手段。

六、诱导多能干细胞

诱导多能干细胞（induced pluripotent stem cell，iPSC）是通过体外基因转染技术将已分化的成体细胞重编程所获得的一类干细胞。该细胞的形态、生长特性、表面标志物、形成畸胎瘤等生物学特性与 ESC 相似。iPSC 具有全能性，可分化为神经等多种组织的细胞，适合于干细胞移植、组织工程、受损组织器官的修复等个体化治疗。

与 ESC 不同，人们可以在不损毁胚胎或不用卵母细胞的前提下获取 iPSC 以制备用于疾病研究和治疗的 ESC 样细胞。这样不仅成功避免了伦理问题的困扰，而且为获得具有患者自身遗传背景的 ESC 样细胞增加了新的途径。同时在理论上证实了人类已分化成熟的体细胞可以被重编程转化为更幼稚、具有高度增殖和分化潜能的 ESC 样细胞，这为干细胞的基础研究和实际应用开辟了广阔的领域。

使用源于患者体细胞的 iPSC 研究疾病病理特征和阐明疾病的分子机制。通过转录因子过表达在体细胞中，特别是那些从患者的体细胞培养得到的 iPSC，可制备一个极有前途的疾病早期阶段的模型，用于体外筛选新型生物标志物和治疗性药物。最近，许多研究团队分别报道，针对特定疾病的病理事件中多个特征来复制患者 iPSC，利用 iPSC 提供的实验模型研究疾病病因等，重新评估目前的疗法。例如，使用源于 Klinefelter 综合征和 AD 患者的 iPSC，探索使用这些 iPSC 复制这些疾病病理特征的可能。结果表明，患者的特定 iPSC 系提供良好的研究疾病发展和治疗的模型。

干细胞的研究及应用离不开其正确的体外培养及分化。而干细胞的自我更新、定向分化及 iPSC 的诱导等都离不开特定的培养环境。小分子化合物是组成这种培养环境不可或缺的重要部分。利用小分子化合物，不仅可以维持干细胞的体外增殖，也可以提高 iPSC 的诱导效率。这些小分子化合物有助于了解干细胞命运决定过程中重要的信号机制。

第四节　肿瘤干细胞

肿瘤干细胞（cancer stem cell，CSC）被定义为具有干细胞样属性的肿瘤细胞亚群，即存在于肿瘤组织中的一小部分细胞，具有自我更新能力，不定向分化潜能，高致瘤性、耐药性，对肿瘤的发生、发展、复发、转移起重要作用。CSC 的定义并没有确定 CSC 和生理干细胞之间的特定关系。

针对 CSC 的研究进展：①人类白血病干细胞。早在 20 世纪 70 年代，科学家们就发现许多白血病，如急性髓细胞性白血病（AMI）的特点是细胞单克隆的增殖，这些白血病细胞包括不同程度分化的血细胞[1]。直到 1997 年 Bonnet 等发现了人类白血病干细胞[2]，才真正揭开了人类对 CSC 研究的序幕，它开创性地发现人类 AMI 中白血病干细胞的存在，通过对不同表型的白血病细胞进行原代克隆培养，从而发现了大部分的白血病细胞不能有效增殖，仅有少数细胞有稳定持续的形成肿瘤克隆的能力，这些细胞的表型为 $CD34^+CD38^-Thy-1^-$。尽管 $CD34^+$ $CD38^-Thy-1^-$ 这类细胞所占比例很少（大约仅为 0.2%），但把它们移植到糖尿病重症联合免疫缺陷小鼠（NOD/SCID 小鼠）之后却能形成类似于 AMI 的肿瘤细胞。通过对 AMI 的进一步研究发现绝大部分 AMI 是处于细胞周期的静止期，这一点对于治疗非常重要，因为大部分白血病的治疗方法是直接针对活化期的细胞，这就意味着 AMI 中干细胞对于普通化疗是耐药的。②乳腺 CSC。对乳腺癌的研究进一步证实了实体瘤中有 CSC 的存在。2003 年 Al-hajj 等[3, 4]利用流式细胞分选技术，首次成功地从人类乳腺中分离出 CSC，极大地推动了对实体瘤 CSC 的研究。它通过细胞表面标志物在乳腺癌患者切除标本制成的单细胞悬液中分选出不同的乳腺癌细胞亚群，乳腺癌初始细胞的特征细胞表型为 $Lin-ESA CD44^+ CD24^-/kw$，此类细胞虽然只占乳腺癌的 2%，但只要约 200 个细胞即可在小鼠乳腺中形成肿瘤，而其他表型的肿瘤细胞则无致瘤能力。而这些表型不同的细胞在形态上没有明显的差别。他们还将 $Lin-ESA CD44^+ CD24^-/kw$ 原发的肿瘤细胞接种到免疫缺陷 NOD/SCID 小鼠，也可以形成肿瘤，且新形成的肿瘤与原来肿瘤的表型异质性相似。而其他的细胞却不能形成肿瘤。更重要的是，仅 200 个纯化的细胞可以在第 2 次接种小鼠形成肿瘤并且能够分化成多种细胞亚群。国内有研究发现 microRNA 分子 let-7 通过负调控下游靶基因 II-Ras 和 II MGA2，而对乳腺 CSC 发挥重要的调控作用[5]。③消化道 CSC。胃肠道经常与食物中的有毒物质直接接触，所以具有较高的癌症发病率。Dick 等将来源于 17 个不同结肠癌患者标本的细胞悬液注射到免疫缺陷的小鼠内，发现只有过度表达 CD133 的少数细胞才能在小鼠内产生与原发肿瘤相似的肿瘤[6, 7]。此外，Haraguchi 等[8]采用 DNA 荧光材料 Hoechst33342 和流式细胞仪在多种人类消化系统肿瘤细胞系中分离到了 SP 细胞，这群细胞占细胞总数的 0.3%～2.2%，均具有干细胞的特性。④肺 CSC。Kim 等从大鼠细支气管-肺泡管结合部分离出 $Sca-1^+ CD45^- Pacam^-$ $CD34^-$ 细胞，具有很强的自我更新和分化能力，称为支气管肺泡干细胞（BASCs）[9]。BASCs 是维持细支气管上皮细胞和肺泡上皮细胞更新的基础，它们表达干细胞抗原 Sca-1 和 CD34，但不表达血小板内皮细胞黏附分子（PECAM）和 CD45。在正常情况下，BASCs 处于静止状态，当体内支气管和肺泡损伤时就会发生增殖，这个发现也进一步支持了 CSC 学说。另外研究者发现，BASCs 在不典型性增生及肺腺癌 K-ras 基因突变活化的终末支气管和肺泡上皮细胞中的数量明显增加，所以认为 BASCs 可能是肺腺癌的起源细胞。虽然 CSC 的概念目前仍存在争议，但是人们不会否认肿瘤细胞中存在对放化疗抵抗的群体，这也是复发转移的根源。如何对抗和消灭 CSC 已成为人们研究的重点。

一、CSC 的理论基础

（一）CSC 的起源

目前对 CSC 的起源仍存在争议，大致有三种：①CSC 可以来源于 ASC，多种因素引起 ASC 更新分化调控机制过度激活而转化为 CSC。②祖细胞在分化过程中发生突变终止分化，转化为 CSC。③成熟终末分化细胞因为突变获得自我更新和分化能力转而形成 CSC。启动突变 CSC 可以自我更新或分化为祖细胞或完全分化的子代细胞[10]（图 7-18）。

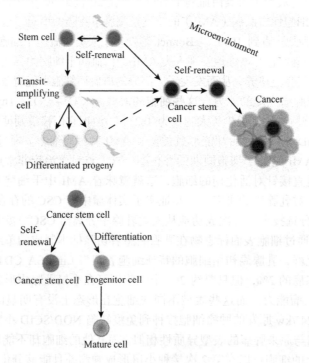

图 7-18　CSC 自我更新和分化；Cancer stem cells are capable of self-renewal and differentiation

（二）CSC 的理论基础

（1）细胞发生癌变必须累积许多突变，干细胞能长时间存活，从而可以接受所有导致肿瘤的突变。

（2）干细胞无限的自我更新为发生基因突变提供了可能。

（3）肿瘤细胞与干细胞一样，具有分裂增殖、迁移、再生长的能力。

（4）肿瘤组织中仅有极小部分细胞（可能干细胞）能通过接种、培养或转移等方式形成新的肿瘤。

干细胞的增殖、自我更新、分化和转化是致瘤性转化的最主要原因（图 7-19）[11]。

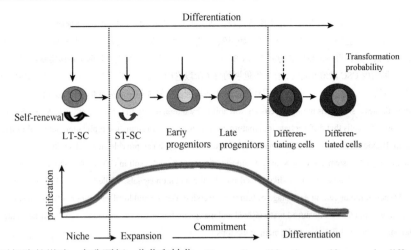

图 7-19 干细胞的增殖、自我更新、分化和转化；Stem cell proliferation, self-renewal, differentiation, and transformation

假设一种长期干细胞（LT-SC）拥有最强的自我更新能力，且在它的生态位中（底部）处于静止期。LT-SC 发展为短期干细胞（ST-SC），表现为自我更新能力减弱而增殖能力增强。进而 ST-SC 形成早期祖细胞，虽已丧失了自我更新能力，但是最具增殖活性的细胞群体。进而早期祖细胞形成晚期祖细胞，开始分化并表达谱系特异性分化标记，这些晚期祖细胞逐渐发展为完全分化细胞而再次丧失分化潜能（即有丝分裂后）。按照转化概率的观点，ST-SC 保留了自我更新能力，而祖细胞更具增殖活性（以两条垂直粗线标记），理论上可以代表致瘤性转化的最好目标；Depicted here is a hypothetical long-term stem cell（LT-SC），which has the greatest self-renewal activity and is quiescent in its niche（bottom）. LT-SC develops into a short-term stem cell（ST-SC），which shows reduced self-renewal activity but increased proliferation. The ST-SC then gives rise to early progenitor cells that may have lost self-renewal capacity, but probably represent the most proliferative cell population. Early progenitors generate late progenitor cells that begin to commit to differentiate by expressing lineage-specific differentiation markers and these late progenitor cells gradually develop into fully differentiated cells that once again lose proliferative potential（i.e., post-mitotic）. From the standpoint of transformation probability, the ST-SC that retains self-renewal activity and progenitor cells that are highly proliferative（demarcated by two vertical thick lines）theoretically could represent the best targets for tumorigenic transformation

在 CSC 假说背景下，包含 CSC 的肿瘤亚群以一种分级和异构的方式生成肿瘤。相反，非致瘤的肿瘤细胞可能不会成功地形成肿瘤（图 7-20）。

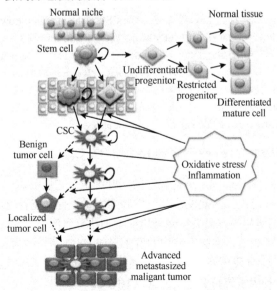

图 7-20 CSC 和肿瘤细胞之间的差异；Potential differences between cancer stem cells（CSCs）and tumor cells

在正常组织中，干细胞通过与组织基质相互作用来维持自我更新的能力。在正常生态位中，干细胞产生能分化为成熟细胞的祖细胞。在细胞分裂期，子细胞的复制潜力逐步降低。如果氧化应激和炎症刺激生态位可以为干细胞提供突变的信号。为应答该突变的信号，干细胞可以获得一种致瘤能力并成为 CSC（星形）。未分化的祖细胞（菱形）在该突变信号的驱动下也可以成为 CSC 样细胞。在肿瘤内 CSC 增殖的同时，在肿瘤进展的每个阶段它们可能产生所有类型的肿瘤细胞。CSC 可生成良性和局限性肿瘤细胞（虚线箭头），也可在进一步突变信号包括附加的表观遗传修饰和基因突变信号的驱动下形成恶性肿瘤及其进展和转移；In normal tissues, stem cells maintain self-renewal ability by interacting with the tissue stroma. Within the normal niche, stem cells generate progenitor cells that differentiate into mature cells. During cell division, the replication potential of daughter cells is decreased at each step. If oxidative stress and inflammation stimulate the niche, it can provide stem cells with mutation signals. In response to the mutation signals, stem cell may acquire a tumorigenic capacity and result in CSCs (star-shape). Undifferentiated progenitor cells (diamond) may also become CSC-like cells driven by the mutation signals. While CSCs proliferate within tumors, they may give a rise to all types of tumor cells at each stage of tumor progression. Benign and localized tumor cells can be potentially (dashed arrow) generated from CSCs. Advanced metastasized and malignant tumor can be formed driven by further mutational signals including additional epigenetic modifications and genetic mutations

（三）CSC 生态位在肿瘤的生长和转移中的作用

CSC 生态位除了使 CSC 维持其干细胞样状态外，生态位具有以下作用：①生态位具有使非致瘤性细胞分化为致瘤性 CSC 的作用。②诱导上皮间质转化，导致肿瘤细胞由原发部位扩散[12-14]。③在转移灶生根发芽。转移前生态位的形成，可能潜在性导致继发性肿瘤启动和生长的生态位，有利于肿瘤细胞在不同器官的植入（图 7-21）。

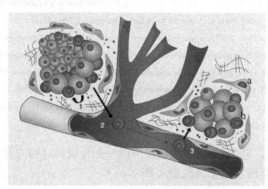

图 7-21　肿瘤生长和转移的 CSC 生态位；The CSC niche in tumor growth and metastasis

CSC 生态位由血管、基质细胞如肌纤维母细胞（a）和 ECM 成分组成。在肿瘤组织中的 CSC（b）定居其生态位，有利于肿瘤细胞转移。生态位有能力（1）将非致瘤性细胞分化为致瘤性 CSCs 和（2）诱导 EMT，从而导致肿瘤细胞从原发肿瘤中播散，（3）在转移灶处播种。The CSC niche is composed of blood vessels, stromal cells such as myofibroblasts (a), and extracellular matrix components. Tumors are organized in such a way that CSCs (b) reside close to their niche, and facilitated to metastasis. The niche has the ability to (1) dedifferentiate nontumorigenic cells into tumorigenic CSCs and to (2) induce the EMT, leading to dissemination of tumor cells from the primary tumor and (3) seeding at the metastatic place

（四）肿瘤微环境中的各种因子维持和扩增 CSC

肿瘤微环境由癌细胞及其周围组织特异性的间叶细胞及它们的表达产物、代谢物质等成分构成。一些慢性组织炎症可以作为癌前病变引发肿瘤发生。有研究者也用炎症损伤修复模式来解释 CSC 的形成，他们认为一方面炎症微环境能增加招募血源性 MSC，当与局部环境中的某种细胞发生融合后，有可能导致细胞重编程的发生形成 CSC；另一方面炎症微环境中细胞因子能够持续激活与细胞增殖/自我更新有关的信号通路导致正常组织干细胞与分化细胞形成肿瘤，如卵巢癌微环境中的各种因子维持和扩增 CSC（图 7-22）[15, 16]。

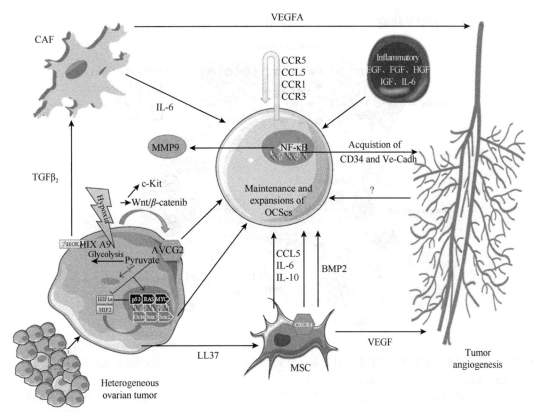

图 7-22　肿瘤微环境中的调控因子维持卵巢癌中 CSC 的可能作用；Schematic of the potential regulatory actors of the tumor microenvironment in the maintenance of ovarian cancer stem cells

二、CSC 的特征

除了具备干细胞的特征：自我更新和分化能力；具有很强的成瘤能力外，在特定组织的肿瘤中还应具备以下特征：

（1）具备一定的正常组织干细胞的特征或标志。

（2）存在其特有的分化增殖倾向。

（3）具备该组织的肿瘤特征。

例如，胰腺 CSC 的标志分子可能为 PDX-1、Ptf-1 等，同时也可能表达一些干细胞共同的表面分子，如 CD34、CD44 等。基于肿瘤的突变性质，也有可能表达胰腺癌高表达的一些产物分子，如 k-ras 或 Ki-67 等。但值得注意的是这些标志具有相对性：①同一 CSC 可能有不同的表面标志分子，如肝癌 CSC 可表达 CD33$^+$也可表达 CD90$^+$CD44$^+$。②一种表面标志是某种 CSC 的标志，但不是另一种 CSC 的标志，如胰腺癌 CSC 标志为 CD24$^+$，而乳腺癌 CSC 标志为 CD24$^-$/10w。③同一 CSC 标志在不同肿瘤的不同细胞系中所占比例差异较大，如喉癌 Hep22 细胞系中只有＜5%的 CD33$^+$的 CSC。

（4）耐药性强：CSC 细胞膜上多数表达 ABC（ATP-binding cassette）转运蛋白。这是代谢物排出的泵，具有保护自身不受外源性物质侵犯的作用，更是参与形成部分的血脑屏障、血睾屏障、胎盘屏障，对 ABC 的耐药性已经成为众多抗癌学者研究的一个重要靶点。

（5）CSC 在表型及功能方面具有多样性（图 7-23）。

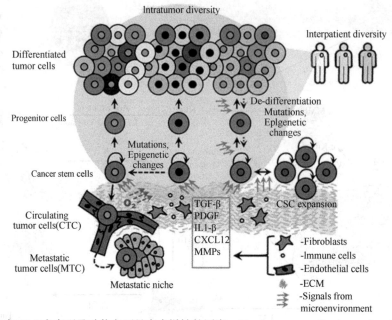

图 7-23　造成 CSC 在表型及功能方面具有多样性的因素；The factors contributing to the phenotypic and functional diversity of CSC populations

不同患者表达不同的 CSC 亚群，造成了它们在遗传及表观遗传学上的差异。异质型 CSC 通过在各肿瘤内建立不同的克隆造成肿瘤异质性。在肿瘤内，CSC 在特定的解剖位置聚集，旁分泌和自分泌不同的信号分子，与周围的基质成纤维细胞、免疫细胞、内皮细胞和细胞外基质的成分（如纤维连接蛋白、层粘连蛋白、蛋白聚糖和胶原纤维）及气体、营养供应、组织酸化和能量状态直接接触。各种微环境影响，包括氧张力、生长因子、细胞因子（如 PDGF，IL1-β，TGF-β，CXCL12）均能调节 CSC 的分化、自我更新等属性；CSC subsets vary from patient to patient due to genetic and epigenetic differences. Heterogenic CSCs contribute to intratumor heterogeneity by establishing distinct clones within an individual tumor. Within tumor mass, CSC populations are enriched in specific anatomic locations defined by various factors such as specific paracrine and autocrine signaling, direct contact with surrounding stromal fibroblasts, immune cells, endothelial cells and components of the ECM (e.g. fibronectin, laminin, proteoglycans and collagen fibers) as well as gas and nutrient supply, and tissue acidification and bioenergetic status. The influences of various microenvironments, including oxygen tension and growth factors and cytokines, such as PDGF, IL1-β, TGF-β, CXCL12 may regulate CSC properties, such as differentiation, self-renewal, invasiveness and tumorigenicity and contribute to CSC reprogramming

三、肿瘤中 CSC 的作用

已知肿瘤可来自于癌症关键基因突变的体细胞，也可来自于由微环境因子失调发生的致癌过程。癌形成中可能主要影响的是寿命长的成体干细胞。因此祖细胞或终末分化的体细胞都可作为恶性转化细胞的来源。CSC 的免疫逃逸特点可能有助于肿瘤的发生与发展。CSC 增加对化疗剂和（或）电离辐射的抵抗。CSC 可能也具有抗免疫介导排斥的能力。如果 CSC 确实代表人类癌症中的抗性细胞，它们就可能促使肿瘤进展、复发和转移（图 7-24）。

CSC 像正常干细胞一样形成分化等级，伴随着长期自我更新，CSC 可分化形成低自我更新潜能细胞。

（1）CSC 及其子细胞的可塑性见图 7-25。

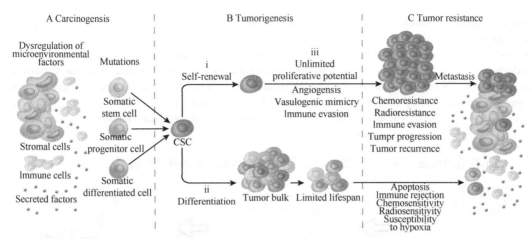

图 7-24 CSC 在癌变、肿瘤和肿瘤抵抗中的作用；The roles of CSCs in carcinogenesis, tumorigenesis and tumor resistance

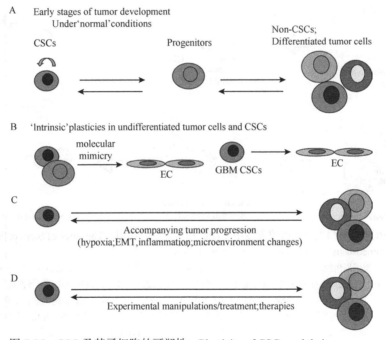

图 7-25 CSC 及其子细胞的可塑性；Plasticity of CSCs and their progeny

A. 在未经治疗的或早期肿瘤中，自我更新的 CSC 及其子细胞的可塑性使其快速生成增殖性肿瘤细胞，继而形成分化肿瘤细胞或非肿瘤干细胞。这种假设的发展过程可能代表了最主要的肿瘤发展过程（以粗箭头表示），尽管可能发生低水平自发的（或内在的）去分化（以细箭头表示）。在未经治疗的或早期肿瘤中，大多数肿瘤细胞将分化为肿瘤祖细胞和分化型肿瘤细胞，而未分化细胞只占少数。例如，绝大多数未经治疗的早期乳腺癌和前列腺癌都符合这种模式。B. CSC 的固有可塑性以"分子模拟"或胶质母细胞瘤中 CSC 转分化为内皮细胞（EC）表示。C. 肿瘤进展过程中，微环境的改变、缺氧、炎症介质的积聚与上皮间质转化（EMT）结果都可能促进非肿瘤干细胞的去分化（以加粗反向箭头表示）。本例结果表示在晚期肿瘤，富含 CSC 的未分化肿瘤细胞与分化型肿瘤细胞将处于一个动态平衡之中。D. 体外实验（如模拟缺氧条件、治疗伴 EMT 诱导剂细胞如使用细胞因子或抗癌药物、致癌分子的过表达等）或体内持续肿瘤治疗会加重非肿瘤干细胞的去分化而形成干细胞样癌细胞（更粗反向箭头表示），导致 CSC 数量的大量增长；A. In untreated or early-stage tumors, self-renewing CSCs generate rapidly proliferating tumor progenitors, which may in turn develop into differentiated tumor cells or non-CSCs. This hypothetical developmenttal pathway perhaps represents the major pathway（indicated by thick arrows）although low levels of spontaneous（or intrinsic）dedifferentiation（indicated by thin arrows）may occur. This model predicts that in the untreated or early-stage tumors, most tumor cells will be partially differentiated tumor progenitors and differentiated tumor cells, with undifferentiated cells representing a minority. The great majority of untreated low-grade breast and prostate cancers, for example, fit this model. B. Intrinsic plasticity in CSCs manifested as 'molecular mimicry' or GBM CSC transdifferentiation into endothelial cells (EC). C. During tumor progression, microenvironmental changes, hypoxia, accumulation of inflammatory mediators, together with resultant EMT, may all promote dedifferentiation of non-CSCs (indicated by the thickened reverse arrow). This scenario predicts that in advanced tumors, the undifferentiated, CSC-enriched tumor cells would be in a dynamic equilibrium with more differentiated tumor cells. D. *In vitro* experimental manipulations (e.g., mimicking hypoxic conditions, treating cells with EMT-inducers such as cytokines or anti-cancer drugs, overexpressing oncogenic molecules, etc) or persistent tumor therapy *in vivo* may accentuate dedifferentiation of non-CSCs to stem-like cancer cells (indicated by further thickened reverse arrow) resulting in increased abundance of CSCs

（2）在组织恒态、肿瘤发生和肿瘤复发中 CSC 和祖细胞的作用见图 7-26。

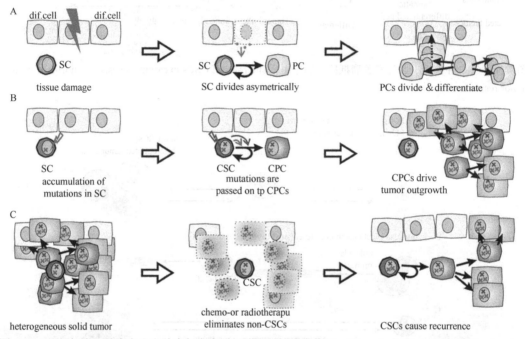

图 7-26　组织恒态、肿瘤发生和肿瘤复发中干细胞和祖细胞的作用；The roles of Stem cells and progenitor cells in tissue homeostasis, tumorigenesis and tumor recurrence

A. 在器官发生或对组织损伤的反应过程中，静止期的干细胞（SCs）经诱导发生不对称分裂，从而进一步分化为祖细胞（PCs）。祖细胞首先进行数量有限的对称细胞分裂快速重建组织。产生的子细胞进一步分化以修复器官特异性功能，同时丧失其重回细胞周期的功能。B. 干细胞长寿、多能，并无限地进行细胞分裂，因此它们容易比其他细胞积累更多的突变，从而更可能随机地触发肿瘤。这些突变传递给祖细胞后，其周期加快可能驱动肿瘤产生。C. 干细胞和 CSC 对化疗和放疗高度耐受，这解释了为什么它们能在减少细胞的治疗中选择性的存活。因此它们能在数年或几十年之后仍可引起癌症复发；A. During organogenesis or in response to tissue damage, resting stem cells (SCs) are induced to undergo asymmetric divisions that produce further differentiated progenitor cells (PCs). Progenitor cells can quickly regenerate tissue by first undergoing a limited number of symmetric cell divisions. The generated daughter cells can then further differentiate to acquire organ-specific functions while generally losing the ability to reenter the cell cycle.B. Stem cells are exceptionally long-lived, pluripotent, and can undergo an unlimited number of cell divisions. Therefore, they may accumulate more mutations than other cells and are thus stochastically more likely to initiate a tumor. These mutations are passed onto progenitor cells, which may drive tumor outgrowth as they cycle much faster by nature.C. Stem cells and CSCs are highly resistant to chemotherapeutic agents and irradiation, which explains why these cells might selectively survive to reductive therapy. Therefore, these cells may cause cancer recurrence years or decades later

（3）肿瘤恶性程度可能与 CSC 数量相关，因为其驱动着肿瘤的生长和复发。

（4）CSC/肿瘤永存细胞（TPC）特征和分化能力影响肿瘤的组织形态学，胃肠道肿瘤相关模型见图 7-27[17]。

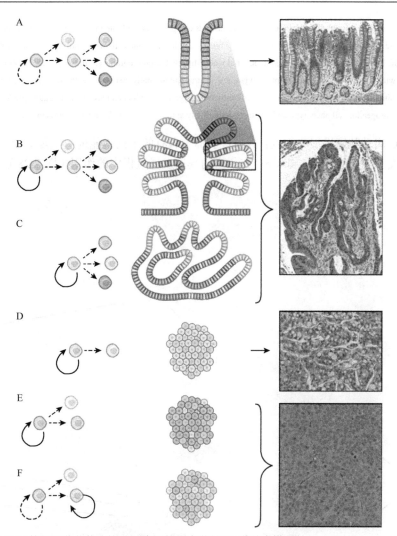

图 7-27 CSC-TPC 特征和分化能力影响肿瘤组织形态学(胃肠道肿瘤模型); The cancer stem cell(CSC)/tumor perpetuating cell（TPC）identity and differentiation capacity likely influence tumor histomorphology：a gastrointestional model

A. 正常肠化是干细胞的后代通过分裂而达到的适应平衡状态，能产生额外的干细胞（红）、帕内特细胞（蓝）或祖细胞（绿）。正常情况下，祖细胞可以分化为三种子细胞：杯状细胞（蓝）、肠内分泌细胞（褐）或肠上皮吸收细胞（紫）。B. 干细胞中致癌事件的增多导致 CSC 池扩大，所有分化的子代细胞也扩增。在实体组织背景中，其结果常导致异常的高位隐窝结构的出现（如息肉）。C. 伴有祖细胞特征的 CSC 在保持正常分化是由直肠中被累及的大量终末分化细胞组成，因此这些细胞结构中大多缺乏正常干细胞表型。D. 伴有祖细胞特征的 CSC，如果正常分化指向某一特定细胞，那么将导致肿瘤含有一种主要的细胞表型（如杯状细胞）而缺乏其他成熟细胞谱系和具有正常干细胞表型的细胞。E. 肿瘤中即使有正常干细胞表型 CSC，但正常分化受损，也可导致仅由一种具有干细胞和祖细胞表型的细胞组成的肿瘤，结构与分化性子代细胞无关。F. 伴有祖细胞特征的 CSC，如果正常分化过程被阻断，肿瘤则主要由具有祖细胞表型的细胞构成。结构与分化性后代细胞无关；A． Normal intestinal differentiation，where progeny of stem cell divisions are appropriately balanced to produce additional stem cells（red）paneth cells（yellow），or progenitor cells（green）.Normal differentiation of progenitor cells results in progeny with one of three cell fates secretory goblet（blue）. enteroendocrine cells（brown），or absorptive enterocytes（purple）；B． Oncogenic events arising in stem cells may results in an amplified pool of CSCs，wherein the CSC have a normal stem cell phenotype and the entire tree of differentiated progeny is also amplified. In the context to solid tissues，the resultant overcrowding causes aberrant higher-order crypt structures（eg. polyps）；C. CSC with a progenitor cell identity，wherein normal differentiation is maintained，may result in tumor largely comprised of teminally differentiated cells with involuting structures，but largely devoid of cells with a normal stem cell phenotype；D. CSC with a progenitor cell identity, wherein normal differentiation is skewed towards one particular cell fate may result in tumors containing one predominant cell type (ie, goblet cells) and devoid of both other mature cell lineages and cells with a normal stem cell phenotype; E. Tumors where CSC have a normal stem cell phenotype, but where differentiation programs are impaired may result in tumors comprised of only cells with stem and progenitor cell phenotypes and no structure normally associated with differentiated progeny; F. (The CSC with a progenitor cell identity, wherein normal differentiation programs are blocked may result in tumors predominantly comprised of cells with a progenitor cell phenotype and no structure normally associated with differentiated progeny

（5）CSC 启动肿瘤进展和复发：异质性肿瘤中含有的干细胞能逃避正规治疗，并继续分裂成为肿瘤复发和转移的基础，如 CSC 在子宫内膜癌发展过程中的作用（图 7-28）。

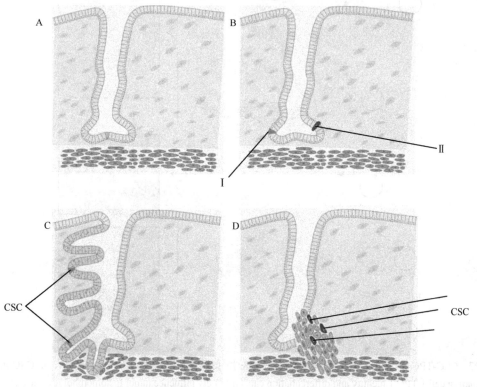

图 7-28　CSC 在子宫内膜癌发展过程中的作用；The role of CSCs in the development of endometrial carcinoma

A. 正常子宫内膜腺体中的潜在上皮干（祖）细胞位于腺体的基底部（黄色）；B. 上皮祖细胞通过基因突变导致 CSC 发展为 I 型或 II 型上皮细胞；CSC 克隆的扩增生成异质性的肿瘤性上皮细胞 I 型（C）或 II 型（D），其中含有少量 CSC 和大量分化型肿瘤细胞；A. Normal endometrial gland with a potential epithelial stem/ progenitor cell located at the base of the gland; B. Epithelial progenitor cell acquires genetic mutations resulting in the development of the CSCs in either type I (left, orange)or type II (right, dark blue) EC. Expansion of the CSC clone producing heterogeneous neoplastic epithelial cells in type I (C) and type II (D) ECs, comprising a small number of CSCs (C, orange; D, dark blue) and numerous differentiated tumour cells (C, light orange; D, light blue)

过度增殖的实体性肿瘤中央总是缺氧环境，HIF-α 的稳定性和缺氧反应可以刺激 CSC 的聚集，导致转移和新肿瘤的产生（图 7-29）[18-20]。

在原发性肝细胞癌中 CSC 是肿瘤形成和转移的基础（图 7-30）[21]。

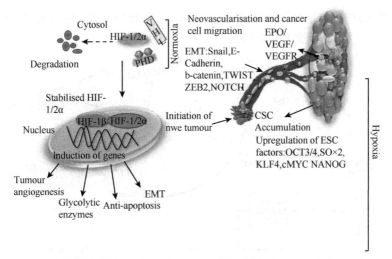

图 7-29　HIF-α 刺激 CSC 聚集和转移；HIF-α triggers CSC accumulation and metastasis

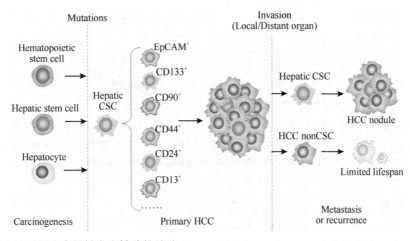

图 7-30　CSC 是肝细胞癌的触发和转移的基础；Tumor initiation and metastasis in HCC based on cancer stem cell model

肝癌 CSC 可起源于 HSC 和体内癌基因、抑癌基因引起的体细胞基因突变而获得致瘤潜能的肝脏干细胞，或通过突变获得干细胞样自我更新和分化功能，使分化肝细胞重新编程转变为去分化的肿瘤细胞。这些肝脏 CSC 通过自我更新和分化最终发展为一个具有异质性的肝细胞癌。而且，肝脏 CSC 因为对治疗的耐受和具有在局部或远处转移形成新肿瘤的能力被认为是肿瘤切除后转移和复发的主要因素；Hepatic CSCs could be derived from hematopoietic stem cells, hepatic stem cells upon somatic mutate- onns of oncogenes and tumor suppressor genes to acquire a tumorigenic potential, or reprogrammed from differentiated hepatic cells to be de-differentiated tumor cells by mutations to acquire the stem cell-like capacity to self-renew and differentiate. These hepatic CSCs eventually expand to a HCC bulk with heterogeneity through self-renewal and differentiation. Moreover, the existence of hepatic CSCs is considered to be responsible to metastasis and recurrence after resection due to its resistance to conventional therapies and its ability of giving rise to a new tumor in local or distant organs

（6）肝癌 CSC 中信号通路的改变：①Wnt 通路的激活导致 β-catenin 在细胞质中积聚，进而易位至细胞核。在核内 β-catenin 转录激活其靶分子的表达，如 cyclin D1、EpCAM 和 miR-181[22]。Akt 通过两个磷酸化位点 Thr308 和 Ser473 被激活。P13K 促进 Thr308 的磷酸化而 PTEN 抑制 Thr308 的磷酸化。②活化的 Akt 通过调控 Bcl-2 和 ABCG2 以避免化疗引起的细胞凋亡，来保护 CSC。活化的 Akt 还可以与 HIF-1α 相互作用，诱导 VEGF 和 PDGF-BB 表达，以调节组织稳态和肝癌 CSC 的耐药性。③受损的 TGF-β 信号与活化的 IL-6/STAT3 通路对调节

EpCAM⁺的肝癌 CSC 的分化和化疗耐药都是十分重要的。研究发现，这些通路相互作用将促进干细胞扩增和肝细胞癌的形成（图 7-31）。

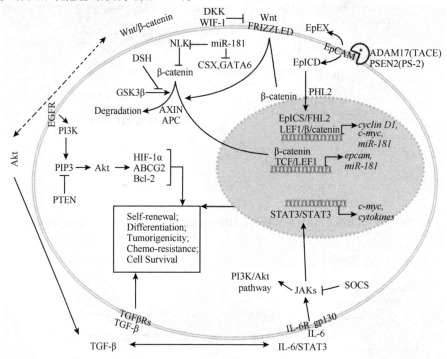

图 7-31 肝癌 CSC 中的 Wnt/β-catenin、Akt、TGF-β 和 IL-6/STAT3 信号通路异常，这些通路相互作用将促进干细胞和肝细胞癌的形成；Wnt/β-catenin，Akt，TGF-β and IL-6/STAT3 signaling pathways are deregulated in hepatic CSCs. These pathways are interconnected，which may further promote stem cells and carcinogenesis in HCC

（7）CSC 在肿瘤免疫逃逸中的作用见图 7-32。

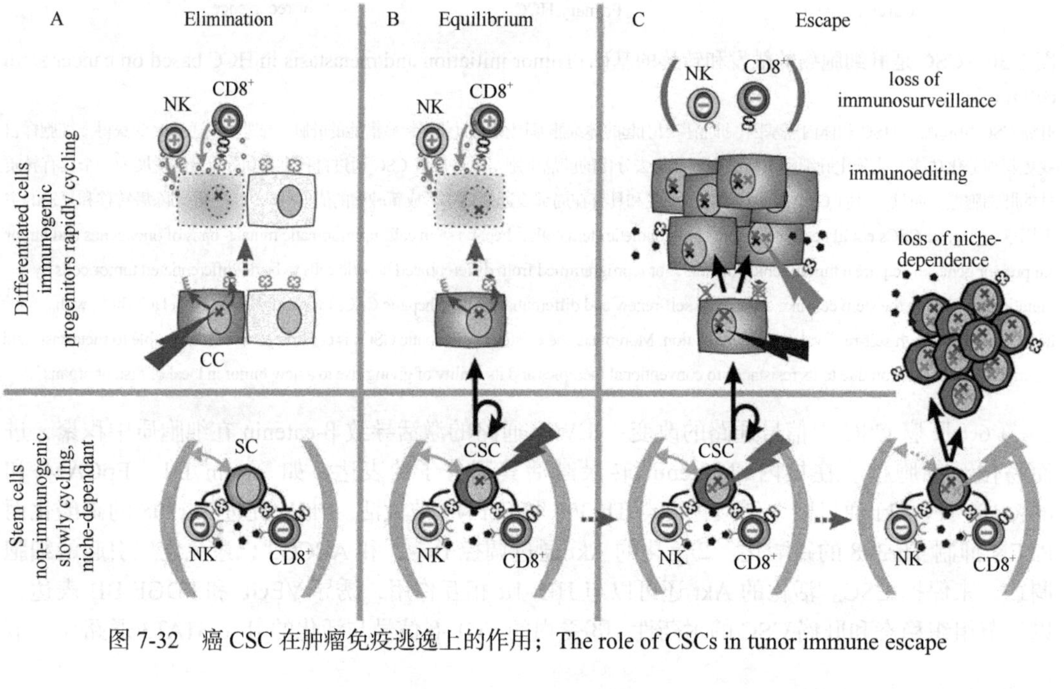

图 7-32 癌 CSC 在肿瘤免疫逃逸上的作用；The role of CSCs in tunor immune escape

清除（A）：恶性转化需要单个细胞内致瘤基因突变（闪光）的积累。如果这种突变发生在分化的细胞，它会上调活化 NK 细胞受体的配体和通过 MHC 类Ⅰa 分子呈递肿瘤特异性多肽。这样，这些细胞可被免疫系统发现并清除，从而恢复正常组织。平衡（B）：干细胞生命周期长且能表达多数免疫抑制因子，因此，它们能积累致瘤基因的突变而免于被免疫系统清除。然而，CSC 最初被局限于干细胞生态位内，只能发生不对称分裂。许多分化的子细胞继承了所有的恶性突变，但是它们具有更强的免疫原性以便被适应性免疫系统清除。因此出现一个稳态。逃逸（C）：肿瘤免疫逃逸的机制包括肿瘤免疫监视、免疫编辑的缺陷或 CSC 的扩增。由于老化、免疫抑制治疗、疾病或其他因素的作用下免疫系统丧失其限制肿瘤的功能。免疫编辑指的是个体肿瘤亚克隆对免疫系统施加的选择压力产生的进化性适应。它将最终导致低免疫原性或高免疫抑制性亚克隆的扩增。无免疫原性 CSC 可能更具有独立扩增其干细胞生态位的功能，这将可能导致低分化肿瘤的发生；Elimination（A）: malignant transformation requires oncogenic mutations（flash）to accumulate within an individual cell. If such mutations occur in a differentiated cell, this cell will upregulate activatory NK cell receptor ligands and present tumor-specific peptides via MHC class Ⅰa molecules. Thus, these cells can be detected and eliminated by the immune system, leading to restoration of normal tissue. Equilibrium（B）: stem cells（SC）are long-lived and express a multitude of immunosuppressive factors. Hence, they may accumulate oncogenic mutations without being cleared by the immune system. However, CSCs are initially confined to stem cell niches and limited to asymmetric divisions. More differentiated daughter cells inherit all malignant mutations, but are more immunogenic and could thus be eliminated by the adaptive immune system. Thus, a robust equilibrium may emerge. Escape（C）: mechanisms contributing to tumor immune escape include defects in tumor immunosurveillance, immunoediting, or the expansion of CSCs. The immune system may lose its ability to constrain tumors due to aging, immunosuppressive therapies, diseases or other factors. Immunoediting describes the evolutionary adaptation of individual tumor subclones to the selection pressure exerted by the immune system. It will ultimately lead to expansion of less-immunogenic or more immunosuppressive subclones. Non-immunogenic CSCs may further acquire the ability to expand independently of their niches, which may lead to the outgrowth of poorly differentiated tumors

来自美国克利夫兰医学中心凯斯西储大学的研究人员的证实，胶质瘤 CSC 通过分泌 Periostin 招募了 M2 型肿瘤相关巨噬细胞，促进其恶性生长[23, 24]。

与 CSC 低免疫原性有关的因素和通路见图 7-33。

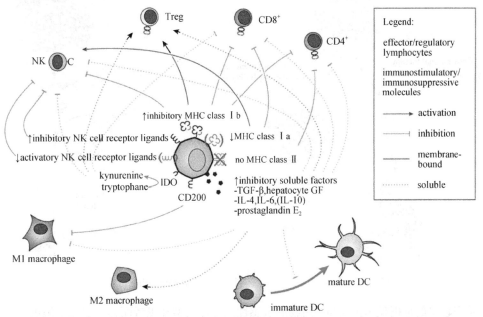

图 7-33　膜结合（实线）和可溶性因子（虚线）与 CSC 的免疫耐受密切相关；Membrane-bound（solid line）and soluble factors（dotted lines）implicated in immunotolerance toward stem cells and CSCs are schematically depicted 抗原提呈分子和免疫刺激分子的低水平表达和免疫抑制因子的高表达。这些信号使免疫效应细胞受损而免疫耐受细胞被激活；These include antigen-presenting and immunostimulatory molecules expressed at low levels and abundantly expressed immunosuppressive factors Immune effector cells impaired by these signals whereas tolerogenic immune cells, which may be stimulated

四、针对 CSC 的靶向性治疗

随着对 CSC 的研究深入，CSC 的应用也越来越广泛，CSC 学说认为 CSC 是肿瘤的起源，因而检测 CSC 表面标志物将会提高癌症的早期诊断率。急性髓性白血病的 CSC 标志物最早发现，随后很多实体肿瘤 CSC 标志物陆续被鉴定出来，这在很大程度上提高了肿瘤诊断的特异性。现有研究表明 CSC 的自我更新、高增殖和耐放化疗等特性，使得常规手段难以清除组织、血液等机体内残留的 CSC，成为肿瘤复发和转移的隐患。

目前抗癌药物主要杀伤增殖期的肿瘤细胞，而对 CSC 的杀伤效果不佳。CSC 产生耐药的机制是由于其主要处于静止期，能够通过改变细胞周期调控点减弱凋亡途径，增强 DNA 损伤修复能力，以及高表达 ABC 将把药物转运至细胞外，降低细胞内药物积累导致治疗失败。肿瘤生物学研究的最新观点认为治愈肿瘤的关键在于杀灭 CSC，因此研发针对 CSC 的特异性药物，将是肿瘤治疗的重大突破。

随着生物学技术的发展，人们对肿瘤细胞和分子水平上的发病机制有了进一步认识，肿瘤靶向的治疗已经进入了一个全新时代，针对 CSC 靶向治疗的研究也取得重大进步，主要集中于以下几个方面：凋亡 CSC、改变 CSC 生长的微环境、逆转 CSC 抗放化疗特性、靶向作用于 CSC 的特异性分子标志及信号通路、促进放化疗法、CSC 特异性免疫治疗等。

肿瘤由 CSC、祖细胞样细胞和分化型肿瘤细胞混合组成。传统治疗方法杀死大多数祖细胞样细胞和肿瘤细胞，而抗药性癌干细胞得以存活并继续增殖导致复发。CSC 特异性治疗方法可以杀死 CSC 或促进其分化，使 CSC 失去自我更新能力，从而不能驱动肿瘤进展，肿瘤逐渐缩小而最终获得治疗效果（图 7-34）。

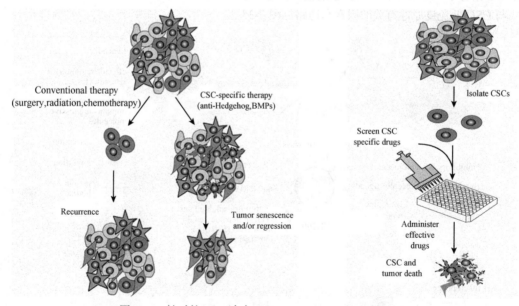

图 7-34 针对的 CSC 治疗；The trentments targeting to CSC

越来越多的证据显示抗 CSC 药物的敏感性因肿瘤类型和患者而异，因此必须进行个性化治疗。经表面标记、功能测定分离 CSC，然后通过高通量药物筛选敏感药。将明确的 CSC 特异性药物用于患者，使肿瘤缩小和死亡，达到个性化靶向 CSC 特异性治疗的目的。

　　针对 CSC 的治疗策略可以增加目前抗癌治疗方案的靶向性，并可能减少复发和转移的风险。例如，针对肝癌 CSC 的特性（自我更新和分化的能力、致瘤性及对化疗/放疗的耐受性），按照不同的功能特点，肝癌 CSC 的信号通路分为 Wnt/β-catenin、AKT、TGF-β 和 IL-6，这些通路在调节肝脏 CSC 方面发挥重要作用。基于这些分子机制的深入研究提供了针对 CSC 的治疗策略[25-27]。

　　随着美国前列腺癌疫苗（povenge）的上市，目前肿瘤疫苗已成为肿瘤治疗的正规手段。近两年针对 CSC 疫苗的研究也在快速发展，应用微球体培养技术，富集 CSC，用干细胞相关标志分离干细胞，以及化疗药物富集慢周期细胞。人们用这些细胞富集的 CSC 制备疫苗，或将其与树突状细胞融合后制备疫苗，也有提取或合成干细胞相关分子的多肽和编码基因制备疫苗，甚至利用和 CSC 存在共同抗原的 ESC 制作肿瘤疫苗。这些研究结果显示：CSC 具有免疫原性，其相关疫苗可以诱导 CSC 特异性细胞毒性 T 细胞和抗体；体内治疗效果显著优于普通肿瘤疫苗，而且对于化疗抵抗的肿瘤仍可产生疗效。靶向 CSC 的治疗是今后发展的重要方向之一。但 CSC 疫苗治疗肿瘤仍存在许多问题。其主要来自肿瘤自身和肿瘤微环境涉及的逃逸机制。靶向 CSC 的疗法联合常规疗法和对抗肿瘤微环境的逃逸因素，可能会大幅度提高肿瘤的治疗的效果。

　　针对 CSC 靶向免疫治疗主要有两种方式：①以单克隆抗体为基础的靶向治疗，通过作用于 CSC 表面特异的抗原分子，清除 CSC；②过继性细胞免疫治疗，主要是 CSC 抗原致敏的 DC 或 T 细胞过继免疫疗法。尽管上述靶向免疫疗法在实验室取得了一定的效果，然而，目前面临的挑战也是明显的，如抗体治疗的抗原调变和修饰，更多高特异性 CSC 标志物还有待发现，设计出能同时清除 CSC 和肿瘤细胞的治疗策略。上述关键问题的解决，将会推进以 CSC 为靶点的免疫治疗进入临床。

　　许多针对 CSC 的治疗策略也开始进行实验验证。这些方法可以增加目前抗癌治疗方案的针对性，并可能减少复发和扩散的风险，包括使用靶向 CSC 的潜在标志物（如单克隆抗体和活化的免疫细胞）的抗肿瘤作用、恢复在 CSC 中的化疗或放疗作用机制、干扰 CSC 通路、诱导分化的治疗、中断原癌基因与微环境的相互作用、抗血管生成治疗和破坏免疫逃逸的途径等（图 7-35）。

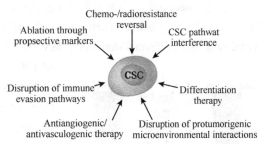

图 7-35　靶向 CSC 部位治疗策略；The therapeutic promise of CSC-directed targeting strategies

挑战与展望

　　近年来，研究者花费了大量精力分离干细胞和研究干细胞表型特征。尽管发现识别干细胞的特定标记将是一个持续的挑战，但一系列新的观测已经彻底改变和充实了对干细胞的研究。其中包括：①干细胞的鉴定和其在不同组织中的生态位，包括曾被认为是一个永久的静止器官大脑；②认识不同组织来源的干细胞，特别是从骨髓来源的干细胞有广泛的发育可塑性；③认识存在于人类和老鼠组织中的某些干细胞可能类似于 ESC；④使用干细胞来修复人体损伤组织中的治疗性克隆；⑤对 CSC 进行研究，并开展针对 CSC 治疗的探索[28]。

与基因治疗相比，用干细胞生物工程治疗疾病的最显著特点就是利用干细胞技术，可以再造多种正常的甚至更年轻的组织器官。这种再造组织器官的新医疗技术，将使任何人都能用上自己（或他人）的干细胞和干细胞衍生的新组织器官，来替代病变或衰老的组织器官，并可以广泛涉及用传统医学方法难以医治的多种顽症，如癌症、心肌坏死性疾病、自身免疫疾病、肝脏病、肾脏病和帕金森病、AD、脊髓损伤、皮肤烧伤等修复与治疗等。如果和基因治疗相结合，还可以治疗众多遗传性疾病。

同时，无论是自体来源或异体来源的干细胞治疗，较传统方法相比都具有很多优点：①具有安全性、有效性和可控性，优于现有的临床治疗方法；②不需要完全了解疾病发病的确切机制；③还可能应用自身干细胞移植，避免产生免疫排斥反应。

虽然有越来越多的证据支持 CSC 学说，然而在肿瘤生物学中仍存在很多问题：①是否所有肿瘤均存在 CSC；②所有 CSC 是否具有一些相同的表型；③由于正常干细胞与 CSC 具有相似的表型及信号转导通路，在针对 CSC 治疗时如何保护骨髓及胃肠道中的正常干细胞不受损害等。探索从肿瘤组织分离 CSC 及体外培养扩增建系的方法，建立合理的体外模型也是需要考虑的问题。通过鉴定肿瘤组织中的 CSC，寻找调节 CSC 生物行为的因子将会推动临床肿瘤治疗，为人类控制肿瘤，改善肿瘤预后增加希望。总之，每个具体干细胞制剂的制备和使用过程，必须有严格的标准操作程序，确保干细胞临床研究符合科学、安全、有效及社会伦理，才能使干细胞与再生医学健康发展。

思 考 题

1. 本章基本概念

干细胞（stem cell），胚胎干细胞（embryonic stem cell，EC），成体肝细胞（adult stem cell，ASC），造血干细胞（hematopoietic stem cell，HSC），骨髓间质细胞/间充质干细胞（bone marrow stromal cells /Mesenchymal stem cell，MSC），多能前体细胞（multipotent adult progenitor cell，MAPC），神经干细胞（neural stem cell），诱导性多能干细胞（induced pluripotent stem cell，iPSC），肿瘤干细胞（cancer stem cell，CSC），治疗性克隆（therapeutic cloning），再生医学（regenerative medicine），可塑性（plasticity），横向分化 transdifferentiation）。

2. 总结干细胞的特征。

3. 简述干细胞分裂的特点。

4. 简述 ESC 对生物学和医学产生的影响。

5. 简述角膜干细胞正常生理功能的意义。

6. 肝干细胞增生有什么意义？

7. 概述 CSC 的理论基础。

8. 什么是 CSC 生态位，其在肿瘤的生长和转移中有哪些作用？

9. CSC 如何逃避肿瘤免疫？

10. 列举干细胞在医学研究中的案例。

11. 干细胞研究的意义和前景？

12. 分析图 7-36 和图 7-37。

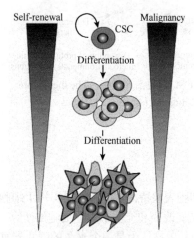

图 7-36　肿瘤恶性程度可能与 CSC 更新和数量相关；The malignancy of the tumor may be related to the renewal and quantity of CSC

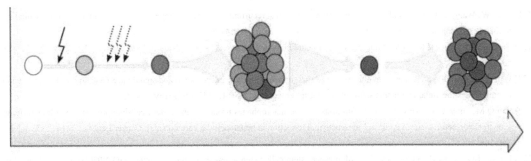

图 7-37　肿瘤进展和复发启动的 CSC 理论；The CSC theory of tumor progression and recurrencestarting

参 考 文 献

[1] Lapidot T，Sirard C，Vormoor J，et al. A cell initiating human acute myeloid leukaemia after transplantation into SCID mice[J]. Nature，1994，367（6464）：645-648.

[2] Bonnet D，Dick J E. Human acute myeloid leukemia is organized as a hierarchy that originates from a primitive hematopoietic cell[J]. Nature Medicine，1997，3（7）：730-737.

[3] Al-Hajj M，Wicha M S，Benito-Hernandez A，et al. Prospective Identification of Tumorigenic Breast Cancer Cells[J]. Proceedings of the National Academy of Sciences of the United States of America，2003，100（7）：3983-3988.

[4] Clarke M F. Self-renewal and solid tumor stem cells[J]. Biology of Blood & Marrow Transplantation，2005，11（2）：14-16.

[5] Yu F，Yao H，Zhu P，et al. let-7 Regulates self renewaland tumorigenicity of breast cancer cells[J].Cell，2007，131（6）：1109-1123.

[6] Kuperwasser C，Chavarria T，Wu M，Kuperwasser C，et al. Reconstruction of functionally normal and malignant human breast tissues in mice[J]. Proceedings of the National Academy of Sciences，2004，101（14）：4966-4971.

[7] Houghton J M，Stoivov C，Nomura S. Gastric cancer originating from bone marrow derived cells[J]. Science，2004，306（5701）：1568-1571.

[8] Haraguchi N，Utsunomiya T，Inoue H，et al. Characterization of aside population of cancer cells from human gastroin testinal system[J]. Stem cells，2006，24：506-513.

[9] Kimc F，Jackson E L，Woolfendon AE，et al. Identification of born. chioalveolar stem cells sin normal lung and lung cancer[J]. Cell，2005，121（6）：823-835.

[10] Zhen Y，Zhao S，Li Q，et al. Arsenic trioxide-mediated Notch path way in hibition depletes the cancer stem like cell population in gliomas[J]. Cancer letters，2010，292（1）：64-72.

[11] 王耀烙，张培彤. 影响肿瘤干细胞侵袭转移的相关机制[J]. 中国肿瘤，2016，25（9）：699-705.

[12] Kennecke H，Yerushalmi R，Woods R，et al. Metastatic behavior of breast cancer subtypes[J]. Journal of Clinical Oncology，2010，28（20）：3271-3277.

[13] Jemal A，Bray F，Center M M，et al. Global cancer statistics[J]. Cancer Journal for Clinicians，2011，61（2）：69-90.

[14] Tran D D，Corsa C A，Biswas H，et al. Temporal and spatial cooperation of Snail1 and Twist1 during epithelial-mesenchymal transition predicts for human breast cancer recurrence[J]. Molecular Cancer Research，2011，9（12）：1644-1657.

[15] Guo J，Niu R，Huang W，et al. Growth factors from tumor microenvironment possibly promote the proliferation of glioblastoma-derived stem-like cells in vitro[J]. Pathology & Oncology Research，2012，18（4）：1047-1057.

[16] Yasuda K，Torigoe T，Mariya T，et al. Fibroblasts induce expression of FGF4 in ovarian cancer stem-like cells|[sol]|cancer-initiating cells and upregulate their tumor initiation capacity[J]. Laboratory Investigation，2014，94（12）：1355-1369.

[17] Yan B，Liu L，Zhao Y，et al. Xiaotan Sanjie decoction attenuates tumor angiogenesis by manipulating Notch-1-regulated proliferation of gastric cancer stem-like cells[J]. World Journal of Gastroenterology，2014，20（36）：13105-13118.

[18] Guo J，Wang B，Fu Z，et al. Hypoxic Microenvironment Induces EMT and Upgrades Stem-Like Properties of Gastric Cancer Cells[J]. Technology in Cancer Research & Treatment，2016，15（1）：60-68.

[19] Xiang L，Gilkes D M，Hu H，et al. Hypoxia-inducible factor 1 mediates TAZ expression and nuclear localization to induce the breast cancer stem cell phenotype[J]. Oncotarget，2014，5（24）：12509-12527.

[20] Zhu H，Wang D，Zhang L，et al. Upregulation of autophagy by hypoxia-inducible factor-1α promotes EMT and metastatic ability of CD133+ pancreatic cancer stem-like cells during intermittent hypoxia[J]. Oncology Reports，2014，32（3）：935-942.

[21] Zhao W, Wang L, Han H, et al. 1B50-1, a mAb raised against recurrent tumor cells, targets liver tumor-initiating cells by binding to the calcium channel α2δ1 subunit[J]. Cancer cell, 2013, 23（4）: 541-556.

[22] Garofalo M, Croce C M. Role of microRNAs in maintaining cancer stem cells [J]. Advanced Drug Delivery Reviews, 2015, 81: 53-61.

[23] Wan S, Zhao E, Kryczek I, et al. tumor-associated macrophages produce interleukin 6 and signal via STAT3 to promote expansion of human hepatocellular carcinoma stem cells[J]. Gastroenterology, 2014, 147（6）: 1393-1404.

[24] Fan Q M, Jing Y Y, Yu G F, et al. Tumor-associated macrophages promote cancer stem cell-like properties via transforming growth factor-beta1-induced epithelial-mesenchymal transition in hepatocellular carcinoma[J]. Cancer Letters, 2014, 352（2）: 160-168.

[25] Lin L, Liu Y, Li H, et al. Targeting colon cancer stem cells using a new curcumin analogue, GO-Y030[J]. British Journal of Cancer, 2011, 105（2）: 212-220.

[26] Q Li. Arsenic trioxide-mediated Notch pathway inhibition depletes the cancer stem-like cell population in gliomas[J]. Cancer Lett, 2010, 292 (1): 64-72.

[27] Sun H, Zhang S. Arsenic trioxide regulates the apoptosis of glioma cell and glioma stem cell via down-regulation of stem cell marker Sox2[J]. Biochemical & Biophysical Research Communications, 2011, 410（3）: 692-697.

[28] Pattabiraman D R, Weinberg R A. Tackling the cancer stem cells - what challenges do they pose?[J]. Nature Reviews Drug Discovery, 2014, 13（7）: 497-512.

（秦　婧　陈春华　陈　莉）

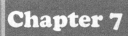

Chapter 7　Cancer Stem Cells

Section 1　Introduction for Stem Cells
　1. Definition
　2. Characteristics of Stem Cells
　3. Stem Cell Developments
　4. Markers of Stem Cells
　5. Classifications
Section 2　Embryonic Stem Cells
　1. Characteristics of ESCs
　2. Potential Sources and Treatment Possibilities
　　of ESCs
　3. An Enormous Impact on Biology and
　　Medicine Using ESCs
Section 3　Adult Stem Cells

　1. Hemotopoietic Stem Cells(HSCs)
　2. Bone Marrow Stromal Cells /Mesenchymal
　　Stem Cells (MSC)
　3. Multi-potent Adult Progenitor Cells (MAPCs)
　4. Neural Stem Cells (NSC)
　5. Other Tissue Stem Cells
　6. Induced Pluripotent Stem Cell (iPSC)
Section 4　Cancer Stem Cells
　1. Basic Theories of CSCs
　2. Characteristics of CSCs Expression
　3. Roles of CSCs
　4. Therapy Targeting CSCs
Challenges and Prospects

Stem cell research is one of the most attractive topics in modern biomedical research, regenerative medicine is the representative core in the stem cell research field. Now use of stem cells hold relatively an open view, that stem cells may be following the drugs, surgery and physical therapy the fourth treatment, have high hopes. A series of clinical research and preliminary results are exciting, the resistance to immune rejection after organ transplantation and treating autoimmune disease, diabetes, cancer, etc have been exciting results, there is no doubt that the future clinical applications provide huge imaginary space, not only in traumatic disease, genetic disease, degenerative diseases, and could be widely used in regenerative medicine. And it will also accelerate scientists to expose the basic law of life and the mechanism of the cell growth, differentiation, biological development.

Stem cell research is one of the most exciting topics in modern-day biomedical investigation and stands at the core of a new field called regenerative medicine .There is two challenges in stem cells research: ①Establishing biological concepts; ②We hope that stem cells may be used to cell-based therapies for diseases (such as cancer and neurodegenerative,) and　repair injury in human tissues (including heart, brain, and skeletal muscle).

Section 1　Introduction for Stem Cells

Cell is the basic unit of the body. In the process of differentiation, cells often due to the highly differentiated lose the ability to divide and eventually die off. The body in the process of development, adapts to make up for the shortage, retains the original part of undifferentiated cells, known as stem cells.

1. Definition

Stem cells are a class of undifferentiated primitive cells that can remain with the capacity developing into specialized cell types with specific functions in the body; otherwise the stem cell maintains itself in a state of long-term self renewal via mitotic division, which have two biological characteristics: pluripotent differentiation and self-renewal proliferation.

Stem cells exist in human and animal (including early embryo and mature organization) different stages of the development, on the one hand to update myself (self-renew), producing daughter cells with the same parents, in order to maintain a constant number of stem cells. On the other hand, under certain conditions stem cells can enter the differentiation process, producing differentiated daughter cells with asymmetric division, eventually forming specific tissue types with function.

It is now clear that stem cells are also presented in many tissues in adult animals and they contribute to the maintenance of tissue homeostasis. Cell numbers can be altered by increased or decreased rates of stem cell input. That cells lost through damage or normal age are replaced from the stem cell pool that present in many labile and stabile cells populations. Permanent cells may be replaced by new cells arising from stem cells.

Stem cells have defined four criteria: ①stem cells can be carried out repeated, continuous, self renew divisions, this is the first condition of maintaining stem cells social stability; ②The cells originated from a single stem cells can differentiate into more than one kind of cell types, for example, hematopoietic stem cells can differentiate into all kinds of blood cells; Some mature stem cells can only be differentiated into one kind of cell type, such as corneal stem cells; ③when stem cells were transplanted into the damaged parts, it has the function of reconstructing the original organization, it has been confirmed by hematopoietic stem cells, recently discovered the liver stem cells and neural stem cells have the characteristic; ④ is not easy to determine the standard: even if without tissue damage, stem cells can be differentiation and amplification in the body.

In recent years, many efforts has been devoted to the isolation and phenotypic characterization of stem cells. Although the development of specific markers to recognize stem cells is an ongoing challenge, a series of new observations have revolutionized and energized stem cell research. Among them are:

(1) Identifying the stem cells and their niches in various tissues, including the brain, which has been considered a permanent quiescent organ;

(2) Recognizing the stem cells from various tissues, particularly from the bone marrow, may have broad developmental plasticity;

(3) Knowing some stem cells present in tissues of human and mice may be similar to its embryonic stem cells.

2. Characteristics of Stem Cells

Stem cells have a proliferation speed which is relatively slow with pluripotent and cells self-renewal characteristics.

(1) Biochemical characteristics - high telomerase activity.

(2) Stem cells have unlimited proliferation and division with slow and homeostatic (difference from the essential characteristics of tumor cells).

(3) Stem cells itself is not in the terminal differentiation way.

(4) Stem cells can divide continuously for several generations, can also be used for a long time in the quiescent state.

(5) Stem cells growth in two ways, one is symmetrical division - form two of the same stem cells that maintain a parental characteristics, still remain as stem cells. Another asymmetric division, due to the regulating differentiation protein not evenly distributed in the cytoplasm, makes a child cell irreversible polarize terminal become function of specific differentiation cells; The number of differentiated cell are controlled by the number of undifferentiation stem cells and the number of division. Symmetric and

asymmetric replication is a special property of stem cells. One of the cells retains its self-renewing capacity while the other enters a differentiation pathway and is converted to a mature, nondividing population (Fig. 7-1).

3. Stem Cell Developments

Stem cell development under normal (physiological) conditions and different forms of plasticity of the stem cell progeny during injury and upon induction (Fig. 7-2). The multiplicity differentiations of stem cell is known as development plasticity. This progenitor cell may generate different differentiated cells but lose self-renewal capacity.

4. Markers of Stem Cells

SSEA-3, SSEA-4, TRA-1-60, TRA-1-81, OCT-4 protein, CD133, CD44, CD34, has the heterogeneous nature of human stem cell and progenitor cell, eg. human hematopoietic stem(Fig. 7-3).

5. Classifications

In recent years, stem cells has become a focus in the study of life sciences and regenerative medicine, its basic reason is that stem cells and stem cell technology overcome difficult to cure disease and improve the quality of life for people and brought great hope. Stem cells have a lot of in vitro proliferation and differentiation of various cell potential, it can be used as alternative treatment of regenerative medicine provide sufficient source of cells. Embryonic stem cells (ESCs) can also be used for the study of human early development events, deepen our understanding genetic disease, and promote the treatment of disease. In recent years induced pluripotent stem cells (iPS) bypass the embryonic stem cell research faces ethical and legal obstacles, in the medical field is very wide application prospect.

Classifications of stem cells: ① Embryonic Stem Cells (totipotent cells); ② Adult stem cells [pluripotent stem cells, hematopoietic stem cells（HSC)], multipotent adult progenitor cell (MAPCs) and tissue stem cells (epidermal stem cells K5, K14, neural stem cells etc.,) (Fig.7-4).

Section 2   Embryonic Stem Cells

Embryonic stem cells (ESCs) are the undifferentiated cells of blastocyst (about 5 to 7 days after fertilization) in early embryonic development. Blastocyst contains about 140 cells, the cyst ward is a layer of flat cells, says the trophoblast, may develop the support organizations such as the placenta. The center of the blastocyst is called the blastocoel, the cells in blastocyst is inner cell mass. These undifferentiated cells can be further divided, differentiation, and develop into an individual (Fig.7-5). The inner cell mass form the three layer differentiation. Each layer will divide to form a variety of tissues and organs of the body. Such as ectoderm will grow into skin, eyes, and nervous system, etc., mesoderm to form bones, blood and muscle, endoderm will grow into liver, lung and intestine, etc (Fig 6-6). Because the cells can develop into a complex dual, these cells are credited with totipotency. It is first identified as pluripotent cells in embryos, and can give rise to all the tissues of the human body. These were called ESCs.

ESC sare a highly undifferentiated cells, including Germ cells (Embryonic Germ Cell, EGC). It can be derived from the teratoma cells (EC), mulberry ball stem cells (ES), blastocyst inner cell mass (ES), reproductive primordium (EG), etc. It has a developmental totipotency, can differentiate into all tissues and organs of adult animals.

1. Characteristics of ESCs

(1) ESCs can be isolated from normal blastocysts, the structures formed at about the 32-cell stage during embryonic development.

(2) ESCs can be maintained in culture as undifferentiated cell lines or induced to differentiate into many different lineages, and give rise to all the tissues of the human body that is called totipotent stem cells.

The basic characteristic of the vertebrate ESCs are:①It be derived from the third day blastocysts inner cell mass (these cells in the pregnant body will form embryo itself) or primitive germ cells; ②long-term remain undifferentiated proliferation;③even after long-term culture in vitro still has the ability to form three layer cells.

(3) Morphological features round or oval, nuclear-cytoplasmic ratio small, with one or more nucleoli; ESCs clones pack closely without clear boundaries. It looks like a bird nest (Fig.7-7).

(4) The markers of SSEA-3、SSEA-4,TRA-1-60,TRA-1-81, Oct4 expressed on the surface of ESCs

(5) Nuclear types of ESCs with normal types.

2. Potential Sources and Treatment Possibilities of ESCs

ESCs can be derived from early embryo formed by in vitro fertilisation, early embryo formed by cell nuclear replacement (Fig.7-8), umbilical cord blood or fetal tissue, and adult cells

Application of cloning technology employing mature nucleus replacement of the egg cell's genetic material, then develop to the blastocyst stage in vitro, separation of embryonic stem cells, for research and treatment. The embryo differentiation has not yet started, the system has not started, so can't call it the "people", so the technology has the obvious difference from "human cloning". This strategy has great allure, such as in normal cell nuclei into enucleated egg cell receptor, cultivate and separation of embryonic stem cells, directional differentiation in vitro for a variety of specific cell function, used to treat a variety of severe disease (Fig. 7-9).

ESCs cultivation in vitro: cultured blastocyst, isolated inner cell mass, cultured inner cell mass in irradiated mouse fibroblast feeder cells, formed   the first plating, after 9~15 days,the cultured inner cell mass dissociated and replaced onto new feeder cells, form the second plating to establish colonies, after 7~10 days, the cultured colonies dissociated, finally established undifferentiated stem cells, that differentiated to the specialized cells (blood cells, neural cells or muscle cells, etc.) (Fig. 7-10).

3. An Enormous Impact on Biology and Medicine Using ESCs

Also known as immortalized stem cells of the new seed cells for tissue engineering, regenerative medicine, organ transplantation and tissue repair is significant.

(1) ESCs have been used to study the specific signals, differentiation steps and gene control required for the development of many tissues.

(2) ESCs may be used to cells treatment.

(3) ESCs may be used to new drugs development and toxicity tests.

(4) In the future, ESCs may be used to repopulate damaged organs, such as the liver after hepatocyte necrosis and the myocardium after infarction. The generation of some specific cell types from cultured ESCs has already been achieved. Insulin-producing pancreatic cells and nerve cells produced in these cultures have been implanted, respectively, in diabetic animals and in mice with neurologic defects. Using ES cells for cell therapy (therapeutic cloning. Using ESCs therapeutic cloning treated some diseases such

as neural degenerative diseases, liver cirrhosis, severe burns, myocardial infarction.

(5) Producing colonic animals and transform gene animals.

Despite the medical application of human ESCs has huge potential, but also presents the ethical questions. These problems mainly include the source of human ESCs is legal and moral, potential applications will cause the ethical and legal issues. ESCs obtained from in vitro fertilization embryo under appropriate conditions can develop the proper? If stem cells from voluntary terminating pregnancy then how to do? Whether moral in order to obtain ESCs to kill embryo? Isn't it a good desire for evil approach provides grounds for? Whether use cells from the spontaneous miscarriage embryo or accident or not appropriateness?

There is no doubt that ESCs research still faces some problems and obstacles. But it is of great value. With the deepening of human ESCs basic research, be sure in regenerative medicine, early embryonic development, therapeutic drug screening has a broad prospect.

Section 3   Adult Stem Cells

Many tissues in adult animals have been shown to contain reservoirs of stem cells, which are called adult stem cells (ASCs).Compared to ESCs, which are pluripotent, ASCs have a more restricted differentiation capacity and are usually lineage-specific. However, the stem cells in adult bone marrow have broad differentiation potential (Plasticit) and in other tissues,stem cells located outside of the bone marrow is called tissue stem cells.

Stem cells are located in sites called niches, which differ from various tissues.

The stem cells differentiation programs are not fixed. A change in stem cell differentiation from one type to another is called transdifferentiation.

People could be isolated adult stem cells from autologous, directionally differentiated the target tissue in vitro and keep cell proliferation ability, these cells go back to the body, so as to achieve the aim of treatment for a long time. So the discovery of a transdifferentiation has the revolutionary significance in stem cell research, it is widely used in clinical treatment for stem cell biology engineering and laid a foundation. To explore the mechanism of transdifferentiation of ASCs has become another hot issue of stem cell research.

ASCs can be obtained by the following several aspects ①by directed differentiation of ESCs differentiation after transplantation.②by separating the embryo tissue, cells, or culture.③by umbilical cord blood, bone marrow, peripheral blood, bone marrow stroma, fat cells, etc. Using the ASCs obtained from adult patients somatic or different source cells for regenerative cell therapy will be an easier way.

1. Hemotopoietic Stem Cells(HSCs)

(1) Features of HSCs

The bone marrow contains HSCs as well as stromal cells which are capable of differentiation into various lineages. HSCs generate all of the blood cells and can reconstitute the bone marrow after depletion caused by disease or irradiation (Fig.7-11).

HSCs can be collected directly from the bone marrow, from umbilical cord blood, and from circulating blood of individuals receiving cytokines, such as granulocyte-macrophage colony-stimulating factor, which mobilizes HSCs.

(2)Clinical application of HSCs

In the clinical treatment, the applications of HSCs are early, such as HSCs transplantation. In addition to treat acute leukemia (AL) and chronic leukemia (CL), HSCs transplantation can also be used in the treatment of severe aplastic anemia, Mediterranean anemia, malignant lymphoma, multiple myeloma (MM) and hematopoietic system other diseases. It can also be used to treat a variety of solid tumors, small cell lung cancer (SCLC), breast cancer (BC), testicular cancer, ovarian cancer, neuroblastoma and the like. Of acute leukemia with no donor, also can be transplantated with their own HSCs in completing remission after treatment, it calls as an autologous HSCs transplantation.

In injury reparation, the main contribution of HSCs is not the generation of cells for these tissues, instead, stem cells may produce growth factors and cytokines that act on the tissue cells to migrate, promoting injury repair and cell replication.

Although HSCs may be able to replace cells in damaged tissues, they do not appear to play a role in the maintenance of these tissues under physiologic conditions (steady state). Perhaps the generation of tissue cells from HSCs occurs only at sites of injury, where the response to injury recruits stem cells from the bone marrow for local tissue repopulation.

2. Bone Marrow Stromal Cells /Mesenchymal Stem Cells (MSC)

(1) Depending on the tissue microenvironment, differentiation pathways for pluripotent bone marrow MSC (Fig. 7-12), it can generate chondrocytes, osteoblasts, adipocytes, myoblasts, and endothelial cell precursors.

Activation of key regulatory proteins by growth factors, cytokines, or matrix components leads to commitment of stem cells to differentiate into specific cellular lineages. Differentiation of special cells requires different factors.

(2) Features of MSC

1) Strong ability of proliferation and multi-directional differentiation potential, not only in vivo or in vitro appropriating environment can be divided into hematopoietic cells, but also has differentiated into muscle cells, liver cells, osteoblasts, cartilage cells, stromal cells and other cells ability (Fig. 7-13).

2) Immune regulating function, via the interaction between cells and cytokine inhibit T cell proliferation and its immune response, so as to develop the function of immune reconstruction.

3) It is easy to obtain, easy to separate, cultivation, amplification and purification, still keep stem cell properties after multiple amplification, and there are no characteristics of immune rejection. Because of these immunological characteristics, MSC have a broad prospect of clinical application in autoimmune diseases as well as a variety of replace therapy. By autologous transplantation can rebuild the structure and function of tissues and organs, and can avoid immune rejection.

3. Multi-potent Adult Progenitor Cells (MAPCs)

The adult bone marrow also harbors a heterogeneous population of stem cells, which appear to have very broad developmental capabilities. They proliferate in culture without senescence, and can differentiate into mesodermal, endodermal, and neuroectodermal cell types. These cells are called multipotent adult progenitor cells (MAPCs).

MAPCs are not confined to the bone marrow. They have been isolated from muscle, brain, and skin, and they are similar to bone marrow MAPCs, can be made to differentiate into endothelium, neurons, hepatocytes and other cell types.

MAPCs isolated from bone marrow, muscle, and brain have very similar gene expression profiles, suggesting that they may have a common origin. It has been proposed that MAPCs constitute a population of stem cells derived from, or closely related to ESCs (i.e., they may be the adult counterparts of ESCs). If this view is correct, what has been referred to as "transdifferentiation" and "plasticity" of stem cells in adult tissues may actually represent the process of differentiation of multipotent ESC-like cells into specific lineages. Indeed, mouse bone marrow MAPCs, injected into blastocysts, contribute to all somatic cell types, a demonstration of their pluripotency.

4. Neural Stem Cells (NSC)

NSC can differentiate into neurons, astrocytes and oligodendrocytes, can renew itself and to provide a large number of brain cells. Once thinking that neurons in the central nervous system loses its regenerating ability before or shortly after birth. But in recent years, some studies show that the adult mammalian brain can continue to produce new neurons, also found the NSC present in the adult brain, mainly in the lower lateral ventricle (SVZ) (olfactory bulb) and hippocampal dentate gyrus.

(1) Features of NSC

1) Self-renewal: Neural stem cells has two division ways, symmetrical division and asymmetric division, so as to maintain stability of the stem cell bank.

2) The potential of multi-directional differentiation: NSCs may different into neurons, astrocytes and oligodendrocytes.

The differentiation capacity of NSCs is not limited to the nervous system, neural stem cells in the appropriation microenvironment also has the ability of multi-directional differentiation to other tissues and cells29.

NSCs implanted into muscle to differentiate into muscle cells and implanted bone marrow can differentiate into blood cells.

3) Low immune: NSCs are undifferentiated primitive cells, not expressed the mature cells antigen, not identified by the immune system.

4) Good organization integration, can fusion with the host nervous tissue, and survival in the host for the long-term.

(2) Regenerative Medicine for Brain and Nerve Repair

Stem cell research offers innovative therapy to functional recovery from brain trauma and optic nerve injury and long term neural repair. Stem cells are present in the developing brain and eye nervous systems, but also in the adult human nervous system. Open head injury often causes damage to brain and optic nerve tissue. If neural tissue is out of the brain, it is generally discarded. We investigated whether such tissue could be used as a source for isolation of neural stem cells and the cultured neural stem cells could be implanted into patients for treatment of neurological deficits caused by trauma. We isolated and propagated neural stem cells from the exposed brain tissue of the patients with open brain trauma, and then implanted neural stem cells with MRI-guided stereotactic device for the patients. Within 2-years follow-ups, the patients were investigated for functional recovery. Contrast to the case control group, implantation of neural stem cells was associated with a significant improvement in patient's neurological function. Investigations of stem cell therapy have required analysis of the fate and migration of implanted neural stem cells. Here, we demonstrate the feasibility of labeling human neural stem cells and retinal stem cells with nanoparticle and tracking of implanted cells in monkey and human central nervous system (CNS). This data demonstrates the possibility of stem cell therapy in CNS and collectively provide necessary foundation for overcoming challenges to the enhancement of translational regenerative medicine of brain and optic nerve injury.

5. Other Tissue Stem Cells

In addition to bone marrow cells that may migrate to various tissues after injury, adult stem cells reside permanently in most organs. These cells (known as tissue stem cells) can generate the mature cells of the organs in which they reside.

(1) Epidermal Stem Cells

Epidermal stem cells are important source of epidermogenesis, repair, reconstruction.

Epidermal stem cells in fetal period focus on primary epidermal ridge, in adult patchily distribute in epidermal basal layer. The sebaceous glands opening and standing hair follicles muscle between the hair follicle outer root sheath have rich stem cells (Fig. 7-14), and in the absence of hair parts such as the palm, hand, foot, epidermal stem cells located in the base layer connected the top of the dermal papilla. Epidermal stem cells can be used in the autograft and allograft transplantation to treat the severe burn, chronic ulcer, etc. It may trandifferentiated into neurons, glial cells, smooth muscle cells and fat cells.

After injury, self-renewing epithelia reconstitute themselves by following three nonmutually exclusive strategies: ①Increasing the number of actively dividing stem cells; ②Increasing the number of replications of cells in the amplifying compartment; ③Decreasing the cell-cycle time for cell replication

(2) Intestinal Stem Cells (Fig. 7-15)

(3) Liver Stem Cells (Fig. 7-16)

Liver stem cells (oval cells) are bipotential progenitors, capable of differentiating into hepatocytes and biliary cells. Liver stem cells function as a secondary or reserve compartment activated only when hepatocyte proliferation is blocked. In hepatic growth processes such as liver regeneration after partial hepatectomy, and in liver growth after most types of acute necrotizing injury, hepatocytes themselves readily replicate and the stem cell compartment is not activated. On the other hand, oval cell proliferation and differentiation are prominent in that hepatocyte proliferation may be slow or blocked. Such as the livers of patients recovering from fulminant hepatic failure, in liver carcinogenesis, and in some cases of chronic hepatitis and advanced liver cirrhosis. Stem cells do not play a major role in the compensatory hyperplasia following hepatectomy, but give rise to the proliferating "oval cells" that arise after some forms of toxic liver injury, which may induce cancer transformation.

(4) Corneal Stem Cells（Fig.7-17）

Corneal stem cell is the source of corneal epithelial cell regeneration, continue division of a lifetime, and migrate to the corneal center, to supplement the epithelial cells with injury and apoptosis. It has an important role in maintaining the cornea physiological and biochemical environment, integrity, local immune response. In addition, corneal stem cells can prevent conjunctival epithelial cell migrating to the surface of the cornea, to keep the cornea transparency and normal physiological function is of great significance.

(5) Stem Cell of Skeletal Muscle

The myocytes of skeletal muscle do not divide, even after injury. Growth and regeneration of injury skeletal muscle occur instead by replication of satellite cells. These cells, located beneath the myocyte basal lamina, constitute a reserve pool of stem cells that can generate differentiated myocytes after injury. Placed its in different tissue environments, satellite cells can differentiate to osteogenic and adipogenic cells. The stem cells have not been found in cardiac muscle although it has been proposed that the heart may contain progenitor-like cells.

Cardiovascular disease is one of the most serious diseases in today's threating human health. In myocardial infarction caused by coronary artery pathological changes the ischemic myocardial cells are replaced by fibrous scar. Heart failure is a major cause of cardiovascular disease. Its high incidence, high morbidity and high mortality has become a major health problem in our country, and showed a trend of increasing incidence, younger, etc, bring to our families and society an increasingly heavy burden.

Drugs and interventional treatment of ischemic heart disease and heart failure can increase blood and strengthen heart's systolic function, but is unable to repair necrotic myocardial cell and reverse fibrous scar, can slow and prevent the occurrence of heart failure; Heart transplant can effect a radical cure in heart failure patients, however, limited by lack of donor heart. Therefore, looking for more effective and widely applied methods in the treatment of heart failure, especially for the transformation of fibrous scar to healthy heart muscle cells treatment is a hot spot in the forefront of the field and exploration target.

Stem cell biology opened up a wide space for myocardial regenerative medicine, also shows the hope in order to solve the problem of heart failure treatment. Recent advances in stem cell biology and medical research shows that the following three categories of myocardial cells can form new starting cells with the prospect of clinical application, namely human pluripotent stem cells (including human embryonic stem cells and induced pluripotent stem cells), the adult heart source precursor cells and fibroblasts reprogramming.

Stem cell therapy for myocardial infarction is becoming a hot spot in recent years, the research and development direction in the future. The world has hundreds of clinical trials of stem cell therapy for myocardial infarction, although these results proved that stem cell transplants have certain curative effect, but the effector is not ideal. One of the important reasons is that the transplantation of stem cells arelow survival rate and function in the ischemic anoxia, super oxygen stress of microenvironment, it is also a problem which needs to be urgently solved in this field.

In a word, stem cells play an important role in tissue repair and regeneration. Using stem cells to repair or replace the imperfection of the tissues and organs caused by illness, accident or genetic factors has become possible. The application of stem cells and its derived tissues and organs in life science and medicine has broad prospects, will bring new concepts and methods of medical treatments.

6. Induced Pluripotent Stem Cell (iPSC)

iPSC is through the in vitro gene transfection technology will have differentiated somatic cell reprogramming into a kind of stem cells. The cells are similar to the ESCs in the cell morphology, growth characteristics, surface markers, biological characteristics. iPSC has totipotency, can differentiate into a variety of organizations such as nerve cells, It is suitable for individualized treatment with stem cell transplants, tissue engineering, restoration of damaged tissues and organs etc.

Unlike ESCs, iPSC can be got without destroying the embryo or not used oocyte to prepare ESC like cells for the research and treatment of diseases. So not only managed to avoid the ethical problems, and to increase the new way for obtaining a patient's own genetic background of ESC like cells. In theory, it is confirmed that the human race has mature differentiated somatic cells which can be reprogrammed into more naive, higher proliferation and differentiation potential ESC like cells, that opens up broad prospects for stem cell research and practical application.

Study the pathological features of diseases using iPSC derived from patient's somatic cells: The limited experimental access to disease-affected human tissues has severely impeded the elucidating of molecular mechanisms underlying disease development. Generation of induced iPSCs by over-expression of defined transcription factors in somatic cells, in particular in those from patient somatic cells, presents an attractive and promising approach to model the early stages of diseases in vitro and to screen novel biomarkers as well as therapeutic medicines. Recently, many research groups have independently reported that patient-specific iPSC-derived cells recapitulated multiple features of pathological events of a particular disease, offering experimental evidence of utilizing patient-specific iPSCs to model diseases and reevaluate the current therapies. We have derived iPSC lines using somatic cells of patients suffering from

Klinefelter's Syndrome (KS) and Alzheimer's Disease (AD) and explored the possibility to use these iPSC lines to recapitulate the pathological features of the diseases. Our results show that patient's specific iPSC lines provide good opportunity to study the development and treatment of diseases.

Research and application of stem cells need to have the correct cultivation and differentiation in vitro. The self-renewal stem cells, directional differentiation and induction of iPSC dependent the specific culture microenvironments. Small molecule compounds are indispensable important part of the culture microenvironments. Using small molecule compounds, we can not only maintain the stem cells proliferation in vitro, also can improve the induction efficiency of iPSC. These small molecules can also help us to understand the important signal mechanism deciding stem cell fate.

Section 4   Cancer Stem Cells

Cancer stem cells (CSCs) have been defined as a subset of tumor cells with stem cell like properties. CSCs features include the abilities to self-renew and differentiate, higher tumorigenicity, and chemo/radio-therapeutic resistance, which are responsible for the growth, progression, recurrence and metastasis of tumor. The CSCs definition does not imply a specific relationship between CSCs and physiological stem cells.

1. Basic Theories of CSCs

(1) Source of CSC

It can be derived from the stem cells, transit amplifying .progenitor cells, as well as in fully differentiated daughter cells. Promoting mutation, cancer stem cells are capable of self-renewal and different to the progenitor cells and possibly even their fully differentiated progeny cells (Fig. 7-18).

(2) Theoretical Hypothesis of CSCs

1) Cancerous cells must accumulate many mutations, stem cells can survive for a long time, which can accepted that all mutations lead to cancer

2) Unlimited self-renewal of stem cells may provide an opportunity for the gene mutation.

3) CSCs are similar to tumor cells both have proliferation, migration and re-growing abilities.

4) Only a very small fraction of cells (possibly stem cells)of the tumor tissue can be inoculated cultured or transfer, etc. to form a new tumor.

Stem cell proliferation, self-renewal, differentiation, and transformation theoretically could represent the best targets for tumorigenic transformation (Fig. 7-19).

In the context of CSC hypothesis, the subset of tumor cells containing CSCs may grow to tumor in a manner that is hierarchical and heterogeneous. In contrast, nontumorigenic cancer cell may not form tumor successfully (Fig. 7-20).

(3) CSC Niche in Tumor Growth and Metastasis

The CSC niche is composed of blood vessels, stromal cells such as myofibroblasts, and ECM components. Tumors are organized in such a way that CSCs reside close to their niche. In addition to maintaining CSCs in a stem like state,①the CSC niche has the ability to dedifferentiate nontumorigenic cells into tumorigenic CSCs,②to induce the EMT, leading to dissemination of tumor cells from the primary tumor and,③seeding at the metastatic place. Furthermore, tumor cell engraftment in different organs is suggested to be facilitated by the formation of a premetastatic niche that potentially enables the initiation and outgrowth of secondary tumors (Fig. 7-21).

(4) Maintenance and expansion of CSCs by the tumor microenvironment, a ovarian cancer model (Fig.

7-22)

The tumor microenvironment composed by the cancer cells and the surrounding tissue specificity of mesenchymal cells and their expression products, metabolites or others.

Some chronic inflammatory tissues, as a precancerous lesions can cause tumorigenesis. Researchers also use inflammatory damage model to explain the formation of CSCs. They think on the one hand, inflammatory microenvironment highly recruiting blood-borne mesenchymal stem cell, when being mixed with certain cells in the local environment likely lead to cell reprogramming to form CSCs. On the other hand, activity inflammatory cytokines in microenvironment could continue to cell proliferation/update related signaling pathways that lead to form normal tissue stem cells and differentiated tumor.

2. Characteristics of CSCs Expression

In addition to the characteristics of stem cells ①with self-renewal and differentiation ability; ②has a strong ability of tumorgenesis, tumor in specific organizations also should have:

(1) There are certain characteristics or markers of normal tissue stem cells.

(2) The presence of its unique differentiation and proliferation tendency

(3) With tumor characteristics of the organization

As CSCs in pancreatic cancer may express PDX-1, Ptf-1, as pancreatic CSCs markers, and also express some surface molecules of common stem cell, such as CD34, CD44 and so on. Based on the nature of tumor mutation, cancer stem cells may also highly express some product molecules of pancreatic cancer, such as k-ras or Ki-67 and so on.

Attentionly these markers are related: ①The same CSCs may have different surface molecules, such as CD33$^+$ liver cancer stem cells, but there are also studies considered CD90$^+$ CD44$^+$ liver cancer stem cells. ②A CSC surface marker may be a kind of cancer, but it is not another kind of CSCs. Such as pancreatic CSCs marker is CD24$^+$ and breast cancer stem cells is CD24$^-$/10 w, respectively. ③The proportion of same tumor stem cells markers in different tumor cell lines is differences, such as throat cancer Hep22 cell line only < 5% CD33$^+$CSCs.

(4) Stronger Drugs Resistance

Most CSCs membrane express ABC (ATP binding cassette) Transporter protein is the pump of metabolites discharging, protect itself from the effect of exogenous substances invasion, but also participate in forming part of the blood brain barrier, blood testosterone barrier, placental barrier, the resistance to ABC has become important target in many anticancer study.

(5) The phenotypic and functional diversity of CSCs populations (Fig. 7-23).

3. Roles of CSCs

Tumors can arise from somatic cells through genetic mutations of cancer-critical genes. In addition, dysregulation of microenvironmental factors can contribute to the carcinogenic process. Such events might predominantly affect long-lived somatic stem cells, which can represent the cancer cell of origin. So that progenitors or terminally differentiated somatic cell types as the source of malignant transformation.

CSCs are posited to be exclusively capable of driving tumorigenesis through 3 defining features: ①Their abilities for long-term self-renewal; ②Their capacity to differentiate into tumor bulk populations devoid of CSC characteristics; ③Their unlimited potential for proliferation and tumorigenic growth. In addition, immunoescape features of CSCs might contribute to tumorigenesis and ultimately to tumor progression. Furthermore, CSCs can exhibit increasing resistance to chemotherapeutic agents and/or ionizing radiation. CSCs might also possess a preferential capacity to with stand immune-mediated rejection. If CSCs indeed represent the pool of resistant cells in human cancer patients, they are likely also drive neoplastic progression, tumor recurrence, and metastasis.

The relationship among CSCs, carcinogenesis, tumorigenesis, and tumor resistance (Fig. 7-24).

CSCs are organized into a hierarchy much like normal stem cells, with long-term self-renewing CSCs differentiating into cells with decreasing self-renewal potential.

Plasticity in CSCs and their progeny (Fig. 7-25).

(1) Stem cells and progenitor cells in tissue homeostasis, tumorigenesis, and tumor recurrence (Fig. 7-26).

(2) Clinically, tumor malignancy may be correlated to the number of CSCs, which drive tumor growth and recurrence

(3) CSC and tumor perpetuating cells (TPC) identity and differentiation capacity likely influence tumor histomorphology, a gastrointestinal model (Fig. 7-27).

(4) The CSCs theory of tumor development and relapse initiation.

The heterogeneous tumor contains their stem cell, Which may be able to evade standard therapy. Any CSCs evading therapy are able to divide and differentiate to repopulate the tumor.

As the hypothesised role of CSCs in the development of endometrial carcinoma (Fig. 7-28).

The centrel of solid tumor with overproliferation is always hypoxia, HIF-α stabilization and the hypoxic response trigger CSCs accumulation, leading to metastasis and the development of new tumors (Fig. 7-29).

Tumor initiation and metastasis based on CSCs, a HCC model (Fig. 7-30).

(5) Signaling Pathways Altered in Hepatic CSCs

①Activation of the Wnt pathway results in β-catenin accumulation in the cytosol and translocation into the nucleus, where β-catenin transcriptional activates the expression of its targets, such as cyclinD1, EpCAM, and miR-181. ② AKT is activated by two phosphorylation sites Thr308 and Ser473. Phosphorylation of Thr308 is promoted by PI3K and suppressed by PTEN. Activated AKT protect hepatic CSCs from apoptosis through the induction of BCL-2 and ABCG2 under the pressure of chemotherapy. Activated AKT could also interact with HIF-1α to induce VEGF and PDGF-BB expression for regulating the homeostasis and drug resistance of hepatic CSCs. ③Impaired TGF TGF-β signaling together with activation of IL-6/STAT3 pathway is important to regulate the differentiation and chemoresistance of EpCAM+ hepatic CSCs. Studies have shown that these pathways are interconnected, which may further promote stem cells and carcinogenesis in HCC (Fig. 7-31).

(6) Proposed role of CSCs in Tumor Immune Escape (Fig. 7-32).

The researchers, from the Cleveland medical center, confirmed glioma stem cells recruited M2 type tumor associated macrophage through secrete Periostin, promote the growth of malignant

Factors and pathways contributing to the low immunogenicity of stem cells and CSCs (Fig. 7-33)

4. Therapy Targeting CSCs

Existing research shows that characteristics of CSC self-renewal, proliferation and high resistance to radiotherapy and chemotherapy, making conventional means are difficult to remove tissue, blood and other body residual CSCs to become tumor recurrence and metastasis risk. Therefore, the latest cancer research point of view that the key to cure cancer biology that kill CSCs, and thus set off a craze for CSCs targeted therapy.

Tumors contain a mix of CSCs, progenitor-like cells, and differentiated tumor mass. Conventional therapies kill mostly progenitor-like and tumor mass cells, while therapy-resistant CSCs survive and continue to proliferate leading to recurrence. CSC-specific therapies kill or differentiate the CSCs. Without the self-renewing CSCs to drive tumor progression, the tumor shrinks and eventually dies (Fig. 7-34, left).

Increasing evidence is revealing that drug sensitivity of CSCs may be patient as well as tumor specific, which will require personalized therapies. CSCs are isolated via surface marker or functional assays and subjected to high-throughput drug screening. The identified CSC-specific drug(s) are then administered to the patient, resulting in tumor shrinkage and death, leading to personalized CSC-specific therapies. (Fig. 7-34 right).

Treatment strategy for CSC to increase targeted anti-cancer therapy programs currently, and may reduce the risk of recurrence and metastasis. Similar to other tumors, CSCs in HCC also possess three CSC features which include the abilities to self-renew and differentiate, tumorigenicity, and chemo/radio-therapeutic resistance. Functional characterization of hepatic CSCs have identified several signaling pathways including Wnt/β-catenin, AKT, TGF-β and IL6 pathways to be important in regulating hepatic CSCs. Further studies based on these identified molecular mechanisms have revealed potential therapeutic strategies by targeting the abilities of CSCs to self-renew, to be tumorigenic and to develop chemoresistance.

Currently targeted immunotherapy for CSCs have two main ways: ①Targeted therapy based on the monoclonal antibody, by acting antigen molecules on surface of specific CSCs, removal CSCs; ②The adoptive cellular immunotherapy, mainly in the CSCs antigen sensitization of DC and T cells adoptive immunotherapy. Although targeted immunotherapy has obtained certain effect in the laboratory, however, the challenge now is also obvious, such as the antigen modulated and decorate by antibody therapy, more high specific CSCs markers to be discovered, the design of treatment strategies can remove CSCs and tumor cells in same time. Solving these key problems, will push to immunotherapy targeting CSCs into clinical.

A number of therapeutic strategies at CSCs are beginning to be experimentally validated. These approaches could potentially enhance responsiveness to current anticancer treatment regimens and might reduce the risk of relapse and dissemination. The approaches include ablation using antitumor agents that target prospective markers of CSCs (e.g., monoclonal antibodies and activated immune cells); reversal of chemo or radioresistance mechanisms operative in CSCs; CSCs pathway interference; differentiation therapy; disruption of protumorigenic CSC-microenvironment interactions; antiangiogenic or antivasculogenic therapy; and disruption of immunoevasion pathways (Fig. 7-35) .

Challenges and Prospects

Though there is more and more evidence to support the CSC theory, however, there are still many problems in tumor biology: ①Whether all tumor present CSC? ②All CSC has the same phenotype? ③ Because the normal stem cells and CSC has similar phenotypes and signal transduction pathway, when for CSC treatment how to protect the normal stem cells in bone marrow and gastrointestinal tract intact, and so on. ④Explore the CSC isolation from tumor tissue and in vitro culture amplification system, the method of building reasonable in vitro model is also need to consider the problem.

In recent years, much effort has been devoted to the isolation and phenotypeic characterization of stem cells. Although the development of specific markers to recognize stem cells is an ongoing challenge, a series of new observations have revolutionized and energized stem cell research. Among these are: ①the identification of stem cell and their niches in various tissues, including the brain, which has been considered a permanent quiescent organ; ②the recognition that stem cells from various tissues and particularly from the bone marrow may have broad developmental plasticity; ③the realization that some stem cells present in tissues of human and mice may be similar to ESCs; ④Using stem cells to repair the damage of human body tissue(therapeutic cloning); ⑤Researching the CSCs, and exploring in the cancer therapy.

Compared with gene therapy, the most remarkable characteristic of biological engineering with stem cells to treat disease is: the use of stem cell technology, can rebuild a variety of normal even more young tissues and organs. The new medical technology of reconstructing tissues and organs of will make everyone can use on yourself (and others) new tissues and organs derived from stem cells and its derivatives, to replace tissues and organs with diseased or aging, and can care widely a variety of problems i that use traditional medicine method is difficult to cure, such as cancer, heart necrotic disease, autoimmune disease, liver disease, kidney disease, and Parkinson's disease, alzheimer's disease and spinal cord injury, burns and other skin repair and treatment, etc. If combined with gene therapy, but also can treat many genetic diseases. Application of stem cells to treat disease is many advantages and security more than the traditional method: and don't need to fully understand the exact mechanism of the disease; Application of autologous stem cell transplantation may also avoid to produce immune rejection.

Of cause, the stem cell therapy of both autologous sources and foreign sources, shall have security, effectiveness and controllability, and is superior to the existing methods of clinical treatment. Each specific stem cell preparation and use process must have a strict standard operating procedures, to ensure that the stem cells in clinical research conforms to the scientific, safe, effective and social ethics, to make the healthy development of stem cell and regenerative medicine.

Through identify the CSCs in tumor tissue, looking for regulating CSCs biological behavior factors will play a huge role in clinical therapy, and increasing hope for controlling human tumor, improving the prognosis of tumor.

Consider/Questions

1. Basic concepts in this chapter

stem cell, embryonic stem cell(EC), adult stem cell(ASC), hematopoietic stem cell (HSC), bone marrow stromal cells /Mesenchymal stem cells (MSC), multipotent adult progenitor cell (MAPCs), neural stem cells, induced pluripotent stem cell(iPSC), cancer stem cell (CSC), therapeutic cloning, regenerative medicine, the tumor microenvironment, plasticity, transdifferentiation.

2. Summary the main characteristics of stem cells.

3. Briefly descript the characteristics of stem cells replication.

4. Briefly descript the ESCs impact on biology and medicine.

5. Briefly descript the normal physiological function and significance of corneal stem cells.

6. Which significance is there in the replication of liver stem cell (oval cell)?

7. Briefly descript the biological characteristics of CSCs.

8. What is CSC niches? Which roles of CSC niches are there in tumor growth and metastasis?

9. How do CSCs escape in tumor immune?

10. Give a case of stem cells application in medical research.

11. What is the significance and promise of stem cell research?

12. Analyze the following fig7-36, 7-37.

第八章 细胞信号转导途径

　　生物与非生物物质最显著的区别在于生物有一个完整的、自然的信息处理系统。一方面生物信息系统的存在使有机体得以适应其内、外环境的变化，维持个体的生存；另一方面信息物质如核酸和蛋白质在不同世代间传递，维持了种族的延续。生物现象就是信息在同一时空或不同时空传递的现象，生物的进化实质上就是信息系统的进化。

　　一切生物现象，都是机体内细胞对胞外信息的转导，并最终在胞内产生特定效应的一系列复杂的信息传导和调控的过程。一切生命现象的物质是蛋白质，蛋白质的新陈代谢是生物现象的本质。信息、物质、能量三者，都属于生物的基本要素。生物体在新陈代谢中，不但存在物质流和能量流，还存在信息流。物质、能量和信息在生物系统中不间断地运动、相互影响、有序地活动即为生命现象。在信息、物质、能量三者中信息流是生物活动的主导，起着调控物质和能量代谢的作用。这种复杂而微妙的信息传递和调控确保着生物的存在，其中任何一个环节出现障碍或发生信息传递的时、空、量三维上的倒错，都会导致病理过程而引发疾病。

　　细胞是生物活动的基本单位，细胞的代谢、分裂、分化、生长和死亡等生命活动受到细胞信号转导途径的作用机制调控。在一条信号转导途径中某一环节上的分子或基因，同时又参与另一条信号转导途径的组成或调控。因此信号转导是一个十分复杂的网络。

　　20 世纪 90 年代以来信号转导研究领域获诺贝尔奖的科学家及其研究：1991 年 Nelzer 和 Sokmann 研究的离子通道；1992 年 Edmond H. Fischer 和 Edwin G. Krebs 研究的糖原代谢中蛋白质的可逆磷酸化；1994 年 Gilman 和 Rodbell 研究的 G 蛋白信号传导；1998 年 Palmer 研究的 NO 的信号传导；2013 年 Randy W. Schekman、James E. Rothman 和 Thomas C. Südhof 研究的囊泡运输（vesicle transport）的调节机制。

　　单细胞生物通过反馈调节，适应环境的变化。多细胞生物则是由各种细胞组成的细胞社会，除了反馈调节外，更主要的是通过内分泌、旁分泌和自分泌一些信息分子来进行协调，更有赖于细胞间的通信与信号转导，以协调不同细胞的行为，如①调节代谢，通过对代谢相关酶活性的调节，控制细胞的物质和能量代谢；②实现细胞功能，如肌肉的收缩和舒张，腺体分泌物的释放；③调节细胞周期，使 DNA 复制相关的基因表达，细胞进入分裂和增殖阶段；④控制细胞分化，使基因有选择性地表达，细胞不可逆地分化为有特定功能的成熟细胞；⑤影响细胞的存活。不同细胞之间需要协调互相关系，共同应对环境信号。这些需求通过细胞通信和信号转导实现。

细胞通过位于胞膜或胞内的受体感受胞外信息分子的刺激，经复杂的细胞内信号转导系统的转换而影响其生物学功能。各类信号通过细胞膜和细胞内信使分子引起细胞基因表达改变的过程称为细胞信号转导（cellular signal transduction）[1]。这是细胞对外界刺激做出应答反应的基本生物学方式，即细胞对环境做出反应及细胞之间相互通信、调控的手段。细胞之间通过细胞表面的信息分子相互作用，从而引起细胞反应的现象称为细胞识别（cell recognition）。一个细胞发出的信息通过介质传递到另一个细胞产生相应反应的过程称为细胞通信（cell communication），如心肌细胞的同步跳动、运动神经末梢对肌肉的支配、雄激素对靶细胞的作用、白细胞的趋化运动等。

细胞通信的分类（信号发放细胞-靶细胞）如下。

（1）接触依赖型（contact dependent type）：锚定于质膜上的信号分子直接接触靶细胞质膜受体，如膜抗原提呈分子被免疫细胞识别。

（2）旁分泌型（paracrine type）：信号释放至附近基质，作用于局部，如生长因子（growth factor，GF）。

（3）突触型（synaptic type）：信号为神经递质，释放至突触间隙，作用于突触后膜（另一个神经元），如乙酰胆碱与其受体。

（4）内分泌型（endocrine type）：信号为激素，经血液作用于全身靶细胞，如性激素与其受体。

（5）自分泌型（autocrine type）：信号释放至周围基质，又作用于自身，如细胞因子（cytokines）。

（6）间隙连接型（gap junction type）：信号经缝隙连接作用于相邻细胞，如 cAMP。

第一节　构成细胞信号转导系统的要素

信号转导的基本模式：接收—转导—输出。细胞外信号分子被细胞的信号接收装置（受体）所感知，然后细胞内的信号转导装置转换为细胞内信号，有序激活信号通路传递信号，最后，特定的靶蛋白被激活，使细胞响应产生的各种反应。

一、细胞信号转导系统的构成

构成信号转导系统的各种要素必须具有识别进入信号、对信号做出响应，并发挥其生物学作用的功能，它们的任务比接力赛的传棒手更多，即不仅仅是将棒接过来，传下去，还需要具有识别、筛选、变换、集合、放大、传递、发散、调节信号等功能。这些功能常需要有一个体系，由一些蛋白质协同作用。细胞内的信号转导系统主要功能包括①信号接收装置：受体（膜、胞内）；②信号转导装置：G 蛋白、蛋白激酶、接合蛋白；③细胞内信使：cAMP、cGMP、IP3、DG、Ca^{2+} 等；④效应分子：转导蛋白或信使靶分子；⑤靶蛋白：代谢酶、基因调控蛋白（转录因子）等（图 8-1）。

二、信号转导中的信息物质

（1）细胞外信息物质包括①物理性：光、温度、压力、辐射等；②化学性：激素、生长因子、细胞因子、神经递质；③气体、其他（抗原 TNF、黏附分子）等。

（2）细胞内信息物质包括无机离子、脂类衍生物、糖类衍生物、核苷酸、信号蛋白分子、第二信使的小分子化合物等。

（3）细胞间信息物质分为三大类：①局部化学介质，包括旁分泌信号和自分泌信号。前者的特点是不进入血循环，而是通过扩散作用到达附近的靶细胞，除生长因子外，一般作用时间较短。自分泌信号是能对同种细胞或分泌细胞自身起调节作用。②激素主要是内分泌信号：由特殊分化的内分泌细胞释放经血液循环到达靶细胞，大多数对靶细胞作用时间较长。③神经递质是突触分泌信号，由神经元突触前膜释放，作用时间较短。

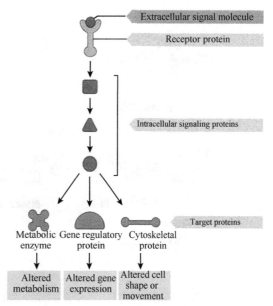

图 8-1　细胞信号转导系统的构成；The various elements of signal transduction systems

三、信号接收装置——受体

受体：位于细胞膜表面或细胞内部的一类特殊蛋白质，能特异地识别信号分子（配体，ligand），并以很高的亲和力与之结合，从而启动细胞内信号转导通路。配体是能和某一结构互补位置相结合的分子。

受体类型

（1）细胞表面受体（膜受体，membrane receptors）：其配体为水溶性分子（图 8-2）。由细胞表面受体介导的信号转导称为跨膜信号转导（transmembrane signal transduction）。

膜受体的分类：①离子通道偶联受体（ion-coupled receptor），存在于电兴奋性细胞（神经、肌肉细胞）之间的突触部位，是神经递质的受体，将化学信号转变为电信号，如乙酰胆碱受体。②G 蛋白偶联受体（G protein coupled receptor，GPCR），许多激素和神经递质的受体，如肾上腺素受体。③酶联受体（enzyme-linked receptor），生长因子和细胞因子的受体，其胞内结构域本身具有酶活性或与酶偶联（图 8-3）；后者进一步分为酪氨酸激酶偶联受体（tyrosine kinase coupled receptor）、受体酪氨酸激酶（receptor tyrosine kinase，RTK）和其他酶活性受体三类。

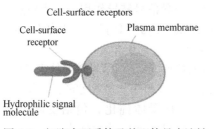

图 8-2　细胞表面受体及其配体是水溶性；Membrane receptors and its ligand is hydrophilic

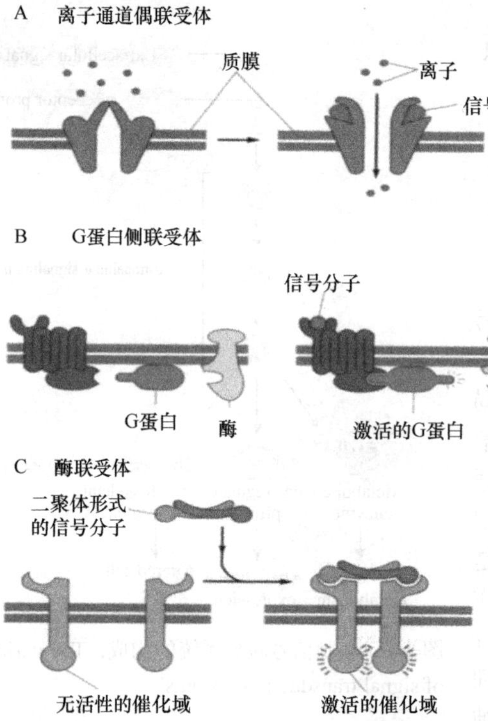

A 离子通道偶联受体

质膜

离子

信号分子

B G蛋白侧联受体

信号分子

G蛋白　酶　　　激活的G蛋白　　　激活的酶

C 酶联受体

二聚体形式
的信号分子

无活性的催化域　　激活的催化域

图 8-3 膜受体分类；Types of membrane receptors

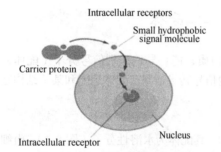

Intracellular receptors

Small hydrophobic
signal molecule

Carrier protein

Intracellular receptor

Nucleus

图 8-4 细胞内受体（核受体）及其脂溶性配
体；Intracellular receptors（nuclear receptors）
and its ligand is lipophilic

（2）细胞内受体——核受体（nuclear receptors）：其配体为脂溶性分子（图 8-4）。

细胞内受体位于胞质或核内，本质上都是配体调控的转录因子，分为两类：①类固醇激素受体家族——糖盐性激素受体，配体是脂溶性分子如类固醇激素（雄激素、孕激素、雌激素等）胞质受体与热休克蛋白（heat shock protein，HSP）结合。②甲状腺激素受体家族，配体是 T_3、维生素 D_3（Vit D_3）、维 A 酸，不与 HSP 结合，以同源（或异源）二聚体与 DNA 或其他蛋白质结合。

（3）胞内受体介导信号转导作用的三个位点：①位于 C 端的激素结合位点；②位于中部富含半胱氨酸（cysteine，Cys）、具有锌指结构的 DNA 或 HSP90 结合位点；③位于 N 端的转录激活结构域（图 8-5）。

受体与配体间的作用特征有①特异性：这是受体最基本的特点，保证了信号转导的正确性。配体和受体分子空间结构的互补性是特异性结合的主要因素。②饱和性。③高度的亲和力。

细胞持续处于信号分子刺激时，细胞可通过多种途径使受体钝化，包括受体失活（inactivation）、受体隐蔽（sequestration）和受体下调（down-regulation），产生适应。

四、信号转导装置——转导蛋白（transduction protein）

信号转导装置是一系列蛋白质依次经历活化—失活，构成从膜受体到细胞核之间的信号转导链（图 8-6）。

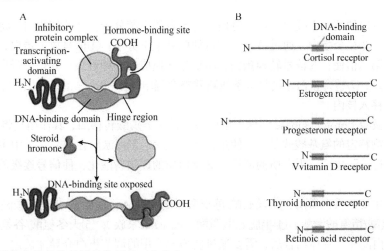

图 8-5　胞内受体介导的信号转导作用的三个位点；Three sites function as signal transduction mediated by intracellular receptors

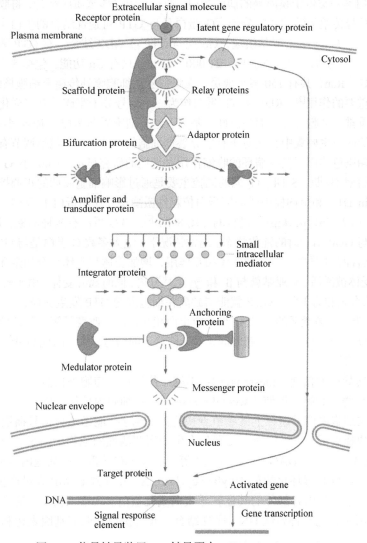

图 8-6　信号转导装置——转导蛋白；Transduction proteins

（1）转导蛋白种类：①接力蛋白，将信号传至相邻下游分子；②信使蛋白，将信号传至细胞内另一亚区；③接合蛋白，通过特定结构域偶联其上下分子；④信号放大蛋白，生成大量调节性小分子即第二信使；⑤信号转换蛋白，将信号转换成另一种形式；⑥切分蛋白，接收一条线路输出至多条；⑦整合蛋白，接收多条线路并整合/输出至一条；⑧潜在基因调节蛋白，膜受体自身活化后移入核内。

（2）蛋白激酶（protein kinase，PK）蛋白激酶是一类磷酸转移酶，其作用是将 ATP 的 γ 磷酸基转移到底物特定的氨基酸残基上，使蛋白质磷酸化。蛋白激酶在信号转导中主要有两方面的作用：①通过磷酸化调节蛋白质的活性。②蛋白质的逐级磷酸化，使信号逐级放大，引起细胞反应。

（3）五类主要的蛋白激酶：①丝氨酸/苏氨酸激酶（PKA、JAK）；②酪氨酸激酶（TPK）；③组氨酸/赖氨酸/精氨酸激酶、④半胱氨酸激酶（caspase 家族）；⑤天冬氨酸/谷氨酸激酶。

（4）G 蛋白配体与受体结合后，需要通过转换器作用的调节蛋白介导才被进一步激活。起着转换器作用的蛋白质是与鸟嘌呤核苷酸（GTP）结合的蛋白质称为 G 蛋白（GTP binding protein）。G 蛋白是一类位于膜内侧的偶联蛋白，通过与膜受体胞质区结合，将膜受体与配体结合的刺激信号特异传给下游的效应分子。G 蛋白是与 GTP 可逆性结合的蛋白质家族，包括：①"大 G"：由 α、β、γ 三个亚基组成，Gα 能与 GTP 或 GDP 结合，有 GTP 酶活性，起"分子开关"作用。②"小 G"位于细胞内，21 000～28 000 只有 Gα 功能，包括 5 个亚家族：Ras、Rho、Rab、ARF、Ran，共有 150 多个成员，在将信号从细胞膜外传递至细胞核的过程中，Ras 蛋白起着非常重要的作用[2]。Rho 小 G 蛋白作为一个信号分子家族具有多样化的功能，可以调节细胞骨架重排、细胞迁移、细胞极性、基因表达、细胞周期调控等 Rho 小 G 蛋白家族对细胞周期调控的研究主要集中在其对于有丝分裂期细胞的调节作用，包括调节有丝分裂前期细胞趋圆化、后期染色体排列及收缩环的收缩作用。近期的研究显示，Rho 小 G 蛋白及其效应分子对于细胞周期 G_1 期、S 期、G_2 期的调控主要是通过影响细胞周期的正调控因子细胞周期蛋白 D1（cyclin D1）和负调控因子周期蛋白依赖性激酶相互作用蛋白 1 及周期蛋白依赖性激酶抑制蛋白 27（p21cip1 /p27kip1）进行的（图 8-7）[3]。③G 蛋白有两种构象，即与 GTP 结合时的激活态和与 GDP 结合时的钝化状态。通常情况下，绝大多数 G 蛋白是与 GDP 结合的钝化型。与 GDP 结合的 G 蛋白能与各种受体相互作用，增加受体与配体结合的亲和力。一旦受体与配体结合，受体被激活，α 亚基就与 β 和 γ 亚基分离，同时离开受体。由于解离下来的 α 亚基与 GDP 的结合亲和力下降，GDP 就能与游离在细胞内的 GTP 发生交换，产生与 GTP 结合的激活型的 G 蛋白。被激活的 G 蛋白与效应蛋白相互作用，改变了第二信使的浓度，从而发生信号转导响应。使配体与受体接触时间延长，使输入的信号放大。因此 G 蛋白的主要功能是转变信号和放大信号。

（5）信号转导中的信使（messenger）：①第一信使：一切胞外信息分子、外来信号，如生长因子或诱导物。②第二信使（second messenger）：细胞内信使，即细胞内传递信息的小分子化合物，在细胞内信号途径上某些节点快速大量增多、能迅速将信号播散至各个下游通路、然后又被快速灭活。第二信使主要有具有生理调节活性的细胞内因子、cAMP、cGMP 、IP3（三磷酸肌醇）、Ca^{2+}、DAG（二酰甘油）等。信号从转导蛋白经细胞内信使向下游扩散：G 蛋白激活后激活腺苷酸环化酶（adenylate cyclase，AC），导致 cAMP 大量产生。大量 cAMP 迅速扩散，作用于细胞内各部分的其他转导蛋白或靶蛋白。③第三信使：信息分子级联传递后激活的转录因子，能与特异性 DNA 序列结合，起着诱导并调节基因表达和引起生理反应的作用。

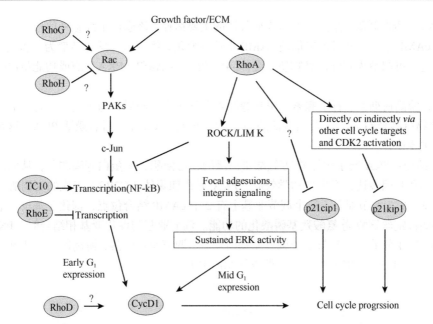

图 8-7 Rho 小 G 蛋白正调控细胞周期的进展；Rho 小 G 蛋白正调控的主要信号通路和促进 G_1/S 期进展的作用；Small Rho GTPases regulate eukaryotic cell cycle progression；The diagram shows the major signalling pathways whereby the small Rho GTPases and their effectors contribute to G_1/S progression

（6）转录因子（transcriptor）：是基因调控蛋白，通过与 DNA 上基因调控序列结合调节基因转录，如在 GPCR-cAMP-PKA 途径中有 CREB（cAMP response element binding protein），在 RTK-Ras-MAPK 途径中有 c-myc，c-Jun，c-Fos；在受调蛋白水解依赖的信号转导途径中核受体信号途径，如 NF-κB、核受体自身为转录因子等。

因此信号转导系统可以概括为四个组分。

（1）检测器：受体的接受和检出，这是受体的主要任务。

（2）效应器：使信号产生最终的效果，起到这种作用的主要有 AC 或磷脂酶 C。

（3）转换器：控制着信号的时间和空间，如 G 蛋白，它决定了 GTP 水解的速度，还决定了效应物被激活时间。其结果不仅使输入的信号被放大，也起到信号计时器的作用。

（4）调谐器：主要修饰信号转导通路，如磷酸化能协调多条信号转导通路的相互关系，在配体存在的情况下使信号转导通路保持连续畅通。

第二节 细胞膜表面受体介导的信号转导途径

亲水性化学信号分子（包括神经递质、蛋白激素、生长因子等）不能直接进入细胞，只能通过膜表面的特异受体传递信号，使靶细胞产生效应。膜表面受体介导的信号转导途径中在信号转导的早期表现为激酶级联（kinase cascade）事件，即为一系列蛋白质的逐级磷酸化，借此使信号逐级传送和放大。本节主要介绍膜受体介导信号转导的五条途径。这五条途径之间既相对独立又存在一定联系。

一、环腺苷酸-蛋白激酶 A 途径（cAMP-PKA 途径）

cAMP 信号途径以 cAMP 浓度改变和激活 PKA 为主要特征，PKA 是 cAMP 依赖性蛋白激酶又称 cAMP 蛋白激酶，是激素调节物质代谢的主要途径。该途径中细胞外信号与相应受体结合，调节 cAMP 活性，通过第二信使 cAMP 水平的变化，将细胞外信号转变为细胞内信号。其信息传递过程可归纳为胞外信息物质→受体→G 蛋白→cAMP→PKA→酶或功能蛋白→生物学效应。

例如，胰高血糖素、肾上腺素、甲状旁腺素等到达靶细胞后，与膜受体结合。活化的激素-受体复合物可结合 G 蛋白，释出激活的 G 蛋白，再激活 Camp，后者激活 PKA。这是激素调节代谢的主要途径。

PKA 结构：PKA 属于丝氨酸/苏氨酸蛋白激酶，可使酶、靶蛋白等磷酸化，从而调节细胞的物质代谢和基因表达，产生生物学效应。PKA 是由四聚体（C2R2）组成的变构酶。其中 C 为催化亚基，R 为调节亚基。每个调节亚基上有 2 个 cAMP 结合位点，催化亚基具有催化底物蛋白质某些特定丝氨酸/苏氨酸残基磷酸化的功能。调节亚基与催化亚基相结合时，PKA 呈无活性状态。当 4 分子 cAMP 与 2 个调节亚基结合后，调节亚基脱落，游离的催化亚基具有蛋白激酶活性（图 8-8）。PKA 的激活过程需要 Mg^{2+} 作用。

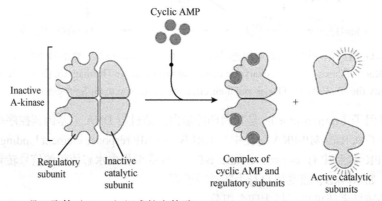

图 8-8　PKA 是四聚体（C2R2）组成的变构酶；PKA is composed of four polymers（C2R2）

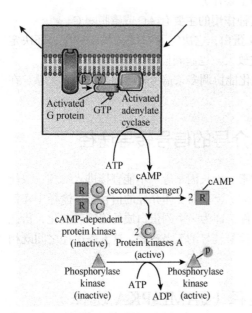

图 8-9　cAMP-PKA 信号转导通路；cAMP-PKA sinaling pathway

活化的 PKA 在 ATP 存在的情况下，①使多种蛋白质特定的丝氨酸和（或）苏氨酸残基磷酸化，从而调节代谢。②当 PKA 的催化亚基进入细胞核后，可催化反式作用因子——CREB 中特定的丝氨酸和（或）苏氨酸残基磷酸化，磷酸化的 CREB 形成同源二聚体，与 DNA 上的 CRE（cAMP 应答元件）结合，进一步激活受 CRE 调控的基因转录。③使细胞核内的组蛋白、酸性蛋白及胞质内的核蛋白体蛋白、膜蛋白、微管蛋白与受体蛋白等磷酸化，从而影响这些蛋白质的功能（图 8-9）。

二、Ca^{2+}-依赖性蛋白激酶途径

以细胞内 Ca^{2+} 浓度变化为共同特征，Ca^{2+} 为第二信使有两种不同的受体参与了这个过程（双信号途径）：①通过多种钙结合蛋白直接或间接影响

酶活性和离子通道的开关，而产生生理效应。胞外信号分子与细胞膜表面的受体结合，激活了 Ca^{2+} 信号传导途径，具有内在酪氨酸蛋白激酶（tyrosine protein kinase，TPK）活性的生长因子受体通过直接的酪氨酸磷酸化激活磷脂酰肌醇与磷脂酶 C 形成磷脂酰肌醇特异性磷脂酶 C（PI-PLC）复合物。②许多 G 蛋白（Gp）偶联的受体通过与异源性 Gp 的相互作用激活 PI-PLC。活化的 PI-PLC 导致三磷酸肌醇（IP3）及二酰甘油（DAG）的产生，它们分别刺激胞内 Ca^{2+} 释放及磷脂依赖性丝氨酸/苏氨酸蛋白激酶（PKC）的激活。例如，当去甲肾上腺素、抗利尿激素等与靶细胞膜上的受体结合后，通过特定 Gp 介导 PI-PLC，催化膜磷脂（PIP2）水解生成 IP3 和 DAG，IP3 和 DAG 分别通过两条途径参与信号转导。

（一）Ca^{2+}-磷脂依赖性蛋白激酶途径

该信号途径是以 IP3、DAG 为第二信使的双信号途径（图 8-10）。

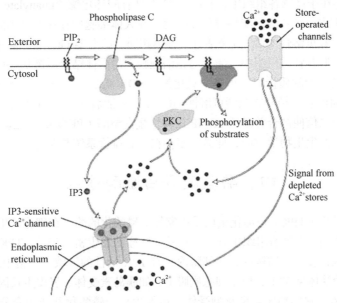

图 8-10　Ca^{2+}-磷脂依赖性蛋白激酶途径（IP3 和 DAG 的作用）；Ca^{2+}-phospholipids dependent protein kinase pathway

PKC 广泛地存在于机体的组织细胞内，含一个催化结构域和一个调节结构域，它们作用于机体的代谢、基因表达、细胞分化和增殖等。PKC 调节结构域常与催化结构域的活性中心部分贴近或嵌合，一旦 PKC 的调节结构域与 DAG、磷脂酰丝氨酸和 Ca^{2+} 结合并聚集至质膜，PKC 即发生构象改变而暴露出活性中心，催化细胞内各底物磷酸化。

（二）Ca^{2+}-调节蛋白依赖性蛋白激酶途径

IP3 为水溶性小分子进入胞质内，与胞质受体结合，释放细胞内储存的 Ca^{2+}，可促进 Ca^{2+} 通道开放，胞质 Ca^{2+} 浓度升高，然后通过该调节蛋白系统影响细胞功能。

（1）钙调蛋白（calmodulin，CaM）是一种普遍存在的多肽链组成的 Ca^{2+} 依赖性蛋白。人体的 CaM 有 4 个 Ca^{2+} 结合位点，当胞质的 Ca^{2+} 浓度 $>10^{-2}$ mmol/L 时，Ca^{2+} 与 CaM 结合，其构象发生改变而激活 Ca^{2+}-CaM 激酶。CaM 调控了真核生物中许多进程，包括细胞骨架组织、囊泡运输及有丝分裂等。同时 CaM 也可能参与到某些激酶的活化途径，如 PI3 激酶。在 Ca^{2+} 依赖的情况下，CaM 通过与某些酪氨酸磷酸化蛋白竞争结合到 p85（PI3 激酶中 85 kU 的调控亚基）的 SH2 区，直接激活 PI3 激酶或调控增强 PI3 激酶的活性。而 CaM 拮抗剂 CGS9343B，能抑制细胞中 Ca^{2+} 刺激的 PI 磷酸化的作用[2]。CaM 还能激活 Ca^{2+} 泵，调控胞内的 Ca^{2+} 浓度. 质膜 Ca^{2+} 泵在运输 Ca^{2+} 及维持细胞溶质低 Ca^{2+} 浓度的过程中起到重要作用。

（2）Ca^{2+}-CaM 激酶在细胞信号传递中起非常重要的作用。Ca^{2+}-CaM 激酶的底物谱非常广，可以磷酸化许多蛋白质的丝氨酸和（或）苏氨酸残基，使之激活或失活。Ca^{2+}-CaM 激酶既能激活 cAMP 又能激活磷酸二酯酶，即它既加速 cAMP 的生成又加速 cAMP 的降解，使信号迅速传至细胞内，又迅速消失。Ca^{2+}-CaM 激酶不仅参与调节 PKA 的激活和抑制，还能激活胰岛素受体 TPK 活性。

三、cGMP-蛋白激酶途径（PKG 途径）

cGMP 广泛存在于动物各组织中，它由 GTP 在鸟苷酸环化酶（guanylate cyclase，GC）的催化下经环化而生成，经磷酸二酯酶催化而降解。在人体细胞中存在两种不同类型的 cGMP，分别为结合型 GC 和可溶性 GC，其激活方式各不相同。结合型 GC 是质膜整合蛋白，大部分存在于在脑、肺、肝及肾等组织中，激素与靶细胞膜上的受体结合后激活 GC。可溶性 GC 是与亚铁血红蛋白结合的胞质蛋白，可被一氧化氮（NO）激活。一氧化氮合酶催化精氨酸生成 NO，NO 与亚铁血红蛋白结合并激活可溶性 GC。GC 激活后再催化 GTP 生成 cGMP，cGMP 水平升高可作为第二信使结合并激活 cGMP 依赖性蛋白激酶（PKG），导致靶蛋白的丝氨酸/苏氨酸残基磷酸化，产生生物学效应，此途径多存在于心血管系统与及组织。

四、酪氨酸蛋白激酶途径

酪氨酸蛋白激酶（TPK）是催化蛋白质中酪氨酸磷酸化的酶，在细胞的生长、增殖、分化等过程中起重要作用，在肿瘤组织中含量增高并与肿瘤的发生密切相关。TPK 的结构为：①细胞外的配体结合区；②跨膜结构区；③细胞内具有 TPK 活性的区域。细胞中的 TPK 分为两大类：第一类是称为受体型 TPK，位于细胞质膜上，如胰岛素受体、表皮生长因子受体及某些原癌基因编码的受体，它们均属于催化型受体，可发生自身磷酸化并使中介分子磷酸化，通过 MAPK 系统调节转录，也可通过激活 AC、多种磷脂酶起作用；第二类称为非受体型 TPK，位于胞质中，其受体本身并不具有 TPK 活性，但能借助细胞内连接蛋白（具有激酶结构）而完成信号传导，如 JAKs 和某些原癌基因编码的 TPK。受体型 TPK 和非受体 TPK 虽都能使蛋白质底物的酪氨酸残基磷酸化，但它们的信号传递途径有所不同。

（一）受体型 TPK-Ras-MAPK 途径

该途径位于细胞膜上，如 EGFR 等，属于催化型受体，可自身磷酸化，并使中介分子磷酸化，通过 MAPK 系统，调节转录，也可以激活 AC，与多种磷脂酶起作用。

1. Ras 基因 其在进化中相当保守，广泛存在于各种真核生物，对细胞生长、增殖、发育分化及癌细胞行为起重要作用。其表达产物是由一条多肽链组成的单体蛋白，相对分子量为 21kDa，故又名 P21 蛋白。因其分子量小于与七个跨膜螺旋受体偶联的 G 蛋白，表达产物被称作小 G 蛋白，具有弱的 GTP 酶活性。它有两种构象：与有活性的 GTP 结合构象和与无活性 GDP 结合构象。这两种构象在一定条件下可以互变，构成 Ras 循环，并受细胞质中 GTP/GDP 影响。Ras 与 GDP 结合时无活性，但磷酸化的鸟苷酸交换因子 SOS 可促进 GDP 从 Ras 脱落，使 Ras 转变成与 GTP 结合状态而活化。活化 Ras 蛋白可进一步活化 Raf 蛋白。Raf 蛋白具有丝氨酸/苏氨酸蛋白激酶活性，它可激活 MAPK 系统。

2. MAPK 通路 该通路的核心是由 3 种蛋白激酶构成的蛋白激酶反应链，即 MAPK 激酶的激酶（MAPKKK 或 MEKK）、MAPK 激酶（MAPKK，MEK 或 MKK）和 MAPK。它们是一组酶兼底物的蛋白分子。其中，MAPKKK（MAPK kinases kinases），是一类丝氨酸/苏氨酸蛋白激酶，Hal 为其中重要的一员，其作用是磷酸化并激活下游底物 MAPKK（MAPK kinase）。MAPKK 具有磷酸化苏氯酸/酪氨酸残基的双特异功能。MEK（MAPK/Erk kinase）为其中重要的成员。其作用是磷酸化并激活下游底物 MAPK。MAPK 是一类丝/苏氨酸蛋白激酶，细胞外信号调节激酶（extracellutar signal regulated kinases，Erk）为其中重要的一员。与 MAPKKK 和 MAPKK 不同，MAPK 的作用是磷酸化并激活多种下游底物，因此可以引发多种细胞反应。MAPK 可被特定的 MEK 在苏氨酸/酪氨酸双位点上磷酸化激活，MEK 又可被特定的 MEKK 在苏氨酸/丝氨酸双位点磷酸化激活。每一种 MEK 可被至少一种 MEKK 所激活，每一种 MAPK 又可被不同的 MEK 激活，构成了 MAPK 复杂的调节网络。MAPK 被激活后可停留在胞质中激活一系列其他蛋白激酶，使细胞骨架成分磷酸化，亦可转位进入细胞核激活各自的核内转录因子如 Elk-1、e-Jun、e-Fos、ATP-2、MEF 等，再调节转录因子的靶基因如即早期基因、后期效应基因和热休克蛋白基因的表达，促进有关蛋白质的合成和通路改变，完成对细胞外刺激的反应（图 8-11）。

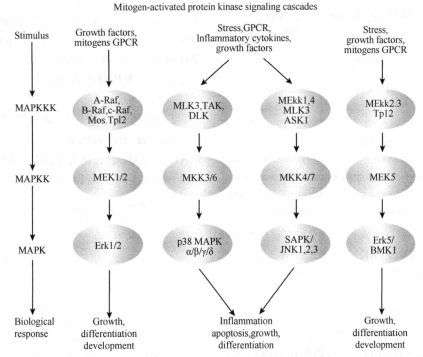

图 8-11 MAPK 及其蛋白激酶反应激活下游多种底物、转录因子，调节基因表达；MAPK and its protein kinases activate a variety of downstream substrates，Transcription factors，Regulate gene expression

3. Ras-MAPK 途径 Ras-MEK 通路是 MAPK 众多途径中的一条。该途径的信号转导为生长因子→生长因子受体（具有 TPK 活性）→含有 SH2 结构域的接头蛋白（如 Grb2）→SOS →Ras-GTP →Raf→MAPKK（MEK）→MAPK→转录因子→调节基因表达（图 8-12）。

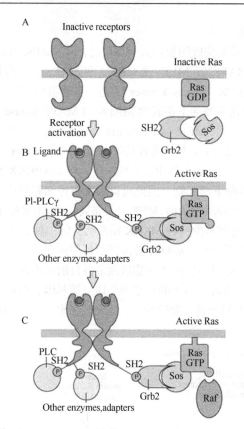

图 8-12 Ras-MAPK 途径；Ras-MAPK signal pathway
通过配体结合后蛋白构象的变化，使位于胞质激酶活性区的酪氨酸残基磷酸化，形成 SH2 结合位点的空间结构，可与具有 SH2 结构域的蛋白结合；The changes of the protein conformation after the ligand and receptor binding make tyrosine residues autophosphorylation which locate on the kinase activity district in the cytoplasm and compose the space structure of SH2 binding sites that can combine with protein which has SH2 domain structure

蛋白质结合。STAT 成员超过 7 种，每种都由特殊系列的 JAK 激酶（JAK1、JAK2、JAK3 及 TYK2）磷酸化。磷酸化在 JAK 与受体在质膜上结合时发生。一对 JAK 激酶与活化的受体作用，对保证该途径的正常功能很重要。例如，应答干扰素（interferon, IFNγ）刺激同时需要 JAK1 和 JAK2。其结构 C 端具有两个相连的激酶区，可磷酸化 STAT。STAT 被 JAK 磷酸化后形成同源二聚体（homodimer）和异源二聚体，然后穿过核膜进入核内，结合到靶基因特异性识别成分上，从而激活靶基因转录，调节相关基因的表达。

3. JAK- STAT 信号传递的基本过程[4]（图 8-13）
其过程可概括为：①细胞因子与其相应配体结合使受体二聚化；②受体和 JAK 发生聚集，邻近的 JAK

（二）非受体型 JAK-STAT 信号途径

JNK 位于细胞质中，借助细胞内连接蛋白（具有激酶结构）完成信息转导。受体本身无酪氨酸蛋白激酶活性，常见的配体为一些细胞因子，如白介素（IL）、干扰素（IFN）、红细胞生成素等，与配体结合能引起受体二聚化，提供激活 JAK 激酶的信号。

1. JAK（c-Jun NH2-terminal kinases） 属于丝氨酸/苏氨酸激酶家族，是一类丝氨酸/苏氨酸激酶，也被称为应激活化的蛋白激酶（stress-activated MAPkinases，SAPK）。已发现四个成员，即 JAK1、JAK2、JAK3 和 TYK1，其结构不含 SH2、SH3，C 端具有两个相连的激酶区。每一个成员与特异性的细胞因子受体结合。活化的（二聚体）细胞因子受体和 JAK 激酶作用，能产生与配体诱导 TPK 受体二聚化相同的效果。其不同点是，受体和激酶活性由不同的蛋白质提供。在转导胞外信号至核时起着重要作用，并可以提高转录能力。

2. 信号转导子和转录激活子（signal transdu- cer and activator of transcription，STAT） JAK 的底物为 STAT，具有 SH2 和 SH3 两类结构域，可以与具有 SH2 结构域的

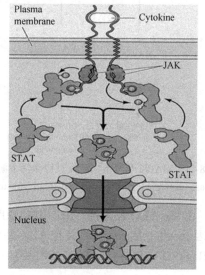

图 8-13 JAK-STAT 信号途径；JAK-STAT signal pathway

相互磷酸化而被活化；③JAK 的 JH1 结构域催化 STAT 上相应部位的酪氨酸残基磷酸化；④同时 STAT 的 SH2 功能区与受体中磷酸化的酪氨酸残基作用而使 STAT 形成二聚体而活化；⑤STAT 进入核内同其他一些转录因子相互作用调控基因转录。

JAK-STAT 信号途径与细胞生长、癌基因转化、细胞分化和细胞死亡有关。多种刺激信号都可介导 JNK 的活化，如生长因子、细胞因子和环境应激（图 8-14）。近来研究表明，JAK-STAT 信号途径与多种疾病发生机制有关，从而使该途径在临床上可作为一个潜在的分子治疗靶标[5]。例如，在霍奇金淋巴瘤（Hodgkin lymphoma，HL）和原发性纵隔大 B 细胞淋巴瘤（primary mediastinal large B-cell lymphoma, PMLBCL）细胞系中，染色体 9p24.1 的结构性放大导致 PDL1 表达增加，激活 JAK–STAT 信号通路，引起失控性的细胞增殖。PD-1 是 CD28 共刺激受体超家族的膜蛋白，表达于免疫调节性 T 细胞，通过与其配体（PD-1ligand，PDL1）结合抑制 T 细胞的激活[6]。淋巴瘤细胞表面表达 PD-1，抑制 T 细胞而逃避免疫监视[7]。

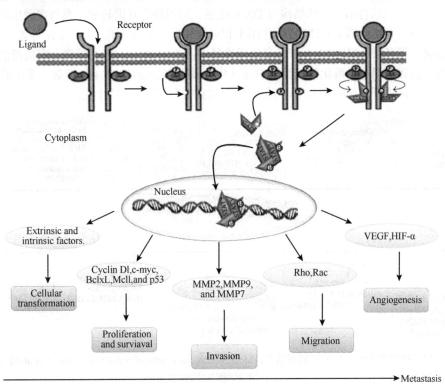

图 8-14　JAK-STAT 信号途径各种配体与其同源性细胞表面受体结合，导致磷酸化 STAT3 分子彼此在 SH$_2$ 结构域进一步二聚化及被易位至细胞核。随后该分子结合到靶基因的启动子并激活其转录。STAT3 调控细胞周期蛋白 D1，c-myc，抗凋亡蛋白 Bcl-xL，Mcd1 及 P53，从而调控细胞增殖和存活。STAT3 蛋白直接结合 MMP2 的启动子并上调其表达。此外，STAT3 还能调节 MMP9 和 MMP7 活动。STAT3 通过调节 Rho 及 Rac 的活性来调控细胞的迁移。STAT3 也可通过上调 VEGF 和 HIF-α 的活性来调节血管生成；JAK-STAT signal pathway Binding of various ligands to their cognate cell surface receptors, results in phosphorylation of STAT3 molecules that further dimerizes with each other at SH$_2$ domain and gets translocated to the nucleus. Following translocation, the dimerized STAT3 molecule binds to the promoter of target genes and activates their transcription. STAT3 regulates cyclin D1, c-Myc, BclxL, Mcl1 and P53, thereby regulating cellular proliferation and survival. STAT3 directly binds to the promoter of MMP2 and upregulates its expression. Additionally, STAT3 also regulate activity of MMP9 and MMP7. STAT3 regulates cellular migration by modulating the activity of Rho and Rac. Angiogenesis required for tumor growth and metastasis. STAT3 is seen to regulate angiogenesis by upregulating the activity of VEGF and HIF-α

五、NF-κB 途径

NF-κB（nuclear factor-κB）属于 Rel 蛋白家族成员，主要参与调节与机体免疫、炎症反应及包括白细胞黏附有关的蛋白质分子的基因转录。哺乳动物细胞中有五种 NF-κB/Rel：RelA（p65），RelB，C-Rel，NF-κB1（p50）、NF-κB2（p52），它们的 N 端都拥有一个由 300 个氨基酸组成的 Rel 同源区（Rel homology domain，RHD），能形成同源或异源二聚体，启动不同的基因转录。典型的 NF-κB 是由 p65 和 p50 蛋白亚基组成的同源或异源二聚体，其中异源二聚体活性较强。在胞质中，NF-2κB 与抑制性蛋白（I-κB）结合，以无活性的形式存在。许多诱导急性反应的因素如 IL-1、IL-2、TNFα、LPS、病毒感染、双链 RNA 和 PKC 的激活均可活化 NF-κB[8]。外界信号可以通过磷酸化 I-κB 激活 NF-κB 使其构象发生改变，NF-κB 进入核内与靶基因 κB 部位结合形成环状结构与 DNA 接触，调控特定基因转录，参与多种生物学反应（图 8-15）。当肿瘤坏死因子（TNF）等作用于相应受体后，可通过第二信使 Cer 等激活此系统。而病毒感染、脂多糖、双链 RNA 等信息传递途径中活化的 PKC、PKA 等则可直接激活 NF-κB 系统。激活过程是通过磷酸化抑制性蛋白使其构象发生改变而从 NF-κB 脱落，活化的 NF-κB 进入细胞核，形成环状结构与 DNA 接触，并启动或抑制有关基因的转录。

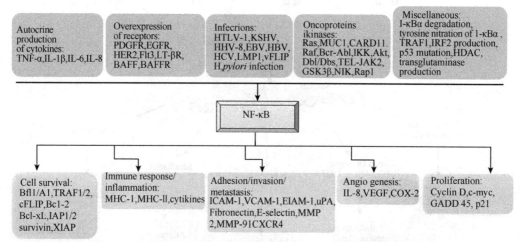

图 8-15　持续激活 NF-κB 的机制和结果；Mechanisms and results of constitutive activation of NF-κB

BAFF：属于 TNF 家族的 B 细胞活化因子；BAFFR：属于 TNF 家族的 B 细胞活化受体；CARD11：胱天蛋白酶募集域家族 11；Dbl/Dbs：弥漫性 B 细胞淋巴瘤中分离的转化型蛋白；ELAM-1：内皮细胞白细胞黏附分子-1；Flt3：FMS 相关酪氨酸激酶 3；GADD：生长停滞及 DNA 的损伤诱导；GSK3β：糖原合酶激酶 3β；HDAC：组蛋白去乙酰化酶；HER2：红细胞白血病病毒癌基因；HHV-8：人类疱疹病毒 8；HTLV-1：人 T 细胞白血病病毒 1 型；ICAM-1：细胞内粘附分子 1；IRF2：干扰素调节因子 2 KSHV：卡波西肉瘤相关疱疹病毒；LT-βR：淋巴毒素 β 受体；MUC1：黏蛋白 1；TEL-JAK2：Janus 维持性端粒激酶 2；TRAF：肿瘤坏死因子受体相关因子；uPA：尿激酶型纤溶酶原激活剂；vFLIP：病毒 FADD 样白细胞介素-1β 转化酶（FLICE）/半胱天冬酶-8-抑制蛋白；XIAP：X 连锁凋亡抑制；BAFF, B-cell activating factor belonging to the TNF family；BAFFR, B-cell activating factor belonging to the TNF family receptor；CARD11, caspase recruitment domain family 11；Dbl/Dbs, transforming protein isolated from diffuse B-cell lymphoma；EBV, Epstein Bar virus；ELAM-1, endothelial cell leucocyte adhesion molecule 1；Flt3, fms-related tyrosine kinase 3；GADD, growth arrest and DNA-damage inducible；GSK3β, glycogen synthase kinase 3β；HBV, hepatitis B virus；HCV, hepatitis C virus；HDAC, histone deacetylase；HER2, erythroblastic leukaemia viral oncogene；HHV-8, human herpes virus 8；HTLV-1, human T-cell leukaemia virus type 1；ICAM-1, intracellular adhesion molecule 1；IRF2, interferon regulatory factor 2；KSHV, Kaposi's sarcoma-associated herpes virus；LMP1, latent membrane protein 1；LT-βR, lymph- otoxin β receptor；MUC1, mucin 1；PDGFR, platelet-derived growth factor receptor；TEL-JAK2, telomere maintenance-Janus kinase2；TRAF, TNF-receptor-associated factor；uPA, urokinase plasminogen activator；VCAM-1, vascular cell adhesion molecule 1；vFLIP, viral FADD-like interleukin-1β-converting enzyme（FLICE）/caspase- 8-inhibitory protein；XIAP, X-linked inhibitor of apoptosis

第三节　细胞胞内受体介导的信号转导途径

胞内受体位于细胞核或细胞质，属于配体诱导型转录因子。其配体为疏水性信号分子：如甾体类激素、甲状腺素、Vit D₃、维 A 酸等，受体与 DNA 结合造成靶基因活化。其过程为①激素与胞质受体结合，形成激素-胞质受体复合物。②激素-受体复合物进入细胞核后结合于染色质的非组蛋白特异位点上，启动或抑制该部位的 DNA 转录过程，进而促进或抑制 mRNA 的形成，诱导或减少某种蛋白质（主要是酶）的合成（图 8-16）。

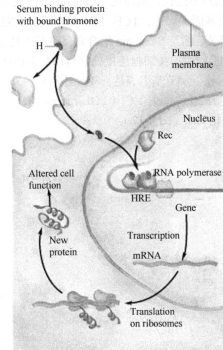

图 8-16　类固醇激素作用机制；Mechanisms of hormone activation

①血清连接蛋白将激素递达靶组织，通过质膜弥散到核内与特异性受体蛋白结合；②激素结合改变受体蛋白的构象，形成同源性或异源性激素受体复合物二聚体连接到 DNA 附近特异性基因的特异性调节区，称为激素应答元件（hormone response elements，HREs）；③连接后调节附近基因转录，增加或减少 mRNA 的生成；④改变激素调节基因产物的水平，引起细胞对激素的反应

第四节　可控性蛋白降解的信号转导途径

可控性蛋白水解相关的信号途径主要有 Wnt、Hedgehog、Notch 等，这些信号途径往往影响相邻细胞的分化，又称为侧向信号发放（lateral signaling）途径。

一、Wnt 信号途径

Wnt 是一类分子量约 40 000kDa 的分泌型糖蛋白，通过自分泌或旁分泌发挥作用。该途径存在于各种属生物中，对动物的早期发育及形态形成具有重要作用。另外，还参与出生后细胞的增殖、分化。Wnt 在各种生物中具有保守性，构成 Wnt 的细胞内信号转导通路的分子在机能、结构上也具有保守性。Wnt 信号途径像其他细胞间信号转导途径一样，也是由一种分泌的信号蛋白（Wnt）、跨膜受体蛋白（Frizzled）及复杂的细胞内多种蛋白机制将信号由细胞表面传至细胞核内。在哺乳动物细胞中 Wnt 信号途径的主要成分包括 Wnt 家族分泌蛋白、frizzled 蛋白（Frz）家族跨膜受体蛋白、细胞内蛋白——酪蛋白激酶 IE（CKIE）、蓬乱蛋白（dishevelled，Dsh 或 Dvl）、GBP-Frat、糖原合成酶激酶 3（GSK3）、APC、Axin、β-钙黏着蛋白（β-catenin）及 T 细胞因子（T cell factor / lymphoid enhancer factor，TCF/LEF）家族转录因子。

　　Wnt 的受体是 Frz[9-10]，为 7 次跨膜蛋白，结构类似于 G 蛋白偶联受体，Frz 胞外 N 端具有富含半胱氨酸的结构域（cysteine rich domain，CRD），能与 Wnt 结合。Frz 作用于胞质内的 Dsh，Dsh 能切断胞内 β-catenin 的降解途径，从而使 β-catenin 在细胞质中积累，并进入细胞核，与 TCF/LEF 相互作用，调节靶基因的表达，TCF/ LEF 是一类具有双向调节功能的转录因子，它与 Groucho 结合抑制基因转录，而与 β-catenin 结合则促进基因转录。β-catenin（在果蝇中称为 armadillo）是一种多功能的蛋白质，在细胞连接处它与钙黏素相互作用，参与形成黏合带，而游离的 β-catenin 可进入细胞核，调节基因表达。Wnt 还需要另外一个合作受体（co-receptor），即 LRP5/6，属于低密度脂蛋白受体相关蛋白（LDL-receptor-related protein，LRP），但至今还不清楚它如何与 Frz 一起活化 Dsh（图 8-17）。

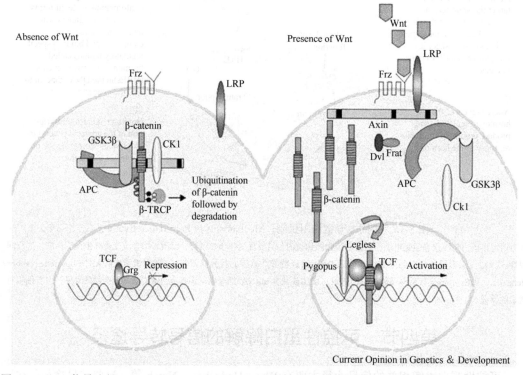

图 8-17　Wnt 信号途径；Wnt→Frz→Dsh→β-catenin 的降解复合体解散→β-catenin 积累，进入细胞核→TCF/LEF→基因转录（如 c-myc、cyclin D1）；Wnt signaling pathways

　　Wnt 信号途径能引起胞内 β-catenin 积累。Wnt 信号传递分子的基因异常与癌变关系的研究显示人类癌组织中存在 β-catenin、APC、Axin 的基因异常。APC 变异几乎都是由于含 Axin 结合部位的 C 端缺损，不能形成 APC/Axin 复合体，不能有效地引起 β-catenin 磷酸化。由于不能形成正常的 Axin 复合体而造成 β-catenin 蓄积。由此可以推断，β-catenin 是作为癌基因的产物，而 APC 及 Axin 是作为抑癌基因的产物发挥作用。

二、Notch 信号途径

Notch 信号介导相邻细胞之间通信进而调控细胞发育的经典型信号。Notch 基因最早发现于果蝇，部分功能缺失导致翅缘缺刻（notches）[11, 12]。由 Notch、Notch 配体（DSL 蛋白）和 CSL（一类 DNA 结合蛋白）等组成。Notch 及其配体均为单次跨膜蛋白，当配体（如 Delta）和相邻细胞的 Notch 结合后，Notch 被蛋白酶切割，释放出具有核定位信号的胞质区（intracellular domain of Notch, ICN），进入细胞核与 CLS 结合，调节基因表达（图 8-18）。

Notch 为分子量约 300kDa 的蛋白质，果蝇只有 1 个 Notch 基因，人类有 4 个（Notch1～4）。同一物种的不同 Notch 成员之间结构都有高度的同源性。Notch 的胞外区是结合配体的区域，包括不同数量的 EGF 样重复序列（tandem epidermal growth factor-lik erepeats，EGF-R）和 3 个 LNR（Lin/Notch repeats），人 Notch1 和 Notch2 各含有 36 个 EGF-R，Notch3 和 Notch4 分别含有 34 个和 29

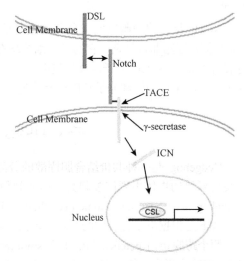

图 8-18 Delta→Notch→酶切→ICN→进入细胞核→CLS-ICN 复合体→基因转录；Delta→Notch →enzyme cut →ICN→in nucleus→CLS-ICN complex→gene transcription

个 EGF-R。Notch 受体可能是通过 LNR 与跨膜区（TM）之间的二硫键形成异源二聚体。Notch 胞内区由 RAM（RBP-Jκ associated molecular）结构域、6 个锚蛋白（Cdc10/ ankyrin，ANK）重复序列、2 个核定位信号（NLS）（Notch4 只有 1 个 NLS）和 PEST 结构域组成。RAM 结构域是 CBF1/RBPJκ（C promoter binding factor-1/ recombination signal binding protein-J kappa）主要的结合部位，CBF1 是 Su（H）蛋白在人或哺乳动物的同源蛋白。CBF1 也能与 ANK 重复序列结构域相互作用。ANK 重复序列结构域也是其他一些蛋白如 deltex、mastermind 等的结合部位，这些蛋白对 Notch 信号通路有修饰作用。RAM 结构域是与 CSL 结合的区域，PEST 结构域与 Notch 的降解有关。Notch 蛋白要经过三次切割，第一次在高尔基体内被 furin 切割为 2 个片断，转运到细胞膜形成异源二聚体。当配体结合到胞外区，Notch 蛋白又发生两次断裂，先是被肿瘤坏死因子-α-转化酶（TNF-α-converting enzyme，TACE）切割，然后被 γ-促分泌酶（γ-secretase）切割，后者需要衰老蛋白（presenilin，PS）参与。酶切以后释放 Notch 胞内区 ICN，进入细胞核发挥生物学作用[12, 13]。

Notch 配体在果蝇中有 2 个配体为 delta 和 serrate，它们行使的功能不同，但也有部分重叠。Notch 的配体又被称为 DSL 蛋白（在哺乳动物中叫做 jagged），都是单次跨膜糖蛋白，其胞外区含有数量不等的 EGF 样重复区，N 端有一个结合 Notch 必需的 DSL 基序。DSL 结构域在配体家族中高度保守，是与 Notch 结合并激活 Notch 所必需的。serrate 和 jagged 胞外区靠近细胞膜的部位有一个含保守半胱氨酸的结构域，Delta 中没有这个结构域。配体的胞内区较短，功能不明。目前发现的人 DSL 蛋白包括 jagged1、jagged2、delta1、delta3 和 delta4[14]。

CSL 为转录因子，在哺乳动物中称为 CBF1，在果蝇中称为 suppressor of hairless，在线虫中称为 Lag-1，取三者首写字母，故名。CSL 能识别并结合特定的 DNA 序列（GTGGGAA），这个序列位于 Notch 诱导基因的启动子上。ICN 不存在时，CSL 为转录抑制因子。当结合 ICN 时，CSL 能诱导相关基因的表达。Notch 信号的靶基因多为碱性螺旋-环-螺旋类转录因子（basic helix-loop-helix，bHLH），它们又调节其他与细胞分化直接相关的基因转录，如哺乳动物中的 HES（hairy/enhancer of split）、果蝇中的 E（spl）（enhancer of split）及非洲爪蟾中的 XHey-1 等[14]。

Notch 是影响细胞决定和分化的重要信号通路，它的某些分子的突变会造成各种疾病，Notch 信号通路非常复杂，它的各个细节均存在一些未解决的问题。在 Notch 受体方面，未经过裂解的完整 Notch 分子或仅经过第一、二次断裂的膜结合 Notch 分子也可以传递信号[15]，这种信号的生理功能和分子基础还有待进一步研究[15, 16]。

三、Hedgehog 信号途径

Hedgehog 是一种共价结合胆固醇的分泌性蛋白，在动物发育中起重要作用。果蝇的该基因突变导致幼虫体出现许多刺突，形似刺猬（Hedgehog）。脊椎动物中至少有 3 个基因编码 Hedgehog 蛋白，即 Shh（sonic hedgehog）、Ihh（indian hedgehog）和 Dhh（desert hedgehog），其中 Shh 是根据电子游戏中的角色命名的，后两者的命名与刺猬有关。

两个跨膜蛋白 patched（Ptc）和 smoothened（Smo）介导 Hedgehog 信号向胞内传递。Ptc 是 12 次跨膜蛋白，能与 Hedgehog 结合；Smo 为 7 次跨膜蛋白，与 G 蛋白偶联受体同源。在无 Hedgehog 的情况下，Ptc 抑制 Smo。当 Hedgehog 与 Ptc 结合时，则解除了 Ptc 对 Smo 的抑制作用，引发下游事件。

Hedgehog 信号通路的转录因子是 Ci（cubitus interruptus），在脊椎动物中为 Gli，具有锌指结构，分子量 155kDa。在胞质中 Ci 与其他蛋白形成复合体，这些蛋白包括 Fu（fused，一种丝氨酸/苏氨酸激酶），Cos（costal，一种能将复合体锚定在微管上的蛋白）和 Su（suppressor of fused 适配蛋白）。在没有 Hedgehog 信号时，Ci 被水解为 75kDa 的片段进入细胞核，抑制 Hedgehog 信号响应基因。当 Hedgehog 与 Ptc 结合时，Ci 的降解被抑制，全长的 Ci 进入细胞核中，启动相关基因表达，这些基因包括 Wnt 和 Ptc。Ptc 的表达，又会抑制 Smo，从而抑制 Hedgehog 信号，是一种反馈性调节[16]（图 8-19）。

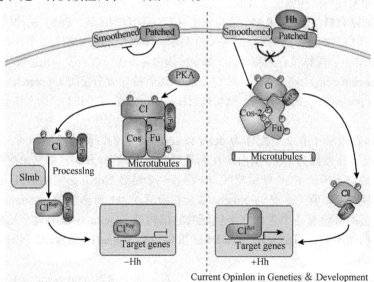

图 8-19　Hedgehog 信号通路；Hedgehog signaling pathway

第五节　细胞信号转导的特点及其相互作用

一、细胞信号转导的特点

细胞信号转导的特点主要有：①信号转导的一过性。②信号转导的记忆性。③信号转导的放大效应，少量胞外信号分子激活大量胞内效应分子。放大效应受到严格调控（图 8-20）。④信号转导的负性调节。⑤信号转导通路特异性。

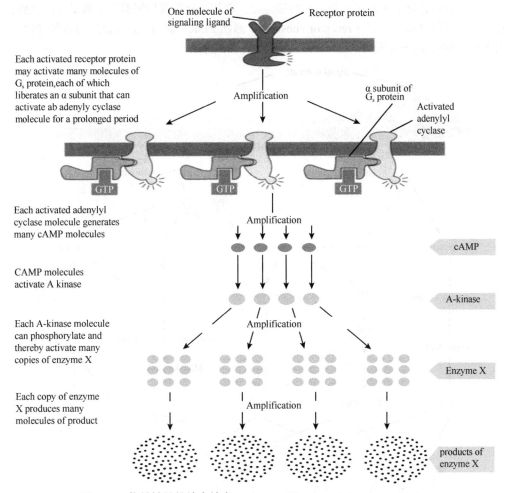

图 8-20　信号转导的放大效应；The amplification of signal transduction

二、细胞信号转导途径之间的相互作用

通过进行细胞信号转导途径之间的串流（cross talk）和细胞信号转导网络的形成导致细胞信号转导途径之间的相互作用。

（1）一条信息途径的成员，可参与激活或抑制另一条信息途径。例如，促甲状腺素释放激素与靶细胞膜的特异性受体结合后，通过 Ca^{2+}-磷脂依赖性蛋白激酶系统可激活 PKC，同时细胞内 Ca^{2+} 浓度增高还可激活 CA，生成 cAMP 进而激活 PKA。又如，EGF 受体是具 TPK 活性的催化型受体。佛波酯能激活 PKC，活化的 PKC 能催化 EGF 受体第 654 位 Thr 磷酸化，此磷酸化受体降低了 EGF 受体对 EGF 的亲和力和它的 TPK 活性。

（2）两种不同的信号途径可共同作用于同一种效应蛋白或同一基因调控区而协同发挥作用（图 8-21）。例如，糖原磷酸化酶为多亚基蛋白质（αβγδ）4，其中 αβ 亚基是 PKA 的底物，PKA 通过催化 αβ 亚基磷酸化而使其活化。该酶的 δ 亚基是钙调蛋白，Ca^{2+}-磷脂依赖性蛋白激酶系统的第二信使——Ca^{2+}能与 δ 亚基结合而使之活化。上述两条途径在细胞核内都可使转录因子 CREB 的 Ser133 磷酸化而激活。活化的 CREB 可与 DNA 上的顺式作用元件结合而启动多种基因的转录。

（3）一种信息分子可作用几条信息传递途径。例如，胰岛素与细胞膜上的受体结合后，可通过胰岛素受体底物（insulin receptor substrate）激活 PI3K。亦可激活 PLCγ 而水解 PIP2，产生 IP3 和 DAG，进一步激活 PKC；另外还可激活 Ras 途径。

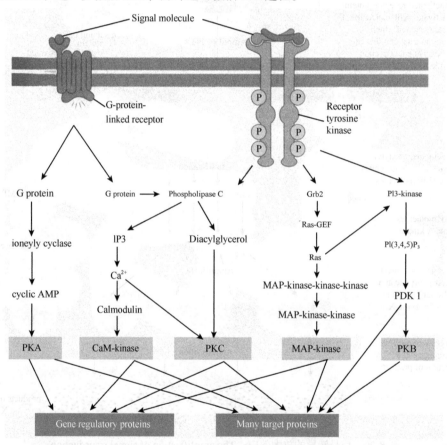

图 8-21　细胞信号转导途径之间的相互作用；The interaction between cellular signal transduction pathways

三、信号蛋白通过特定结构域相互作用

　　许多信号转导蛋白之间可以通过能互相识别的特定结构域，这些结构域有相似结构，发生直接的相互作用，发生聚合，形成三维网络，由此决定信号的传递途径。各条途径有相互作用，甚至形成网络以互相协调，但又保持特异性。

第六节 细胞信号转导障碍与肿瘤

细胞依靠各种信号转导途径中的信号分子的活化来完成其增殖、分化、发挥功能和凋亡的生命过程，因此认识信号传递过程和相互关系不仅对了解疾病的发生、发展、转归和预防有重要意义，而且有望通过干扰细胞内的信号转导，特异地控制细胞生长、分化和凋亡来达到在分子水平治疗疾病的目的。正常细胞的生长分化受到精细的网络调节。近年来人们意识到绝大多数的癌基因表达产物都是细胞信号转导系统的组成成分，它们可以从多个环节干扰细胞信号转导过程，导致肿瘤形成。在肿瘤发生中细胞信号转导起重要作用，同时为肿瘤治疗提供了重要靶标。

一、信号转导障碍引发肿瘤的原因

（1）表达 GF 样物质：sis 癌基因的表达产物与 PDGF-β 链高度同源，int-2 癌基因蛋白与 bFGF 结构相似。

（2）表达 GFR 类蛋白：在卵巢肿瘤中亦可见 PDGFR 高表达，与预后呈负相关。

（3）表达蛋白激酶类：src 癌基因产物具有较高的 TPK 活性，在某些肿瘤中其表达增加，可催化下游信号转导分子的酪氨酸磷酸化，促进细胞异常增殖。

（4）表达信号转导分子类：在 30%的人肿瘤组织有 Ras 基因突变，变异的 Ras 与 GDP 解离速率增加或 GTP 酶活性降低，均可导致 Ras 持续活化，促增殖信号增强而发生肿瘤。

（5）表达核内蛋白类：高表达的 Jun 蛋白与 Fos 蛋白与 DNA 上的 AP-1 位点结合，激活基因转录，促进肿瘤发生。

例如，Hedgehog 信号通路中 Ptch1、Smo、Su 的突变或 Gli1 的放大均已在多种人类癌症中报道[16]。其作用模式包括突变活化、配体介导的自分泌信号和旁分泌信号（图 8-22）。又如，在多发性骨髓瘤中的 Hedgehog 信号可诱导上皮间质转化(EMT)和肿瘤转移的形成(图 8-23, 图 8-24)。

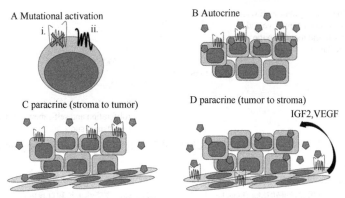

图 8-22　癌症中的 Hedgehog 信号模式；Models of Hedgehog signaling in cancer

A. 无配体介导的信号（突变活化）。Ptch1 活性的丢失和 Smo 的过表达或活跃突变可能增强 Hh 通路的活性。B. 配体介导的自分泌信号。肿瘤细胞生成 Hh 配体，在肿瘤细胞内刺激 Hh 通路活性。C. 配体介导的旁分泌信号。非恶性基质细胞生成 Hh 配体是肿瘤细胞生长和生存所必需的。D. 配体介导的旁分泌信号。肿瘤细胞生成 Hh 配体，在非恶性基质和内皮细胞内激活 Hh 信号，导致在微环境内产生不同的因子，最终同新生血管一起支持肿瘤细胞的生长与存活；A. Non-ligand mediated signaling (mutational activation). i. Loss of PTCH1 activity may increase Hedgehog pathway activity. ii. Overexpression or activating mutations in SMO are also depicted. B. Ligand mediated autocrine signaling. Tumor cells produce Hedgehog ligand that stimulates Hedgehog pathway activity in tumor cells. C. Ligand mediated paracrine signaling. Non-malignant stromal cells produces Hh ligand required by tumor cells for growth and survival. D. Ligand mediated paracrine signaling. Tumor cells produce Hedgehog ligand that activates Hedgehog signaling in non-malignant stromal and endothelial cells. This results in the production of unknown factors within the microenvironment that ultimately supports tumor cell growth and survival as well as angiogenesis

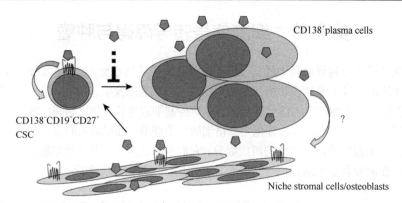

图 8-23　多发性骨髓瘤中的 Hedgehog 信号；Hedgehog signaling in multiple myeloma

通过 Hedgehog 信号通路调节多发性骨髓瘤的肿瘤干细胞。Hedgehog 信号的抑制可抑制多发性骨髓瘤肿瘤干细胞侧群细胞表型，通过诱导多发性骨髓瘤肿瘤干细胞的终末 CD138 表达的浆细胞分化，多发性骨髓瘤的多种信号模式较为活跃。实验数据显示分化性浆细胞能生成肿瘤干细胞存活和增殖所必需的配体。信号阻断导致肿瘤干细胞分化。正常骨髓间质细胞亦能为多发性骨髓瘤细胞生成配体和信号，以支持其生长和存活。肿瘤对间质的旁分泌信号作用也会促进肿瘤生长；Regulation of multiple myeloma（MM）CSC by the Hedgehog signaling pathway. The inhibition of Hedgehog signaling inhibits MM CSC displaying the side population phenotype by inducing terminal plasma cells differentiation of MM CSC as indicated by the expression of CD138. Multiple modes of signaling appear to be active in MM. Experimental data suggest that differentiated plasma cells can produce the ligand necessary for CSC survival and proliferation. Blocking signaling leads to CSC differentiation. Normal bone marrow stromal cells can also produce ligand and signal to myeloma cells to support their growth and survival. A possible role fort umor-to-stoma paracrine signaling may also take occur

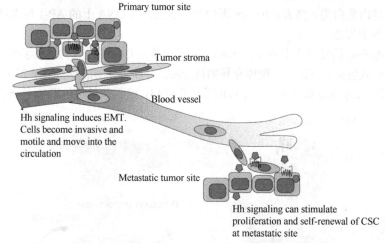

图 8-24　Hedgehog 信号可诱导上皮间质转化（EMT）和肿瘤转移的形成；Hedgehog signaling induces EMT and metastasis formation

在 Hedgehog 信号通路活化，肿瘤发生 EMT，由于其获得间质细胞特性使其有较强的运动和浸润能力，易使癌细胞脱离原发瘤经循环发生远处转移，一旦形成远处转移瘤 Hedgehog 信号可能对于转移瘤的克隆性生长和自我更新是必需的；Cells undergoing EMT under the influence of Hh signaling and become more motile and invasive as they acquire mesenchymal cell properties. This allows cells to escape from the primary tumor and circulate to distant sites. Once established at a distant site，Hh may be required for the clonogenic growth and self-renewal

NF-κB 及其调节的基因产物在癌症发展中的作用如图 8-25 所示。

二、针对信号转导通路的靶向性治疗

信号转导是细胞通过位于胞膜或胞内的受体感受胞外信息分子的刺激，经复杂的细胞内信号转导系统的转换而影响其生物学功能的过程。例如，淋巴细胞在正常环境下的生长通过一系列受体的级联活化和细胞内控制转录机制的下游激酶严格调控，如果信号转导通路异常会引发肿瘤。癌症治疗中靶向 NF-κB 的作用如图 8-26 所示。

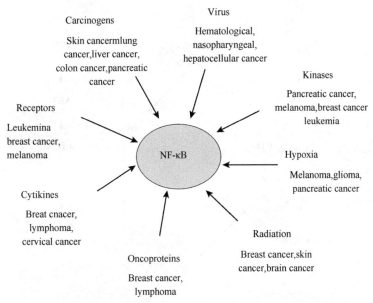

图 8-25　NF-κB 及其调节的基因产物在癌症发展中的作用；The roles of NF-κB and its regulating gene products in cancer development

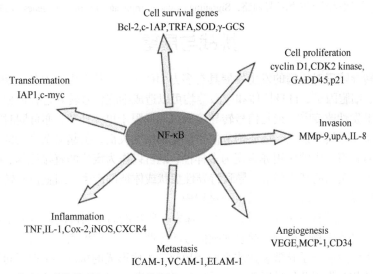

图 8-26　癌症治疗中靶向 NF-κB 的作用；The roles of targeting NF-κB in cancer treatment

与淋巴瘤病因学发生有关的信号级联通路见图 8-27。许多异常基因的突变或分子事件导致一系列最终的控制细胞增殖、迁移、血管形成和凋亡的蛋白转录事件，这些信号通路都是潜在的治疗靶点。

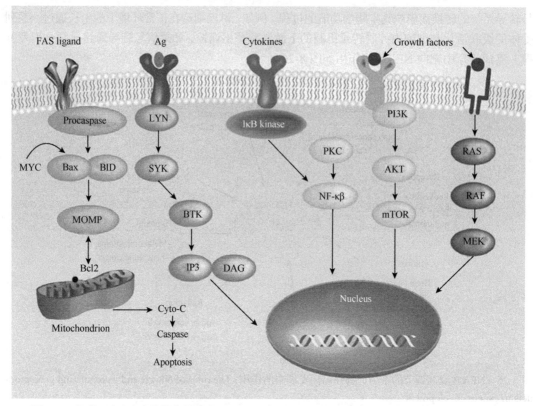

图 8-27　与淋巴瘤发生有关的信号通路；Signaling cascades implicated in etiopathogenesis of lymphomas

挑战与展望

　　细胞信号转导障碍对疾病的发生发展具有多方面的影响，其发生原因各不相同，如基因突变、细菌毒素、细胞因子、自身抗体和应激等均可以造成细胞信号转导过程的原发性损伤，或可引起它们的继发性改变[17]。细胞信号转导障碍可以局限于单一环节，亦可同时或先后累及多个环节甚至多条信号转导途径，造成调节信号转导的网络失衡，引起复杂多变的表现形式。细胞信号转导障碍在疾病中的作用亦表现为多样性，既可以作为疾病的直接原因，引起特定疾病的发生；亦可干扰疾病的某个环节，导致特异性症状或体征的产生。细胞信号转导障碍还可介导某些非特异性反应，出现在不同的疾病过程中。

　　目前还有很多问题有待深入探讨，例如，探索一些功能尚不明确的信号分子对于细胞生物学行为的影响及具体生物学机制；探索细胞信号转导调控对特定疾病发生的影响，以及由特定信号蛋白及其下游效应分子异常表达或突变所导致的肿瘤形成的机制；探索不同信号与其他信号途径彼此间的相互作用及信号通路下游效应分子之间的信号交汇与串扰等。

　　随着研究的不断深入，已经发现越来越多的疾病或病理过程中存在着信号转导异常，认识其变化规律及其在疾病发生、发展中的病理生理意义，不但可以揭示疾病发生的分子机制，而且可以利用特异性的信号蛋白及其效应因子抑制剂开发为新型的抗病靶向药物，为疾病的防治提出了新的方向。

思　考　题

　　1. 本章基本概念：细胞信号转导（cellular signal transduction），生物现象（biological

phenomenon），细胞识别（cell recognition），细胞通信（cell communication），受体（receptor），配体（ligand），跨膜信号转导（transmembrane signal transduction），蛋白激酶（protein kinase，PK），第二信使（second messenger），Ras 基因，转录因子（transcription factor），串流交叉对话（cross-talk）。

  2. 细胞间信号转导调控哪些细胞行为？

  3. 简述细胞通信的种类。

  4. 简述构成信号转导系统的要素。

  5. 简述信号转导中的三种信使。

  6. 简述细胞信号转导的特点。

  7. 为什么说细胞信号转导障碍是引发肿瘤的原因？

  8. 举例说明细胞信号转导障碍与疾病的关系分析可能的机制。

参 考 文 献

[1] Shi Ying. Progress in the studies of intracellular signal transduction and transcription regulation[J]. Foreign Medical Science：Molecular Biology，1997，19（5）：203.

[2] David M，Petit D，Bertoglio J. Cell cycle regulation of Rho signaling pathways[J]. Cell Cycle，2012，11（16）：3003-3010.

[3] Villalonga P，Ridley A J. Rho GTPases and cell cycle control[J]. Growth Factors，2006，24（3）：159-164.

[4] Liongue C，Ward A C. Evolution of the JAK-STAT pathway[J]. JAK-STAT，2013，2（1）：e22756.

[5] Rui L. The JAK-STAT pathway and hematological malignancy：beyond Stats[J]. Journal of Hematology & Transfusion，2013，1（1）：1002-1003.

[6] Flies D B，Sandler B J，Sznol M，et al. Blockade of the B7-H1/PD-1 Pathway for Cancer Immunotherapy[J]. Yale Journal of Biology & Medicine，2011，84（4）：409-421.

[7] Cetinözman F，Jansen P M，Willemze R. Expression of programmed death-1 in primary cutaneous CD4-positive small/medium-sized pleomorphic T-cell lymphoma，cutaneous pseudo-T-cell lymphoma，and other types of cutaneous T-cell lymphoma[J]. American Journal of Surgical Pathology，2012，36（1）：109-116.

[8] Zhang X P，Jiang J，Yu Y P，et al. Effect of Danshen on apoptosis and NF-κB protein expression of the intestinal mucosa of rats with severe acute pancreatitis or obstructive jaundice[J]. Hepatobiliary & Pancreatic Diseases International：HBPD INT，2010，9（5）：537-546.

[9] Miao C G，Yang Y Y，He X，et al. Wnt signaling pathway in rheumatoid arthritis，with special emphasis on the different roles in synovial inflammation and bone remodeling[J]. Cellular Signalling，2013，25（10）：2069-2078.

[10] Miller J R，Hocking A M，Brown J D，et al. Mechanism and function of signal transduction by the Wnt/beta-catenin and Wnt/Ca^{2+} pathways[J]. Oncogene，1999，18（55）：7860-7872.

[11] Artavanis-Tsakonas S，Rand M D，Lake R J. Notch signaling：cell fate control and signal integration in development[J]. Science，1999，284（5415）：770-776.

[12] Pires-Dasilva A，Sommer R J. The evolution of signalling pathways in animal development[J]. Nature Reviews Genetics，2003，4（1）：39-49.

[13] Arias A M，Zecchini V，Brennan K. CSL-independent Notch signalling：a checkpoint in cell fate decisions during development?[J]. Current Opinion in Genetics & Development，2002，12（5）：524-533.

[14] Milner L A，Bigas A. Notch as a mediator of cell fate determination in hematopoiesis：evidence and speculation[J]. Blood，1999，93（8）：2431.

[15] Shimizu K，Chiba S，Saito T，et al. Integrity of intracellular domain of Notch ligand is indispensable for cleavage required for release of the Notch2 intracellular domain[J]. EMBO Journal，2002，21（3）：294-302.

[16] Osipo C，Miele L. Hedgehog signaling in hepatocellular carcinoma：novel therapeutic strategy targeting hedgehog signaling in HCC[J]. Cancer Biology & Therapy，2006，5（2）：238-239.

[17] 陈莉，程纯. 现代病理学临床研究的基本问题[M]. 北京：科学出版社，2007.

（李杏玉　孙　艳　陈　莉）

Chapter 8 Cell Communication & Signaling

The most obvious difference between living and nonliving organism is a complete natural information processing system. The existence of biological information system enables organisms to adapt to the internal and external changes in the environment, maintain the survival of the individual; On the other hand information material such as nucleic acids and proteins to maintain the transmission between the different generations of the continuation of race. Biological phenomenon is messages in the same or different time and space, the biological evolution is essentially the evolution of the information system. All biological phenomenonare the cell transductions of extracellular information within the body and series of complicated process of information transmission which finally produce certain effects in the intracellular.

The material of all biological phenomenonis protein and metabolism is the essence of life. Information, material and energy are the basic elements of life. There are not only material flow and energy flow, but also information flow during the metabolism. Constant motion, interplay, and orderly activities of material, energy and information in the life system are the phenomenon of biological phenomenon.

Among the information, material and energy, information flow is the dominant in life activity and it controls metabolism of material and energy. This kind of complex and subtle information transmission and control can ensure the existence of life, pathological process would be happened and that leads to disease if any link in this process has disorder or perversion in three-dimensional perversion on the time, space, amount of information transmission.

Scientists in field of signal transduction who won the Nobel Prize since the 1990s:1991, Nelzer & sokmann: Ion channels 1992, Krebs &Fisher: The reversible phosphorylation of proteins in glycogen metabolism 1994,Gilman &Rodbell: G protein signal transduction 1998, Palmer, NO signal transduction 2013,Randy W Schekman, James E Rothman&Thomas C Südhof:The adjustment mechanism of the vesicle transportation. The winning reason is "Discover the main transportation system in cells-regulatory mechanisms of vesicle transportation".

Single-celled creatures through feedback adjustment, to adapt to the change in the environment. Multicellular organisms are in a community, in addition to feedback regulation, more important is through the endocrine, paracrine and autocrine some information molecules to coordinate. More depends on communication between cells and signal transduction, to coordinate the behavior of the different cell, such as: ①Regulate metabolism, based on the regulation of metabolism related enzyme activity, control cells material and energy metabolism; ② The function of cells such as muscle contraction and relaxation, the release of the gland secretion; ③ Regulating the cell cycle, DNA replication related gene expression, cells entered the stage of division and proliferation; ④ Control cells differentiation, selective expression of gene, cellsare irreversible to differentiate into adult cells with specific function;⑤Affect the survival of cells. Different cells need to coordinate the relationship witheach other, andjointly cope with environmental signals. These requirementare done by cells communication and signal transduction.

The process of all kinds of signals causing cell gene expression change through the cell membrane and intracellular messenger molecules is known as cell signal transduction.In other wordsthe extracellular information molecule stimulated cells through the cell membrane or intracellular receptors, then influence cells biological functions by the complex intracellular signal transduction, this process is called cellular signal transduction.It's the basic biology action of cells response to external stimuli, and the way cells respond to the environment,and mutual communication and regulation between cells.

Cell Recognition: The interactions of surface molecular information between cells cause the phenomenon of cellular responses.

Cell Communication: That cell messages from one cell transfer to another cell through medium produces the corresponding reaction process of cells.For Instance,the synchronization of myocardial cells, motor nerve endings dominant muscle, androgen effects on target cells and leukocyte chemotactic movement,etc.

Classification of Cell Communication

1. Contact dependent type: The target signal molecules anchor on the plasma membrane directly contacting with cytoplasm membrane receptor. For Instance, membrane antigen presented molecules are recognized by immune cells.

2. Paracrine type: Signals are released to the nearby matrixand act on the local. For Instance, growth factor (GF).

3. Synaptic type: Signal is the neurotransmitter, and it is released to the synaptic cleft, and acted on (another) the postsynaptic membrane. For instance, acetylcholine receptors.

4. Endocrine type: Hormone signal acts on whole target cells through blood. For Instance, the sex hormone and its receptors.

5. Autocrine type: Signal is released to the surrounding matrixand is acted on itself. For Instance, cytokines.

6. Gap junction type: Signal works on the adjacent cells through the gap junctions.

Section 1　Elements of Cell Signal Transduction System

The basic mode of signal transduction: Reception—transduction—export.

Cell signal receiving device (receptor) accepts extracellular signaling stimuli, then intracellular signal transduction devices transfer signal by activating signaling pathways orderly, finally specific target protein is activated, and produces a variety of cell reactions.

1. Composition of Cell Signal Transduction Systems

The various elements in signal transduction systems must be identificate to enter the signal, response to the signal and play the role of its biological function. its tasks,more than the hand of relay, namely is not only the great took it and pass it on, its also need to have identification, selection, transformation, collection, amplification, transmission, divergent, control signal, and other functions. These functions need to have a system, often by some protein synergy effect. Intracellular signal transduction system has main functions include: ①Reception apparatus: receptor (membrane, intracellular); ②Signal transduction device: G protein, protein kinase, joint protein; ③Intracellular messenger:cAMP, cGMP, IP3, DG, Ca^{2+}; ④Effector molecule: target molecular of transduction protein or messenger; ⑤Target protein: metabolic enzymes and gene regulatory proteins (transcription factors), etc (Fig. 8-1)

2. Information Material in Cell Signal Transduction

(1) Extracellular information material ①Physical: Light, temperature, pressure, radiation, etc.; ②Chemical: Hormones, growth factors, cytokines, neurotransmitter; ③ Gas and others (antigen, TNF, adhesion molecule), etc.

(2) Intracellular information material including inorganic ions, lipid derivatives, sugar derivatives, nucleotide, signal protein molecules, the second messenger of small molecular compounds.

(3) Intercellular information material: ①local chemical medium (paracrine signals), Features: Do not enter blood circulation, but through diffusely arrived near the target cells, in addition to the growth factor, general effect time is shorter. And some autocrine signals can regulate the same cell or secretory cells themselves. ② hormone (endocrine signal) : Released by the special differentiation of endocrine cells, though blood circulation reaches the target cells, most effect on target cells is longer time. ③ neurotransmitter secretion signal (synapses) : The presynaptic membrane of neurons release. Duration is shorter. ④ autocrine signal, can regulate the same cells or secretor cells themselves.

3. Aecepting Apparatus—Receptors

Receptor: one kind of special protein located on the cell membrane surface or in cells, identify the signal molecules specifically (the ligand), binding it with high affinity, then start the intracellular signal transduction pathways.

(1) Types of Receptors

1) Cell surface receptors (membrane receptors) its ligand is hydrophilic (Fig. 8-2). The signal transduction mediated by cell surface receptors is known as cell transmembrane signal transduction.

Types of membrane receptors

a. Ion-coupled receptor: Neurotransmitter receptors exist between electrically excitable cells (nerve and muscle cells), which transfer the chemical signals into electrical signals, like acetylcholine receptors.

b. G protein coupled receptor (GPCR):There are many receptors of hormones and neurotransmitters, for example, adrenaline receptors.

c. Enzyme-linked receptor: Receptors of growth factors and cytokineshave the enzyme activity or coupling with enzymes in the intracellular domain structure of itself (Fig. 8-3). The latter including (i) Tyrosine kinase coupled receptor, (ii) Receptor tyrosine protein, RTK, and (iii) Active receptors of other enzymes.

2) Intracellular Receprors (Nuclear receptors)

Its ligand is lipophilic (Fig. 8-4). Intracellular receptors are located in the cytoplasm or nucleus essentially transcription factors under the regulation of ligand. They can be divided into two categories.① Steroid hormone receptor family: Glucocorticoids, mineralocorticoid, sex hormones receptors, cytoplasm receptor combine with heat shock protein (HSP). ②Thyroid hormone receptor family: T3, VitD and retinoic acid, they donot combine with HSP, homogenous or heterogeneous dimers combined with DNA or other proteins.

3) Three Sites Function, as signal transduction mediated by intracellular receptor:

a. Located in the hormone binding sites on C end;

b. Located in the central where rich Cysare, with zinc finger structure of DNA or Hsp90 binding sites;

c. Located in the N end the transcriptional activation domain structure (Fig.8-5).

(2) Interaction between Receptors and Its Ligands: ①specificity: it is the most basic characteristics of receptor, ensure the validity of the signal transduction. The main reasons of specificity is the complementarity binding between ligand and receptor molecules in space structure. ②saturability and ③the high affinity.

(3) When Cell Continously Stimulating by Signaling Molecule, its Passivate Receptor Through Various Patterns (①receptor inactivation,②receptor concealmentor sequestration and ③receptor down - regulation) lead to adoption.

4. Transduction Proteins

①a series of proteins and ②they undergo the activation and inactivation in turn,and make the signal transduction chain between the membrane receptor into the nucleus (Fig.8-6).

(1) Species of Transduction Proteins

1) Relay protein - would transmit the signals to the downstream adjacent molecules;

2) Messenger proteins - would transmit the signals to a subregion in the cell;

3) Joint protein - coupling to upstream and downstream molecules by the structure of a specific field;

4) Signal amplification protein - generated a large number of small molecules of regulatory namely second messengers;

5) Signal transduction protein - convert the signal into another form;

6) Segmentation protein - receive a line of signal, output up to multiple lines of signals;

7) Integrated protein - receiving multiple lines and output to a integration;

8) Potential gene regulatory proteins- membrane receptors transfer into nuclear after its activation.

(2) Protein Kinase (PK)

Protein kinase (PK) is a kind of phosphoric acid transferase, which role is transfering gamma phosphate group from ATP to the substrate which content specific amino acid residues, and makes the protein phosphorylation. PK acts mainly two aspects in signal transduction:

1) Control the activity of protein through phosphorylation.

2) Protein phosphorylation step by step and the signal amplification step by step cause cell reactions.

Five types of protein kinase ①Serine /threonine protein kinase (PKA, JAK) ; ②Protein tyrosine kinase (TPK); ③Histidine /lysine /arginine kinase protein group; ④Cysteine protein kinase (Caspase family); ⑤Aspartic acid / glutamate kinase.

(3) GTP Binding Proteins

After bind of ligand and receptor, needs regulatory proteins mediated with converter effect to further activation. The protein with converter effect is GTP combinating proteinas called G protein (GTP binding protein). G protein is a kind of intramembrane coupling protein, through combined with membrane receptor cytoplasm area, specifically transform the signal combining the membrane receptor and ligands to the downstream effecter molecule.

GTP binding protein is the protein family reversiblely bind with GTP: ①The"big G" : it consists of the three subunits of alpha (α), beta (β) and gamma (γ), Gα can combine with GTP or GDP, and it has inherent GTP enzyme activity, and acts as the "molecular switch". ②The"small G" is located in the cell, only $21000\sim28000$, only has Gα functions (including 5 subunits: Ras、Rho、Rab、Arf、Ran, total more than 150 members). In the process of transfer signals from outside the cell membrane to the nucleus, Ras protein plays a very important role. The small Rho GTPases cycle between GDP-bound inactive forms and GTP-bound active form, and act as the molecular switches to regulate the processes of actin cytoskeleton dynamics, cell migration, cell motility, cell polarization, gene expression and control of cell cycles. The proliferation of eukaryotic cells is a tightly regulated process in which the cells sense both of intracellular and extracellular environments in each cell-cycle phases. Rho GTPases and their effectors are able to regulate the G_1 /S transition(Fig.8-7), cell rounding at mitosis onset, chromosomal alignment and actomyosin ring contraction at the end of mitosis.

(4) Messenger

1) The first messenger: All extracellular information molecules, external signal.

2) The second messenger (intracellular messenger): Small molecule compounds passing information in the cell, fast increase on some stages of the intracellular signaling pathways, quickly spread the signals to the downstream channel, and then be inactivated quickly.

The second messenger mainly include cytokines with physiologic regulating activity, cAMP, cGMP, IP3, Ca^{2+}, DAG, and soon on. Signal spreads downstream from transduction proteins by intracellular messenger: activated G proteins activated adenylate cyclase (AC) leading to the production of large numbers of cAMP, more messenger molecule cAMP quickly spreads, acting on other transduction proteins or target proteins in the other parts of cells.

3) The third messenger: Transcription factors are activated by cascade passed messages molecular, can combine with DNA sequences specifically and play a role in regulating and inducing gene expression and cause physiological reactions (effect molecules and produce the effect).

Transcriptor, gene regulating proteins through combining with gene regulation sequence on DNA, regulated gene transcription. For instance, in GPCR - cAMP - PKA way: CREB (cAMP response element binding protein), in RTK - Ras - MAPK pathway: c-Myc, cJun, cFos, in proteolytic dependent signal transduction pathways: NF-κB, in the nuclear receptor signaling pathways: nuclear receptor is the transcription factors, etc.

5. Cell Signal Transduction System

Signal transduction system is responsible for signal transduction function can be summarized as four components

(1) Detector: acceptance and receptor detection, the main task of the receptors.

(2) Effecter: make the signal to produce the final effect, mainly have the effect is adenylate cyclase (AC) or phospholipase C.

(3) Converter: controlling the time and space of the signal.

(4) Tuner: mainly modify signal transduction pathways, such as the phosphorylation.

Section 2   Cell Signal Transduction Mediated by Membrane Surface Receptor

Hydrophilic chemical signaling molecules (including neurotransmitters, hormones, growth factors, etc.) cannot be directly into the cell, only through specific receptors on the surface of the membrane, produce   the effect of target cells. Membrane surface receptor mediated signal transduction pathways in the early stages of the signal transduction show the   kinase cascade events, as a series of protein phosphorylation step by step, this signal transmission and amplification step by step.

Membrane receptor mediated signal transmission is at least the following five pathways. This five pathways are relatively independent and a certain relationship between them. To facilitate the narrative and understanding, we are respectively introduced the various information transmission pathway.

1. cAMP-PKA Pathway

cAMP-PKA pathway is the main way which regulates hormones metabolism and its main character is regulating cAMP concentration and activating protein kinase A (PKA). The structure of PKA: it belongs to the serine/threonine protein kinase and can make the enzymes, target protein phosphorylation and regulate cell metabolism and gene expression, produces biological effect. It's the allosteric enzymes which is composed of four polymers (C2R2) (Fig. 8-8).

The   information   transfer   process   can   be   summarized   as: Extracellular   information material--receptor-G-protein-Adenylate cyclase (AC)--protein kinase (PKA- function of enzyme or protein -biological effects(Fig.8-9).

2. Ca^{2+} - Dependent Protein Kinase Pathway

Changing intracellular Ca^{2+} concentration as the common characteristic. Ca^{2+}, as the second messenger, is doublesignaling pathways:

(1) Ca^{2+} - phospholipids dependent protein kinase pathway (Fig.8-10).

(2) Ca^{2+} - calcium regulatory proteins dependent protein kinase pathway.

IP3 is water-soluble small molecules, combining with receptor in the cytosol, releasing stored Ca^{2+} in cells. It promotes Ca^{2+} channels open, and increases cytosol Ca^{2+} concentration, and it affects cell function through the regulatory protein system.

3. CGMP (PKG way) - Protein Kinase Pathway

This way most exists in the cardiovascular system and brain.

4. Tyrosine Protein Kinase (TPK) Pathway

TPK is an enzyme catalyzing tyrosine phosphorylation, in cell growth, proliferation and differentiation, playing an important role, such as high content in tumor tissues and having close relationship with the incidence of tumor. TPK structure:①extracellular ligand-binding domain, ② transmembrane region, and ③intracellular activity TPK domain.

(1) TPK-Ras—MAPK Pathways (Receptor Pattern)

It is located in the cell membrane (EGFR), and belongs to the catalytic receptor, it can phosphorylate itself and intermediary molecules, and activate protein kinase MAPK system through the mitogen, transcriptional regulation, and PK - Ras and MAPK pathway also activates the AC and acts with a variety of phospholipase.

1) Ras gene is quite conservative in evolution, and widely exists in all eukaryotes, It plays a significant role on cell growth, proliferation, differentiation and development in cancer cell behavior. The expression product is small protein G.

2) Mitogen Activated Protein Kinases (MAPK pathway)

A reaction chain of MAPK and protein kinase. At the key of the MAPK pathway is composed of a reaction chain by three kinds of protein kinase, namely the MAPK kinase kinase (MAPKKK or MEKK), MAPK kinase (MAPKK, MEK or MKK) and MAPK. They are a group of protein molecules with enzyme and substrate. Each kind of MEK can be activated by at least one MEKK, each kind of MAPK can be activated by different MEK, constitutes the regulatory network of complex MAPK. Activated MAPKs can stay in the cytoplasm to activate a series of other protein kinase, make cytoskeletal component phosphorylation, and also translocate into the nucleus be then activate their respective nuclear transcription factors, such as Elk-1 e-Jun, e-fos, ATP-2, MEF, etc, to adjust the target genes of transcription factors, such as immediate early genes, late effect genes and the expression of heat shock protein genes, promote protein synthesis and signal pathways change, complete the response to extracellular stimuli (Fig.8-11).

3) Ras-MAPK Pathways

Ras-MEK pathway is "MAPK (Mitogen Activated Protein Kinases)" one of the numerous pathways. Growth factor→ growth factor receptor (with tyrosine kinase activity) →joint protein containing SH_2 domain structure (such as Grb2) →SOS→Ras-GTP→Rafl→MAPKK (MEK) →MAPK→transcription factor → regulating gene expression (Fig. 8-12).

(2) JAK-STAT Pathway (Non-Receptor Pattern)

It is located in the cytoplasm, with helping join protein in the cell (kinase structure) completes the information transduction. Receptor has no tyrosine protein kinase activity by itself, their common ligands are some cytokines, such as interleukin (IL), interferon (IFN), erythropoietin, etc.

1) JAK (c-JunNH2-terminal kinases) belongs to serine/threonine kinase family, located in the cytoplasm. The help of linking protein in the cell (kinase structure) to complete information transduction, and JAK plays an important role in the process of extracellular signals transducting to nuclear.

2) SATA (signal transducer and activator or transcription) is substrate of JAK with SH2, SH3 domain structure can be combined with the protein which have SH_2 domain structure.It has two connected kinase zone at C end structure which can phosphorylate STAT. STAT phosphorylated by JAK (JAK1、JAK2、JAK3 and TYK2) form dimers which go into the core through the nuclear membrane, combines and activates the transcription of target gene, regulate gene expression.

3) The basic process of JAK - STAT signal transmission can be summarized as: ①cytokines binding their corresponding ligand making receptor dimer; ② receptors and JAKs aggregation, neighboring JAKs

mutual phosphorylation and activation; ③JH1 structure domain in JAKs catalytic tyrosine residues phosphorylation on STATs corresponding part; ④at the same time the SH2function domain of STATs acting with tyrosine residues with receptor phosphorylation action, then make the STATs form dimers and activation; ⑤STATs enter to nucleus and play interactions with other transcription factors to regulate the genes transcription (Fig. 8-13).

JAK- STAT pathway exists in many life processes, such as cell growth, oncogene transformation, cell differentiation and cell death. JAK-STAT activation can be mediated by many factors, such as growth factors, cytokines, and environmental stress (Fig. 8-14). Recent studies have shown that JAK-STAT is associated with a variety of diseases mechanism, so that JAK - STAT pathway in clinical can treat as a potential molecular target.

For instance, In Hodgkin's lymphoma (HL) and primary mediastinal large B-cell lymphoma (PMLBCL) cell lines, a structural amplification in chromosome 9p24.1 leads to abundant PDL1 expression and JAK–STAT pathway activation, that manifests as uncontrolled cell proliferation. PD-1 is a membrane protein of the CD28 co-stimulatory receptor superfamily expressed on immune regulatory T cells, which inhibits T-cell activation upon binding to its ligand (PDL1). Neoplastic lymphoma cells express PD-1 on their surface and can evade immune surveillance by exploiting the immune suppressive role of PD-1 on T cells.

5. NF-κB Pathway

Nuclear factor-Kb (NF-κB) is mainly involved in regulating gene transcription of protein molecule that involved in the body's immune, inflammatory reaction and leukocyte adhesion. External signals phosphorylated and inhibited IκB activate NF-κB and make its conformation changed, the NF-κB goes into the nucleus and combine with target genes κB predominate parts to form ring structure that contact with the DNA, regulating the specific gene transcription, participating in a variety of biological reactions. Mechanisms of constitutive activation of NF-κB show in Fig. 8-15.

Section 3   Cell Signal Transduction Mediated by Intracellular Receptor

The receptor located in cytoplasm or nucleus. Receptor itself is a transcription factor. Its ligands are hydrophobic signal molecules: steroid hormone, thyroid hormone, vitamin D3, retinoic acid combination of receptor and DNA activate target gene.

Hormone combines with receptors, then forms hormones-cytoplasm receptor complexes in cytoplasm. Hormone-receptor complexes transfer into the nucleus, combine on nonhistone specific site of chromatin, staring or inhibiting the process of DNA transcription, then promote or inhibit the formation of the mRNA, inducing or reducing the synthesis of a protein (mianly enzyme) (Fig. 8-16). Early primary response and delayed secondary response to steroid hormone.

Section 4   Controllable Protein Degradation and Cell Signal Transduction

These signaling pathways often affect adjacent cell differentiation, also known as the lateral signal distributing (lateral signaling).

1. Wnt Signaling Pathway

Wnt is a kind of secreted glycoprotein which molecular weight is about 40000, and it plays some function by way of autocrine or paracrine. Its exits in various genera and plays an important role on early development and morphogenesis of animals. In addition, it also participated in the cell proliferation and differentiation after birth.

Wnt is conservative in all kinds of biological constitute. The molecules of intracellular Wnt signaling pathways are also conservative in the function and structure. Wnt signaling pathways, like other intercellular signal transduction pathways, also is composed of a kind of secreting signal proteins (Wnt), transmembrane receptors (Frizzled), and the complex mechanism of intracellular proteins transmits the signal from the cell surface to the nucleus.

In mammalian cells, the main components of the Wnt signaling pathways include: Wnt family secreted proteins, Frizzled (Frz curly) family of transmembrane receptor protein, intracellular protein---casein kinase IE(C KlE), Dishevelled (loose), GBP-Frat, glycogen synthases kinase 3 (GSK3), APC, Axin, p-serial protein and TCF/LEF transcriptional regulatory factor family (Fig.8-17).

2. Notch Signaling Pathway

It is composed of Notch, Notch ligands (DSL protein) and CSL (a class of DNA-binding proteins). Notch and its ligands are single-pass transmembrane protein, when the ligand (such as Delta) binding (binds) to the adjacent cell Notch, Notch protease cleavage, and release cytoplasmic domain (intracellular domain of Notch, ICN) which has nuclear localization signal, after that, it goes into the nucleus and combines with CLS to regulate gene expression (Fig.8-18).

3. Hedgehog Signaling Pathway

The transcription factor of hedgehog signaling pathways are Ci, Ci forms complex with other proteins in the cytoplasm, these proteins include: Fu (Fused), Cos (Costal) and Su (suppressor of Fused). When no Hedgehog signal, the Ci hydrolyze into 75 KD pieces, go into the nucleus, inhibit hedgehog signal response gene. When the Hedgehog combined with Ptc, the degradation of Ci is inhibited, the total length of Ci into the nucleus, and starts the related gene expression, these genes including Wnt and Ptc. The expression of Ptc suppresses the Smo, thus inhibiting the Hedgehog signal, this is a kind of feedback control（Fig.8-19）.

Section 5　Characteristics of Cell Signal Transduction

1. The characteristics of Cell Signal Transduction

1) Transient of signal transduction;

2) Memory of the signal transduction;

3) The scale of signal transduction, Amplification effect: A small amount of extracellular signaling molecules-many effective intracellular molecules. Amplification effect is also strictly controlled (Fig.8-20).

4) Negative regulation of signal transduction.

5) The specificity of signal transduction.

2. Interaction of Cellular Signal Transduction Pathways

Though the crposs-talk between the cell signal transduction pathways and the formation of cellular signal transduction network result in the interaction between cellular signal transduction pathways.

(1) A member of the signal transduction pathway can be involved in activating or inhibiting another signal pathway.

(2) Two different signaling pathways can work together in the same kind of effect protein or gene regulation zone and collaboratively work (Fig.8-21).

(3) Asignal molecule can effect some pieces of signal transmissions.

3. Interactions of Signal Protein in Specific Structure Domain

Many signal transduction proteins can directly interact each other by recognizing the specific domain structure, aggregation, and forming the three-dimensional network, which decides the way of signal transmission. The domain structure has similar structures. Not only different signal pathways crossing with each other, worked interaction, and even coordinate with each other through the network but also keep the specificity of signal transduction in signal network.

Section 6   Signal Transduction Disorders and Tumors

Cells rely on the activation of a variety of signaling molecules in signal transmission ways to complete its life process of proliferation, differentiation, function and apoptosis, so knowing the process of signal transmission and mutual relations not only is to understand the occurrence, development and outcome of diseases and prevention of diseases is important, but also is expected by interfering with the cell signal transduction, specifically control cell growth, differentiation and apoptosis to achieve the goal of treatment at molecular level.

The growth and differentiation of normal cells are regulated by network finely. In recent years, people have realized that the vast majority of cancer gene expression products are the components of cellular signal transduction systems. They can interfere with the cell signal transduction process from multiple links, leads to the formation of a tumor. Cell signal transduction plays an important role in tumorigenesis, and provides an important way for tumor treatment.

1. Reasons of Signal Transduction Disorder Causing Tumor

(1) The expression of GF material: sis cancer gene expression product is highly homologous with PDGF-beta chain, int-2 oncogene protein and bFGF structure is similar.

(2) Expressing GFR protein: PDGFR highly expresses in ovarian tumors, and negatively correlated with prognosis.

(3) The expression of protein kinase: src carcinoma gene product has the high activity of TPK, its expression increases in some tumors, catalyzes tyrosine phosphorylation of downstream signal transduction molecules, promote cell abnormal proliferation.

(4) The expression of signal transduction molecules: ras gene mutate in 30% human tumor tissues, variation of the ras and increased GDP dissociation rate or decreased GTP enzyme activity, can all lead to

the ras continuous activation, promoting proliferation signal enhanced and oncogenesis.

(5) The expression of nuclear protein: high expressed jun and fos protein combine with DNA AP-1sites, activating transcription, promoting tumorigenesis.

For instance, in Hh signaling pathway, mutations in *PTCH1, SMO,SUFU* or amplification of *GLI1* have all been reported in human various canccers(Fig. 8-22). Hedgehog signaling in multiple myeloma induces EMT and metastasis formation (Fig. 8-23 and 8-24).

The roles of NF-κB and its regulating gene products in cancer development (Fig. 8-25).

2. Intervention of Cell Signal Pathways in Cancers Treatments

Signal transduction is a process wherein an extracellular signal activates cell bound receptors to elicit a physiologic response intracellularly. For instance, the growth of lymphocytes under normal conditions is tightly regulated by a cascade of activated receptors and downstream kinases controlling transcription machinery within a cell and aberrancy. The roles of NF-κB and its regulating gene products in cancer treatment (Fig. 8-26).

Many aberrant genetic mutations or molecular events drive a sequence of events that ultimately lead to transcription of proteins controlling cell proliferation, migration, angiogenesis and apoptosis. These pathways are potential therapeutic targets. Signaling cascades implicated in etiopathogenesis of lymphomas (Fig. 8-27).

Challenges and Prospects

Sum up, the disorder of cell signal transduction has various effects on disease development, its reasons are various, gene mutation, bacterial toxin, cytokines, antibodies and other stress all can cause the primary injury of cell signal transduction process, or cause their secondary change. Cell signal transduction disorder can be limited to a single link, or simultaneously involving multiple signal transduction pathways, and even lead to regulate signal transduction network imbalance, caused the complex forms. The role of cell signal transduction disorder in disease is characterized by diversity, either as a direct cause of the disease, cause a particular disease; Can also interfere with a link of the disease, lead to specific signs or symptoms. Cell signal transduction disorder can also be mediated some nonspecific reaction, appeared in the process of different diseases. With the deepening of the research, has found more and more diseases or pathological process there exists abnormal signal transduction, recognizeing the change rule of signal transduction and its pathophysiological significances in disease development, can not only reveal the molecular mechanism of disease development, and puts forward in a new direction for disease prevention and control.

Consider/Questions

1. Basic concepts in this chapter

cellular signal ransduction, biological phenomenon, cell recognition, cell communication, receptor, ligant, transmembrane signal transduction, protein kinase (PK), second messenger, ras gene, transcription factor (transdactor), Cross-talk.

2. Which cells behaiviors were regulated by cellular signals?

3. Summarized the classification of cell communication.

4. Summarized the elements of a signal transduction system.

5. Briefly describes the roles of three kinds of messengers in signal transduction.

6. State the characteristics of cell signal transduction.

7. Which reasons are cancer caused by signal transduction disorder?

8. Giving an example, describe a disease related to cell signal transduction disorder, and analysis its mechanismes.

本章彩图

第九章 肿瘤血管形成

血管系统分布血液、氧气和营养物质到全身各组织。该系统由动脉、小动脉、毛细血管、小静脉和静脉组成。最小血管：微血管是循环系统的一部分，由最小的血管毛细血管、小动脉和小静脉组成。微血管是一个非常动态和复杂的系统，它具有不断变化的能力。较大的血管具有比较稳定的结构，可塑性不强。

动脉和静脉管壁厚度不同，最大的血管包括内膜、中膜和外膜。动脉、小动脉、小静脉和静脉以输送管道的功能为主。毛细血管由内皮细胞（endothelial cells，ECs）组成中空管腔，由周围细胞支持。毛细血管是心血管系统中最重要的通道，其薄壁允许血液与组织之间进行氧气和养分的交换。

血管形成是一个非常重要的过程，它涉及从先前存在的血管形成新血管。在胎儿发育、伤口愈合、排卵及生长发育过程中，正常血管形成是体内必需的重要过程[1]。血管形成是胚胎、胎儿正常发育的必要生理过程，血管形成为组织生长和发育提供了重要的营养物质和氧气[2]。正常成人血管不新生（非致病性血管生成可在成人卵巢周期中看到，在康复训练时或伤口愈合过程中在骨骼肌和心肌中也可看到）。

当血管形成异常时，病理问题往往随之而来。多种疾病病程伴有血管新生的病理过程：如恶性肿瘤、牛皮癣、子宫内膜异位症、关节炎、局灶性回肠炎和眼黄斑变性；因此提出了"血管新生依赖性疾病"（angiogenic-dependent disease）的概念。也有些疾病伴有血管减少，如阻塞性心脑血管病（动脉粥样硬化、心肌梗死）等。因此血管形成是一柄"双刃剑"，它既是生命之脉，又是死亡之脉。

对正常和病理血管形成的了解一直是过去数十年来癌症生物学和临床医学研究的焦点。21世纪，基于血管新生的治疗将成为多种疾病治疗的共同途径，如同 20 世纪抗生素治疗的作用一样，是医学创新的内容之一。

第一节 正常血管形成

成年人体内通过两种不同的机制发生血管形成，即血管发生（vasculogenesis）和血管生成（angiogenesis）。这两个过程通常都发生在胚胎发育期，然而特殊情况时这些过程可以在成年人中启动，这些过程均受到生理条件的严密调控。血管发生这种方式特别在胚胎发育时血管系统的形成（即从无到有）。从造血干细胞（hematopoietic stem cells，HSCs）转化为成血管细胞（angioblasts），进一步分化为血管内皮细胞，形成一种原始的小毛细血管[3]。血管生成指在原有血管的基础上再长出新的血管，即ECs从原有的血管壁以出芽和分化成新血管，这一方式常是损伤组织的修复机制。现今常用"angiogenesis"一词代表不同类型的血管生成过程。

一、胎儿血管建立

胎儿血管建立始于中胚层起源的原始细胞——HSCs和成血管细胞形成的"血岛"（特定的空间结构），位于血岛中心的HSCs分化为造血细胞，在血岛周边成血管细胞分化成ECs（图9-1）。

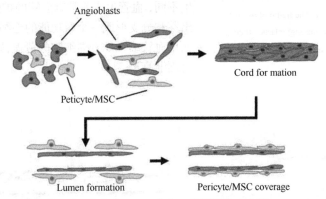

图9-1　由HSCs转化为成血管细胞，分化为ECs，形成一种原始的小血管；Only original vascular structures form in the early embryonic development by an angioblast and endothelial cell-derived HSCs

二、成人血管发生

目前认为，血管发生源于骨髓多能成体祖细胞（multipotent adult progenitor cells，MAPCs）[4]，由其分化成早期内皮祖细胞（endothelial progenitor cells，EPCs）。当MAPCs演变成EPCs，它们获得造血和内皮系特异性标志物，如血管内皮生长因子受体2（VEGFR-2）和CD34。骨髓中的EPCs在两区中的一区保持未分化状态。第一个区域被称为血管区，它由处于细胞周期S期或G_2/M期的EPCs组成。这些细胞在收到正确的信号后能分化和进入外周循环。第二个区域被称为成骨区，EPCs在那里处于细胞周期G_0期，不能释放入循环。这两个功能区之间的平衡是由存在于骨髓细胞外基质（ECM）和骨髓基质细胞的细胞因子所维持[5]（图9-2）。

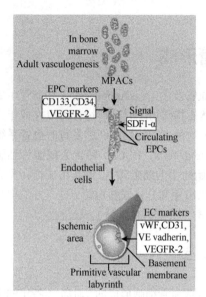

图 9-2　成人血管发生；Adult vasculogenesis.
MAPCs 分化为成血管细胞，然后在循环中分化为原始血管中的 EPCs 和 ECs；The figure illustrates the process where MAPCs become angioblasts, then circulating EPCs and ECs as part of the primitive vascular labyrinth

从骨髓来源的 MAPCs 有较大的可塑性，其与纤维连接蛋白（fibronectin, FN）和 VEGF-A 培养时能分化为 ECs。此外，在骨髓移植后 MAPCs 能分化成骨骼肌、心肌和 ECs。在病理情况下，如烧伤患者或接受冠状动脉搭桥术的患者循环中 EPCs 浓度在疾病发生后第一个 6 小时内提高了 60 倍，在 72 小时内回归到正常水平。这是由于血管和组织损伤诱导了几种细胞因子（包括 VEGF）的释放，促进了 EPCs 的动员使 EPCs 水平短暂提高，并启动血管发生。

三、血 管 再 生

与血管发生一样，血管生成通常在胚胎发育期发生，然而在受到特定刺激时它也可在成人期发生。非致病性血管生成可在成人卵巢周期中、在康复训练时或伤口愈合过程中的骨骼肌和心肌中见到。与血管发生不同，血管生成前常有血管的扩张，而后血管通过出芽和分支形成一个有功能的毛细血管床（图 9-3）。如果血管形成没有周细胞的覆盖，则该血管不稳定并会逐渐衰退。

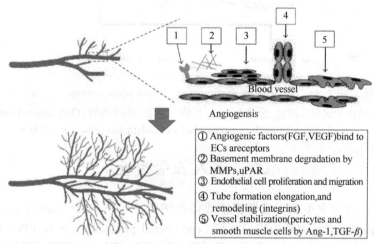

图 9-3　血管生成的过程；The process of angiogenesis
1. 血管形成因子在 EC 上与受体结合后，激活信号转导途径
2. 基质金属蛋白酶活化降解 ECM
3. EC 迁移、增殖
4. EC 表达的整合素促进其黏附于 ECM 并迁移形成管腔
5. 血管生成素（angiopoietin）1 与 Tie-2 受体结合，招募周细胞使血管稳定
①Angiogenic factors bind to their receptors on endothelial cells and activate the signal transduction pathways
②Matrix metalloproteinases are activated, and they degrade the extracellular matrix
③Endothelial cells migrate out of the preexisting capillary wall and proliferate
④Integrins are expressed by endothelial cells, facilitating their adhesion to the extracellular matrix and their migration for tube formation
⑤Angiopoietin 1 binds to TIE-2 receptors and stimulates pericyte recruitment and vessel stabilization

四、其他血管形成的模式

（1）套叠式血管形成（Intussusception angiogenesis）：并不是 ECs 增生而是 EC 突进血管，由周细胞、平滑肌细胞、成纤维细胞协助形成连接 EC 的桥分隔成两个血管（图 9-4）。

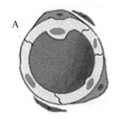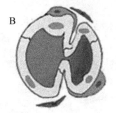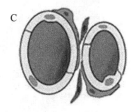

图 9-4　套叠式血管形成；Intussusception angiogenesis

（2）侧支小动脉形成（collateral arteriogenesis）：由 ECs 招募巨噬细胞和淋巴细胞，巨噬细胞降解 ECM 通过旁分泌信号调控 ECs、周细胞/平滑肌细胞的相互作用，导致小动脉生长和稳定（图 9-5）。

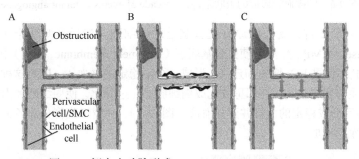

图 9-5　侧支小动脉形成；Collateral arteriogenesis

第二节　肿瘤血管形成

血管形成与癌症生物学研究总是紧密交织。在肿瘤发生中关于血管形成的假设由 Judah Folkman 在 1971 年首先提出[6]，当时他认为实体肿瘤中活跃增殖的癌细胞会争夺肿瘤所拥有的有限资源。肿瘤内细胞间的压力增加抑制了对肿瘤细胞生长和存活至关重要的代谢和营养物质的扩散。这种环境导致肿瘤细胞诱导从既定血管出芽形成新生血管，在肿瘤内部形成血管系统，从而使肿瘤细胞获得它们生存和增殖必需的氧气和营养。因此，抑制肿瘤血管形成可能是一种有价值的治疗肿瘤的方法[7]。因而引发对调节这一过程中蛋白质的研究，包括血管形成抑制剂和促进剂。自此，发现和了解了许多蛋白质和血管形成调节因子及其作用。

一、肿瘤血管形成过程

肿瘤始于宿主来源的无血管细胞团，因为失控性的生长常呈不典型增生。肿瘤最初赖以生存和发展依靠宿主周围环境中现成可使用的血管，通过血管中营养成分的渗透作用。此时肿瘤生长缓慢，直径常小于 1~2mm。当肿瘤生长超过 2~3mm^3，它们需要持续的血液供应以除去废物，输送养分[7]。如果肿瘤生长超过了局部血管供应的最大距离（大约 200μm），会引起肿瘤细胞缺氧[8]。为了对抗这种缺氧，肿瘤细胞会尝试创建新的血管，肿瘤血管形成是一个复杂得多步骤和多信号过程（图 9-6）。

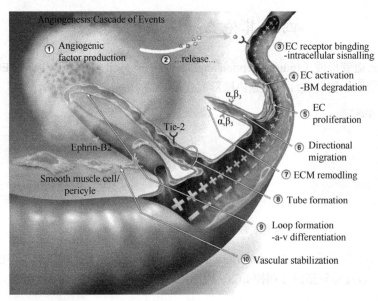

图 9-6 肿瘤血管形成的级联事件；Cascade of events in tumor angiogenesis

在肿瘤血管形成首先要去除原有血管壁上的周细胞，然后在基质金属蛋白酶（matrix metalloproteinase，MMP）作用下使血管基底膜（basement membrane，BM）和 ECM 降解，此时 VEGF、FGF 等促进 ECs 增殖和迁移，形成一个不稳定的微血管。随着这种血管的形成，间质细胞向这些血管聚集，随后在那里分化成周细胞。经过分化，使周细胞和内皮细胞发生细胞-细胞接触，然后形成稳定的血管并建立血流（图 9-7）。肿瘤细胞将分泌各种因子以保证在肿瘤组织中的新血管形成。

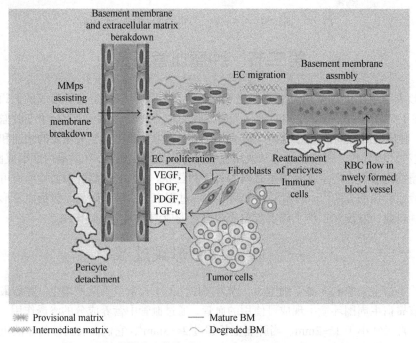

图 9-7 肿瘤影响血管生成；Tumor influenced angiogenesis

血管形成始于 BM 和 ECM，随后 ECs 增殖和迁移，最终形成稳定的血管；The stepwise process of angiogenesis begins with ECM and BM breakdown，followed by EC proliferation，EC migration and finally re-formation of stable blood vessel

二、血管生成与肿瘤（实体瘤）的关系

无血管形成的肿瘤是"没有危险的癌症"，即"无血管期"癌瘤无危险性（如直径<1mm 或<0.5cm^3，圆珠笔尖大小）。一旦肿瘤伴有血管形成后，癌瘤细胞呈指数生长，表现恶性生物学行为。癌瘤生长与转移依赖于血管新生（供氧，营养物）。血管形成是肿瘤演进的基础。

三、肿瘤血管形成与肿瘤浸润转移的关系

对于绝大多数肿瘤来说，仅约 1/1000 的肿瘤细胞具备浸润转移能力。原发肿瘤细胞必须获得进入血管系统的途径，能够在循环中生存、在靶器官微血管内着床、进入靶器官和诱发靶器官内的血管形成，才能完成转移；而且，转移瘤的细胞扩散再导致新的转移瘤的形成，同样需要经过这一连锁过程。

（一）肿瘤血管有利于肿瘤细胞转移

（1）新生肿瘤血管由于基底膜不完整且存在渗漏现象，为肿瘤转移提供了阻力最小的通道。

（2）内皮细胞分泌的胶原酶和纤维蛋白溶酶原激活物加强了肿瘤血管突起部的浸润趋化行为。这些"浸润性"毛细血管"吞噬"肿瘤细胞的行为，使肿瘤细胞更容易转移而扩散。

（3）肿瘤血管形成能增加周围生长活跃的肿瘤细胞与淋巴管的密切接触；或者增加淋巴静脉管的数量，使更多的血管内微转移细胞团进入淋巴系统。

（二）新生血管生成参与肿瘤浸润转移的全程

当休眠的肿瘤细胞达到临界体积（通常 1~2mm），并从肿瘤微环境（如缺氧）接收到细胞内信号时，肿瘤细胞开始分泌生长因子、细胞因子和其他信号分子。这些因素可影响基质细胞也产生上述因子，并使信号血管扩张，朝向肿瘤细胞生长。微血管在肿瘤中萌生，输送的营养、生长因子和氧气使其生存和增殖。最终在肿瘤中形成复杂的血管网，并有利于肿瘤细胞浸润至 BM 外和转移到其他组织，形成转移瘤（图 9-8）。

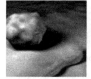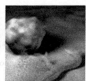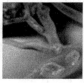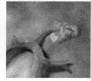

图 9-8　新生血管生成在肿瘤发展过程的不同阶段的作用；Angiogenesis plays various roles in stages of tumor development

尽管癌瘤具有"异质性"，但血管新生是各种肿瘤的共性（图 9-9）。

四、肿瘤血管形成模式

正常血管形成后很少延伸，但在肿瘤中通过多种机制导致血管形成。已观察到肿瘤血管形成的几种模式（图 9-10），如出芽、套叠、染色体异常的 CSCs 也能够分化为 ECs，或 EPCs 能分化成 ECs，促进血管形成，它可以驻留在血管壁，也可以在肿瘤细胞趋化因子作用下从骨髓迁移。当肿瘤细胞替代 ECs 发生血管生成拟态（vasculogenic mimicry）[9]。

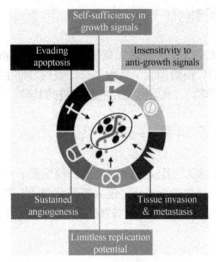

图 9-9　肿瘤中血管形成对其生长的意义；The significance of tumors angiogenesis

血管生成拟态是一种与经典的肿瘤血管生成途径完全不同的、不依赖 ECs 的肿瘤血管生成。肿瘤细胞通过自身变形和基质重塑产生血管样通道，通道内无内皮细胞衬覆，通道外基底膜 PAS 染色为阳性，形成可输送血液的管道系统，并在某个环节与宿主血管相连使肿瘤获得血供，重建肿瘤的微循环。

（一）血管生成拟态的特点

（1）一层厚薄不一 PAS 阳性物质将瘤细胞和血流分开（红细胞在 PAS 阳性物质形成的管道中流动），血管生成拟态有不同形状的 PAS 阳性图案。

（2）由高度侵袭性肿瘤细胞以无 ECs 衬覆的形式主动形成，并非是在血流冲力下被动形成，或由 ECs 增生形成。

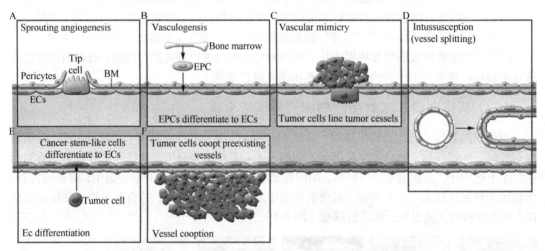

图 9-10　肿瘤血管形成模式；Angiogenesis mode

A. 肿瘤细胞释放 VEGF 引起血管形成；B. 三种血管祖细胞分化成内皮细胞协同形成肿瘤血管；C. 肿瘤细胞血管拟态的发生；D. 肿瘤插入或套叠分隔原有血管；E. 肿瘤干细胞也能够分化为内皮细胞；F. 肿瘤吸附于原来血管；A. Tumor cells release VEGF causing the sprouting angiogenesis. B. Three angiogenic progenitor cells differentiate to ECs induce the formation of tumor angiogenesis C. Tumor cell occurs vascular mimicry. D. Tumor separately insert or overlay existing vessels，intussusception between the spliffing of original tumor blood vessels. E. CSCs are able to differentiate into endothelial cells F. Tumor cell suck in original tumor blood vessels（vessel cooption）

（3）血管生成拟态中基质衬覆的血管无红细胞漏出，相反，毛细血管通过出芽的方式进入肿瘤组织内，可以见到在瘤细胞之间漏出的红细胞。

（4）很少有微血栓，推测瘤细胞或血管外基质有抗凝功能。

（5）对肿瘤血管的标志物均为阴性（无 ECs）。

（二）血管生成拟态的意义

（1）不同肿瘤可以获得不同的血管形成机制，或同种肿瘤有多种血管形成机制。

（2）肿瘤恶性度与血管生成拟态反相关；具有血管生成拟态的肿瘤内常无中央坏死灶。

（3）PAS 阳性物可能是机体对肿瘤的基质反应，即所谓纤维化血管化。

体外研究结果也显示不仅葡萄膜黑色素瘤的血管生成拟态微循环有侵袭性的瘤细胞构成，而且在成纤维细胞、其他基质细胞和 ECs 不存在时，这些血管生成拟态也可能出现。

五、肿瘤血管形成的分子机制

已知肿瘤血管形成是肿瘤发生、发展和浸润与转移的重要条件。肿瘤血管生成过程受到各种血管生成因子和抗血管生成因子的共同调控。

（一）有关血管出芽性生长的机制

（1）由促血管生成因子（如 VEGF）启动血管出芽。

管芽前沿的 ECs 为芽尖细胞（tip cell）伸出丝状伪足并朝向血管生成信号迁移。VEGF 激活 VEGFR2 以刺激芽尖细胞迁移。辅助受体 Nrp1 联合并增强 VEGFR2 信号。ECs 既是芽尖细胞又是增殖的芽柄细胞（stalk cell），Notch 调节 ECs 的表型变化。伴有 VEGFR2 信号活性的 ECs 通过增加 DLL4 的表达来争夺的芽尖细胞的位置，而在相邻的 ECs 上 DLL4 与 Notch 受体结合，可释放转录调节受体 NICD。NICD 转录性的下调 VEGFR2 和 Nrp1 表达，同时增加 VEGFR1（另一种 VEGF 受体），从而抑制了芽柄细胞对 VEGF 反应。

芽尖细胞在出芽的前端位置并不固定，它根据 VEGFR1/ VEGFR2 不同的比例向前方移动。芽尖细胞迁移需要 BM 降解（部分由 MMPS 作用）、ECs 连接的松动（由 VE-钙黏着蛋白、ZO-1 及其他因素调节）和周细胞脱离（由 Ang2 调节）。VEGF 增加血管的渗透性，使已沉积为临时基质层的血浆蛋白外渗（如纤连蛋白和纤维蛋白原），而原有的 ECM 被蛋白酶改造，这些因素均导致芽尖细胞的迁移（图 9-11）。

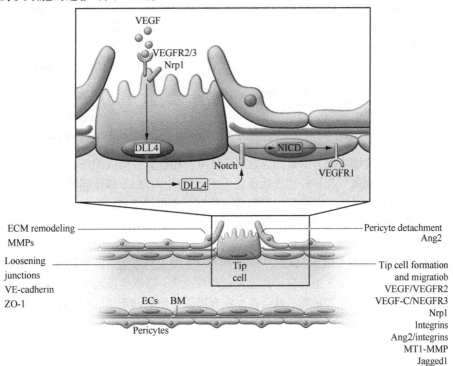

图 9-11　芽尖细胞选择性启动步骤；Initial steps of tip cell selection

（2）芽尖细胞导向和芽柄细胞延伸：芽尖细胞黏附到 ECM，通过整合素介导向信号分子方向迁移。虽然 Notch 信号抑制细胞增殖，但在信号交汇点上 Nrarp 的表达保证了 Wnt 信号使芽柄细胞增殖。这个系统通过芽尖细胞保证了血管迁移的方向，通过柄细胞增殖使血管芽延伸。当两个芽尖细胞相遇，他们互相融合（吻合），该机制由巨噬细胞辅助完成。巨噬细胞在血管吻合处积聚，作为接应芽尖细胞丝状伪足互动的桥梁细胞，通过产生血管生成因子或释放蛋白酶降解 ECM 进一步受刺激血管芽生成。一旦芽尖细胞之间的连接建立，VE-钙黏着蛋白将进一步加强它们的连接。随后芽尖细胞沉积于 BM，并招募周细胞。MAPCs 被 ECs 表达的 PDGF 吸引到新血管分化为周细胞，并对 TGF-β 做出反应，抑制 ECs 的迁移、增殖和血管渗漏，使新生血管稳定（图 9-12）。

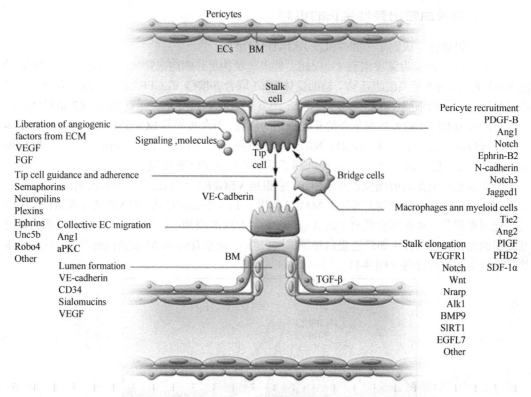

图 9-12　芽尖细胞导向和芽柄细胞延伸；Tip cell guidance and stalk elongation

（3）通过静态指骨细胞的分解达到成熟：一旦融合相连管腔形成的新血管中血流通过，缺氧组织得到灌注。得到氧气和营养输送后血管生成信号减少，ECs 氧传感器失活，促静态分子增加，致 ECs 恢复静态分布，在血流表面形成流线型紧密单层排列，其表面与血液接触调节组织灌注。在血流的建立中通过应激反应转录因子 KLF2 调节，重塑血管间的连接，周细胞成熟和 BM 沉积使血管成熟（图 9-13）。

来自 ECs 和周围含有 VEGF、FGF、Ang1 和 Notch 的支持细胞，以及其他一些细胞的自分泌和旁分泌，维持静态 ECs 表型和保护血管免受环境应力。降低生长因子信号可导致血管收缩和 ECs 凋亡。一旦血管稳定和成熟，就会在血液和周围组织之间形成屏障，控制液体和溶质的交换。

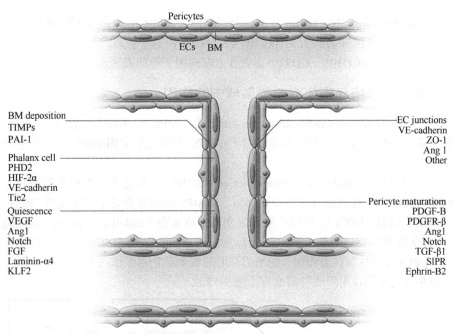

图 9-13　通过静态连接细胞的分布使血管成熟；Maturation through resolution of quiescent phalanx cells

血管出芽方式的生成过程如图 9-14 所示。

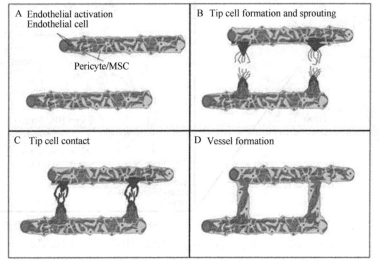

图 9-14　出芽方式的血管生成；Sprouting angiogenesis

（二）肿瘤干细胞驱动肿瘤血管形成

肿瘤干细胞（cancer stem cells，CSCs）在某些恶性肿瘤具有驱动肿瘤血管形成和（或）参与血管生成拟态，促进肿瘤生长的潜在能力。

CSCs 和血管生成信号通路的关系如下。

（1）BMP-9 通过 BMP-9/ALK1 途径抑制 VEGF 的表达，与 TGFB1/ALK5 途径相反，其可以增强 VEGF 的表达和血管生成的效果。在这两种途径之间，平衡的关键作用是 BMP-4，其可以保持血管完整性。

（2）Notch 通过 Notch/NICD/Hes/Hey 信号通路诱导血管发育与正常干细胞的存活。Notch 抑制剂 DAPT（G-分泌酶抑制剂），不仅降低 CSCs 的自我更新能力，和 CD133⁺细胞的数目，也降低了血管标志物如 CD105、CD31、血管性血友病因子等的表达。

（三）血管干细胞在实体瘤血管形成中的作用

（1）间充质祖细胞（mesenchymal progenitor cells，MPC）：来源于骨髓或附近的组织能分泌 VEGF，是一种有效的 ECs 存活和运动因子。MPC 可分化形成周细胞以提供新生血管结构支撑。

（2）造血祖细胞（hematopoietic progenitor cells，HPC）：通过表达组织重塑和 ECs 存活因子如 VEGF 和 MMP9，提供旁分泌给芽尖细胞，与 MPC 相似在血管生成中充当"附件"细胞。

（3）内皮祖细胞（EPCs）：可以产生 ECs 集落形成细胞（endothelial colony-forming cells，ECFC）和分化成 ECs 促进血管形成。ECFC 为周边成熟 ECs 或 HPC 的招募池提供独特的旁分泌物质。EPCs 可以驻留在血管壁，也可以在肿瘤细胞趋化因子作用下迁移出骨髓。

这三种祖细胞协同作用形成肿瘤血管（图 9-15）。

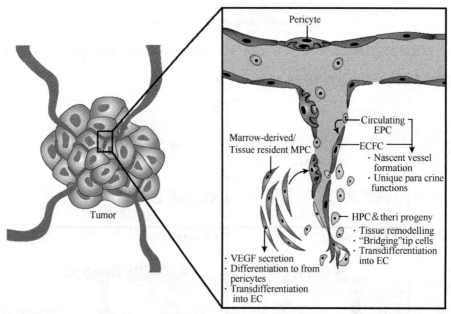

图 9-15　ECFC 和 MPC 形成管腔和周围细胞，HPC 直接引导和（或）协调血管芽形成及血管吻合；ECFC and MPC form lumens and perivascular cells, respectively, whereas HPC direct and or chestrate vessel sprouting and anastomosis

第三节　肿瘤新生血管的特点

肿瘤血管的特点主要表现为失控性生长、不成熟性的管壁结构、异常的分布与密度和异质性的生物学作用。

一、血　管　结　构

由于肿瘤组织中血管生成生长因子持续高水平释放使肿瘤新生血管出现迅速，生长快，并呈持续性的特点，10%～20%的肿瘤血管 ECs 始终处于 DNA 合成状态。肿瘤血管扩张、囊状、曲折，以混乱的方式互连。正常的血管的特点是二叉分枝，但肿瘤血管可呈现三分叉或不均匀直径的分支。而且在肿瘤中血管分布不均，一般认为外周血管丰富时中央血管少，而中央血管丰富时外围血管则少。新生血管可从肿瘤外围围绕肿瘤生长，亦可以直接进入肿瘤中央，呈树状向外分支性生长。较大的癌块中间动、静脉分支吻合可形成血管湖，这些统称为肿瘤相关性血管病变。

造成这种异常血管结构的分子机制还不是很清楚，但失控制的 VEGF 信号可能是一个关键因素。通过干扰 VEGF 可观察到肿瘤血管的"正常化"，即直接靶向 VEGF 或 VEGF 受体减少 VEGF 的治疗（如激素依赖性肿瘤中激素撤退），或模仿抗血管生成的一种鸡尾酒试剂（如曲妥珠单抗治疗 HER2 过度表达的肿瘤）。瘤细胞增殖产生的实体（机械）性应力也将压迫血管。因此，分子和力学两因素的结合使肿瘤血管异常，在设计新的癌症治疗策略时应考虑这两类因素。

二、血流量与微循环

无论是正常还是异常，均由动静脉压差和流体阻力控制血管网中血流。流体阻力是血管结构（简称几何电阻）和全血黏度（流变学，称为黏性阻力）的作用结果。血管结构和黏度的异常增加肿瘤中血流阻力。导致肿瘤的整体灌注率（单位体积的血流量）低于许多正常组织，平均 RBC 速率可以低于正常一个数量级。此外，肿瘤血流量分布不均，随时间波动，甚至可以在某些血管逆流，常见于灌注差或根本没有灌注的区域。肿瘤中表现为不适当的血供和血流速度。

肿瘤中有细胞丰富区、边缘区、半坏死区和坏死区，各区血供不尽相同，半坏死区与坏死区血流明显减少减慢，非坏死区血流速度可以快于正常组织。大肿瘤血流速度的均值低于小肿瘤。在大肿瘤中实际增加的效应血管管径小，血流慢，营养供给少。在肿瘤中 ECs 增生指数为 2.2%，肿瘤细胞增生指数为 7.3%。同样小鼠瘤细胞 22 小时更新一代，ECs 是 50 小时更新一代。用显微分光光度计研究肿瘤血流的质与量，其中红细胞常出现完全性脱氧，瘤内 10%～40% 仅为 ECs 所构成的血管，无相应的营养血流，氧利用率很低。癌细胞增生、癌内缺乏淋巴管网、瘤体间流体静脉压升高、压迫小血管，使瘤内血流量仅为正常的 1%～10%。肿瘤微循环较肿瘤生长表现出低效和相对不足，肿瘤组织特别是中心部位常因为缺血、缺氧而坏死。瘤细胞无氧酵解产生大量 H^+，使肿瘤中存在着不同程度的低营养、低 pH、低氧的三低细胞群。肿瘤血流量的异质性是肿瘤急性和慢性缺氧的一个重要因素，还是抗放疗和其他疗法的主要原因。

三、血管通透性

血液分子外渗发生扩散、对流，并在一定程度上通过血管物质交换的转胞作用。扩散被认为是肿瘤血管交换运输主要形式。一个分子的扩散渗透性取决于它的大小、形状、电荷、可塑性及血管转运途径。内皮细胞间隙增宽，窗孔数量增加，囊泡和液泡通道出现，以及在肿瘤血管缺乏正常的基底膜和血管周细胞。这些超微结构改变使实体肿瘤血管通透性一般高于在各种正常组织。

肿瘤血管壁通常不规则，窦状壁薄，由肿瘤细胞和 ECs 组成，外周常缺乏功能性周细胞，并且 BM 不完整，导致这些血管渗漏。同时实体性肿瘤中心缺氧性坏死刺激 VEGF 活化也增加了血管通透性，加重了肿瘤血管渗漏。但是缺乏周细胞的肿瘤血管更易受到抗 VEGF 治疗的攻击。由于很少进化为成熟的小动脉或小静脉，不具收缩功能，不受神经体液调节，正常血管有活性的物质对该血管不起作用（乙酰胆碱、血管紧张素Ⅱ、温度）。

尽管大部分肿瘤中血管通透性增加，但并非所有肿瘤血管都如此。不仅在不同肿瘤中血管通透性不同，即使在同一肿瘤在其生长、退化或复发过程的不同空间和时间中也不同。局部微环境在控制血管通透性中起重要的作用。例如，人脑胶质瘤（hgl21）生长在免疫缺陷小鼠皮下时有血管透漏，但生长在颅窗的肿瘤中显示血脑屏障存在的特性。肿瘤-宿主相互作用可能控制与通透性增加（如 VEGF）和减少（如血管生成素 1）相关细胞因子的产生和分泌。此外，血管对刺激的反应取决于宿主器官的部位和宿主-肿瘤相互作用。

四、血管内皮细胞的异质性

肿瘤血管 ECs 的异质性是其突出的生物学特性，主要表现在 ECs 的结构、功能、抗原成分、代谢特点上。某些器官肿瘤组织中 ECs 具有这些肿瘤细胞表达的抗原性（如脑、卵巢、肺癌的血管 ECs），这可能在肿瘤转移时的选择性黏附、体液因子的区域性释放中发挥作用。如在胰腺癌中，癌细胞和肿瘤增殖血管 ECs 均高表达巢蛋白（nestin），后者促进胰腺癌的肝转移（图 9-16）。在肿瘤血管周细胞的形态异常也与血管异质性有关（表 9-1）。

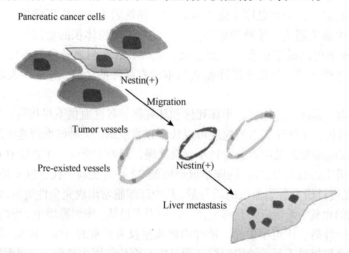

图 9-16　高表达巢蛋白的胰腺癌经高表达巢蛋白的肿瘤增殖血管转移到肝；The pancreatic cancer with highly expressing nestin metastasis to liver through the small proliferating tumor vessels with highly expressing nestin

表 9-1　肿瘤血管结构和功能异常的关系

结构异常（血管紊乱）	功能异常（循环紊乱）
1.管壁异常 内皮细胞不完整或缺如，基底膜中断或缺如。肿瘤细胞排列形成血道外膜细胞、有收缩性的管壁成分及药理学/生理学受体缺如	1. 形态学变化结果 动静脉短路开放，血液反流或中断，血流速度或方向不稳定，血管舒缩性能丧失，血管壁脆性增高，微血管被白细胞和（或）肿瘤细胞阻塞，肿瘤血管阻力增大
2.血管构筑异常 外形不规则（窦状或囊腔样血管形成），血管壁盘绕、扭曲、拉长。动静脉短路存在（肿瘤团块血流＞起营养作用血流）血管分级不明显	2. 流变学变化结果 红细胞沉积，白细胞黏附，血小板聚集，微血小板或巨血小板形成，血液黏度增加
3.血管密度异常 血管形成不均匀分布（混乱的血管网和无血管区域出现），毛细血管间距扩大	3. 血管通透性增加结果 血液浓缩，间质内液体增多，间质流体压力增高（由于肿瘤微血管压迫所致），血细胞外渗、出血，黏性阻力增加

第四节 调控肿瘤血管形成的因素

肿瘤血管形成由血管生成因子和抗血管生成因子相互作用来调节，既受机体神经内分泌因素影响，又受肿瘤细胞和肿瘤基质细胞表达的生长因子调控。许多蛋白质和血管生成调节因子已被发现，它们的作用也被了解。已经报道的有30多种血管生长因子和抑制因子。

一、促肿瘤血管生成因子

多种生长因子参与了促进肿瘤血管形成。这些因子与其受体或蛋白与蛋白的结合，导致下游信号传导途径激活，以促进ECs增殖、迁移及血管生成和血管通透性增加。

（一）VEGF和VEGFR

VEGF是一种重要的调节血管发生和血管生成的因子，也是一种可以促进内皮细胞和血管发生的促有丝分裂因子。在肿瘤中VEGF被认为是最强的促血管形成因子，分别与肿瘤生长、血管密度和转移有关。几种正常的细胞，包括成纤维细胞、ECs和角质形成细胞在整个生命过程中释放少量的VEGF。

1. VEGF的结构 目前有6种已知的VEGF单体，它们来源于由8个外显子组成的单一基因。异构体包含121、145、165、183、189或206基因。其中一些亚型与细胞或膜连接，而另一些则释放到细胞外。除了这些区别，它们都具有相同的生物学行为。

2. VEGF的作用 ①血管形成的启动子；②刺激微血管ECs增殖；③促进ECs迁移和出芽；④抑制ECs凋亡；⑤增加ECs渗透性[10, 11]。

3. VEGFR VEGF与两种不同的酪氨酸激酶受体作用来改变血管生成，它们分别是VEGFR1（Flt-1）和VEGFR2（Flk-1）。VEGFR1与VEGF的相互作用非常强烈，但这种相互作用在血管生成中扮演次要角色。VEGFR1是VEGF活性的一个抑制因子，负性调节VEGF的功能。VEGFR2与VEGF的相互作用促进ECs有丝分裂、趋化、血管生成和增加VEGF的血管通透性作用。在ECs和EPCs上可观察到VEGFR2的表达。

4. 与肿瘤的相关性研究 目前在VEGF引起的肿瘤血管形成与干预性的研究主要在四个方面。

（1）在mRNA和蛋白质水平上研究原发与转移性肿瘤中VEGF/VPF的过表达（胃肠道癌、胰腺癌、乳腺癌、肾癌、膀胱癌和胶质母细胞瘤等的研究）。

（2）肿瘤微血管ECs上受体过表达与肿瘤发生的关系。

（3）与肿瘤血管显著相关的血浆蛋白、纤维蛋白原渗出与血管外纤维蛋白的交联和沉积，促进肿瘤、肿瘤微环境间质成分形成的研究。

（4）人源化的抗VEGF抗体的可行性与安全性研究。

笔者曾经的研究显示：胶质瘤中VEGF蛋白阳性染色主要定位于肿瘤细胞的胞质，内皮细胞也可呈阳性表达。43例脑星形细胞瘤组织中肿瘤细胞VEGF阳性表达率为77.0%。Ⅰ、Ⅱ级组VEGF阳性表达率和表达强度均显著低于Ⅲ、Ⅳ级组，VEGF表达强度与MVD呈等级正相关。肿瘤血管主要呈三种形态：①芽状血管；②囊状血管；③丛状血管。在恶性程度低的肿瘤（Ⅰ级和Ⅱ级）内增生的血管以芽状和囊状血管为主，丛状血管不多见，恶性程度高的肿瘤（Ⅲ级和Ⅳ级）内增生的微血管中含有较多的丛状血管。VEGF表达情况和MVD及肿瘤微血管形态可能有助于判断星形细胞瘤的恶性程度[12]。

　　抗 VEGF 信号通路药也进行了大量的临床测试和实验室研究,旨在抑制与癌症有关的血管生成。这些药物的目标是 VEGF(avastin),或 VEGFRs(nexavar and sutent)。虽然这些药物在动物模型上有显著的结果,但在临床试验中结果却不一。已有临床试验显示多达 94% 的侵袭性癌症和 88% 的原位癌有较好的疗效。这些患者 5 年内随访未见复发[13]。然而许多以血管生成通路为目标的其他血管生成抑制剂在部分患者身上并没有产生同样的长期反应。

(二)碱性成纤维细胞生长因子

　　碱性成纤维细胞生长因子(basic fibroblast growth factor,bFGF)对维护肿瘤血管生成过程有重要作用,但不像 VEGF 能启动肿瘤血管生成。bFGF 也能促进 VEGF 的产生,上调血管平滑肌中 VEGF mRNA 水平,增加微血管 ECs 上 VEGFR 的含量。

　　bFGF 的作用:①刺激 ECs 增殖;②促进微血管管道形成;③促进 ECs 迁移;④组织损伤后血管重塑的重要启动子[14]。

(三)内皮蛋白

　　内皮蛋白(endoglin,Eng)是一种细胞表面的二聚体糖蛋白,是 TGF-β 的辅助受体。Eng(CD105)可见于增殖 ECs,是一种 EPC 的标志物[15]。在血管生成和炎症过程中 Eng 表达显著增加。在不同肿瘤中使用抗-Eng 治疗有希望能防止肿瘤血管生成。

　　CD105 在肿瘤血管生成中的作用:①CD105 拮抗 TGF-β 及其受体对血管 ECs 的抑制作用,促进肿瘤血管生成。②CD105 是 ECs 增殖的标志仅在处于增殖状态的肿瘤组织中血管 ECs 上高表达。血清 CD105 水平可以用来对实体肿瘤患者长期随访,预测疾病复发、转移的风险。

　　笔者比较了乳腺良性病变与癌中 CD105 标记的微血管密度(MVD),发现乳腺癌组明显增高。MVD 值与肿瘤淋巴结转移相关。乳腺癌中 P53 蛋白表达与 CD105 呈正相关。单因素(Log rank)检验结果显示乳腺癌 CD105 标记的 MVD、P53 表达、淋巴结转移、TNM 分期与 ER 是影响预后的因素。多因素(Cox 比例风险模型)生存分析显示乳腺癌 CD105 标记的 MVD 是独立的预后因素[16]。

(四)血管生成素受体

　　血管生成素受体(angiopoietin receptor)属于酪氨酸蛋白激酶家族,由 ECs 表达与 VEGFR 功能相仿。迄今为止,已确定酪氨酸蛋白激酶-1(Tie1)和酪氨酸蛋白激酶-2(Tie2)的作用机制,Tie1 和 Tie2 受体主要对血管完整性发挥调节作用,Tie2 对血管生成时的血管出芽和分支也有重要作用。

(五)血管生成素

　　血管生成素(angiopoietin)是蛋白生长因子(一种小多肽),是 ECs 上 Tie 受体的配体。有两种重要的血管生成素在血管生成中发挥作用,Ang-1 和 Ang-2。

　　(1)Ang-1 是一种已经定性清楚的血管生成调节因子。①Ang-1 是 Tie2 受体的激动剂和配体。在体内招募周细胞至新血管,加强新血管的稳定性,降低新血管的通透性。②Ang-1 有利于促进 ECs 生存和出芽。③Ang-1 增加血管 ECs 直径[17]。

　　(2)Ang-2:①Tie-2 受体拮抗剂,降低周细胞水平,导致血管不稳定或破裂;②早期肿瘤血管 ECs 高表达 Ang-2,Ang-2 与血管降解有关,可作为肿瘤诱导性血管生成的早期生物标志物;③增加新形成血管的可塑性[8]。

（六）促血管素

促血管素（angiotropin）是最初从外周单核细胞中分离出来的一种多聚核酸肽。在肿瘤血管形成中的作用：①在伤口愈合过程中帮助激活微血管 ECs；②在体内刺激血管生成；③随机诱导毛细血管 ECs 迁移[18, 19]。

（七）血小板衍生生长因子

血小板衍生生长因子（platelet-derived growth factor，PDGF）是另一种重要的信号分子，它在血管生成中发挥几种不同的作用。尽管最初由血小板纯化而来，但它也出现在成纤维细胞、星形胶质细胞、ECs 和其他一些类型的细胞中。PDGF 在肿瘤血管形成中的主要作用：①增加毛细血管壁的稳定性；②刺激培养的周细胞和平滑肌细胞增殖；③增加毛细血管 ECs DNA 的合成；④促进体外血管出芽[2, 18, 19]。

PDGF 与周细胞上 PDGF 受体相互作用增加了 Ang-1 的表达。Ang-1 的增加导致了信号级联反应，有助于周细胞和 ECs 相互作用，这种相互作用对维持新形成毛细血管管壁的稳定性非常重要，是新血管形成的重要组成部分。阻断 PDGF 与其受体的结合会减少毛细血管生长的稳定性，使其无法为癌细胞提供养分。

（八）转化生长因子-β

转化生长因子-β（transforming growth factor-β，TGF-β）是一个二聚体细胞因子家族，调控体内许多生物学进程，包括血管生成。TGF-β 通常出现在许多不同类型细胞和 ECM 中。在微血管内，ECs 和周细胞都产生和表达 TGF-β。目前认为，TGF-β 具有促进和抗血管生成的两种特性：①低剂量上调血管生成因子和蛋白酶帮助启动血管生成转化。②高剂量抑制 ECs 生长，促进骨髓再生，刺激平滑肌细胞再生。③刺激和抑制 ECs 管芽的生长。④炎症细胞（如成纤维细胞和单核细胞 TGF-β）释放炎症介质信号，介质到达血管生成区释放促血管生成因子（如 VEGF、FGC 和 PDGF）。⑤加强血管壁完整性[20]。肿瘤细胞表达 TGF-β 能诱导间质反应，导致反应性基质微环境的形成，促进血管生成和肿瘤生长。

（九）整合素

整合素（Integrin）作为黏附分子在细胞与细胞接触中发挥重要作用。它们含有多种 α-和 β-亚单位，由已知亚单位组成的复合物已有 20 多种。整合素是许多不同细胞过程（包括血管形成）的重要的调节因子。在所有整合素中，$\alpha_V\beta_5$ 与 VEGF 相互作用[21]，促进血管生成。$\alpha_V\beta_3$ 是研究最广泛的一种，它在血管生成中有重要作用。在肿瘤血管形成中 $\alpha_V\beta_3$ 的作用：①结合并激活 MMP-2 帮助降解 ECM；②帮助调节细胞的黏附、伸展和迁移；③增加伤口附近 ECs 活化；④在 ECs 发芽期定位于正在生长的血管末端 ECs 上[21, 22]。

（十）血管内皮细胞钙黏着蛋白

钙黏着蛋白（vascular endothelial Cadherin）是一类钙结合跨膜蛋白，在细胞间相互作用中发挥重要作用。几项研究都强调了一种 VE cadherin 在新生血管中的重要作用。VE cadherin 特异性定位于 ECs 间黏着连接处，使血管壁 ECs 连接处保持稳定。VE cadherin 在肿瘤血管形成中的作用：①通过介质促进分子跨过 ECs；②通过接触抑制调节 ECs 生长；③通过促进 VEGF 信号防止 ECs 凋亡；④有助于稳定在血管生成阶段产生的血管分支和血管芽[10, 11, 23]。

（十一）白细胞介素

白细胞介素（interleukins，ILs）是一组由白细胞释放的细胞因子，调控广泛的生物学活性。少数 ILs 影响血管的生长[24]。无论是增强或抑制血管生成的能力均基于谷氨酸-亮氨酸-精氨酸（ELR）是否存在于氨基端。IL-8 拥有这个序列能增强血管生成，而 IL-4 不含这个序列，则是一个血管生成抑制剂。

IL-8 由巨噬细胞产生，在正常血管生成中不发挥重要作用。但作为一个肿瘤性血管生成的调控中心。已经证实，在几种肿瘤组织中 IL-8 水平升高。增加 IL-8 的表达与新生血管密度增加和肿瘤生长增加有关。IL-8 的一个重要特性是它能够增加 MMP-2 的水平，MMP-2 能降解 BM 和重塑 ECM，启动肿瘤血管生成早期阶段。

（十二）其他因素

许多其他因子也被证明在血管发生中发挥作用，但它们对脉管系统的影响没有上述因子广泛，也没有上述因子研究的透彻。

（1）肿瘤坏死因子-α（tumor necrosis factor-α，TNF-α）是由激活巨噬细胞分泌的一种细胞因子。在肿瘤血管形成中的作用：①在体内刺激血管生成；②在体外刺激 ECs 管形成[25]。

（2）TGF-α 是巨噬细胞分泌的另一种细胞因子。在肿瘤血管形成中的作用：①促进 ECs 增殖；②在体内刺激血管生成[26]。

（3）MMP-9 在肿瘤血管形成中有助于裂解 ECM 来调动 EPC[5, 27]。最近的一项研究证实早期乳腺癌和大肠癌患者基质金属蛋白酶-9 和血管内皮生长因子- A 的水平与普通患者相比有变化[28]。

（4）基质细胞衍生因子-1（stromal cell-derived factor-1，SDF - 1）在肿瘤血管形成中帮助引导 EPC 到缺血区[29]。

二、肿瘤血管生成抑制因子

（一）血管抑素

血管抑制素（angiostatin）是一种 38 kDa 的纤溶酶原内部片段，对肿瘤血管形成的抑制作用：①血管抑制素通过增加转移性肿瘤细胞凋亡率来减少远处转移。②抑制体外毛细血管 ECs 生长[30]。

（二）内皮细胞抑制素

内皮细胞抑制素（endostatin）是 18 胶原蛋白羧基端 20kDa 内部片段，是一种重要的 BM 蛋白多糖，抑制血管的作用：①抑制迁移、增殖和管形成，通过下调 cyclin-D1 启动子的转录活性，阻断 ECs 的细胞周期，抑制 ECs 增殖；通过诱导 caspase-9 活化促进凋亡通路，导致抗凋亡蛋白 Bcl-2、Bcl-xL 和 Bad 的减少；②阻断 VEGF 与 VEGFR2 相互作用[31]。

通过研究唐氏综合征患者获得了血管抑素的重要证据。唐氏综合征患者由于有 21 号染色体三体，而有三个 18 号胶原蛋白。这些患者内皮细胞抑制素水平增加 1.6～2 倍，并显著降低了与新生血管有关的肿瘤（除睾丸癌和巨核细胞性白血病外）、动脉粥样硬化和糖尿病性视网膜病变的严重程度。肿瘤、动脉粥样硬化和糖尿病性视网膜病变这三种疾病都是血管生成依赖性疾病，内皮细胞抑制素在抑制人类不必要的病理性血管生成中发挥重要的作用[32]。

（三）抑瘤蛋白

已知Ⅳ型胶原蛋白降解释放出 28kDa 的片段为抑瘤蛋白（tumstatin），这种化合物显示抗血管生成的特性。抑瘤蛋白绑定在整合素 αVβ3 上，导致 ECs 在 G_1 期阻滞并被诱导凋亡[33]。

（四）血小板因子 4

血小板活化因子 4（platelet factor-4，PF4）是由活化血小板 α-颗粒分泌的趋化因子，通常促进血液凝固。此外，PF4 还是一种血管生成抑制剂。其作用：①PF4 高亲和性的与 ECs 表面肝素样黏多糖结合，阻断它们的活性。②PF4 抑制 MMP-1 和 MMP-3 上调，抑制 ECs 迁移。③PF4 破坏 pRB 磷酸化抑制 ECs 的细胞周期[34]。

（五）血小板反应蛋白

血小板反应蛋白（thrombospondin-1，TSP-1）是第一个被发现的天然生成的血管抑制蛋白，是一种多域基质糖蛋白，即一种天然的全长蛋白。TSP-1 与 TGF-β1 结合存储在血小板 α-颗粒，当 TSP-1 与 TGF-β1 解离时可从血小板释放。TSP-1 抑制 ECs 增殖，诱导 ECs 凋亡。其作用：①诱导 ECs 与其调控几种重要的细胞凋亡因子的浓度有关。TSP-1 上调 Bax，下调 Bcl-2，并激活 caspase3 通路，导致程序性 ECs 死亡。②减缓 ECs 迁移，TSP-1 与 ECs 表面接受促进迁移信号的受体结合[35]。

（六）组织金属蛋白酶组织抑制剂

组织金属蛋白酶（tissue inhibitor of metalloproteinase，TIMPs）来自软骨蛋白水解酶家族，能抑制 MMPs。正如前面提到，MMPs 在启动血管形成中发挥不可或缺的作用，它们负责 BM 降解和 ECM 重塑。在血管生成反应中由 MMPs 介导形成的 ECM 为 ECs 黏附、迁移和管形成传递养分提供了一个支架。TIMPs 对 MMPs 的抑制降低了 ECs 血管形成的能力。高水平的 TIMP-1 显著抑制了体外 ECs 在明胶中的迁移[36]。

（七）IL-4

IL-4 为一种肿瘤生长抑制因子，但它的作用随不同肿瘤细胞而改变。例如，在结肠肿瘤、头颈部肿瘤、胶质母细胞瘤中，IL-4 能直接抑制癌症细胞增殖；而在另一些情况下，如 B 细胞淋巴瘤和黑色素瘤中，IL-4 能诱导对抗肿瘤的宿主免疫反应。还有证据表明，IL-4 抑制血管新生，从而抑制肿瘤的生长[37]。

在体外研究中，IL-4 抑制 ECs 趋向 bFGF 的迁移。在体内已证实 IL-4 能抑制由高浓度 bFGF 诱导的大鼠角膜血管新生。这些实验表明，IL-4 抑制肿瘤生长，可能是由于 IL-4 抑制血管生成的过程。在其他非癌症相关动物研究也表明 IL-4 具有体内抗血管生成的能力。

（八）干扰素

干扰素（interferons，IFNs）作为一种细胞因子属于分泌性糖蛋白的大家族。它们是由各种免疫细胞产生和分泌。IFN-α 和 IFN-β 都能通过抑制 b-FGF mRNA 和蛋白水平来抑制血管生成。除了下调关键的血管生成信号因子，IFN-α 也能抑制体内 ECs 迁移[38]。

第五节　抗肿瘤血管形成的研究

随着对肿瘤发生机制研究的不断深入，肿瘤血管形成在肿瘤发展中的重要地位及抗血管治疗肿瘤的作用已成为肿瘤治疗的一个全新领域。这引起了对调节血管生成过程的蛋白质的研究，包括血管生成抑制剂和促进剂。血管生成抑制剂有可能成为抗肿瘤的主要药物，并为最终治愈肿瘤提供有效手段。

对癌症血管生成抑制机制的研究是一个重要的并充满希望的领域。在分子层面了解血管生成所取得的重要进展，即从整体更好地了解血管生成和目前使用的抗血管生成药物的机制。抑制血管生成是一种重要治疗方法，可对抗癌症，降低动脉粥样硬化，预防糖尿病患者因视网膜新生血管引起的失明等。

近年来，一些新的血管抑制疗法已经被美国食品药品监督管理局（food and drug administration，FDA）测试和批准；包括贝伐珠单抗（Avastin）、厄洛替尼（Tarceva）和雷珠单抗（Lucentis），其余几种正在进行Ⅲ期试验，有望用于癌症治疗[12]，包括食管癌、胰腺癌、淋巴瘤、肾细胞癌、胃癌及许多其他癌症。但是肿瘤可以通过有几种不同的适应机制来克服抗血管生成疗法，这也正是为什么单独抗VEGF治疗在临床试验中的效果有限，必须联合多靶点干预。

一、抗血管形成靶向治疗的优点

（1）不良反应少，除对某些生理及创伤情况下的血管形成具有一定程度的抑制作用外，还可避免骨髓抑制、胃肠道及心脏损害等毒性反应。

（2）避免导致基因突变，主要通过细胞因子、受体及信号传导过程发挥作用，避免影响遗传物质而导致基因突变的继发性癌症。

（3）不诱导肿瘤细胞的耐药性，该方法作用于具有遗传稳定性的ECs，不易发生耐药；但是许多肿瘤仍然可以克服血管生成抑制剂的作用，因而需要联合治疗的方法。

（4）作用广泛：血管生成与肿瘤的生长、浸润、转移密切相关，抗血管生成治疗具有广谱作用。

（5）协同放、化疗作用并可多次重复应用，并减轻后者的毒副反应。

二、血管生成抑制剂

最近，已经开发出针对多种血管生成调节因子的新药。还有许多其他药物在后期临床试验。对一些重要的血管生成促进剂和抑制剂，以及涉及肿瘤学的最新研究进展进行深入理解将促进更有效地针对肿瘤血管生成疗法的发展。

（一）对抗血管生成的因子

通过选择性地抑制一种或几种血管生成因子或通过阻断其受体而发挥作用。

VEGF是目前影响血管形成最重要的因素。抗VEGF及其信号通路药物已被应用于临床，如靶向VEGF的药物avastin，可安全有效地用于治疗大肠癌、肺癌和视网膜黄斑变性（age-related macular degeneration，AMD）。靶向VEGFRs的药物Nexavar和Sutent，也已临床应用。缺乏周细胞的肿瘤血管对抗VEGF治疗更敏感。

（1）avastin 是一种重组人单克隆抗体，能抗血管新生。2004 年 2 月份，美国 FDA 以快速通道的方式，批准该药作为转移性结-直肠癌联合用于化疗的第一线药物。2004 年 10 月欧洲人类医学产品委员会（European society of human medicine products council，CHMP）也批准该药应用于临床[13]。临床结果表明转移性结直肠癌患者经 avastin 联合化疗后效果明显。该药对其他癌，如非小细胞性肺癌、胰腺癌、肾细胞癌也有一定疗效。avastin 和抑瘤蛋白联合治疗能显著抑制肿瘤生长。IFN-α 与 avastin 联合使用可能是肾细胞癌较好的治疗方法。特别在治疗转移性肾细胞癌中效果明显。

（2）β-2 糖蛋白 1（β-2 glycoprotein 1），能抑制人类脐静脉内皮细胞（HUVEC）增殖、迁移和管形成的作用，并呈剂量依赖性。这是由下调 VEGFR2 实现的。

（3）番茄红素（lycopene）是在西红柿中发现的一种类胡萝卜素，可能抑制 PDGF-B 的诱导信号，降低多余血管形成的水平。

（4）CD105 抗体为载体结合化疗药物、生物毒素、放射性核素等形成的复合物，能特异地靶向肿瘤部位，直接杀伤肿瘤细胞。与其他抑制肿瘤血管生成的药物相比，CD105 抗体特异性地与增殖的 ECs 结合，减少了对全身其他部位的损伤。其治疗效果可靠，副作用小。

（5）使用 TGF-β 反义寡核苷酸（AP12009），减少血管生成作为恶性脑胶质瘤患者一种治疗方法。对晚期患者仍观察到积极的疗效。

（6）将抗-Eng 单克隆抗体（TRC105）与毒性分子结合以确保靶向的 ECs 死亡。这一模式已在小鼠乳腺癌中获得成功，并且未检测到任何毒性。在晚期或转移癌患者使用不加修饰的抗-Eng 单克隆抗体（TRC105）有一定的临床效果[39]。

在缺血区如慢性伤口和心肌梗死区诱导新生血管形成也是一个非常活跃的研究领域。通过增加 VEGF 基因或蛋白来诱导缺血区血管生成的临床试验中，增加局部 VEGF 诱发缺血组织较低水平的血管新生。然而作为一种单独的治疗方法，这些血管生成的数量是不够的。这个结果表明 VEGF 是血管生成的重要成分，但仅仅控制其浓度水平仍不足以来调节血管的生成。

（二）直接抑制 ECs

直接作用于 ECs 的抑制剂，以血管抑素、内皮细胞抑制素较为重要。

（1）皮下注射重组人血管抑素在 I 期临床试验显示很少或几乎无毒性。Ⅱ 期试验联合紫杉醇和卡铂已在非小细胞肺癌（NSCLC）患者身上完成，疗效好于单独化学疗法，但低于预期水平。采用静脉注射血管抑素基因络合阳离子脂质体的实验正在进行。

（2）动物实验在肝细胞癌（HCC）移植瘤内注射抑瘤蛋白片段（pSecTag2B-Tum-1）显著抑制了癌的生长，减少了肿瘤中 CD34 阳性的血管数量。

（三）内皮细胞抑制素的研究

（1）内皮细胞抑制素治疗骨肉瘤患者可以提高患者预后，抗血管生成治疗是否可以帮助预防骨肉瘤的肺转移，这是骨肉瘤患者手术后的继发问题。

（2）对于类癌和胰腺神经内分泌肿瘤，在目前的化疗中加入内皮细胞抑制素可提高疗效。使用新的重组内皮细胞抑制素（YH-16，也称为"恩度"endostar）治疗晚期 NSCLC 患者正在进行 Ⅲ 期试验[40]。研究发现长春瑞滨和顺铂加恩度的联合治疗能改善病情并有显著的临床意义。

（3）使用一种内皮细胞抑制素和血管抑素融合蛋白治疗肾细胞癌的动物实验结果显示该融合蛋白抑制肿瘤血管生成，肿瘤生长和转移能力降低。

（四）聚乙二醇 IFN-α

聚乙二醇 IFN-α（polyethylene glycol IFN-α，PEGIFN-α）是经过修饰、有较长半衰期的抑制血管剂。转移性肾癌患者皮下注射 PEGIFN-α 和重组 IL-2 在大多数情况下几乎无毒性。

三、抗肿瘤血管形成的基因治疗

基因治疗即通过载体将目的基因导入体内，通过作用于 mRNA 或表达特定的蛋白质而发挥其抗血管生成作用。

其主要作用机制：①抑制血管生成因子基因的表达；②干扰 ECs 信号的转导；③直接导入抑制血管生成基因；④表达特定的血管生成抑制因子。

注射抗血管生成药物如 VEGF-TRAP、贝伐珠单抗，载体（聚乙二醇化纳米）可通过肿瘤血管（渗漏血管）靶向性进入肿瘤组织，而不能跨越正常组织的成熟血管壁（图 9-17）。

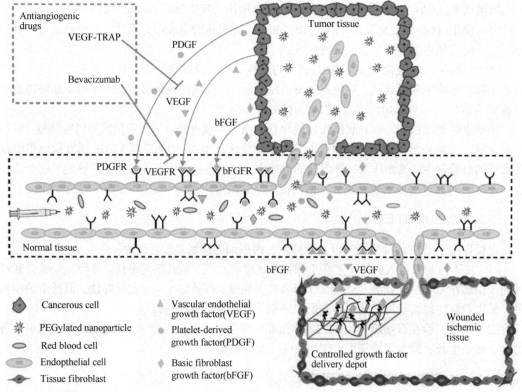

图 9-17　抗血管生成药物作用机制肿瘤组织中，癌细胞能分泌血管生成因子与毛细管血管 ECs 上各自的受体结合，导致紊乱的血管进入浸润性肿瘤中。利用渗漏血管可以使全身注射载体（如聚乙二醇化纳米）进入到肿瘤组织，而载体不能跨越正常组织的成熟血管壁。增强渗透性和滞留作用是被动性的靶向肿瘤。抗血管生成药物，如 VEGF-TRAP 和贝伐珠单抗，阻断了生长因子对血管生成的作用；Mechanism of angiogenesis of the anti angiogenic drugs, The cancer cells in tumor tissue secrete angiogenic growth factors that bind to their respective receptors on the endothelial cells lining the capillaries, leading to recruitment of disorganized blood vessels infiltrating the tumor. This leaky vasculature allows entry of the systemically injected vector (e.g., a Pegylated nanoparticle)into tumor tissue, whereas the vector cannot pass across the mature walls of normal tissue vessels. This results in passive targeting of the tumor by the enhanced permeability and retention effect. Antiangiogenic drugs, such as VEGF-TRAP and bevacizumab, block the angiogenic effect of the growth factors

对于缺血性疾病需要治疗性血管生成时可通过利用合成递送支架（如装载有非共价或共价结合的生长因子，纤维蛋白水凝胶），以增加局部递送促血管生成因子的目的。

四、核酶在抗肿瘤血管形成中的应用

核酶（ribozyme，Rz）是一类具有生物催化活性的 RNA 分子，能够定点切割特定的 mRNA 靶分子，从而有效地阻断特定基因的表达，发挥其生物学作用。利用化学性质稳定的核酶特异性地剪切 VEGF-R2mRNA 对晚期恶性肿瘤干预的初步结果显示了良好的耐受性和较小的毒副作用。

五、以血管生成拟态为靶向的治疗途径

干扰或诱导基质对肿瘤细胞的反应是靶向血管生成拟态治疗的关键。抑制血管生成拟态产生和维持抑制的分子机制可达到治疗目的。例如，将一个或多个侵袭性肿瘤细胞表达相关分子基因作为治疗的靶点，也许可作为针对血管生成和血管生成拟态治疗的通用靶点。

六、抗癌干细胞生态位治疗

肿瘤异质性中包括存在 CSCs 依赖于血管和具有生态位独特的微环境。CSCs 驻留在血管生态位时成为"CSCs 生态位（CSCs niche）"。CSCs 和它们的生态位之间的关系可以是双向的：CSCs 产生的血管生成因子（如 VEGF）刺激血管生成，而肿瘤血管维持 CSCs 的自我更新和维护。抗血管生成治疗剂与其他化疗药物结合会破坏血管生成和中断血管对 CSCs 的维持（图 9-18）。

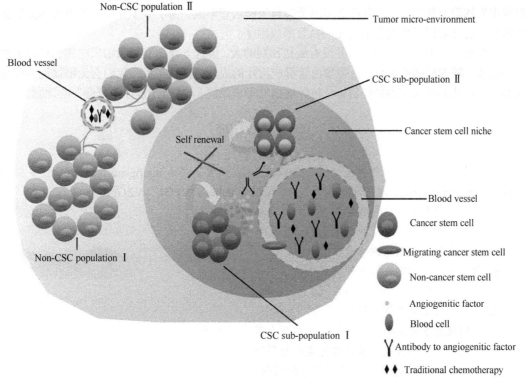

图 9-18　抗 CSCs 生态位治疗模型；Model of anti- CSCs niche therapy in tumor

挑战与展望

当我们寻求针对这些肿瘤发生过程的治疗方法时，肿瘤细胞与血管 ECs 间、肿瘤与 ECM 及肿瘤与非内皮细胞基质的促血管生成和淋巴管间复杂的相互作用，以及同时存在的促血管生成与淋巴管生成的多条分子通路，这些都是肿瘤微环境中同时出现的信号机制，是我们面临的最大挑战。

（1）为什么肿瘤能够抵抗抗 VEGF 治疗？

肿瘤能够抵抗抗 VEGF 治疗是因为耐药性肿瘤中增加了周细胞对肿瘤血管的支持。周细胞被认为能保护残余血管，抵御抗 VEGF 治疗。肿瘤周细胞最有可能表达高水平的 VEGF 及其他可能的促血管形成因子。此外，周细胞能减少 ECs 增殖率，让新形成血管的 ECs 成熟和稳定。因此通过共同抑制肿瘤血管的周细胞和血管生成因子来阻止肿瘤血管生成，解决对抗 VEGF 治疗的抵抗。

（2）为什么有些药物在动物模型上有较好的效果，但在临床试验中却结果不一？

只针对一种血管生成因子是不能阻止大部分肿瘤血管新生的。虽然这些结论最初令人沮丧，但它们还是开辟了其他的血管抑制疗法。许多临床试验使用现有化疗药物或放射疗法联合抗血管药物，对大多数的患者，这种两方面攻击比单用抗血管生成药物或单用化疗的效果更好。

总之，这些研究已经阐明了为什么单独抗 VEGF 治疗在临床试验中只看到有限的效果。

血管形成具有重要生理、病理意义，随着研究深入，将发现更多关于血管生成通路的信息，有助于理解肿瘤发生、发展的机制，确定治疗靶点，发展和使用可以同时针对一些血管形成因子的药物，产生对血管形成更有效的抑制剂，增加治疗成功的可能性。

很明显，在肿瘤血管生成中有很多不同的因子发挥了重要的作用。迄今为止，VEGF 被证明是最主要的因子，但许多其他因子，如 IL-8、MMP-2、类肝素酶、TGF-β 和 bFGF 也在血管形成中发挥重要作用。由于有这么多因子参与肿瘤血管形成，为了减少肿瘤血管形成和抑制肿瘤转移，有必要同时抑制几个关键的血管形成因子。

虽然抗血管形成治疗的利益并没有最初预期的大，但这方面的发展和临床应用仍获得了很大的进步。随着时间的推移，抗肿瘤血管形成治疗的成效将继续扩大，我们会无限接近治疗癌症和血管形成相关疾病的最终目标。抗肿瘤血管形成始终是 21 世纪医学"革命"的课题之一。

思 考 题

1. 本章基本概念：血管发生（vasculogenesis），血管生成（angiogenesis），血管生成拟态（vasculogenic mimicry），肿瘤干细胞生态位（CSCs niche），VEGF，VEGFR。

2. 简述肿瘤血管生成中的主要事件。

3. 为什么说血管形成是肿瘤发生所必需？

4. 简述血管生成拟态的特点和意义。

5. 血管干细胞在实体瘤血管形成中的作用是什么？

6. 描述肿瘤血管生成的几种模式。

7. 总结肿瘤新生血管的特点。

8. 分别简述 5 种促血管生成因子和抑制血管生成因子。

9. 阐述抗血管形成靶向治疗的优点与局限性。

10. 简述抗肿瘤血管形成的基因治疗的机制。

参 考 文 献

[1] Folkman J, Shing Y. Angiogenesis[J]. Journal of Biological Chemistry. 1992, 267 (16): 10931-10934.

[2] Papetti M, Herman IM. Mechanisms of normal and tumor-derived angiogenesis[J]. American Journal of Physiology, 2002, 282 (5): C947-C970.

[3] Carmeliet P. Angiogenesis in life, disease and medicine[J], Nature, 2005, 438 (7070): 932-936.

[4] Jackson K A, Majka S M, Wang H, et al. Regeneration of ischemic cardiac muscle and vascular endothelium by adult stem cells[J]. Journal of Clinical Investigation, 2001, 107 (11): 1395-1402.

[5] Rafii S, Avecilla S, Shmelkov S, et al. Angiogenic factors reconstitute hematopoiesis by recruiting stem cells from bone marrow microenvironment[J]. Annals of the New York Academy of Sciences, 2003, 996 (1): 49-60.

[6] Folkman J. Angiogenesis[J].Annual review of medicine. 2006, 57: 1-18.

[7] Folkman J. Tumor angiogenesis: therapeutic implications[J]. New England Journal of Medicine, 1971, 285 (21): 1182-1186.

[8] van Kempen L C, Leenders W P. Tumours can adapt to anti-angiogenic therapy depending on the stromal context: lessons from endothelial cell biology[J]. European Journal of Cell Biology, 2006, 85 (2): 61-68.

[9] 张诗武, 高欣, 孙保存. 血管生成拟态和血管生成及其意义[J]. 国际肿瘤学杂志, 2003, 30 (3): 180-182.

[10] Gerber HP, McMurtrey A, Kowalski J, et al. Vascular endothelial growth factor regulates endothelial cell survival through the phosphatidylinositol 3'-kinase/Akt signal transduction pathway. Requirement for Flk-1/KDR activation [J]. The Journal of Biology Chemistry. 1998, 273 (46): 30336-30343.

[11] Esser S, Lampugnani M G, Corada M, et al. Vascular endothelial growth factor induces VE-cadherin tyrosine phosphorylation in endothelial cells[J]. Journal of Cell Science, 1998, 111 (Part 13): 1853-1865.

[12] 汪怡, 陈莉, 鄂群.脑星形细胞肿瘤中 PTEN、血管内皮细胞生长因子表达与微血管密度[J]. 中华病理学杂志, 2003, 32 (3): 260-261.

[13] Tabruyn S P, Griffioen A W. Molecular pathways of angiogenesis inhibition[J]. Biochemical and Biohysincal Research Communications, 2007, 355 (1): 1-5.

[14] Miller D L, Ortega S, Bashayan O, et al. Compensation by fibroblast growth factor 1 (FGF1) does not account for the mild phenotypic defects observed in FGF2 null mice[J]. Molecular & Cellular Biology, 2000, 20 (6): 2260-2268.

[15] Pizarro C B, Oliveira M C, Pereira-Lima J F, et al. Evaluation of angiogenesis in 77 pituitary adenomas using endoglin as a marker[J]. Neuropathology, 2009, 29 (1): 40-44.

[16] 刘宏斌, 杨其昌, 陈莉, 等. 乳腺癌中 CD105 的表达及其预后意义[J]. 南通大学学报（医学版）, 2006, 26 (6): 435-437.

[17] Yancopoulos G D, Klagsbrun M, Folkman J. Vasculogenesis, angiogenesis, and growth factors: ephrins enter the fray at the border[J]. Cell, 1998, 93 (5): 661-664.

[18] Soncin F. Angiogenin supports endothelial and fibroblast cell adhesion[J]. Proceedings of the National Academy of Sciences of the United States of America, 1992, 89 (6): 2232-2236.

[19] Otrock Z K, Mahfouz R A, Makarem J A, et al. Understanding the biology of angiogenesis: review of the most important molecular mechanisms[J]. Blood Cells Molecules & Diseases, 2007, 39 (2): 212-220.

[20] van den Driesche S, Mummery C L, Westermann C J. Hereditary hemorrhagic telangiectasia: an update on transforming growth factor β signaling in vasculogenesis and angiogenesis[J]. Cardiovascular Research, 2003, 58 (1): 20-31.

[21] Friedlander M, Brooks P C, Shaffer R W, et al. Definition of Two Angiogenic Pathways by Distinct αv Integrins[J]. Science, 1995, 270 (5241): 1500-1502.

[22] Clark R A F, Tonnesen M G, Gailit J, et al. Transient functional expression of $\alpha V \beta 3$ on vascular cells during wound repair[J]. 1996, 148 (5): 1407-1421.

[23] Carmeliet P, Lampugnani M G, Moons L, et al. Targeted deficiency or cytosolic truncation of the VE-cadherin gene in mice impairs VEGF-mediated endothelial survival and angiogenesis[J]. Cell, 1999, 98 (2): 147-157.

[24] Strieter R M, Polverini P J, Kunkel S L, et al. The functional role of the ELR motif in CXC chemokine-mediated angiogenesis[J]. The Journal of Biology Chemistry, 1995: 270 (45): 27348-27357.

[25] Leibovich S J, Polverini P J, Shepard H M, et al. Macrophage-induced angiogenesis is mediated by tumour necrosis factor-alpha [J]. Nature, 1987, 329 (6140): 630-632.

[26] Schreiber A B, Winkler M E, Derynck R. Transforming growth factor-alpha: a more potent angiogenic mediator than epidermal growth factor [J]. Science, 1986, 232 (4755): 1250-1253.

[27] Heissig B, Werb Z, Rafii S, et al. Role of c-kit/Kit ligand signaling in regulating vasculogenesis[J]. Thrombosis and Haemostasis. 2003, 90 (4): 570-576.

[28] Zaman K，Driscoll R，Hahn D，et al. Monitoring multiple angiogenesis-related molecules in the blood of cancer patients shows a correlation between VEGF-A and MMP-9 levels before treatment and divergent changes after surgical vs. conservative therapy [J]. International Journal of Cancer. 2006，118（3）：755-764.

[29] Ceradini D J，Kulkarni A R，Callaghan M J，et al. Progenitor cell trafficking is regulated by hypoxic gradients through HIF-1 induction of SDF-1[J].Nature Medicine. 2004，10（8）：858-864.

[30] Wahl M L，Kenan D J，Gonzalez-Gronow M，et al. Angiostatin's molecular mechanism：aspects of specificity and regulation elucidated[J]. Journal of Cellular Biochemistry，2005，96（2）：242-261.

[31] Kang H Y，Shim D，Kang S S，et al. Protein kinase B inhibits endostatin-induced apoptosis in HUVECs[J]. Journal of Biochemistry & Molecular Biology，2006，39（1）：97-104.

[32] Zan M. High serum endostatin levels in Down syndrome：implications for improved treatment and prevention of solid tumours[J]. European Journal of Human Genetics，2001，9（11）：811-814.

[33] Eikesdal H P，Sugimoto H，Birrane G，et al. Identification of amino acids essential for the antiangiogenic activity of tumstatin and its use in combination antitumor activity[J]. Proceedings of the National Academy of Sciences of the United States of America，2008，105（39）：15040-15045.

[34] Li X，Jiang L，Wang Y，et al. Inhibition of angiogenesis by a novel small peptide consisting of the active fragments of platelet factor-4 and vasostatin[J]. Cancer Letters，2007，256（1）：29-32.

[35] Armstrong L C，Bornstein P. Thrombospondins 1 and 2 function as inhibitors of angiogenesis[J]. Matrix Biology，2003，22（1）：63-71.

[36] Chetty C，Lakka S S，Bhoopathi P，et al. Tissue inhibitor of metalloproteinase 3 suppresses tumor angiogenesis in matrix metalloproteinase 2-down-regulated lung cancer[J]. Cancer Research，2008，68（12）：4736-4745.

[37] Haas C S，Amin M A，Allen B B，et al. Inhibition of angiogenesis by interleukin-4 gene therapy in rat adjuvant-induced arthritis[J]. Arthritis and Rheumatism，2006，54（8）：2402-2414.

[38] Melichar B，Koralewski P，Ravaud A，et al. First-line bevacizumab combined with reduced dose interferon-α2a is active in patients with metastatic renal cell carcinoma[J]. Annals of Oncology，2008，19（8）：1470-1476.

[39] Rosen L，Gordon M S，Hurwitz H I，et al. Early evidence of tolerability and clinical activity from a phase I study of TRC105（anti-CD105 antibody）in patients with advanced refractory cancer[J]. Ejc Supplements，2009，6（12）：126.

[40] Kulke M H，Bergsland E K，Ryan D P，et al. Phase II study of recombinant human endostatin in patients with advanced neuroendocrine tumors[J]. Journal of Clinical Oncology Official Journal of the American Society of Clinical Oncology，2006，24（22）：3555-3561.

（周　虹　张丽丽　陈　莉）

Chapter 9　Tumor Angiogenesis

The cardiovascular system distributes blood, and thus oxygen and nutrients throughout the body. This system consists of arteries, arterioles, capillaries, venules, and veins. Minimum vessels: the microvasculature is considered as the portion of the circulatory system composed of the smallest vessels, such as the capillaries, arterioles, and venules. The microvasculature is a very dynamic and complex system. It is capable of constant change, while the larger blood vessels are more permanent structures with very little plasticity.

Arteries and veins have several distinct layers including the tunica intima, the tunica media, and tunica adventitia in the largest vessels. Due to the thickness of these structures, arteries, arterioles, venules, and veins are all considered conduit vessels. Capillaries are hollow tubes composed of endothelial cells (ECs) which are supported by pericytes. Capillaries are the most important vessels in cardiovascular system. The thin walls of these microscopic vessels allow the exchange of oxygen and nutrients between the blood and tissues.

Angiogenesis is a critical process involving the formation of new blood vessels from preexisting vessels. Normal angiogenesis is an essential physiological process that the body employs during fetal development, wound healing, ovulation, as well as growth and development. Angiogenesis provides developing and healing tissues with vital nutrients and oxygen. Normally there is a few angiogenesis (non-pathogenic angiogenesis can be seen in the adult ovary cycle, during the rehabilitation or wound healing process in skeletal and cardiac muscle). When angiogenesis goes awry, pathological problems often ensue. A variety of diseases contain pathological processes of angiogenesis: Cancer, psoriasis, endometriosis, arthritis, focal Crohn's disease and eye disease (macular degeneration); so proposed the concept of "angiogenesis-dependent diseases". Some diseases are also associated with vascular reduction: obstructive cardiovascular disease (atherosclerosis, myocardial infarction) and so on.

Angiogenesis is "The double-edged sword"- life clock, death clock, Angiogenesis is a "common denomination" disease.

The understanding of normal and pathogenic angiogenesis has been a major focus of both cancer biology and clinical medicine for the past few decades. In the 21st century, therapy based on angiogenesis has become a common way to treat a variety of diseases, as the 20th century, the role of antibiotics, is one of the elements of medical innovation.

Section 1　Angiogenesis

Blood vessels comprising the microvasculature are formed in adults via two different mechanisms: vasculogenesis and angiogenesis. Both processes normally occur during embryonic development; however, special circumstances allow these processes to be initiated during adult life. Vasculogenesis: The term is used for spontaneous blood-vessel formation. This form particularly relates to the embryonal development of the vascular system (de novo). Vasculogenesis is the de novo formation of ECs from angioblasts derived Hematopoietic stem cell (HSCs). This process helps to form a primitive vascular labyrinth of small capillaries. Angiogenesis: The physiological process involves the growth of new blood-vessel from pre-existing vessels, which ECs sprout with the degradation of capillaries basement membrane from preexisting blood vessels. The ECs then migrate and proliferate to form a cord-like or tubular structure and blood flows through it. Then budding and differentiation grows more new blood vessels. This form plays an important role during the adult life span, also as "repair mechanism" of damage tissues. This process is tightly controlled under physiological conditions. Now commonly use the term "Angiogenesis" represent different types of blood-vessel formation.

1. Fetal Vasculogenesis

The establishment of fetal vasculature begins with hemangioblasts, primitive cells of mesodermal origin. Hemangioblasts help form "blood islands", which means clusters of cells that have a designated spatial arrangement that facilitates their function. Hematopoietic stem cells (HSCs), which later become hematopoietic cells, are found at the center of these islands. Angioblasts, cells that differentiate into ECs, are found at the periphery of the blood islands (Fig. 9-1).

2. Adult Vasculogenesis

It is currently believed that vasculogenesis originates when multipotent adult progenitor cells (MAPCs). In bone marrow differentiate into early endothelial progenitor cells (EPCs), they gain hematopoietic and endothelial lineage-specific markers such as VEGF receptor-2 (VEGFR-2) and CD34. EPCs in the bone marrow remain undifferentiated in two zones. The first zone is known as the vascular zone, and it consists of EPCs in either the S phase or G2M phase of the cell cycle. These cells are capable of differentiating and entering peripheral circulation upon receiving the correct signals. The second zone is known as the osteoblastic zone, where EPCs are maintained in the G_0 phase of the cell cycle. These cells are not actively divided, and therefore are not readily available for release into circulation. The balance between these two functional compartments is maintained by cytokines presenting in the bone marrow's extracellular matrix (ECM) and on bone marrow stromal cells (Fig.9-2).

The adult stem cells existing within bone marrow (instead of blood islands) are discovered to contain much greater plasticity than originally thought, and are now considered MAPCs. MAPCs are capable of differentiating into ECs when removed from bone marrow and cultured on fibronectin with vascular endothelial growth factor-A (VEGF-A). In addition, MAPCs are capable of differentiating into skeletal muscle, cardiac muscle, and vascular endothelium after bone marrow transplantation.

In pathological conditions, such as burn patients or in patients who undergo coronary artery bypass grafting, circulating EPC concentration increases to 60-fold in the first 6h after the incident, and within 72h it returns to normal levels. This transient increasing is due to vascular and tissue damage increased EPC levels led to several cytokines (including VEGF) released, promote the start of EPC mobilization and angiogenesis.

3. Regeneration(Angiogenesis)

Like vasculogenesis, vessel regeneration(angiogenesis) occurs most often during embryonic development; however, it can also occur in adult life in response to specific stimulations. Nonpathogenic angiogenesis can be seen in adults during the ovarian cycle, in skeletal and cardiac muscle during times of exercise and training, as well as during the process of wound healing.

In contrast to vasculogenesis, angiogenesis is the expansion of preexisting vasculature, such as a vascular labyrinth of capillaries, by means of budding and branching into a functional capillary bed which is illustrated in Fig.9-3. This normally occurs in organized manner form, of which is known as primary vascular trees.

Vessels made from ECs which are not covered with pericytes, are unstable, and undergo regression.

4. Other Patterns of Angiogenesis

(1) Intussusception angiogenesis: No EC proliferation, EC project the lumen of blood vessels, the blood vessels formed the connecting bridge, furthermore divided into two blood vessels by pericytes, smooth muscle cells, fibroblasts EC assisting(Fig. 9-4).

(2) Collateral arteriogenesis: By collateral vascular, ECs recruit macrophage and lymphocytes (LCs), macrophages degrade ECM to allow the interactions of EC and pericytes / smooth muscle cells regulated by paracrine signaling, leading to the growth and stability of arterioles(Fig. 9-5).

Section 2   Tumor Angiogenesis

In the past, research in angiogenesis was closely intertwined with cancer biology. The importance of angiogenesis in tumor growth was initially hypothesized in 1971, when Judah Folkman put forward his theory that solid tumors possess limited resources that many actively proliferating cancer cells fight for. Increased interstitial pressure within the tumor also inhibits the diffusion of metabolites and nutrients essential growth and survival of tumor cells. This environment causes tumor cells to induce the sprouting of new blood vessels from the established vasculature, creating a vascular system within the tumor, thus enabling tumor cells to obtain the oxygen and nutrients they need to survive and multiply.

1. Processes of Tumor Angiogenesis

Tumors begin as an avascular mass of host-derived cells that proliferate atypically because they have lost the ability to control their growth. Tumors initially survive and thrive on vasculature that is already available in the surrounding host environment. In order for tumors to grow beyond 2-3mm^3, they need a continual supply of blood to remove waste and deliver nutrients. Hypoxia of tumor cells will occur if the tumor grows beyond the maximum distance of effusion from local vessels (around 200 μm). In order to counter this lack of oxygen, tumor cells will attempt to create new blood vessels to supply their needs in a mechanism that tumor angiogenesis is a complex multistep and multisignaling process(Fig. 9-6).

Tumor angiogenesis actually begins with the removal of mural cells (pericytes) from preexisting blood vessels. The absence of these pericytes initiates the degradation of the EC basement membrane and extracellular matrix, a process which is aided by MMPs. As the basement membrane and extracellular matrix are being degraded, ECs begin proliferating and migrating with the help of soluble growth factors (such as VEGF and FGF). The ECs will continue to grow until they form an unstable microvessel. Following the formation of this small blood vessel, mesenchymal cells are recruited to the vessel, where they are subsequently differentiated into pericytes. After differentiation, cell to cell contact between pericytes and ECs occurs. Stable blood vessels are then formed and blood flow can be established (Fig. 9-7). Tumor cells will secrete a variety of factors to ensure that the new blood vessels formed are fed directly to the tumor tissue.

2. Relationship between Angiogenesis and Tumors (solid tumors)

"No vessel" no cancer risk (<1mm diameter, <0.5cm^3, like a ballpoint pen tip in avascular stage), after the blood supply, cancer cells grow exponentially. Cancer growth and metastasis depend on angiogenesis (oxygen, nutrients). Angiogenesis is essential to tumor development. Angiogenesis is essential for tumor development.

3. Angiogenesis in Tumor Infiltration and Metastases

Angiogenesis plays a distinct role that uniquely contributes to the process of tumor infiltration and metastases. For the majority of tumors, it is only about 1/1000 of tumor cells with invasion and metastasis. Primary tumor cells must get their way into the vascular system, can survive in a loop within the target organ capillaries implantation into the target organs and induce the formation of blood vessels within the target organ, in order to complete the transfer; moreover, the proliferation of metastatic tumor cells are led to the formation of new metastases, the same need to go through the process chain.

(1) Tumor angiogenesis is favor to tumor metastasis

1) Because neoplastic vascular basement membrane is incomplete and leakage, it provides the path with least resistance for tumor metastasis.

2) Endothelial cells secrete collagenase and plasminogen activator (PA) to strengthen the chemotactic infiltration behavior of tumor cells in tumor blood vessels protrusion. These "invasive" capillaries "swallow" tumor cells, the tumor cells are more easily metastasis and spread.

3) Tumor angiogenesis can enhance peripheral actively growing cancer cells closely contact to lymphatic tube; or increase the number of lymphatic tube led to intravenous micrometastases cells into the lymphatic system.

(2) Angiogenesis play various roles in stages of tumor development

When a dormant tumor reaches critical size (usually 1-2 mm) and receives intracellular signals from the tumor microenvironment (e.g., hypoxia), the tumor cells begin to excrete growth factors, cytokines, and other signaling molecules. These factors can influence the stromal cells to also produce these factors, which signal blood vessels to dilate, and grow towards the tumor cells. Microvessels are sprouted within the tumor, which survive and proliferate due to the new delivery of nutrients, growth factors, and oxygen. Eventually, a complex vascular network has been created within the tumor which promotes invasion beyond the basement membrane and metastasis to other tissues (Fig. 9-8).

Although all cancers are "heterogeneous", an angiogenesis is common in variety of tumors. (Fig.9-9)

4. Tumor Vascularization Models

After development, the vasculature rarely extends, neither so in tumor formation. Tumor angiogenesis occurs via a number of potential mechanisms. Other tumor angiogenesis modes have been observed. Endothelial progenitor cells (EPCs), which can either reside in the vascular wall or migrate from bone marrow in response to chemoattractants from the tumor cell, can differentiate into ECs and contribute to vessel formation.

Vascular mimicry can also occur, whereby tumor cells can act as replacement cells for ECs. Another possibility is that chromosomal abnormalities in putative cancer stem cells allow tumor cells to differentiate into ECs.

Other mechanisms by that tumor cells can obtain a blood flow include vessel cooption, whereby the tumor cell arises near to (or migrates toward) the preexisting blood vessel, by the process of intussusception, where a preformed vessel splits into two daughter vessels by the insertion of a tissue pillar(Fig. 9-10).

Vasculogenic mimicry: One kind of tumor angiogenesis does not rely on the endothelial cells, which is completely different from the classic way of tumor angiogenesis. Tumor cells go through its own deformation and matrix remodeling produces angioid channel, the channel is not lined with endothelial cells the channel outside the basement membrane shows PAS positive staining, pumping blood to form pipeline system and is connected to the host blood vessels in some parts to get blood supply and rebuild the tumor microcirculation.

(1) Features of Vascular Mimicry:

1) With unevenly thickened walls, PAS positive material separates tumor cells and blood flow (RBC flows in pipe formed by PAS positive material);

2) It is active formed by highly aggressive tumor cells without lined by endothelial cells, not formed by passive blood flow momentum, or by endothelial cells proliferation;

3) There are no leaking red blood cells in matrix lined blood vessels of vascular mimicry, the opposite way by budding capillaries into the tumor tissue, can be seen leaking red blood cells between the tumor cells.

4) The fact of few microthrombi is speculated an anticoagulant function of tumor cells or vascular extracellular matrix;

5) There are different shapes of PAS-positive pattern in vascular mimicry;

6) The markers of tumor blood vessels all were negative (no endothelial cells).

(2) Significance of vascular mimicry

1) Different tumors can get different mechanisms of angiogenesis. Or with a variety of angiogenesis mechanisms in same tumor.

2) Malignant tumors are inversely related to vascular mimicry; There is no central necrosis in tumor with vascular mimicry.

3) PAS positive substance may be the body's response to a tumor stroma, called fibrotic vascularization.

However, Maniotis and other did not support this conclusion by in vitro studies. His results showed that not only in uveal melanoma angiogenesis mimicry microcirculation was consisted by invasive tumor cells, but also in the fibroblasts, endothelial cells and other stromal cells it did not exist, these kind of vascular mimicry may also occur.

5. Molecular Mechanisms of Tumor Angiogenesis

It is expound that tumor angiogenesis is an important condition for tumor development, invasion and metastasis by angiogenic factors and anti-angiogenic factor common regulation. The process of tumor angiogenesis is very closely regulated.

(1) The mechanisms of sprouting angiogenesis

1) Vascular Sprouting

It is initiated by proangiogenic factors (e.g., VEGF). ECs at the leading edge of the vascular sprout extend filopodia and migrate toward angiogenic signals. VEGF activates VEGFR2 to stimulate tip cell migration. The coreceptor Nrp1 complexes with and enhances VEGFR2 signaling. ECs become either the migratory vessel-leading tip cell or the proliferating stalk cell, but their phenotype is fluid; Notch regulates this specification. ECs with activated VEGFR2 signaling compete for the tip cell position by increasing their expression of DLL4, which binds to Notch receptors on neighboring ECs, releasing the transcription regulator NICD. NICD transcriptionally downregulates VEGFR2 and Nrp1 expression while increasing VEGFR1, a VEGF trap, thus enhancing the stalk cells' unresponsiveness to VEGF.

The tip cell is not a fixed position, and its fluidity at the front occurs depending on the VEGFR1/VEGFR2 ratio. Tip cell migration requires BM degradation (in part due to MMP), EC junction loosening (caused by VE-cadherin, ZO-1, and others), and pericyte detachment (regulated by Ang2). VEGF increases the permeability of the vessel, allowing the extravasation of plasma proteins (e.g., fibronectin and fibrinogen) that are deposited as a provisional matrix layer while the preexisting interstitial matrix is remodeled by proteases; these events enable tip cell migration. Initial steps of tip cell selection (Fig.9-11).

2) Tip Cell Guidance and Stalk Elongation Tip cells adhere to the ECM, mediated by integrins, and migrate toward guidance signal molecules (e.g., semaphorins and ephrins). Stalk cells trail behind the tip cell and proliferate to allow sprout elongation and lumen formation. While Notch signaling inhibits proliferation, expression of Nrarp at branch points allows Wnt signaling to maintain stalk cell proliferation. This system allows vascular migration/directionality (by tip cells) and elongation of the shaft (by proliferating stalk cells).

When two tip cells meet, they fuse (anastomose); this mechanism is assisted by macrophages, which accumulate at sites of vascular anastomosis to act as bridge cells by interacting with the neighboring tip cells' filopodia. Once contact between the tip cells has been established, VE-cadherin–containing junctions further strengthen the connection. Perivascular macrophages further stimulate sprouting by producing angiogenic factors or proteolytically liberating them from the ECM.

The stalk cells also deposit BM and recruit pericytes, thus stabilizing the forming vessel. Pericyte precursors are attracted to vessels by EC-expressed PDGF. Once at the vessel, these mesenchymal precursor cells differentiate to pericytes in response to TGF-β and decrease EC migration, proliferation, and vascular leakage, resulting in nascent vessel stabilization(Fig. 9-12).

3) Maturation through Resolution of Quiescent Phalanx Cells Once fusion occurs, a connected lumen is forced to allow blood flow through the new vessel. This perfuses the hypoxic tissue, and the resultant oxygen and nutrient delivery leads to decreased levels of angiogenic signals, inactivation of EC oxygen sensors, and increased proquiescent molecules that lead to EC quiescence. Establishment of the blood flow remodels vessel connections, which are regulated by the shear stress–responsive transcription factor KLF2. ECs resume a quiescent phalanx phenotype in a tightly opposed monolayer with a streamlined surface that conducts the blood flow and regulates tissue perfusion. Perfusion induces vascular maturation by reestablishment of cell-cell junctions, pericytes maturation, and BM deposition(Fig. 9-13).

Autocrine and paracrine signaling from ECs and surrounding support cells by VEGF, FGF, Ang1, and Notch, among others, maintain a quiescent EC phenotype and protect the vessel from environmental stresses. Reduced growth factor signaling can lead to vessel retraction and EC apoptosis. Once stabilized and matured, the vessel forms a barrier between the blood and surrounding tissue, controlling the exchange of fluids and solutes.

Summary the process of sprouting angiogenesis is shown in Fig. 9-14.

(2) Cancer Stem Cells Driving Tumor Angiogenesis

Cancer stem cells (CSCs) in certain malignancies possess the capacity to drive tumor angiogenic responses and/or to engage in vasculogenic mimicry, potential means of promoting tumor growth.

1) BMP-9 suppresses VEGF expression by the BMP (bone morphogenetic protein)-9/ALK (activin-like kinase) 1 pathway against the effect of the TGF-β1/ALK5 pathway which can enhance VEGF expression and angiogenesis. In between these two pathways, the key role of the balance is BMP-4, which can keep the vascular integrity.

2) Notch induces vascular development and normal stem cell survival through the Notch/NICD (Notch intracellular domain) /Hes/Heysignaling pathway. Notch inhibitor DAPT (gsecretase inhibitor) not only decreases the self-renewal ability of tumor cells and the number of CD133+ cells, but it also decreases the expression of vascular markers like CD105, CD31, von Willebrand factor, etc..

(3) Functions of Vascular Stem Cells in Solid Tumors

1) Mesenchymal progenitor cells (MPC) derived from the bone marrow or nearby tissues are a source of vascular endothelial growth factor (VEGF), a potent endothelial cell survival and motility factor. MPC may also differentiate to form pericytes that provide structural support the nascent vasculature.

2) Hematopoietic progenitor cells (HPC) and their progeny act as "accessory" cells during angiogenesis by expressing tissue remodeling and endothelial survival factors such as MMP9 and VEGF. Similar to MPC, they may provide paracrine instructions to sprouting tip cells during anastomosis.

3) Endothelial progenitor cells (EPC) may give rise to endothelial colony-forming cells (ECFC) and constitute the primary lumen-forming cells of angiogenic sprouts. ECFC may also provide unique paracrine cues to neighboring "adult" endothelium or the recruited pool of HPC.

Taken together, these three populations of progenitors work in concert to form the building blocks of tumor blood vessels (Fig. 9-15).

Section 3　Characteristics of Tumor Angiogenesis

Tumor vessels have uncontrollable growth, immaturity Vascular Architecture, abnormal distribution and density, as well as heterogeneous biological behavior.

1. Vascular Architecture

A tumor vasculature occurs rapidly, grows fast, and is sustained, 10% to 20% of the tumor vascular endothelial cells always are in DNA synthesis state that sustain angiogenesis due to the vascular growth factors released persistently high level by tumor. Tumor vessels are dilated, saccular, tortuous, and disorganized in their patterns of interconnection. Normal vasculature is characterized by dichotomous branching, but tumor vasculature is unorganized and can present trifurcations and branches with uneven diameters. It is generally believed that when peripheral vessels are richer, central vessels are less, whereas when central vesselsare richer, peripheral blood vessels are less. Blood vessel-rich area is as a hot point.The new vessels grow from the tumor periphery or directly into the center of the tumor, then the tree branches out in tumor angiogenesis. In the early avascular stage of tumor, tumor cells and body blood vessels take a symbiotic way.In large nest of tumor, the vascular branches anastomosis of artery and vein can form blood lake, which is collectively referred to as tumor-associated vascular diseases.

The molecular mechanisms causing this abnormal vascular architecture are not well understood, but the uncontrolled VEGF signaling may be a key contributor. "Normalization" of the tumor vasculature has been observed by interfering with VEGF signaling: that is, treatments directly targeting VEGF or VEGF receptor, therapies that reduce VEGF (e.g., hormone withdrawal from a hormone-dependent tumor), or agents mimicking an anti-angiogenic cocktail (e.g., Herceptin treatment of a HER2 overexpressing tumor). Solid (mechanical) stress generated by proliferating tumor cells also compresses vessels in tumors. Thus, the combination of both molecular and mechanical factors renders the tumor vasculature abnormal, and both types of factors must be taken into account when designing novel strategies for cancer treatment.

2. Blood Flow and Microcirculation

Whether normal or abnormal, arterio-venous pressure difference and flow resistance govern blood flow in a vascular network. Flow resistance is a function of the vascular architecture (referred to as geometric resistance) and of the blood viscosity (rheology, referred to as viscous resistance). Abnormalities in both vasculature and viscosity increase the resistance to blood flow in tumors. As a result, overall perfusion rates (blood flowrate per unit volume) in tumors are lower than in many normal tissues and the average RBC velocity can be an order of magnitude lower than normal. Furthermore, tumor blood flow is unevenly distributed, fluctuates with time and can even reverse its direction in some vessels-therefore, regions with poor perfusion, or none at all, are commonly seen. There is inequality blood supply and blood flow velocity in the tumor.

Because presenting different blood supply lead to the cell rich regions, half necrotic and necrotic regions in tumor. In semi-necrosis and necrosis regions, the blood flow is significantly reduced and is slowed down, but in non-necrotic area blood flow velocity is faster than normal tissue. Mean value of tumor blood flow velocity in the big tumor is lower than that in small tumor. In a large tumor vascular endothelial cells with less nutrition supply, the diameter of actual effect vessels is small, blood flow is slow and there is nutrient depletion. The cancer cells with hypoxic necrosis are owing to update faster than the endothelial cells. The proliferation index endothelial cells around the tumor is 2.2%, tumor cells is 7.3%. Meanwhile, in mice tumor cells grow within 22 hours into a newer generation, the endothelial cells grow within 50 hours or more in a new generation.

According to research on the quality and quantity of tumor blood flow with microscopic spectrophotometer, in which red blood cells often appear completely deoxygenated, the tumor is only about 10 to 40 percent of vascular endothelial cells constituted without corresponding nutritional blood flow. The utilization of oxygen is lower. Cancer tissues lack lymphatic tuber, the hydrostatic pressure in the tumor tissues increases, oppressing small blood vessels so that blood flow in the tumor only is 1 to 10% of normal. Tumor cells with anaerobic glycolysis produce large amounts of H^+, there are three low cell populations (low-nutrient, low PH value and hypoxia) in tumor. Tumor microcirculation, compared with tumor growth, is relatively inefficient and insufficient, especially in the central part of the tumor tissue, which there often occurs ischemia, hypoxia and necrosis. The heterogeneity of tumor blood flow is an important contributor to both acute and chronic hypoxia in tumors—which in turn is a major cause of resistance to radiation and other therapies.

3. Vascular Permeability

Extravasation of molecules from the bloodstream occurs by diffusion, convection, and to some extent, by transcytosis in an exchange vessel. Diffusion is considered to be the major form of transvascular transport in tumors. The diffusive permeability of a molecule depends on its size, shape, charge, and flexibility as well as the transvascular transport pathway. Widened inter-endothelial junctions, increased numbers of fenestrations, vesicles and vesico-vacuolar channels, and a lack of normal basement membrane and perivascular cells were found in tumor vessels. In agreement with these ultrastructural alterations, vascular permeability in solid tumors is generally higher than that in various normal tissues.

The tumor-induced angiogenesis are abnormal with irregular, antral and thin wall. The walls of tumor vessels are usually absent functional pericytes, leaving an incomplete basement membrane, which causes those vessels to be especially leaky and passive dilatation. The endovascular stimulation attributed to VEGF can also increase vascular permeability. Some parts of the capillary wall lack endothelial cells, which rarely evolve into mature small arteries and small veins, having non-contractile function without neurohumoral regulation. Normal vascular active substances (acetylcholine, angiotensin II, temperature) do not work for the tumor vessels.

Despite increased overall permeability, not all blood vessels of a tumor are leaky. Not only does the vascular permeability vary from one tumor to the next, but it also varies spatially and temporally within the same tumor as well as during tumor growth, regression, and relapse.The local microenvironment plays an important role in controlling vascular permeability. For example, a human glioma (HGL21) has fairly leaky vessels when grown subcutaneously in immunodeficient mice, but it exhibits blood-brain barrier properties in the cranial window. The host-tumor interactions may control the production and secretion of cytokines associated with permeability increase (e.g.,VEGF) and decrease (e.g., angiopoietin 1). Furthermore, the response of the blood vessels to a given stimuli may also vary depending on the host organ site and host–tumor interaction.

4. Heterogeneity of Vascular Endothelial Cells

The heterogeneity of vascular endothelial cells is tumor outstanding biological characteristics, mainly in the structure, function, antigen components or / and metabolic characteristics of endothelial cells. In tumor tissue of certain organs, vascular endothelial cells still retain these organ tumor's antigenic (e.g., the endothelial cells in brain, ovarian, lung cancers present these antigens expressing in tumor cells). That state the surface antigens on endothelial cells may play a role in selectively adhered and regional release humoral factors in tumor metastasis.In pancreatic cancer, Nestin is highly expressed in some pancreatic cancer cells and small proliferating tumor vessels easily metastasis to liver (Fig. 9-16). The abnormal morphology of perivascular cells in tumor is association with vessels heterogeneous.

Table 9-1　Association with abnormal structure and function of tumor vessel

Structural abnormalities (vascular disorders)	Dysfunction (circulation disorders)
1. Vessel wall abnormity The endothelial cell is incomplete or absent, the basement membrane is interrupted or absent, the tumor cells are arranged in the form of blood channel outer membrane cells, contractile components and pharmacological / physiological receptors absent.	1. Morphological changes Arteriovenous shunt is open, blood retrograde flow or interrupted, unstable flow velocity or direction, loss of vasomotor properties, the vessel wall is brittle and the vessels are blocked by leukocytes and / or tumor cells, and the vascular resistance increases.
2. Vascular abnormalities Irregular shape (sinus or cystic like), vessel wall is twisted and elongated. Arteriovenous shunt is present (Tumor mass flow > Nutrient flow), vascular classification is not obvious.	2. Rheological changes Red blood cell deposition, leukocyte adhesion, platelet aggregation, formation of microplatelets or giant platelets, increased blood viscous.
3. Vascular density abnormalities An uneven distribution of blood vessels (chaotic vascular network and no vascular region), increased capillary space between.	3. Increased vascular permeability results Blood concentration, interstitial fluid increased, interstitial fluid pressure increased (as a result of tumor capillary compression), extravasation of blood cells, bleeding, viscous resistance increased

Section 4　Regulating Factors of Angiogenesis

Tumor angiogenesis regulated by the interaction promote angiogenesis and anti-angiogenic factors. It is not only affected by the body's neuroendocrine factors, but is also regulated by growth factors which are expressed in tumor cells and stromal cells. Understanding these principles that led to the idea that the inhibition of tumor angiogenesis could be a valuable therapy against cancer. This sparked research into the proteins that regulate this process, both angiogenesis inhibitors and promoters. Since that time, many proteins and angiogenesis regulatory factors have been discovered, and their role is also to be understood. There have been reported more than 30 kinds of vascular endothelial growth factor and inhibitors.

1. Angiogenic Promoters

Several growth factors are involved in promoting tumor angiogenesis. The most characterized players include ligand-receptor complexes of VEGF-VEGFR-2, RGD (from ECM matrix)-integrin, and TGF-β-endoglin. These, along with other factor-receptor or protein–protein (SLIT and ROBO) binding complexes, result in activation and crosstalk among downstream signaling pathways to promote endothelial cell survival, migration, proliferation, and vascular guidance and increase vascular permeability.

(1) Vascular Endothelial Growth Factor (VEGF) and VEGF Receptors (VEGFR)

VEGF is an important regulator of both vasculogenesis and angiogenesis, a specific mitogen for ECs and angiogenesis. VEGF is considered the most powerful proangiogenic factor in tumors. It associated with tumor growth rate, vessel density, metastases. Several normal cell types including fibroblasts, ECs, and keratinocytes release a small amount of VEGF throughout life.

1) Structure of VEGF

There are currently six known monomers of VEGF that arise from alternative splicing of a single gene with eight exons. The documented isoforms contain 121, 145, 165, 183, 189 or 206 amino acids. Some of these isoforms remain associated with cells or membranes, while others are released extracellularly.

Despite these differences, all of them have identical biological activities.

2) Functions of VEGF

a. Promoting angiogenesis and vasculogenesis

b. Stimulating microvascular EC proliferation

c. Enhancing EC migration and sprouting

d. Inhibiting EC apoptosis

e. Increasing EC permeability

3) VEGF receptors (VEGFR)

VEGF interacts with two different receptor tyrosine kinases, VEGFR-1 (Flt-1) and VEGFR-2 (Flk-1), to alter angiogenesis. VEGFR-1 interacts very strongly with VEGF, but this interaction plays a minor role in the events of angiogenesis. VEGFR-1 is an active inhibitor of VEGF, negatively regulating VEGF function.The interaction of VEGFR-2 with VEGF is a major contributor to the mitogenic, chemotactic, angiogenic, and increased permeability effects of VEGF. VEGFR- 2 expression has been observed on both endothelial and hematopoietic precursors (EPCs).

4) The correlation of cancer research

Currently in VEGF-induced angiogenesis and research intervene mainly in three areas:

a. VEG/VPF at mRNA and protein level overexpressed in primary and metastatic tumors (gastrointestinal cancer, pancreatic cancer, breast cancer, kidney cancer, bladder cancer and glioblastoma and other studies).

b. The relationship between the receptor on tumor microvascular endothelial cell over-expression and tumorigenesis.

c. Exudating plasma protein and fibrinogen in tumor angiogenesis and the extravascular fibrin significantly crosslinking and deposition promote the formation of tumor stroma, and the research of tumor microenvironment.

d. The research of feasibility and safety of anti-VEGF antibody.

We have results display; glioma VEGF protein positive staining in the cytoplasm of tumor cells, is also positive in endothelial cells. In 43 cases of brain astrocytoma tumor cells VEGF positive expression rate is 77.0%. In grade Ⅰ and grade Ⅱ the level of VEGF positive expression and intensity are significantly lower than grade Ⅲ and grade Ⅳ groups. The intensity of VEGF expression level was positively correlated with MVD (microvessels density). They mainly show three patterns of tumor blood vessels: ①Bud-like; ②Cystic; ③Plexiform. In low grade tumor (grade Ⅰ and Ⅱ) blood vessels mainly have hyperplasia and cystic vascular sprout, plexiform vessels are rare. But highly malignant tumor (grade Ⅲ and Ⅳ) within the proliferation of microvessels contains more plexiform vessels. MVD and VEGF expression and tumor microvessels may help to determine the malignant levels of astrocytoma.

Anti-VEGF signaling pathway drugs have also been tested in a large number of clinical and laboratory studies aimed at preventing angiogenesis associated with cancer. Some of these drugs target VEGF (Avastin), while others target the VEGFRs (Nexavar and Sutent). Although these drugs have reached dramatic results in animal models, the results in many of the clinical trials have been mixed. There have been clinical trials which show as many as 94% of invasive carcinomas and 88% of in situ carcinomas having a complete response. These same patients saw no recurrence during the five-year follow up. However, many other angiogenesis inhibitors targeting VEGF signaling pathways have failed to produce the same long-term responses in a majority of their patients.

(2) Basic Fibroblast growth factor (bFGF)

bFGF plays an important role in maintaining tumor angiogenesis, that starting tumor angiogenesis is different from VEGF. bFGF has also been shown to promote VEGF production, up-regulate VEGF mRNA levels in vascular smooth muscle, increasing the density of VEGFR in microvascular endothelial cells.

Function of bFGF

1) Stimulating EC proliferation;

2) Promoting microvessel tube formation;

3) Promoting EC migration;

4) Important promoter of blood vessel remodeling after tissue injury.

(3) Endoglin(Eng, CD105)

Endoglin (Eng, CD-105) is a homodimeric cell surface glycoprotein that serves as a coreceptor for TGF-β. Eng is found on proliferating ECs and also serves as an EPC marker. It has been observed that Eng expression is greatly increased during angiogeneses and inflammation. Studies have shown that Eng can regulate TGF-β, but the mechanism remains unknown. With this function in mind, researchers have investigated the use of anti-Eng based therapies in several different forms of cancer with the hopes of preventing tumor-based angiogenesis. The roles of CD105 in tumor angiogenesis: ①CD105 antagonize TGF-β and its receptors on vascular endothelial cells in vitro, and promote tumor angiogenesis; ②CD105 is a sign of endothelial cells proliferation, which strongly is expressed only in the endothelial cells of proliferative tumor tissue.

Serum levels of CD105 can be used long-term for follow-up of the patients with solid tumors. They predict disease recurrence and metastasis risk.

We compared the MVD markers with CD105 in benign breast disease and cancer, breast cancer with significantly higher. MVD was associated with lymph node metastasis. P53 expression was positively correlated with CD105 in breast cancer. Log rank test showed MVD, P53 marker CD105 expression in breast cancer, lymph node metastasis, TNM staging and prognostic factors ER. Multivariate (Cox proportional hazards model) survival analysis showed that breast cancer markers CD105 MVD, is an independent prognostic factor.

(4) Tie Receptors

The Tie receptors are a family of tyrosine kinases expressed by ECs that mimic the behavior of VEGF receptors. To date, Tie1 and Tie2 have been identified, and their mechanisms of action have been studied. Both Tie1 and Tie2 receptors are important for vascular integrity, only Tie2 appears to be vital to vascular sprout and branch occurring during angiogeneses.

(5) Angiopoieten or Angiogenin(Ang)

Angiopoietins are protein growth factors (a small peptide), which act as ligands for the Tie Receptors on Ecs. There are two important angiopoietins that play a role in angiogenesis, Ang-1 and Ang-2.

1) Ang-1 is a well characterized regulator of angiogenesis. It is an important agonist ligand for Tie2 receptors. ①Ang-1 is Tie2 receptor agonist ligand. In vivo recruit pericytes to new blood vessels, enhance the stability of new blood vessels, reduce new blood vessel permeability. ②Helps promote EC survival and sprout formation. ③Increases the diameter of blood vessels endothelium.

2)Ang-2: ①Agn-2 of Tie-2 receptor, reduces levels of pericytes, leading to instability or rupture of blood vessels. ②Early tumor vascular endothelial cells with high expression Ang-2, and the degradation of blood vessels, can be used as tumor-induced angiogenesis early biomarkers. ③Increases plasticity of newly formed blood vessels.

(6) Angiotropin

An originally isolated from peripheral mononuclear cells out of polynucleic acid peptide. The role of Angiotropin in tumor angiogenesis:①In the wound healing process helps activate microvascular endothelial cells. ②Stimulate angiogenesis in vivo. ③Induce capillary endothelial cell migration at random .

(7) Platelet-derived growth factor (PDGF)

PDGF is another important signaling molecule with several different roles in angiogenesis. Although originally purified from platelets, it has also been identified in fibroblasts, astrocytes, ECs, and several other cell types

The role of PDGF in tumor angiogenesis:

1) Increasing capillary wall stability

2) Stimulating the proliferation of cultured pericytes and SMCs

3) Increasing DNA synthesis on capillary ECs

4) Stimulating formation of angiogenic sprouts in vitro

The interaction of PDGF with its receptor on pericytes increases the expression of Ang-1. This increases in Ang-1 leading to a signaling cascade that helps establish the interaction between pericytes and ECs. This interaction is important for maintaining the stability of newly formed capillary walls, a vital part of new blood vessel formation.

PDGF binds to its receptor blockade reduces the stability of capillary growth, so that they cannot provide nutrients to cancer cells.

(8) Transforming Growth Factor-Betas (TGF-β)

TFG-β's are a family of homodimeric cytokines that help control many different processes in the body, including angiogenesis. TGF-β's are normally found in the ECM of many different cells types. Within the microvasculature, both ECs and pericytes produce and display receptors for TGF-β, illustrating the variety of cells capable TGF-β expression. To date, both pro- and antiangiogenic properties have been ascribed to TGF-β.

1) At low doses, it upregulates angiogenic factors and proteinases.

2) At high doses, it inhibits EC growth, promotes reformation of BM and stimulates SMC reformation

3) Stimulates or inhibits EC tube growth.

4) Signals inflammatory mediators such as fibroblasts and monocytes, media reach angiogenesis district release of pro-angiogenic factors (such as VEGF, FGC and PDGF).

5) Enhances integrity of vessel walls.

Tumor cells expressing TGF-β-induced interstitial reactions leading to the formation of reactive stromal micro-environment, promote angiogenesis and tumor growth.

(9) Integrin

Integrins are heterodimeric cell surface receptors for ECM proteins that also play a role in cell-cell attachment. They contain various α-and β-subunits, with over 20 different combinations of subunits known. Integrins are important regulators for many different cell processes including both vasculogenesis and angiogenesis. Of the integrins, αVβ3 is one of the most extensively studied, and has an important role in angiogenesis.

1) The role of αVβ3 in tumor angiogenesis

a. Binds and activates MMP2 to help break down ECM.

b. Helps regulate cell attachment, spreading, and migration.

c. Shows Increased activity near wound sites.

d. Localized to ECs at ends of growing vessels during EC sprouting.

2) Integrin αVβ5 interacts with VEGF to promote angiogenesis

(10) Vascular endothelial cadherin.

Cadherins is a class of calcium-binding transmembrane proteins that play an important role in cell-cell interactions. Several studies have underlined the important role of one particular cadherin, the vascular endothelial (VE) cadherin, in neovascularization. Vecadherins are localized exclusively to the adherens junctions in ECs VE-cadherin specifically located in junctions of endothelial cell adhesion, keeping stablity of the blood vessel wall endothelial cell junctions. The role of vascular endothelial (VE) cadherin in tumor angiogenesis is to:

1) Thought to mediate passage of molecules across endothelium.

2) Regulates ECs growth through contact inhibition.

3) Helps prevent EC apoptosis by promoting VEGFs signal.

4) Helps stabilize the branches and sprouts produced during angiogenesis.

(11) Interleukins(ILs)

ILs are a group of cytokines that are released by leukocytes and control a wide range of biological activities. A few of these ILs have been shown to affect the growth of blood vessels. The ability to either enhance or suppress angiogenesis is based on a Glu-Leu-Arg (ELR) motif at the NH2 terminus. IL-8 possesses this sequence, and therefore enhances angiogenesis, while IL-4 does not contain the motif, it is an inhibitor of angiogenesis.

IL-8 is produced by macrophages, it does not play an important role in normal angiogenesis. But as a tumor angiogenesis Mediation Center. Have confirmed that the level of IL-8 is elevated in several tumor tissues. Increased expression of IL-8 is associated with increased density of new blood vessels and increased tumor growth.

IL-8 has an important characteristic-ability to increase the levels of MMP-2, MMP-2 can degrade the endothelium basement membrane and remodeling ECM, start early stages of tumor angiogenesis.

(12) Other Factors

Many factors have been shown to play important roles in angiogenesis, but their effects on the vasculature are not as widespread or as understood as the previously mentioned factors.

1) Tumor necrosis factor-α(TNF-α) A cytokine produced by activated macrophages secrete.

a. Stimulating angiogenesis in vivo.

b. Stimulating EC tube formation in vitro.

2) Transforming growth factor-α (TGF-α) another cytokine secreted by macrophages

a. Promoting EC proliferation.

b. Stimulating angiogenesis in vivo.

3) MMP-9 help to mobilize EPCs by cleaving ECM. A recent study verified altered levels of MMP-9 and VEGF-A in patients with early-stage breast and colorectal cancer when compared to normal patients.

4) Stromal-cell-derived factor-1 (SDF-1): Helps guide EPCs to ischemic areas during angiogenesis.

2. Angiogenesis Inhibitors

(1) Angiostatin

Angiostatin is a 38 kDa internal fragment of plasminogen that displays inhibitory effects against tumor angiogenesis:

1) Angiostatin increases the cell apoptosis rate of metastatic tumor to reduce distant metastases.

2) Inhibiting the growth of capillary endothelial cells in vitro.

(2) Endostatin

Endostatin is an angiostatic 20-kD internal fragment of the carboxy terminus of collagen XVIII, an important proteoglycan in basement membranes.

1) Inhibition of endothelial cell migration, proliferation and tube formation by down-regulating the transcriptional activity of cyclin-D1 promoter, blocking the cell cycle of endothelial cells, and inhibiting endothelial cell proliferation. By inducing caspase-9 activation,it induces apoptosis pathway, leading to

reduction anti-apoptotic protein of Bcl-2 and Bcl-XL and Bad.

2) Blocking VEGF interaction with its receptor VEGFR-2

Evidence for endostatin's importance can been seen by studying individuals with Down Syndrome. People with Down Syndrome have a third copy of collagen XVIII due to a trisomy of chromosome 21. These individuals tend to have a 1.6-2 fold elevation of endostatin levels and have greatly reduced levels of malignant tumors (except testicular cancer and megakaryocytic leukemia), atherosclerosis, and diabetic retinopathy due to neovascularization. These three diseases are all angiogenesis-dependent, and they showcase important role that endostatin may play a role in inhibiting unwanted pathogenic angiogenesis in humans.

(3) Tumstatin

Degradation of type IV collagen releases a 28 kDa fragment known as tumstatin, a compound that also displays antiangiogenic properties. Tumstatin binds the $\alpha V\beta 3$ integrin, which results in G_1 arrest and the induction of EC apoptosis.

(4) Platelet Factor-4 (PF4)

Platelet Factor-4 (PF-4) is a chemokine naturally secreted from the alpha-granules of activated platelets that normally promotes blood coagulation. In addition to this role, PF-4 is also known to be an inhibitor of angiogenesis.

1) PF4 binds with high affinity to heparin-like glycosaminoglycans on the surface on ECs blocking them from further activity.

2) PF-4 blocks the upregulation of MMP-1 and MMP-3, inhibiting ECs migration.

3) PF-4 is also capable of inhibiting the ECs cycle by impairing pRB   phosphorylation.

(5) Thrombospondin-1 (TSP-1)

Thrombospondin-1 (TSP-1) was the first natural angiostatic a multidomain matrix glycoprotein that has been shown to be a natural inhibitor of neovascularization. TSP-1 is a native, full length protein. TSP-1 is stored in α-granules of platelets, where it is complexed with TGF-$\beta 1$. When released from the platelets and free from TGF-$\beta 1$, TSP-1 inhibits the migration of ECs and induces ECs apoptosis.

1) The induction of apoptosis in ECs is associated with TSP-1's ability to alter the concentrations of several important apoptotic factors. TSP-1 upregulates Bax, downregulates Bcl-2, and activates the caspase-3 intrinsic pathway, leading to programmed EC death.

2) To slow down migration, TSP-1 binds to EC surface receptors capable of promoting promigratory signals.

(6) Tissue inhibitor of metalloproteinase (TIMPs)

Tissue Inhibitors of Metalloproteinases (TIMPs) are a family of proteases, derived from cartilage, which inhibit MMPs. As previously mentioned, MMPs play an integral role in the initiation of angiogenesis. They are responsible for EC basement membrane degradation and ECs remodeling. The newly formed ECM developed by MMPs during the angiogenic response provides a scaffold for ECs to adhere, migrate, and form tubes for nutrient delivery. The inhibition of MMPs by TIMPs reduces the angiogenic capacity of Ecs. High levels of TIMP-1 greatly inhibit migration of ECs. through gelatin in vitro.

(7) IL-4

IL-4 acts as an inhibitor of tumor growth, but its mechanism of action likely varies with different tumor cells. For example, IL-4 is thought to directly inhibit proliferation of cells from cancers such as colon tumors, head and neck tumors, and glioblastomas, while in other cases it is thought to induce a host immune response against the tumor cells, such as in B-cell lymphomas and melanomas. There is also evidence that IL-4 inhibits neovascularization, thus inhibiting tumor growth.

In vitro, IL-4 inhibits migration of ECs towards bFGF. In vivo, IL-4 has been shown to inhibit neovascularization in rat corneas that should have been induced by the high concentration of bFGF present. These experiments demonstrate that IL-4-mediated suppression of tumor growth may be due to IL-4 ability to inhibit angiogenic processes. Other noncancer-related animal studies have shown IL-4's antiangiogenic capabilities in vivo.

(8) Interferons (IFNs)

Interferons (IFNs) belong to a large family of secreted glycoproteins known as cytokines. They are produced and secreted by a wide variety of immune-related cells. It is thought that both IFN-α and IFN-β are able to inhibit angiogenesis by repressing bFGF mRNA and protein levels. In addition to downregulating the key angiogenesis signaling factors, IFN-α also inhibits the migration of EC cells in vivo.

Section 5 Anti-angiogenesis—Current Research and Clinical Implications

With the deepening of the mechanisms of tumor incidence, tumor angiogenesis play an important role in tumor development and anti-angiogenic therapy have generates a new field in cancer therapy.

This has led to study the protein modulating angiogenesis process, including angiogenesis inhibitors and accelerators. Angiogenesis inhibitors may become the main anti-tumor drugs, and provide an effective mean for the ultimate cure for cancer.

We have made important progress at the molecular level understanding angiogenesis. Overall better understand the mechanism of angiogenesis and anti-angiogenesis drugs currently used to generate. Inhibition of angiogenesis is an important therapeutic approach to fight cancer, reduce atherosclerosis, and to prevent diabetes-induced retinal neovascularization due to blindness.

In recent years, several new antiangiogenic therapies have been tested and approved by the FDA, including Avastin, Tarceva and Lucentis; several ongoing trials Ⅲ remaining expected for cancer treatment. It is expected for the treatment of cancer. Including esophageal cancer, pancreatic cancer, lymphoma, renal cell carcinoma, gastric cancer, and many other cancers.

However, there are several different tumor adaptive mechanisms to overcome the anti-angiogenic therapy, showing why anti-VEGF treatment alone in clinical trials only see a limited effect, the intervention must be combined with multitargets.

1. Advantages of Targeting Angiogenic Therapy

(1) Adverse reactions, with the exception of some physiological and vascular trauma cases with some degree of inhibition of the formation, to avoid bone marrow suppression, gastrointestinal toxicity and heart damage and the like;

(2) Avoid causing gene mutation, mainly by cytokines, receptors and signaling processes play a role, to avoid the impact caused by mutations in the genetic material of secondary cancers;

(3) Not inducing resistance of tumor cells, which operates on the genetic stability of endothelial cells, drug resistance is not easy; but many can still be against the action of tumor angiogenesis inhibitors, and therefore need a method of combination therapy;

(4) Broad role angiogenesis and tumor growth, invasion and metastasis, anti-angiogenic therapy with broad-spectrum effect;

(5) Synergistic effect of radiotherapy and chemotherapy and repeated application anti-angiogenic therapy with chemotherapy and radiotherapy in combination, a synergistic effect and reduce the toxicity of the latter.

2. Angiogenesis Inhibitors

Currently, several drugs have been approved by the FDA for the treatment of angiogenesis-dependent diseases including Avastin for colorectal cancer, Tarceva for lung cancer, and Lucentis for macular degeneration. Many other drugs are in late-stage clinical testing, some important angiogenic promoters and inhibitors, and ongoing research and developments as they relate to oncology. Increasing the mechanistic understanding of these processes will improve the development of more efficient angiostatic treatments in cancers.

Anti-angiogenic factors: by selectively inhibiting one or more angiogenic factors or by blocking its receptors, which plays a role.

VEGF is angiogenesis of the most important factors. Anti-VEGF drugs and signaling pathways have been used clinically, such as targeting VEGF drug Avastin, and the targeting VEGFRs drugs Nexavar and Sutent. AMD has been proven safe and effective for ophthalmic treatment with anti-VEGF drugs. Lack of pericytes tumor vessels are more sensitive to anti-VEGF treatment. Inhibition of VEGF signaling.

(1) Common Angiogenesis Inhibitors

1) Avastin

Avastin is a recombinant human monoclonal antibody, and it can be antiangiogensis. February 2004, the US FDA in its fast-track way, approval of the drug as metastatic colorectal - colorectal cancer used in combination with chemotherapy in first-line drugs. October 2004 European Society of Human Medicine Products Council (CHMP) has approved the drug for clinical application.

The clinical results show that patients with metastatic colorectal cancer Avastin in combination with chemotherapy after the effect is obvious. The drug for other cancers, such as non-small cell lung cancer(NSClC), pancreatic cancer, renal cell carcinoma have a certain effect. Avastin and tumstatin combination therapy can significantly reduce tumor growth. IFN-α in combination with Avastin renal cell carcinoma may be a better treatment. Especially in the treatment of metastatic renal cell carcinoma.It displays as a future cancer treatment method and has better prospects.

2)β-2 glycoprotein 1, can inhibit human umbilical vein endothelial cells (HUVEC) proliferation and tube formation and the role of migration in a dose-dependent manner. This is down VEGFR-2 implementation.

3) Lycopene, found in tomatoes, a carotenoid, may inhibit the PDGF-BB induced signal, reduce the level of unwanted angiogenesis.

4) CD105 antibody as a carrier, combined with chemotherapy drugs, biological toxins, radionuclides with the formation of complexes can be specifically oriented tumor,target therapy directly killing tumor cells. Compared with other drugs to inhibit tumor angiogenesis, CD105 antibody specifically binding to proliferating endothelial cells, reduces the damage to other parts of the body. So reliable treatment, lower side effects, is expected to become a new and effective method of treatment.

5) Using the TGF-β antisense oligonucleotides (AP12009), reducing angiogenesis of malignant glioma from patients is a cure. It is still observed in patients with advanced aggressive treatment.

6) The anti--Eng monoclonal antibody (TRC105) and toxic molecules combine to ensure targeted endothelial cell death. This model has been successful in mice with breast cancer, and there is no measure to any toxicity. Use without modification of the anti--Eng monoclonal antibody (TRC105) in patients with

advanced or metastatic cancer patients have some clinical effects.

In the ischemic area, such as chronic wounds and myocardial infarction induced angiogenesis are a very active area of research. By increasing the VEGF gene or protein to induce angiogenesis in the ischemic area of clinical trials, increasing the local pro-growth factor VEGF-induced ischemic tissue lower levels of angiogenesis. However, as a stand-alone treatment, the number of these angiogenesis is not sufficient. This information indicates that VEGF is an important component of angiogenesis, but only to control the concentration level is in sufficient to regulate angiogenesis.

(2) A direct effect on the endothelial cell inhibitor to angiostatin and endostatin is more important.

1) Subcutaneous injection of recombinant human angiostatin in Ⅰ clinical trials have shown little or no toxicity. Ⅱ trial in combination with paclitaxel and carboplatin was completed in non-small cell lung cancer (NSCLC) patients. More effective than chemotherapy alone, but they are lower than expected. By intravenous injection of angiostatin gene complex experiments underway cationic liposomes.

2) Animal experiments in hepatocellular carcinoma (HCCs) intratumoral injection of Tumstatin fragment (pSec Tag2B-Tum-1) transplant significantly inhibit the growth of HCC. In addition, reducing the number of CD34 positive blood vessel in the tumor.

(3) Endostatin is currently being analyzed for therapeutic potential in several forms of cancer.

1) Endostatin may be used as a possible treatment to boost the post-operative prognosis of osteosarcoma patients antiangiogenic treatment could help to prevent the progression of pulmonary metastasis, a secondary problem often associated with postoperative osteosarcoma.

2) Adding endostatin to current chemotherapeutic strategies may enhance the efficacy of the treatment for carcinoid and pancreatic neuroendocrine tumors. The use of novel recombinant endothelial endostatin (YH-16) also known as "endostar" for advanced NSCLC patients in a phase III trial. The study found that the addition of endostar to the vinorelbine and cisplatin treatment resulted in significant and clinically meaningful improvement.

3) A recently completed animal study has investigated the use of an endostatin-angiostatin fusion protein in Renal Cell Carcinomas (RCCs). The group tested the fusion protein's ability to inhibit tumor angiogenesis, tumor growth, and metastasis. All animals underwent postmortem histopathological analysis of the liver, kidney, lung, spleen, and brain to determine levels of metastasis.

(4) Polyethylene glycol IFN-α (PEGIFN-α)

PEGIFN-α is modified with a long half-life of inhibiting angiogenesis effect. Subcutaneously in patients with metastatic renal cell carcinoma PEGIFN-α and recombinant IL-2 in most cases almost non-toxic.

3. Anti-angiogenesis Gene Therapy

Gene therapy, through vector target gene into the body, or by acting on the mRNA, causes expression of specific proteins exert their anti-angiogenic effect. The main mechanism of action:

1) Inhibition of angiogenesis factor gene expression;
2) Interfere with the signal transduction of endothelial cells;
3) Directly into the inhibition of angiogenesis gene;
4) Expression of a specific angiogenesis inhibitor.

Injection of anti-angiogenic drugs as VEGF-TRAP, bevacizumab, carrier (pegylated nm) can be targeted by the tumor blood vessels into the tumor tissue (leakage of blood vessels), and the carrier cannot cross the blood vessel wall mature normal tissues(Fig. 9-17).

The cancer cells in tumor tissue secrete angiogenic growth factors that bind to their respective receptors on the endothelial cells lining the capillaries, leading to recruitment of disorganized blood vessels infiltrating the tumor. This leaky vasculature allows entry of the systemically injected vector (e.g., a PEGylated nanoparticle) into tumor tissue, whereas the vector cannot pass across the mature walls of normal tissue vessels. This results in passive targeting of the tumor by the enhanced permeability and retention effect. Antiangiogenic drugs, such as VEGF-TRAP and bevacizumab, block the angiogenic effect of the growth factors.

Ischemic diseases requiring treatment for angiogenesis can be delivered by using synthetic support (e.g. loaded with a non-covalent or covalent binding of growth factors, fibrin hydrogel) to increase the local delivery of angiogenic factors to achieve.

4. Using Ribozyme Anti-tumor Angiogenesis

Ribozyme (Rz) is a class of RNA molecules having biocatalytic activity, which can point cut specific mRNA target molecule, thereby effectively blocking the expression of specific genes which exert their biological effects.

The use of chemically stable ribozyme specifically cuts VEGF receptor (VEGFR-2) of the mRNA of the preliminary results of the study of advanced cancer showed good tolerability, low toxicity.

5. Approaching Therapy of Targeting Angiogenic Mimicry

Interference or induced matrix response to tumor cells will be the key target angiogenic therapy mimicry. Inhibition of vascular mimicry generates and maintains the molecular mechanism for therapeutic purposes. The expression of one or more of the invasive tumor cell related signaling molecules as therapeutic targets, perhaps as a general target for mimicry generation treatment for angiogenesis and blood vessels.

6. Anti-Cancer Stem Cell Niches Therapy

The heterogeneity in tumor cells also exists in cancer stem cells(CSC). Tumor cells rely on vasculature and harbor a unique microenvironment. CSCs may reside in a vascular niche named as 'CSCs niche' Relationship between CSCs and their niche may be bidirectional: CSCs generate angiogenic factors (i.e. VEGF) to stimulate angiogenesis and the tumor vasculature supports CSC self-renewal and maintenance Anti-angiogenic therapeutic agents combined with other chemotherapy drugs will disrupt angiogenesis and also interrupt the vasculature-derived CSC maintenance (Fig.9-18).

Challenges and Prospects

When we seek therapies for these tumor processes, the tumor / endothelial cells, tumor / extracellular matrix and tumor / non-angiogenic endothelial cell matrix production and lymphatic interaction between complexity and the simultaneous presence of angiogenic and lymphangiogenesis in multiple molecular pathways, and these are all signaling mechanisms which can occur simultaneously within the tumor microenvironment is our greatest challenge.

1. Why are tumors resistant to anti-VEGF treatment?

The reason why tumors have been able to withstand the anti-VEGF treatment is that resistant tumors have increased pericyte support on their tumor vasculature. The pericytes are believed to protect the remaining vessels and defend against the anti-VEGF treatment. The hypothesis states that tumor pericytes are most likely expressing appreciable levels of VEGF and possibly other proangiogenic factors. In addition, pericytes are capable of reducing the rate of EC proliferation which allows EC maturation and stabilization in newly formed blood vessels.

Therefore, currently, several ongoing clinical trials are attempting to prevent tumor angiogeneses by inhibiting pericyte association with tumor vasculature along with angiogenic factors

2. Why do some drugs achieve dramatic results in animal models, but have mixed results in clinical trials?

Only targeting one angiogenic factor is not enough to permanently halt neovascularization in most tumors. Although these results are initially disheartening, they also open up the possibility of other angiostatic therapies. Many clinical trials now use existing chemotherapeutic drugs or radiation along with antiangiogenic drugs. This two-front attack has had more success than antiangiogenic drugs or chemotherapy alone in a majority of patients, but it needs further study.

In short, these studies have begun to shed light on why anti-VEGF treatments alone may have seen limited results in clinical trials.

3. Prospects

It is obvious that many different factors play an important role in tumor angiogenesis. To date, VEGF has been shown to play the most dominant role, but many other factors such as IL-8, MMP-2, heparanase, TGF-β, and bFGF also play an essential part in the process. Because so many factors are involved with tumor angiogenesis, it is likely that several of these key factors must be inhibited simultaneously in order to significantly reduce the unwanted angiogenesis and eventually reduce tumor metastasis.

Although the benefit of antiangiogenic treatments has not been as great as initially anticipated, many advances have come from their development and clinical use. However, with time, it is likely that the success of angiogenic treatment in cancer will continue to improve and we will come ever closer to the original goal of curing cancer and other angiogenic-related diseases. Anti-angiogenesis has always been one of the topics of the 21st century medicine "revolution".

Consider/Questions

1. Basic concepts in this chapter
vasculogenesis, angiogenesis, vasculogenic mimicry, CSCs niche,VEGF&VEGFR.
2. Summarized the cascade of events in tumor angiogenesis.
3. Why is angiogenesis essential to tumor development?
4. Summarized vascular mimicry significant and characteristics.

5. Described the functions of vascular stem cells in solid tumors.

6. Described the angiogenetic modes of tumor.

7. Summarized the basic characteristics of tumor vessels.

8. Summarized five kinds of angiogenic promoting and inhibiting factors, respectively.

9. Described anti-angiogenic targeted therapy advantages and limitations.

10. Described the mechanism of anti-angiogenic therapy.

第十章　上皮间质转化（EMT）

根据细胞形态，机体的组织器官主要分为上皮细胞和间质细胞两种类型，它们具有不同的细胞表型、结构特点及功能。上皮细胞具有极性，细胞与细胞间存在多种连接，上皮细胞维持多细胞生物的完整性，成为可调节的内环境所需的必要屏障。相比而言间质细胞则无极性，缺少细胞间连接，具有向周边组织浸润和游走的能力，参与机体更复杂的结构及功能的形成。这两种细胞表型并非永久不变，在适当的条件下，上皮细胞和间质细胞可发生相互转变。

上皮间质转化（Epithelial-mesenchymal transition，EMT）（图 10-1）是指上皮细胞失去了

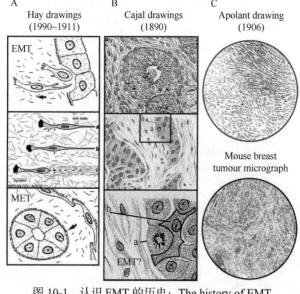

图 10-1　认识 EMT 的历史；The history of EMT

A. 1968 年 Betty Hay 首先设计了"上皮间充质转化"的术语并描述这一过程的瞬态特性。1991 年进一步描述了这是一个可逆的过程，即可发生 MET。2008 年修改该术语为 EMT；B. 100 多年前，圣地亚哥 Ramony Cajal 首先描绘和阐述了乳腺癌形态表现中的 EMT；C. 在 20 世纪（1906 年），Hugo Apolant 也清楚地描述了小鼠乳腺肿瘤中 EMT 改变的形态。显微照片显示，在小鼠乳腺肿瘤诊

断为 EMT 类型中，细胞角蛋白（CK8/18）在上皮和梭形细胞中的分布（该图片由加州大学戴维斯分校的 P. Damonte 博士和 R. 卡迪夫博士提供）；A. Betty Hay coined the term 'epithelial tomesenchymal transformation' (Hay, 1968) and described the transient nature of this process, as well as the reversion to the epithelial character (MET, Hay, 1991). Modified from Acloque et al (2008); B. More than 100 years ago, Santiago Ramony Cajal drew and described the morphological appearance of breast carcinoma so accurately that we can find what we believe to be the first description of EMT. Note the morphology of the cell highlighted as 'b'; C. At the turn of the 20th century, Hugo Apolantalso clearly represented the morphology of EMT-type mouse mammary tumors (Apolant, 1906). The micrograph shows the distribution of cytokeratin 8/18 in both theepithelial and spindle cell populations in a mouse mammary tumour diagnosed as EMT-type (This picture is courtesy of Dr P. Damonte and Dr R. Cardiff, Univ. California at Davis)

上皮极性，细胞紧密连接和黏附连接渐渐丧失，获得间质细胞表型伴有细胞外基质（ECM）成分分泌增加，成为侵袭性和迁移运动能力的细胞的生物学过程（或是细胞动力学程序）EMT 是可逆的，间叶细胞能够转回上皮表型，这一过程被称为间质-上皮转化（mesenchymal epithelial transition，MET）。EMT 和 MET 均可发生在生理、病理及环境等因素作用下。

　　EMT 是一个高度保守的、控制多细胞生物中形态发生的基本过程。EMT 与多种细胞过程有关（图 10-2）。EMT 是一个 E-cadherin 基因的转录抑制过程，导致上皮表型的缺失和对间质表型相关的肌动蛋白细胞骨架重构。EMT 允许癌细胞的扩散，在肿瘤出现及其进展中起重要的作用。这种细胞过程是可逆的；如循环中孤立的癌细胞在转移部位可以外渗并通过 MET 形成新的转移瘤。

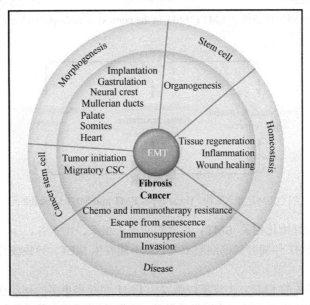

图 10-2　EMT 在多种细胞过程中的交汇作用；EMT at the crossroads of multiple cellular processes

　　EMT 是细胞表型发生转化的复杂过程，即具有极性的上皮细胞转化为在细胞基质中自由移动的间质细胞，在 EMT 功能中基因转录开关连接是复杂或多路径的，后者定义为上皮和间质细胞的行为。

　　EMT 的生物学本质是转向分化，可以发生在胚胎和成熟组织应对损伤时发生的创口修复和器官重塑中，也可以发生在肿瘤进展中，因此认为在胚胎发育、创口修复、器官纤维化性疾病及增加肿瘤浸润表型和转移过程中 EMT 起关键性作用[1]。在损伤组织的修复过程中，组织损伤促进募集间充质干细胞（mesenchymal stem cells，MSCs），可以分泌 EMT-诱导的细胞因子，如转化生长因子 β（TGF-β）等，导致细胞间接触溶解和相应的形态变化，在与其他的 EMT 诱导剂如 Wnt 协同作用下，上皮细胞完全转化成能动性的间质表型（图 10-3）。

　　EMT 和 MET 存在于胚胎发育、器官形成、伤口愈合、组织再生、器官纤维化、肿瘤进展和转移中。根据 EMT 发生的生物学背景，EMT 可以分为三种类型（图 10-4）[2]。

　　（1）胚胎发育、器官形成相关 EMT：在胚胎发生过程中，原始上皮（外胚层）经历 EMT 形成原始间叶，可以迁移和经过 MET 形成能分化成新的上皮组织的上皮细胞。

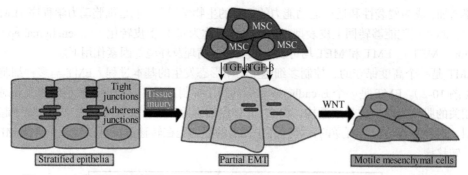

图 10-3　在病理生理条件下 EMT；EMT in the context of pathophysiological conditions

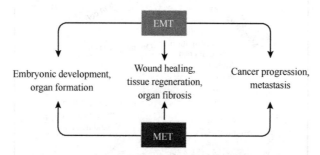

图 10-4　三类 EMT 和 MET；Three types EMT and MET in health and disease

（2）组织损伤和纤维化相关 EMT：在成熟或成人组织，由于各种压力、炎症或创伤，上皮细胞也可以经历 EMT 伴随着局部细胞紊乱，但不能发生 MET，导致成纤维细胞生成和最终纤维化。

（3）肿瘤进展相关的 EMT：上皮癌细胞发生 EMT 而获得更多的移动性间质表型，促使癌细胞入侵继发部位的癌细胞增殖形成继发性肿瘤。在这个过程中，移动性间质细胞必须通过血管和体液迁移入侵到继发组织，经 MET 和增殖形成继发性肿瘤。

EMT 的主要特征是胚胎发育和癌形成中进行性缺失上皮性的特征和获得梭形细胞形态[3]。在癌细胞中 EMT 是保持细胞形态和极性的细胞间黏附和识别机制丧失的结果，因此在发育和细胞分化中理解 EMT 的分子事件有利于深入了解肿瘤浸润过程中发生的基因调节作用和相关的分子事件。

第一节　胚胎发育相关的 EMT

脊椎动物在胚胎发育早期就已经发生了 EMT。EMT 和 MET 对于特殊细胞类型的最终分化和获得体内器官复杂的三围结构是必需的过程。据此 EMT 可分为三个阶段（图 10-5）。第一阶段包括原肠胚的形成，神经嵴形成；第二阶段有腭、肾、胰腺、肝脏及肌肉组织的形成等；第三阶段为心瓣膜的形成[4]。

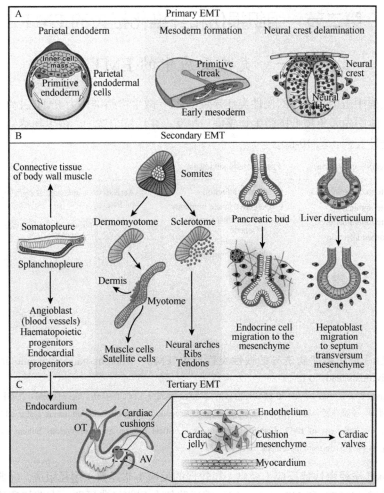

图 10-5　胚胎发育不同阶段 EMT；Primary，secondary，and tertiary EMT during embryonic development

A. 初级 EMT 发生在胚胎发育的早期，甚至是着床时，如小鼠壁层内胚层的形成。着床后第一次 EMT 是原肠胚形成过程中转变为中胚层祖细胞，而来源背神经管的神经嵴细胞脱层是之后的事件；B. 早期中胚层细胞被细分成轴向、轴向平行、中间和侧板中胚层细胞，这些细胞将分别聚结成暂时的上皮结构：脊索、体节、胚体壁和胚脏壁。这些暂时的结构将发生二次 EMT，导致间叶细胞的产生、分化成特定的细胞类型。内胚层组织，包括胰芽和肝憩室，从它们各自的上皮原基诱导解离出内分泌细胞和肝细胞；C. 第三次 EMT 的例子是在心脏从房室腔（AV）或流出管道（OT）中缓冲间质的形成。这些缓冲间质是心脏瓣膜的前体；A. Primary EMT occurs early during embryonic development，even before implantation such as during the formation of the parietal endoderm in mice. The first EMT after implantation is undergone by the mesendodermal progenitors during gastrulation，whereas the delamination of neural crest cells from the dorsal neural tube is a later event；B. Early mesodermal cells are subdivided into axial，paraxial，intermediate，and lateral plate mesodermal cells that will condense into transient epithelial structures：the notochord，the somites，and the somatopleure and splanchnopleure，respectively. These transient structures will undergo secondary EMT，leading to the generation of mesenchymal cells that differentiate into specific cell types. Endodermal tissues，including the pancreas bud and the liver diverticulum，exhibit morphological changes reminiscent of a secondary EMT to induce the dissociation of endocrine cells and hepatoblasts；C. An example of tertiary EMT arises during the formation of the cushion mesenchyme in the heart from the atrioventricular canal（AV）or the outflow tract（OT）. The cushion mesenchyme is the precursor of the cardiac valves

第二节　组织损伤和纤维化相关的 EMT

一、炎症反应中的 EMT

在易感人群中微生物诱导的慢性炎症导致 EMT。微生物感染作为 EMT 启动子起重要的作用。在健康个体中先天免疫抵抗微生物感染。相反，在易感个体中，微生物感染超过了先天免疫水平导致慢性炎症（图 10-6）。

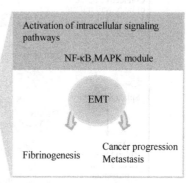

图10-6　易感性人群中微生物诱导的慢性炎症导致 EMT；Microbe-indued chronic inflammation in predisposed individuals leads to EMT

（与慢性感染有关的慢性炎症导致 NF-κB 和 MAPK 信号的持续激活是发生 EMT 的基础。最终使 EMT 在各种人类疾病中起重要作用，如纤维化形成、肿瘤进展和转移）；Chronic inflammation, associated to chronic infection lead to sustained NF-κB and MAPK module activation：the basement of EMT. Finally, EMT plays a critical role in onset of various human pathologies such as fibrinogenesis, cancer progression and metastasis

激活 NF-κB 途径由快速反应（经典）和较慢的反应（非经典）途径组成。经典途径控制炎症反应，并通过 TRAF1 和 NF-κB2 合成反馈通路偶合到非经典通路，在非经典途径中的两个限速因素激活。通过表观遗传修饰及周期蛋白依赖性激酶（CDK）增强转录延伸，限速 TRAF1/NF-κB2 翻译减少，从而增强了 EMT 途径的激活（图 10-7）。

二、纤维化中的 EMT

纤维化是一个进展性的病理过程，以广泛细胞外基质（extracellular matrix，ECM）沉积为特点。EMT 与内脏器官慢性病变发生纤维化过程密切相关。

1. 肝纤维化形式（hepatic fibrogenesis）　肝纤维化中肌成纤维细胞积累和分泌过多的胶原纤维并以纤维方式存储，从而损害器官的功能导致其衰竭。纤维化的起源一直被认为是间质成纤维细胞转换为肌成纤维细胞进而形成肝纤维化胶原网络的病理激活。EMT 在肝纤维化中最明显的特征是受损组织中上皮细胞获得了运动表型[2]。假设这是肝细胞在恶劣生长微环境中的一个整合逃生程序，这个恶劣生长微环境由氧化还原改变所激发，或由改变了的 ECM 复合物的作用所引起，而且还与慢性伤口愈合反应时高浓度生长因子和细胞因子作用有关[2]。这个逃生程序的特点是通过细胞代谢和运动的改变，以达到促进细胞生存选择逃离氧化损伤的目的。逃生程序一般有两个可能的结果：①运动的肝上皮细胞到达一个相对好的微环境，并发生向原始表型的重新分化；②该细胞持续处在恶劣生长微环境中，

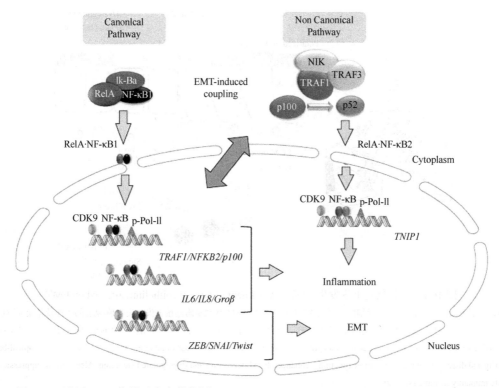

图 10-7　激活 EMT 信号对炎症的作用；Inflammatory consequences of EMT on innate signaling

其逃生表型消耗殆尽使细胞发生凋亡。与非逃生细胞相比，以上两种逃生细胞都有明显的病理优势，非逃生细胞在恶劣生长微环境中发生坏死，并进一步释放活性氧和其他促纤维化、促炎性分子[5]。因此提出了体内肝纤维化时肝细胞通过 EMT 产生 ECM 而获得间质表型的概念。越来越多的证据表明，在慢性炎症和肝纤维化过程中，发生 EMT 可以诱导肌成纤维细胞，促进 Ⅰ型胶原蛋白的合成和沉积[6]。

2. 肺纤维化形式（lung fibrogenesis）　如在哮喘中由于炎症刺激发生 EMT 导致肺纤维化（图 10-8）。

3. 在肾纤维化中上皮和内皮发生 EMT 时 miRNA 的作用（图 10-9）　在心、肾纤维化发生中内皮细胞也因 EMT 转化成间质细胞，在接受固定的腹膜透析和发生腹膜纤维化时间叶细胞也可以转化为不同的间质细胞，此为化生机制。

4. 肾小管基底膜发生 EMT 的关键事件及治疗干预（图 10-10）。

三、EMT 细胞的分子改变

（一）EMT 过程中的分子变化

抑制转录因子 Snail1、Snail2、ZEB1 和 ZEB2 对于上皮细胞形态的维持是重要的。在有炎症时 NF-κB、TGF-β1、BMPs、Wnt 和 Notch 信号蛋白表达上调，可以激活 Snail-Zeb 通路，导致 EMT 表达纤连蛋白（fibronectin，FN），波形蛋白（vimentin，Vim）、成纤维细胞特异性蛋白-1（fibroblast-specific protein-1，FSP-1）等，上皮特征性的标志 E-cadherin 和 ZO-1（zonula occludens-1）的表达减少（图 10-11）。

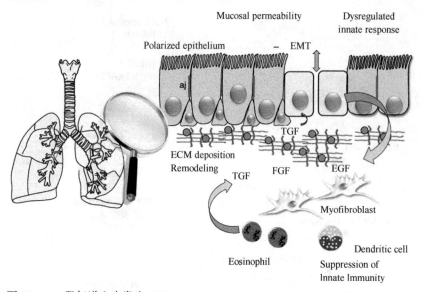

图 10-8　一段气道上皮发生 EMT；A segment of airway epithelium affected by EMT

ECM 和组织存在的白细胞（嗜酸粒细胞）释放的生长因子调控 EMT 导致黏附连接丧失，失去顶-基底的极性及黏膜屏障功能破坏，增加了 ECM 沉积物并使信号失调。在某些哮喘患者中也有抑制内源性免疫的作用；EMT is modulated by growth factors released from the ECM and tissue resident leukocytes（eosinophils）and result in loss of adherens junctions（aj），loss of apical-basal polarity and disruption of mucosal barrier function，enhanced ECM deposition and dysregulated signaling. Also there is suppression of innate immunity in some asthmatics

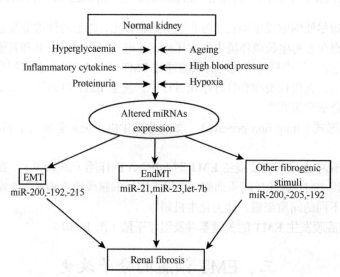

图 10-9　在肾纤维化中上皮和内皮发生 EMT 时 miRNA 的作用；The implications of miRNA in renal fibrosis with epithelium and endothelium cells occur EMT

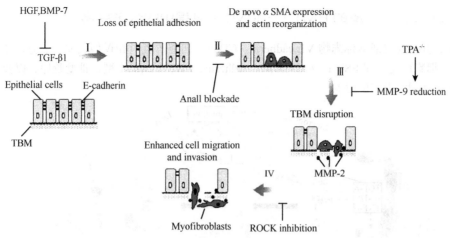

图 10-10　肾小管基底膜 EMT 的关键事件及治疗干预示意图；Schematic illustration of the key events of EMT involving the renal tubular basement membrane（TBM）and possible therapeutic interventions

该图显示完成 EMT 的四个关键事件：上皮细胞的黏附特性丧失；α-平滑肌肌动蛋白（α-SMA）表达和肌动蛋白重组；小管基底膜（tubular basement membrane，TBM）破坏；增强细胞迁移和侵袭能力。TGF-β1 能影响肾小管上皮细胞 EMT 四个步骤。阻止肾纤维化中的任何步骤都会显著影响 EMT。例如，肝细胞生长因子（hepatocyte growth factor，HGF）和骨形态发生蛋白（bone morphogenic protein，BMP）-7 可拮抗 TGF-β1，从而抑制 EMT 的启动（步骤Ⅰ）。通过氯沙坦（losartan）阻断 EMT 启动子血管紧张素（angiotensin，Ang）Ⅱ 的活性以减轻纤维化（步骤Ⅱ）。保持 TBM 完整性的 TPA⁻/⁻小鼠选择性阻断了梗阻性肾病中 EMT（步骤Ⅲ）。最后，ROCK 激酶的药物作用抑制细胞的迁移和减少肾纤维化（步骤Ⅳ）；The diagram illustrates four key events essential for the completion of EMT: loss of epithelial adhesion properties; de novo α-SMA expression and actin reorganization; disruption of TBM; and enhanced cell migration and invasion capacity. Transforming growth factor（TGF）β1 alone is capable of inducing tubular epithelial cells to undergo all four steps. Strategies to block any step during EMT would have a major impact on EMT and, thereby, on renal fibrosis. For instance, hepatocyte growth factor（HGF）and bone morphogenic protein（BMP）-7 could antagonize TGF-β1 and consequently inhibit the initiation of EMT（step Ⅰ）. Blockage of angiotensin（Ang）Ⅱ by losartan abolishes its activity as an EMT promoter and attenuates renal fibrosis（step Ⅱ）. Preservation of TBM integrity in tPA⁻/⁻ mice is selectively blocked EMT in obstructive nephropathy（stepⅢ）. Finally, pharmacological inhibition of ROCK kinase impairs cell migration and reduces renal fibrosis（stepⅣ）

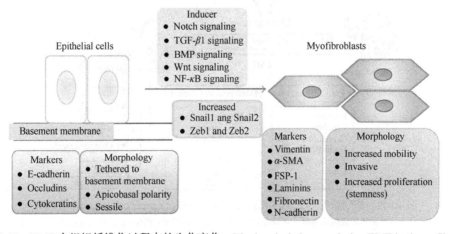

图 10-11　EMT 在组织纤维化过程中的生化变化；Biochemical changes during EMT in tissue fibrosis

（二）在血管内皮的 EMT（EndMT）过程中的分子变化

EMT 引起内皮细胞标志物 VE cadherin、CD31、细胞角蛋白和 IV 型胶原的表达减少，以及获得间质细胞标记，如 FSP-1，α-SMA，N-cadherin，FN，Vim，I 型、III 型胶原，以及 MMP2 和 MMP-9 表达（图 10-12）。

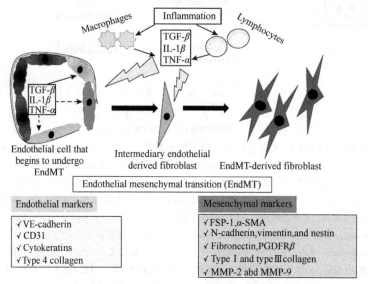

图 10-12　在内皮细胞 EMT 过程中的生化变化；Biochemical changes during EndMT program

第三节　癌进展和转移相关的 EMT

在 EMT 的发生中，肿瘤上皮通过下调上皮标志物，上调间叶标志物，获得了间叶细胞的形态，因此导致迁移、浸润能力增加，并对对化疗耐受，获得癌症干细胞（CSC）的特征。所有癌发生 EMT 后均增加了肿瘤的演进（图 10-13）[6-16]。

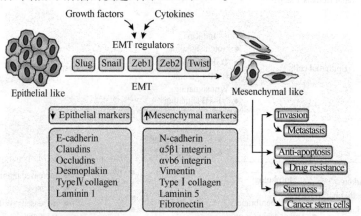

图 10-13　癌细胞发生 EMT 的结果；The results of cancer cells occurring EMT

EMT 调节癌细胞从上皮细胞转化成间质细胞，并抑制上皮细胞标记和表达间叶细胞标记，最终使癌细胞发生转移，产生耐药性和获得癌症干细胞的特征；The EMT regulators transform the cancer cells from epithelial-cell like to mesenchymal-cell like with suppression of epithelial markers and expression of mesenchymal markers. The final effects on cancer cells are cancer metastasis, drug resistance and with features of cancer stem cells

一、EMT 在肿瘤进展中起关键作用

EMT 在肿瘤转移起始阶段起重要作用。EMT 与肿瘤侵袭和转移的相关性是目前研究的热点。固定的、伴有顶-基极性的上皮细胞被转化为能动的、分散的梭形间充质细胞[4]，使肿瘤细胞离开原发部位侵入周围组织。加强肿瘤细胞运动性对转移、侵袭、血管浸润和外渗性的各个步骤至关重要[7]。因此，EMT 是癌症细胞侵袭和转移的先决条件和关键步骤（图 10-14）。

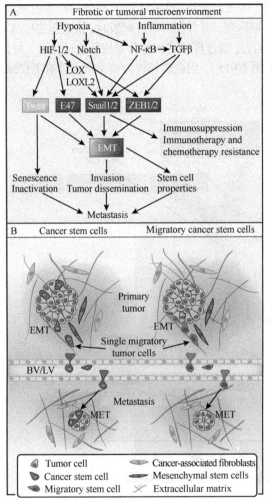

图 10-14　EMT 和肿瘤进展；EMT and Tumor Progression

A. EMT 诱导剂作为迁移促进因素。在纤维化或肿瘤微环境中，缺氧和炎性促进 EMT 诱导剂的激活。除了通过诱导细胞分离，促进肿瘤扩散和在癌旁组织的侵袭，EMT 在转移潜能的发挥上还具有重要意义。Twist 和 Snail 表达干细胞特性，有利于小部分细胞群的自我更新，从而克隆和分化成继发性癌。另外，Twist 也使癌基因触发的细胞衰老的自我保障机制失活，并且 Snail 能够诱导免疫抑制，免疫耐受和化疗耐受；B. 现在认为 EMT 在肿瘤进展和转移形成中起着重要的作用。个体细胞从原始肿瘤分离并且在 ECM 网中迁移。目前相关的研究正集中在分析癌症相关成纤维细胞（cancer-associated fibroblasts，CAF）的作用，包括骨髓原性的间充质干细胞。另一个挑战是了解恶性迁移的细胞是否是 CSC（在原发肿瘤中的肿瘤启动细胞），如果他们是否源于体细胞性上皮细胞，那么该上皮细胞已经经历了 EMT 获得干细胞的特性，或者这两种可能性的结合。BV/LV：血管/淋巴管；

A. EMT inducer as metastasis promoting agents. In the fibrotic or tumoral microen vironment, hypoxia and inflammation favor the activation of EMT inducers. In addition to promoting tumor dissemination by inducing cell delamination and invasion of adjacent tissues, new facets of the EMT have been recently described that help to understand their implication in the metastatic potential. Both Twist and Snail conferred stem cells properties, favo ring the self-renewal of a small population of cells that can colonize and differentiate into secondary carcinomas. In addition , Twist also inactivated the cellular safeguard mechanism of cellular senescence triggered by oncogenes and Snail induced immunesuppre-ssion, immuno-resistance, and chemores- istance;

B. EMT is now thought to play a fundamental role in tumor progression and metastasis formation. Individual cells delaminate from primary tumors and migrate following the extracellular matrix network. Current research is actively analyzing the contributions of cancer-associated fibroblasts(CAF), including bone-marrow derived mesen- chymal stem cells. Another challenge is to understand whether malignant migratory cells are cancer stem cells that act as tumor-initiating cells in the primary tumor, if they are derived from somatic epithelial tumor cells that have undergone EMT to acquire stem cell-like properties , or some combi- nation of these two possibilities. (BV/LV , blood vessels/lymphatic vessels)

在 EMT 诱导信号的应答中，侵袭肿瘤瘤体边缘的细胞亚群可能会失去上皮细胞特性。当这些细胞进一步从瘤体中脱离移出，基质细胞提供 EMT 的信号使上皮细胞亚群较少的暴露在上皮细胞信号中，而获得更多的间叶细胞的特性。转化的间叶细胞更容易浸润到周围组织。伴有完全间叶表型的细胞易于进入毛细血管或引流的淋巴管。在某种情况下，巨噬细胞协助此过程的完成。当然，转移的癌细胞同样也要能抵抗环境和基因毒性的压力，这是癌细胞在血液循环中存活至关重要的特征。在到达远端器官后，间叶细胞的表型有助于转移癌细胞在继发组织中的外渗与侵袭。此处转移细胞暴露在不同于原发肿瘤组织的信号中，并且间叶细胞的状态能授予单个癌细胞生存优势或维持该细胞的长期休眠。当有合适信号刺激时，该细胞将经历 MET 并且逐步再获得上皮的特性，如快速增殖的能力。通过自分泌和旁分泌信号途径增强上皮信号，使其上皮表型稳定，有助于转移瘤的生长（图 10-15），因此转移性肿瘤主要由伴有上皮细胞特性的细胞组成。

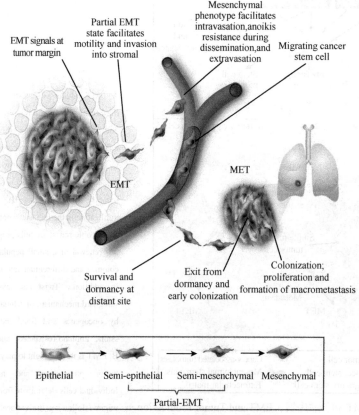

图 10-15　EMT 的可塑性使癌细胞能在侵袭-转移级联反应中获得功能性适应；EMT plasticity allows cancer cells to undergo functional adaptations during the invasion-metastasis cascade

肿瘤转移中转化的间叶细胞浸润到缺乏上皮信号刺激的不利的组织微环境继续 EMT，一旦定居到转移部位将重新获得上皮信号刺激，这些间质细胞特性的细胞可以发生 MET，重新转化成上皮细胞，重建细胞间连接和细胞骨架，形成相对稳定的转移瘤（图 10-16）。因此 MET 对发生 EMT 的肿瘤细胞转移至新部位并长期增殖具有重要意义。

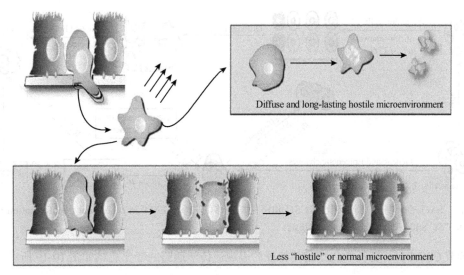

图 10-16 在肿瘤浸润、转移中肿瘤微环境对 EMT 和 MET 的影响；The effect of tumor microenvironment to EMT and MET in tumor invasion and metastasis

二、EMT 与肿瘤干细胞的关系

miRNA 的异常表达与肿瘤干细胞（CSC）的形成和 EMT 表型获得有关。miRNA 可调节 EMT 细胞演化为 CSC，使 EMT 细胞具有了 CSC 样特征，CSC 也表现出间叶表型。进而伴有 EMT 表型的细胞分享 CSC 样细胞（cancer stem-like cell，CSLC）耐药的特征（图 10-17），使肿瘤复发和转移，导致癌进展[8-11]（图 10-18）。

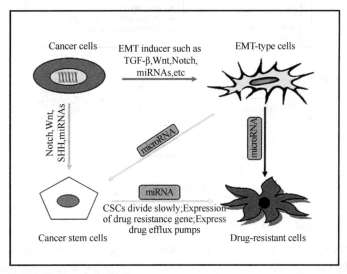

图 10-17 EMT、CSC 和 miRNA 间的联系；The connection between EMT，cancer stem cells and miRNA

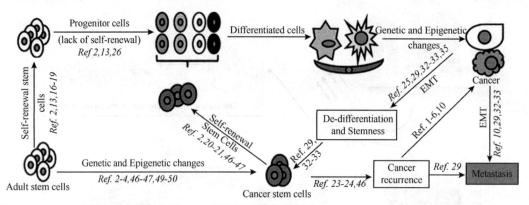

图 10-18　EMT 在干细胞恶性转化为 CSC 和癌复发转移的关系；EMT in malignant transformation of stem cells into CSC and recurrence and metastasis

调节 CSC/EMT 特征和化疗耐药特征的表观遗传学通路的变化总结如图 10-19 所示。

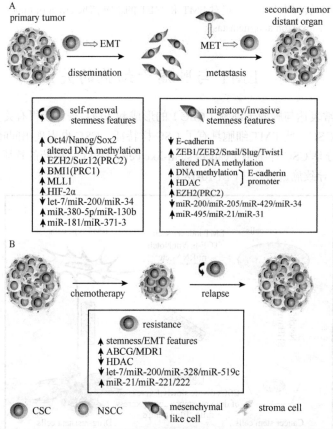

图 10-19　代表调节 CSC/EMT 特征的表观遗传学通路的变化（A）和代表化疗耐药特征的表观遗传学通路的变化（B）总结；Summary representing the most prominent alterations of epigenetic pathways that regulate CSC/EMT features（A）and resistance to chemotherapy（B）

三、针对肿瘤 EMT 的干预

表皮生长因子受体（ErbBs）的信号能通过激活不同的细胞内受体酪氨酸激酶（receptor tyrosine kinase，RTK）刺激癌细胞发生 EMT。这往往是转录因子活性增加所致，如 Snail 抑制细胞内黏附分子 E-cadherin 的表达。因此，这些细胞变得梭状形态更明显，表达间质相关分子，如 Vimentin、N-cadherin 和某些 MMPs，增强了癌细胞迁移和侵袭，恶性程度更高。ErbB 信号的抑制剂能够干扰某些癌细胞 EMT 的进程。在选择性的病例中，逆转 EMT 能增加对 EMT 相关耐药癌细胞的抗癌疗效（图 10-20）。

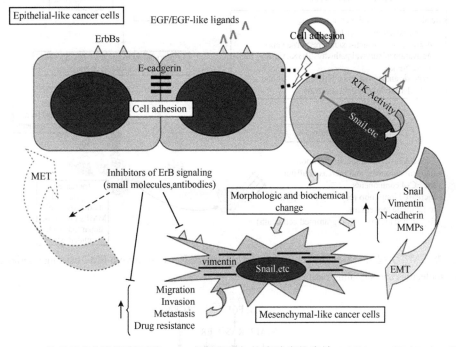

图 10-20 ErbB 信号的抑制剂能够干扰 EMT 的进程增加抗癌治疗的疗效；Inhibitors of ErbB signaling have been able to interfere with the EMT process to result in increased efficacy of anti-cancer therapy in certain cancer cells

第四节 调控 EMT 的分子机制

EMT 是癌演进所必需，当损伤、过量的生长因子和细胞因子刺激、ECM 的质或量的改变，以及缺氧或氧化应激等产生的不利肿瘤微环境促使癌发生 EMT，癌细胞代谢和存活将重新编程，引起一系列基因、分子及信号通路调控的改变（图 10-21）。

肿瘤早期阶段细胞保持上皮特征类似于相邻正常上皮。当癌细胞中 EMT 的主要调控因子额外过表达，如转录因子 Twist、Snail 和 SIP1 将导致基因表达谱和细胞行为的显著改变。Twist、Snail 和 SIP1 以一个尚未知的机制通过启动和触发整个 EMT 转录表达中的 E 盒抑制 E-cadherin（图 10-22）。

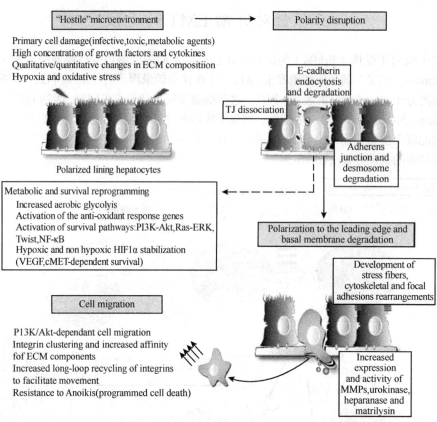

图 10-21　癌 EMT 引起的一系列基因、分子及信号通路的改变；Cancer with EMT causing a series changes of genes，molecules and signaling pathways

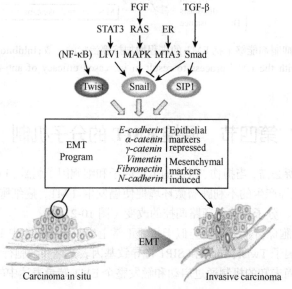

图 10-22　驱动和介导 EMT 因子；Drivers and mediators of EMT

一、TGF-β

在许多组织 EMT 发生中发现有许多细胞因子参与，其中 TGF-β 被认为是主要的开关[14]。TGF-β 超家族成员是一种多功能的多肽类细胞因子[4]。在各种生理和病理事件中发挥关键作用[15]，包括胚胎形成、器官形成、分化、凋亡、免疫调节、纤维化及各种人类疾病[16-17]，如在癌形成中 TGF-β 的分泌抑制细胞增殖[18]、抑制转化[19]、诱导细胞凋亡[20]和促进 ECM 的沉积等，又如在许多肿瘤中 TGF-β 信号紊乱能下调凋亡[21]。另一方面 TGF-β 活化与癌形成的演进有关。例如，EMT 来源的肝肌成纤维细胞的增生，上调其纤维蛋白产物引起纤维化基质沉积的增加[22-24]，使人肝癌中有较强的 TGF-β mRNA 和蛋白的表达[25]，尿中 TGF-β 水平增加与硬化性肝癌的预后差有关[26]，在肝中持续表达成熟的 TGF-β 将加速转基因鼠肝癌的形成[27]，而且 TGF-β 能促进培养肝细胞的自发性转化[28]。

TGF-β 在哺乳类动物中有 3 种亚型，分别为 TGF-β1、TGF-β2 和 TGF-β3。其中 TGF-β1 是含量最丰富、表达最多的亚型。同时细胞膜上存在相应的 3 种跨膜受体，以 Ⅰ、Ⅱ 型受体为主，具有丝氨酸/苏氨酸酶活性，Ⅲ 型受体包括内皮因子和 β 聚糖。

TGF-β 的信号通路主要有两条，分为依赖 Smads 信号通路和非依赖 Smads 信号通路。前者是经典的 TGF-β 信号通路，Smad 家族主要分为受体调节型（receptor-regulated R-Smads）、协同作用型（Co-Smads）和抑制作用型（I-Smads）三种类型。R-Smads 包括 Smad1、Smad2、Smad3、Smad5、Smad8；Co-Smads 包括 Smad4；I-Smads 包括 Smad6、7。其中的 Smad2 和 Smad3 与 TGF-β 信号通路有关。非依赖 Smad 的 TGF-β 信号通路途径有多种。TGF-β 受体复合物可以激活丝裂原活化蛋白激酶（mitogen-activated protein kinase，MAPK），并行的 MAPK 通路包括细胞外信号调节激酶（extracellular signal-regulated kinase，ERK）通路、c-Jun 氨基端激酶（c-Jun N-turminal kinase/stress activated protein kinase，JNK）通路及 p38-MAPK 通路。ERK 是 MAPK 中重要的一员。TGF-β 与细胞膜上受体结合，可使受体形成二聚体，自身酪氨酸激酶残基磷酸化，磷酸化的酪氨酸与细胞膜上的生长因子结合蛋白 2（growth factor receptor binding protein2，Grb2）的 SH2 结构域相结合，而 Grb2 的 SH3 结构域同时与鸟苷酸交换因子 SOS（son of sevenless）结合，后者使小分子鸟苷酸结合蛋白 Ras 的 GDP 解离而结合 GTP，从而激活 Ras；激活的 Ras 进一步与丝氨酸/苏氨酸蛋白激酶 Raf-1 的氨基酸结合，激活 Raf-1 后，可以磷酸化 MEK1/MEK2 的 2 个调节性丝氨酸，从而激活 MEKS；MEKS 为双特异性激酶，可以使丝氨酸/苏氨酸和酪氨酸发生磷酸化，最终高选择性激活 ERK1 和 ERK2。

（一）TGF-β 对 EMT 信号网和转录的调控

TGF-β 是 EMT 的诱导因子，许多肿瘤中均有 TGF-β 的表达增加，因为 TGF-β 诱导 EMT 而促进肿瘤浸润和转移，因此是癌进展的重要指标[29, 30]。很多证据表明 TGF-β 和 EMT 两者均涉及相同的各种生理和病理事件。TGF-β 与其受体结合，使 R-Smad 磷酸化后与 Smad4 形成复合物，进入细胞核内促进 EMT 相关分子的表达。Smad 家族蛋白与其他信号分子合作，如 Ras-MAPK-PI3KZ、NF-κB、Wnt[31]、整合素（integrin）、Notch，以及转录因子 Snail[32]、Slug[33]、Twist[34]和 Zeb1/2[35]作为某些上皮细胞中 TGF-β 诱导 EMT 的重要因子。TGF-β 也可直接刺激 Par6 的磷酸化，降低细胞间紧密连接的稳定性和增加 Snail 的表达，导致 E-cadherin 的减少和黏附连接蛋白的分解并激活 Rho GTP 酶使细胞骨架重组、细胞极性消失而导致 EMT。

1. TGF-β 的信号通路（图 10-23） TGF-β 激活：EMT 主要经过经典的 Smad 依赖机制，需要两种受体激酶和 R-Smads（Smad2 和 Smad3）的信号转导子家族。在磷酸化中 R-Smads

与 Smad4 形成复合物，随后转位进入核内调节 EMT 靶基因的转录，如 Smad7、Snail 和 I 型胶原蛋白[36-38]。

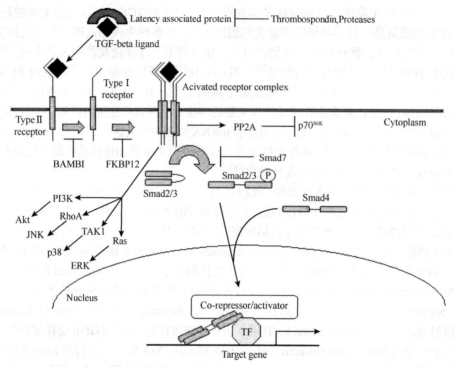

图 10-23　TGF-β 的信号通路；The signal pathways of TGF-β

2. 癌症中 TFG-β 信号调控如图 10-24 所示

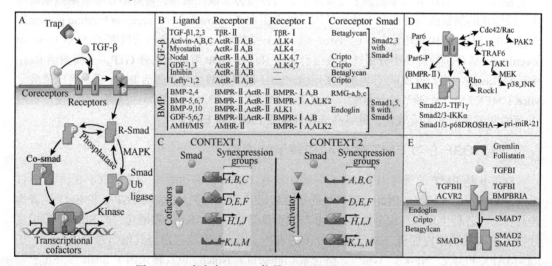

图 10-24　癌症中 TGF-β 信号；TGF-β signaling in cancer

A. 配体 traps 与共受体分子调控 TGF-β 家族配体与信号受体接触。配体聚集成一个 I 型 II 型丝氨酸/苏氨酸激酶的受体四聚体复合物。II 型受体磷酸化和激活 I 型受体，然后磷酸化激活 Smad 转录因子（R-Smads）。激活的 R-Smads 结合 Smad4，进一步组成转录激活和抑制复合物来调控靶细胞中上百个靶基因的表达。MAPK 与其他蛋白激酶磷酸化 Smad 使其被泛素化连接酶和其他灭活机制识别；B. 关于配体-受体-共受体-Smad 在 TGF-β 和 TGF-β 家族 BMP 分支间关系的简略图；C. 不同环境中转录伴侣分子之间的显著结合（如不同细胞类型或环境）通过特异性激活的 Smads 决定了一组基因的靶向。与每个 Smad 伴侣分子结合将协调调节靶基因的下游基因组的表达。Smad 信号作为整合调节信号的节点，影响伴侣分子的作用；D. TGF-β 信号选择性模式包括 Smad4 非依赖性 R-Smad 信号通路（通过 TIF1γ，IKKα，p68DROSHA 相互作用），Smad 非依赖性受体-Ⅰ 信号通路（通过小 G 蛋白和 MAPK 途径），和直接受体-Ⅱ信号通路（通过 Par6，以及在 BMPR-Ⅱ情况下的 LIMK1）；E. 人类癌细胞中 TGF-β 信号通路核心成分受到突变影响（灰）、过表达（黑），或者下调（白）的结果；A. Ligand traps and coreceptor molecules control the access of TGF-β family ligands to signaling receptors. The ligand assembles a tetrameric complex of receptor serine/threonine kinases types I and Ⅱ. Receptor-Ⅱ phosphorylates and activates receptor-I，which then phosphorylates and activates Smad transcription factors（R-Smads）. Activated R-Smads bind Smad4 and further build transcriptional activation and repression complexes to control the expression of hundreds of target genes in a given cell. Mitogen-activated protein kinases（MAPK）and other protein kinases phosphorylate Smads for recognition by ubiquitin ligases and other mechanisms of inactivation；B. An abridged chart of ligand-receptor-coreceptor-Smad relationships in the TGF-β and BMP branches of the TGF-β family；C. Distinct combinations of transcription partner cofactors in different contexts（e.g., different cell types or conditions）determine the set of genes targeted by specific activated Smads. Each Smad-cofactor combination coordinately regulates a synexpression group of target genes. Smad signaling serves as a node for integrating regulatory signals that impinge on partner cofactors；D. Alternative modes of TGF-β signaling include Smad4-independent R-Smad signaling（via interactions with TIF1γ，IKKα，p68DROSHA），Smad-independent receptor-I signaling（via small G proteins and MAPK pathways），and direct receptor-Ⅱ signaling（via Par6，and via LIMK1 in the case of BMPR-Ⅱ）；E. Core TGF-β pathway components that are affected by mutation（gray），overexpression（black），or downregulation（white）in human cancers

3. TGF-β 通路激活诱导 EMT 如图 10-25 所示

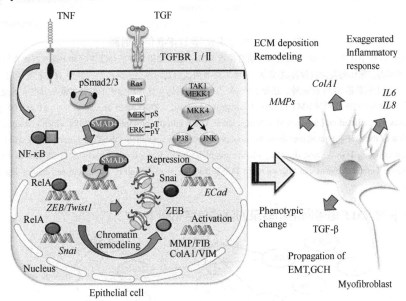

图 10-25　TGF-β 通路激活诱导 EMT；Pathways activated by TGF-β induce EMT

在 EMT 发生之前和之后的一个理想上皮细胞显示了典型（Smad）和非经典 TGF-β 细胞内信号通路模式图。TGF-β 信号是主转录调节因子 Snail（Snail/2）、zebra（ZEB）和 Twist（Twst）的上游分子，通过组蛋白修饰诱导转录重新编程使染色质重塑。已知在炎症反应中 TNF-NF-κB 有相互联系，刺激 TGF-β 信号抑制了 Ecad（CADH1），上调了上皮细胞中的纤连蛋白（FIB）、胶原 1（COL1）和 α-SMA；An ideal epithelial cell before and after EMT showing the canonical（Smad）and non-canonical TGF-β intracellular signaling pathways. The TGF-β signaling is upstream of the master transcriptional regulators，Snail（SNAⅡ/2），Zebra（ZEB）and Twist（Twst）that induce transcriptional reprogramming and chromatin remodeling through histone modification. Stimulation of TGF-β pathways result in repression of E Cad（CADH1）and upregulation of fibronectin（FIB），collagen 1（Cal1）and α-SMA in the epithelial cells known interconnections with the TNF-NF-κB inflammatory response

4. 整合素（integrin）介导 TGF-β 信号通路如图 10-26 所示

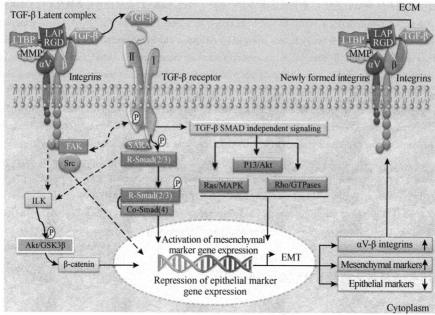

图 10-26　整合素介导 TGF-β 信号通路

αV 整合素识别与结合在 TGF-β 中 LAP 上的整合素结合位点 RGD，诱发黏附介导的细胞连接和（或）TGF-β 与附近 MMPs 连接，导致 TGF-β 经同源二聚体的复杂过程释放/激活。一旦 TGF-β 激活后其同源二聚体将结合 Ⅱ 型 TGF-β 受体启动 TGF-β-Smad 信号，该信号除了能上调其他 EMT 标记外，还能上调 αV 整合素的表达。这些新形成的整合素能从其潜在的复合物中释放更多的 TGF-β，维持和加强 TGF-β 诱导 EMT 过程；αV integrins recognize a RGD motif present in the LAP of TGF-β. This binding induces either adhesion-mediated cell forces and/or brings latent TGFβ into the proximity of MMPs which consequently lead to the liberation/activation of the TGF-β homodimer from its latent complex. Upon activation, the TGF-β homodimer will bind to the Type Ⅱ TGF-β receptor initiating TGF-β-Smad signaling which upregulates the expression of αV integrins in addition to that of other EMT markers. These newly formed integrins can liberate more TGF-β from its latent complex, sustaining and reinforcing TGF-β induced EMT progression

5. TGF-β 对 EMT 信号网络和转录的调控总结见图 10-27

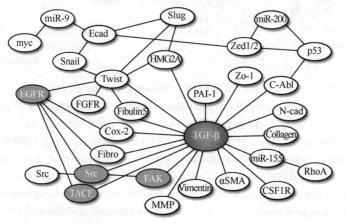

图 10-27　TGF-β 对 EMT 信号网和转录的调控；The EMT signaling network and transcription regulated by TGF-β

黑色代表基因的表达增加，白色代表基因表达降低。灰色代表在 EMT 中 TGF-β 刺激增加了酶活性。线表示 EMT 中这些分子之间的相互作用或相互激活；Black spheres represent genes whose expression is increased, while White spheres signify genes whose expression is decreased. Gray spheres depict increased enzymatic activity stimulated by TGF-β during EMT. Lines between nodes indicate a described interaction or transactivation between those molecules during EMT

（二）TGF-β 在癌症中的作用

在正常和癌变前的细胞中，TGF-β 直接通过细胞自主性肿瘤抑制效应（细胞淤滞、分化、凋亡）或者间接通过对基质的影响（炎症抑制和基质来源分裂素）调节体内平衡和抑制肿瘤。然而，当癌细胞失去 TGF-β 肿瘤抑制性作用而获得 TGF-β，引起免疫逃逸，生长因子的生成、分化成侵袭性表型的优势，将促进转移性克隆的建立和扩张（图 10-28）。

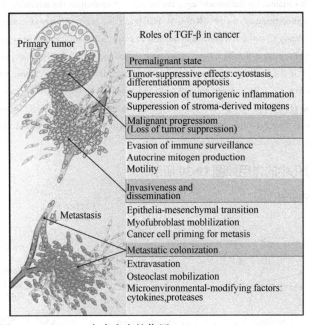

图 10-28　TGF-β 在癌症中的作用；The role of TGF-β in cancer

1. TGF-β 在癌间质中的作用如图 10-29 所示

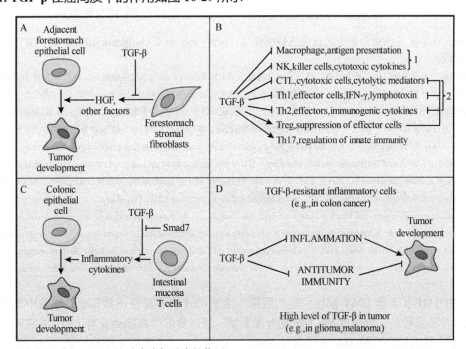

图 10-29　在癌间质中 TGF-β 抗肿瘤或促肿瘤的作用；Anti- and protumorigenic effects of TGF-β in the stroma

A. TGF-β 通过抑制诸如 HGF 等细胞生存和运动因子的产物来抑制某些上皮组织（如前胃上皮）中肿瘤发生；B. TGF-β 作为重要的免疫耐受增强子通过抑制先天性免疫（1）和获得性免疫（2）系统中几乎所有的主要元件的发展和功能来发挥作用。其中一些功效是由 T 细胞严格调控的（调节性 T 细胞），而 T 细胞又限制了其他淋巴细胞的功能；C. 如在结肠上皮细胞中观察到：限制炎症反应，TGF-β 能够避免从慢性炎症而来的原癌基因的促瘤作用。然而，T 细胞在一些炎症性肠疾病的患者中（如结肠癌前驱状态）过表达 Smad7 时对 TGF-β 不敏感；D. 在某些类型的癌症中，在炎症细胞缺陷的 TGF-β 反应可导致过度的炎症，促进肿瘤的生长。在另一些癌症中，肿瘤衍生的 TGF-β 能抑制抗肿瘤免疫反应，此亦能促进肿瘤的进展；A. TGF-β suppresses tumor emergence in certain epithelial tissues (e.g., the forestomach epithelium) by inhibiting the production of cell survival and motility factors such as hepatocyte growth factor (HGF)；B. TGF-β acts as a major enforcer of immune tolerance by inhibiting the development and functions of nearly all major components of the innate (1) and adaptive (2) immune system. Some of these effects are exerted through the activation of regulatory T cells (Treg) that constrain the function of other lymphocytes；C. By imposing limits on the inflammatory response，TGF-β can avert the protumorigenic effect that could derive from chronic inflammation，as observed in colonic epithelial cells. However，T cells in some patients with inflammatory bowel disease (a colon cancer-prone condition) overexpress Smad7 and are not sensitive to TGF-β；D. In some types of cancer，a defective TGF-β response in inflammatory cells can lead to excessive inflammation，favoring tumor progression. In other types of cancer，tumor-derived TGF-β can suppress antitumor immune responses，which also favors tumor progression

2. TGF-β 在癌分化中的作用如图 10-30 所示

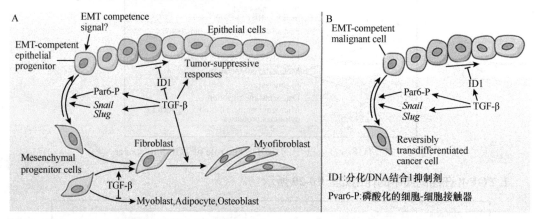

图 10-30　TGF-β 在细胞分化中的致癌或抑癌作用；Anti- and protumorigenic effects of TGF-β on cell differentiation

A. TGF-β 有利于上皮细胞分化、减少增殖，部分原因是通过下调 ID1 来实现。因为上皮祖细胞可以代替成为对 TGF-β 反应的 EMT 细胞。TGF-β 的功能是通过转录因子 Snail 和 Slug 或通过磷酸化的细胞-细胞调节因子 Par6 促进 EMT 的发生。在脂肪细胞和骨骼肌细胞系损伤的条件下，TGF-β 也促进间充质祖细胞向成纤维细胞和肌成纤维细胞谱系分化；B. 乳腺癌细胞中观察到癌细胞可通过激活 ID1 调节 TGF-β 的应答避免分化成低增殖状态。那些经过 EMT 的、对 TGF-β 反应产生高迁移性癌祖细胞侵入间质，其存在与肿瘤的转移有关；A. TGF-β favors epithelial differentiation into less proliferative states partly through the downregulation of Inhibitor of Differentiation/DNA binding 1 (ID1). But because of as yet unknown determinants, epithelial progenitor cells can instead become competent to undergo EMT in response to TGF-β. TGF-β functions through the transcription factors Snail and Slug and through phosphorylation of the cell-cell contact regulator Par6 to stimulate EMT. TGF-β also stimulates the differentiation of mesenchymal progenitor cells toward fibroblast and myofibroblast lineages，at the expense of adipocyte and musculoskeletal lineages；B. Carcinoma cells may avert differentiation into a less proliferative state by switching the *ID1* response to TGF-β from repression to activation，as observed in breast cancer cells. Carcinoma progenitor cells that are competent to undergo EMT in response to TGF-β yield highly motile，invasive mesenchymal derivatives，whose presence in tumors is associated with metastatic dissemination

3. 由 TGF-β 诱导 EMT 编程引起的后果　给予 TGF-β 容易在正常和恶性细胞中形成转移性 EMT 的细胞状态，再通过 MET 恢复上皮表型，这通常发生在胚胎发育 EMT 中或肿瘤转移的情况中。细胞长期接触 TGF-β 或其他 EMT-启动因子有助于癌症干细胞的继续发展和扩增，这些均是化疗耐受和疾病复发的共同基础。在复发性肿瘤的生长中，CSC 怎样、何时、在哪经历 MET 仍有待进一步阐明（图 10-31 ）。

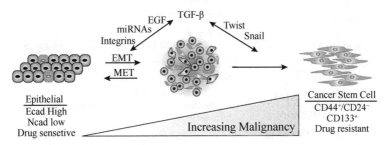

图 10-31　由 TGF-β 诱导 EMT 编程引起的后果；The consequences of EMT programs induced by TGF-β

4. TGF-β 与肿瘤演进　由于 TGF-β 介导肿瘤抑制的效果。癌细胞可以通过两种途径避免 TGF-β 的抑制作用：①受体失活或突变导致的通路失效；②选择性切断肿瘤抑制通路。后者中，癌细胞可以通过参与 TGF-β 应答并从中获得额外收益从而达到促癌的目的。两种情况下，癌细胞均可以通过 TGF-β 来调节微环境，躲避免疫监视，或者诱导促癌因子的产生（图 10-32 ）。

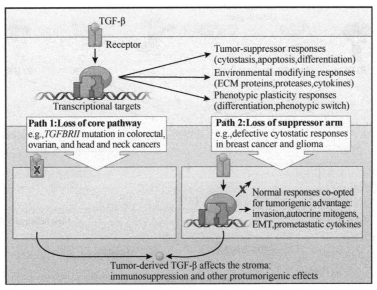

图 10-32　TGF-β 与肿瘤演进；TGF-β and tumor progression

二、其他与 EMT 相关的转录因子

（一）Snail 及其信号调控

Snail 是 Snail 超家族的成员之一,脊柱动物包括 Snail 和 Slug 两个亚家族。哺乳动物 Snail 基因家族包括 Snail1、Snail2 和 Snail3。人 Snail 基因位于第 20 号染色体长臂（20q13）,Snail 蛋白是含有锌指结构的转录因子。

Snail 的结构和 Snail 诱导 EMT 相关信号通路见图 10-33 和图 10-34。

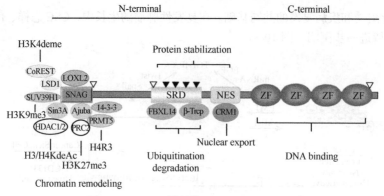

图 10-33　Snail 的结构；Structure of Snail

Snail 含有的 N-端 SNAG 结构域和 C-端的锌指结构域。N-端 SNAG 结构域与几个共同阻遏剂和表观遗传学重塑复合物相互作用，C-端的锌指结构域负责与 DNA 结合。富含丝氨酸的结构域(serine-rich domain，SRD)和核输出序列(nuclear export sequence，NES)控制 Snail 蛋白的稳定性和亚细胞定位(三角形表示磷酸化位点)；Snail contains an N-terminal SNAG domain and C-terminal zinc finger domains. The N-terminal SNAG domain interacts with several co-repressors and epigenetic remodeling complexes，and the C-terminal zinc finger domains are responsible for DNA binding. The serine-rich domain (SRD) and nuclear export sequence (NES) control the Snail protein stability and subcellular localization. Phosphorylation sites are indicated as triangles

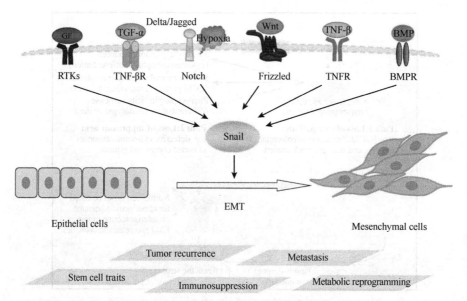

图 10-34　Snail 诱导 EMT 相关信号通路示意图；Schematic diagram of the signaling pathways associated with Snail-induced EMT

Snail 完整和复杂信号通路网络，包括 RTKs、TGF-β、Notch、Wnt、TNF-α 和 BMPs 信号通路，激活转录因子 Snail 诱导 EMT。Snail 的表达引起代谢重编程，赋予肿瘤细胞具有干细胞特性，抗免疫抑制，促进肿瘤的复发和转移；An integrated and complex signaling network，including RTKs，TGF-β，Notch，Wnt，TNF-α，and BMPs signaling pathways，activate the transcription factor Snail，resulting in the induction of EMT. The expression of Snail causes a metabolic reprogramming，confers tumor cells with stem cell-like traits，resistance to immunosuppression，and promotes tumor recurrence and metastasis

　　转染 Snail 基因后具有典型 EMT 的人类黑色素瘤细胞可部分通过血小板反应性蛋白-1（thrombospondin-1，TSP-1）产物诱导肿瘤组织中调节性 T 细胞和树突状细胞受损，从而抑制免疫反应。Snail 阳性的黑色素瘤细胞对免疫治疗不敏感，但当在瘤内注射 Snail 基因特异性的小干扰核糖核酸（small interfering RNA，siRNA）和抗 TSP-1 抗体后，就可通过免疫反应抑制肿瘤的生长和转移，这提示 EMT 和肿瘤细胞的免疫耐受有关。

（二）Twist

Twist 转录因子是一个由 202 个氨基酸残基组成的结合蛋白，含有高度保守的碱性螺旋-环-螺旋结构域。人类 Twist 基因定位于染色体 7p21，包含 2 个外显子和 1 个内含子，其中外显子 1 具有编码功能，mRNA 序列全长 1669 bp，开放阅读框架长 609 bp。该蛋白在小鼠和人之间同源性高达 96%，能够独立下调 E-cadherin 的表达，并上调 FN 和 N-cadherin 表达，诱导 EMT 的发生[34, 39]。有研究表明其还可通过多种信号通路诱导 EMT 表型。Twist1 和 Twist2 通过抑制 p16/ink4a 和 p21/cip 抗癌细胞凋亡，使肿瘤细胞失控性增殖。

（三）Wnt

Wnt 蛋白是一组调控胚胎形成期间细胞间信号转导的、高度保守的、分泌信号分子，其基因最早是由小鼠乳癌原癌基因及果蝇无翅基因整合而成。细胞分泌的 Wnt 蛋白同时与细胞表面 frizzled 受体和 LRP5/6 结合，抑制 GSK-3β 的活性，从而抑制 Axin-APC-GSK-3β 与 β-catenin 形成泛素调节的蛋白降解复合物[42]，使 β-catenin 在细胞质和细胞核内积累。在细胞核内，β-catenin 与 TCF4/LEF 转录因子相互作用，刺激下游靶基因 cyclin D1、c-myc、Slug、FN 和 vimentin 的表达[41]，使上皮细胞向间质样细胞转变。此外，Wnt 可仅和受体结合，通过转录因子、钙依赖性激酶和钙调蛋白发挥作用，或通过 Dsh 激活 Jun-N 端激酶（JNK）调节转录因子 p53、Elk1、DPC4、ATF2、c-Jun 等的活性而起作用。

三、EMT 过程的生物标志物

1. E-钙粘蛋白（E-cadherin）　是黏附连接的主要成分。在 EMT 过程中，TGF-β 抑制 E-cadherin 的表达，以及从质膜诱发其内化，是 EMT 最重要的标志物之一[42-44]。

E-cadherin 作为浸润抑制基因，在 EMT 中下调黏附分子 E-cadherin 的表达使细胞丧失了细胞间的识别和黏附能力，在已知的转录因子中已发现较有价值的 Snail 基因对 E-cadherin 转录的直接抑制[43, 45-47]，在小鼠皮肤肿瘤和人乳腺癌浸润前缘 E-cadherin 表达活性增强[46-49]。图 10-35，图 10-36 分别表示在正常细胞和癌细胞中 E-cadherin 的转录和降解。

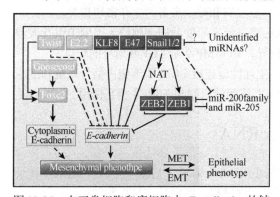

图 10-35　在正常细胞和癌细胞中 E-cadherin 的转录；E-cadherin transcription in normal and cancer cells
在细胞中 Snail、ZEB、E47 和 KLF8 直接抑制 E-cadherin 的转录，而 Twist、Goosecoid、E2.2 和 Foxc2 是 E-cadherin 的间接抑制剂。Snail1 通过不同的机制激活 ZEB 基因表达，包括诱导 ZEB2 的自然反义转录（natural antisense transcript, NAT）。miR-200 家族及某些情况下的 miR-205，抑制 ZEB 基因转录，阻止 EMT 发生。循环 miRNAs 和 ZEB 因子交叉调节增加了几个 EMT 诱导物的协同作用，加强了 EMT 过程的控制。初步数据显示，Snail1 也可能抑制 miR-200 家族的表达。是否 miRNAs 也能控制 snail 表达有待进一步研究；Snail, ZEB, E47 and KLF8 factors directly repress E-cadherin transcription whereas Twist, Goosecoid, E2.2 and Foxc2 are indirect E-cadherin repressors. Snail1 activates the expression of the ZEB genes by different mechanisms, including the induction of a natural antisense transcript for ZEB2（NAT）. The miR-200 family and in some cases also miR-205, represses the transcription of ZEB genes preventing EMT. A loop of miRNAs and ZEB factors cross regulation plus the cooperation of several EMT inducers reinforces the control of the EMT process. Preliminary data indicate that Snail1 may also repress the expression of the miR-200 family. Whether miRNAs can also control Snail expression awaits further investigation

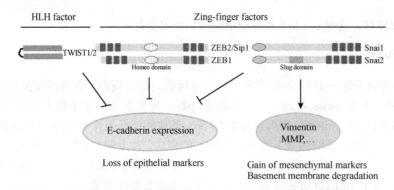

图 10-36　在正常细胞和癌细胞中 E-cadherin 的降解；E-cadherin degradation in normal and cancer cells
EMT 调控的关键因子由螺旋-环-螺旋和锌指 DNA 结合蛋白组成。ZEB 转录因子家族同源结构域被阴影圈表示，Snai2/slug1 的
Slug 结构域被灰色图形表示。这些转录因子一旦入核内就下调 E-cadherin 表达。Snail 转录因子家族也可以激活 FN 和 vimentin
的表达，控制基底膜的降解；The core EMT regulatory factors are composed of Helix Loop Helix and zing-finger DNA binding
proteins. Homeo domains of the ZEB transcription factor family is represented as hatched circle and the Slug domain of SNAI2/Slug1
is represented as a gray motif. Once in the nucleus these transcription factors downregulate E-cadherin expression. The SNAI family of
transcription factors can also activate vimentin and fibronectin expression and control the membrane basement degradation

　　发生 EMT 时，细胞由原先具有极性的整齐排列转变成散在分布，而 E-cadherin 的丢失，导致了细胞黏附度降低，影响了细胞骨架的改变，使细胞极性的变化，细胞形态上由规则的立方形或扁平状转化为不规则的梭形纤维细胞状，细胞的功能也随之改变。这些变化使细胞的运动和迁移能力得到提高。

　　2. N-钙粘蛋白（N-cadherin）　作为黏附分子促进细胞迁移。TGF-β 刺激 EMT 与 N-cadherin 表达增加有关。

　　3. 波形蛋白（vimentin）　是一个中间丝蛋白，表达在所有原始间叶细胞，但在分化上皮细胞不表达。vimentin 可能驱动 EMT 的程序，也可以作为一个典型的检测转向分化间充质细胞类型的标志物。

　　4. 纤连蛋白（fibronectin），（FN）　是一个关键的 ECM 组件，癌细胞能提高其产生与 EMT 相关。TGF-β 是一个强有力促进 FN 产生和沉积到 ECM 的诱导物。

　　5. α-平滑肌动蛋白（α-SMA）　是收缩微丝的主要成分和检测肌成纤维细胞的标志。EMT 中 TGF-β 刺激能提高 α-SMA 的表达，它与增强肿瘤浸润和减少患者的生存密切相关。

　　6. 基质金属蛋白酶（MMP）　催化降解基底膜，促进原发肿瘤细胞侵入周围组织及入侵肿瘤相关的血管。EMT 中，有些 MMP 可以被诱导，如 MMP-9 是 TGF-β 信号的靶点。

　　7. β₃ 整合素　是一种跨膜蛋白，通过黏着斑生理性地连接 ECM 和细胞内信号系统和细胞骨架。β_3 整合素迅速和显著上调 TGF-β，通过 FAK-依赖的机制与 TβR-Ⅱ 相互作用。

四、MicroRNAs

　　MicroRNAs（miRNAs）是高度保守的非编码小 RNAs，在转录后水平上调节 mRNA 转录表达[50]。已经证明 miRNAs 参与调控许多生理和病理过程，特别是 EMT 和肿瘤转移[51-53]。miR-200 家族和 miR-205 通过靶向 ZEB 和 SIP1 介导 EMT，而 ZEB 和 SIP1 调节转移[54]。miR-21、miR-181a、miR-429、miR-137 和 miR-661 也参与 EMT 的过程[55-59]。miR-145 通过抑制连接黏附分子 A（junctional adherin molecule A，JAMA）、fascin 和 mucin1 抑制乳腺癌的迁移[60, 61]。

已经明确了 miR-145 抑制乳腺癌细胞趋化作用，直接抑制乳腺癌移转。在乳腺癌细胞（MDA-MB-231）中 miR-145 的过表达与 EMT 标志物的表达呈负相关提示 miR-145 抑制 EMT。miR-145/Oct4 在 EMT 中发挥平衡调节作用（图 10-37）。

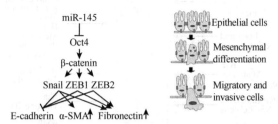

图 10-37　MiR-145 通过 Oct4 调节 EMT 和其下游转录因子 Snail、ZEB1 和 ZEB2；MiR-145 regulated EMT through Oct4 and its downstream transcriptional factors，Snail，ZEB1 and ZEB2

MiR-30 可通过直接靶向预测的 Snail1 mRNA 3'UT R 的 MiR-30 保守序列的结合位点负调控 Snail1 的表达。更重要的是，用 MiR-30b 转染 AML12 细胞后可显著抑制 TGF-β 诱导的 EMT[62]。通过评估细胞形态改变和 Snail1 的表达谱及 E-cadherin 和其他成纤维细胞标志物，证明 TGF-β 诱导 EMT 发生的肝细胞在转染 MiR-30b 后显著抑制了肝细胞迁移。这些研究结果为理解 MiR-30 调控 EMT 的作用提供了新思路。在 EMT 发生时，Snail 家族成员（Snail1 和 Snail2，即 Snail 和 Slug 表达升高）和 ZEB 家族成员（尤其是 ZEB2）过表达[63]。肿瘤抑制基因 p53 是诱导或抑制一系列基因和 miRNAs 的转录因子，先前研究已经显示在肿瘤形成中总是伴有 p53 基因的缺失或突变，而 p53 与肿瘤浸润转移和进展有关。已有报告指出靶向 ZEB1 和 ZEB2 的 miR-200 家族在 TGF-β 诱导的间叶细胞和伴有间叶特征的癌细胞中显著下调。p53 上调 MiR-200 和 MiR-192 家族成员。MiR-200 家族成员抑制 ZEB1/2 的表达，MiR-192 家族成员抑制 ZEB2 的表达。因此抑制 EMT 的过程可由 p53 通过抑制转录因子 ZEB1 和 ZEB2 的表达来实现[64]。

Lee 等研究发现 MiR-122 有较强的肿瘤抑制作用，在肝癌中其表达下降，上调 MiR-122 的表达可逆转肝癌细胞的间质特性，从而降低癌细胞的浸润和转移[6]。因此推测，MiR-122 可作为肝癌 EMT 过程重要的调节器。

概括 EMT 信号通路（图 10-38）。

EMT 是信号通路之间串流的产物，包括 TGF-β、Wnt/β-catenin、Notch、FGF、STAT3 和 EGF。通过调节转录因子（ZEBs、Snail 和 Twist），这些信号通路将上皮表型转变成间质表型。在癌细胞中，KLF4 通过与 TGF-β、Notch 和 Wnt/β-catenin 信号途径相互作用抑制 EMT。通过 UPS 降解 KLF4 对于 TGF-β 诱导的转录激活是必需的。在 Notch 信号通路中，KLF4 负调控 Notch1 的表达，作为 Notch1 靶基因转录的负调控因子。KLF4 还通过抑制 β-cadherin 和转录因子（transcription factors，TCF）结合，从而与 Wnt/β-catenin 相互作用抑制 TCF 转录活性（图 10-39）。

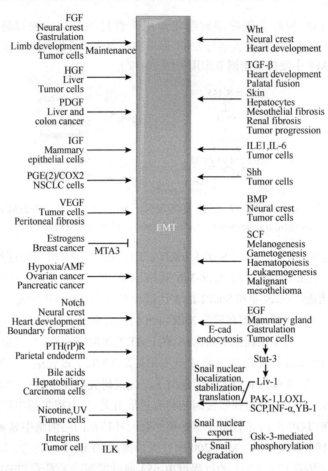

图 10-38　EMT 的信号通路；EMT signaling pathways

在众多细胞环境，包括胚胎发育和人类疾病发生过程中有大量信号通路和药物可诱导 EMT 的发生。图示相应靶组织和促 EMT 相关信号涉及的生物学过程。一些转录因子的表达对 EMT 的发展发挥重要作用，然而它们的亚细胞定位和蛋白酶调节的降解过程可在翻译后水平调控这些转录因子的表达；AMF：自分泌运动因子；EGF：表皮生长因子；FGF：成纤维细胞生长因子；BMP：骨形成蛋白；IGF：胰岛素样生长因子；ILEI：白介素相关蛋白；ILK：整合素链接激酶；IL-6：白介素-6；LOXL：赖氨酰化氧样蛋白质；MTA3：转移相关蛋白 3；PAK-1：p21-活化激酶 2；PTH（rP）R：甲状旁腺激素相关肽受体；SCF：干细胞因子；SCP：小 C 端域磷酸酶；UV：紫外线；YB-1：Y-box 结合蛋白；A plethora of signaling pathways and agents induce EMT in numerous cellular contexts, both during embryonic development and in human pathologies. The figure shows the target tissues and the biological process below the corresponding signal that promotes EMT. Although the expression of several transcription factors is an essential aspect of the EMT program, some of these transcription factors are also regulated at the posttranslational level through their subcellular localization and the regulation of their degradation by the proteasome; AMF, autocrine motility factor; EGF, epidermal growth factor; FGF, fibroblast growth factor; BMP, bone morphogenetic protein; IGF, insulin-like growth factor; ILEI, interleukin-related protein; ILK, integrin-linked kinase; IL-6, interleukin-6; LOXL, lysyl oxidase-like proteins; MTA3, metastasis-associated protein 3; PAK-1, p21-activated kinase 2; PTH（rP）R, parathyroid hormone related peptide receptor; SCF, stem cell factor; SCP, small C-terminal domain phosphatase; UV, ultraviolet light; YB-1, Y-box binding protein

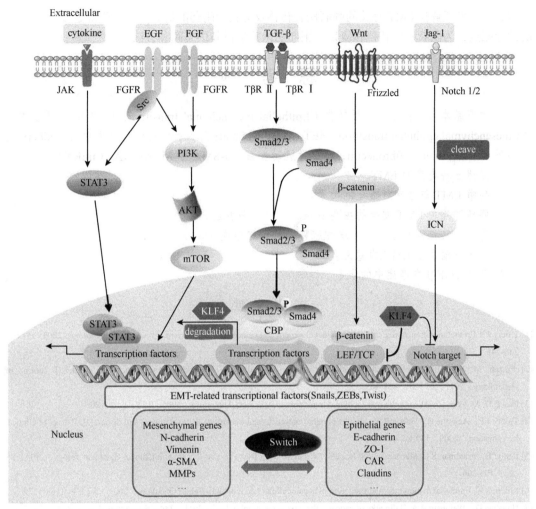

图 10-39　不同因子的功能影响 EMT 的机制；The functions of different factors involved in the mechanism of EMT

挑战与展望

　　EMT 不仅在胚胎发育和正常的生理中起作用，而且在许多病理情况中、在肿瘤侵袭与转移过程中均发挥重要作用，肿瘤细胞借助 EMT 过程增强了细胞的迁移和运动能力。

　　EMT 常是生理和病理的关键过程。EMT 可以视为成人发育程序再激活。EMT 是原发瘤癌细胞离开有序组织结构的初始阶段，是细胞释放以致扩散或远处转移的先决条件，是癌转移程序启动的重要标志。由于 EMT 在癌发生中的重要作用，进一步研究将通过细胞模型和体内实验的共同分析、验证、通过封闭相关信号通路、动态监测 EMT 相关分子 mRNA 和蛋白的表达，以及启动子区甲基化的程度、通过逆转 EMT 事件中的转录调节基因等，在研究过程中将发现更多 EMT 分子标志物，有利于研究 EMT 形成的分子调控机制和功能，有利于深入剖析 EMT 过程与癌进展的关系。由于癌肉瘤是指肿瘤组织中既有恶性上皮细胞，又有恶性梭形成分，有利于 EMT 成为上皮性癌转化为肉瘤的假说的佐证。研究结果将进一步揭示诱导 EMT 和促进癌发生的信号通路，进一步认识肿瘤微环境对 EMT 的作用，进一步明确启动 EMT 的关键因素，进一步理解与 EMT 有关的肿瘤侵袭转移及对化疗耐药的机制，从而获得更多针对 EMT 的治疗靶点，为阻断癌的转移和复发、靶向癌治疗提供新的思路和方法[65]。

思 考 题

1. 本章基本概念：上皮间质转化（Epithelial mesenchymal transition，EMT）；间质上皮转化（mesenchymal epithelial transition，MET）；TGF-β；Snail；Twist；Wnt；E-钙黏蛋白（E-cadherin）；波形蛋白（vimentin），fibronectin；α-平滑肌动蛋白（α-SMA）；MicroRNAs（miRNAs）

2. 描述三种类型的 EMT。

3. 列举 EMT 与器官纤维化的关系。

4. 概括肿瘤中 EMT 发生的主要步骤和相关基因表达。

5. 为什么转移性肿瘤仍由上皮细胞特性的细胞组成？

6. 简述肿瘤发生 EMT 的意义。

7. 简述 TGF-β 在癌症中的作用。

参 考 文 献

[1] Thiery J P. Epithelial-mesenchymal transitions in development and pathologies [J]. Current Opinion in Cell Biology, 2003, 15 (6): 740-746.

[2] Pinzani M. Epithelial-mesenchymal transition in chronic liver disease：fibrogenesis or escape from death?[J]. Journal of Hepatology, 2011, 55 (2): 459-465.

[3] Hay E D. An overview of epithelio-mesenchymal transformation[J]. Acta Anatomica, 1995, 154 (1): 8-20.

[4] Thiery J P, Acloque H, Huang R Y, et al. Epithelial-mesenchymal transitions in development and disease[J]. Journal of Clinical Investigation, 2009, 139 (5): 871-890.

[5] Lee U E, Friedman S L. Mechanisms of Hepatic Fibrogenesis[J]. Best Practice & Research Clinical Gastroenterology, 2011, 25 (2): 195-206.

[6] Mikulits W. Epithelial to mesenchymal transition in hepatocellular carcinoma[J]. Future Oncology, 2009, 5 (8): 1169-1179.

[7] Hanahan D, Weinberg R A. Hallmarks of cancer：the next generation[J]. Cell, 2011, 144 (5): 646-674.

[8] Kong D, Banerjee S, Ahmad A, et al. Epithelial to mesenchymal transition is mechanistically linked with stem cell signatures in prostate cancer cells[J]. PloS One, 2010, 5 (8): e12445.

[9] Kong D, Li Y, Wang Z, et al. Cancer stem cells and epithelial-to-mesenchymal transition(EMT)-phenotypic cells：are they cousins or twins?[J]. Cancers, 2011, 3 (1): 716-729.

[10] Mani S A, Guo W, Liao M J, et al. The epithelial-mesenchymal transition generates cells with properties of stem cells[J]. Cell, 2008, 133 (4): 704-715.

[11] Morel A P, Lièvre M, Thomas C, et al. Generation of breast cancer stem cells through epithelial-mesenchymal transition[J]. PloS One, 2008, 3 (8): e2888.

[12] Kurasawa Y, Kozaki K, Pimkhaokham A, et al. Stabilization of phenotypic plasticity through mesenchymal-specific DNA hypermethylation in cancer cells[J]. Oncogene, 2012, 31 (15): 1963-1974.

[13] Islam A B, Richter W F, Jacobs L A, et al. Co-regulation of histone-modifying enzymes in cancer[J]. PloS One, 2011, 6 (8): e24023.

[14] Zavadil J, Böttinger E P. TGF-beta and epithelial-to-mesenchymal transitions[J]. Oncogene, 2005, 24 (37): 5764-5774.

[15] Derynck R, Akhurst R J, and Balmain A. TGF-beta signaling suppression and cancer progression[J]. Nature Genetics, 2001, 29: 117-129.

[16] Massague J. TGF-b signal transduction[J]. Annual Review of Biochemistry 1998, 67: 753-791.

[17] Shi Y, Massague J. Mechanisms of TGF-beta signaling from cell membrane to the nucleus[J]. Cell, 2003, 113: 685-700.

[18] Wollenberg G K, Semple E, Quinn B A, et al. Inhibition of proliferation of normal, preneoplastic, and neoplastic rat hepatocytes by transforming growth factor-beta[J]. Cancer Research, 1987, 47 (1): 6595-6599.

[19] Serra R, Carbonetto S, Lord M, et al. Transforming growth factor h1 suppresses transformation in hepatocytes by regulating a1h1

integrin expression. Cell Growth & Differ，1984，5：509-517.

[20] Oberhammer F，Fritsch G，Pavelka M，et al. Induction of apoptosis in cultured hepatocytes and in the regressing liver by transforming growth factor-β1 occurs without activation of an endonuclease[J]. Toxicology Letters，1992，64-65 Spec No（12）：701-704.

[21] Thorgeirsson S S，Teramoto T，and Factor V. Regulation of apoptosis inhepatocellular carcinoma[J]. Seminars in Liver Disease，1998，18（12）：115-122.

[22] Blobe G C，Schiemann W P，Lodish H F. Role of transforming growthfactor beta in human disease[J]. The New England Journal of Medicine，2000，342：1350-1358.

[23] Gressner A M，Weiskirchen R，Breitkopf K，et al. Roles of TGF-beta in hepatic fibrosis[J]. Frontiers in Bioscience A Journal & Virtual Library，2002，7（1-3）：d793-d807.

[24] Henderson N C，Forbes S J. Hepatic fibrogenesis：from within and outwith. Toxicology，2008，254：130-135.

[25] Rossmanith W，Schultehermann R. Biology of transforming growth factor beta in hepatocarcinogenesis[J]. Microscopy Research & Technique，2001，52（4）：430-436.

[26] Tsai J F，Jeng J E，Chuang L Y，et al. Elevated urinary transforming growth factor-beta1 level as a tumour marker and predictor of poor survival in cirrhotic hepatocellular carcinoma[J]. British Journal of Cancer，1997，76（2）：244-250.

[27] Factor V M，Kao C Y，Santonirugiu E，et al. Constitutive expression of mature transforming growth factor beta1 in the liver accelerates hepatocarcinogenesis in transgenic mice[J]. Cancer Research，1997，57（11）：2089-2095.

[28] Zhang X，Wang T，Batist G，et al. Transforming growth factor h1 promotes spontaneous transformation of cultured rat liver epithelial cells[J]. Cancer Research，1994，54：6122-6128.

[29] Derynck R，Akhurst R J. Differentiation plasticity regulated by TGF-beta family proteins in development and disease[J]. Nature Cell Biology，2007，9（9）：1000-1004.

[30] Akhurst R J. TGF h signaling in health and disease[J]. Nature Genetics，2004，36：790-792.

[31] Zavadil J，Bottinger E P. TGF-beta and epithelialto-mesenchymal transitions[J]. Oncogene 2005，24：5764-5774.

[32] Batlle E，Sancho E，Francí C，et al. The transcription factor snail is a repressor of E-cadherin gene expression in epithelial tumour cells[J]. Nature Cell Biology，2000，2（2）：84-89.

[33] Hajra K M，Chen D Y，Fearon E R. The SLUG zinc-finger protein represses E-cadherin in breast cancer[J]. Cancer Research，2002，62（6）：1613-1618.

[34] Yang J，Mani S A，Donaher J L，et al. Twist，a master regulator of morphogenesis，plays an essential role in tumor metastasis[J]. Cell，2004，117（7）：927-939.

[35] Eger A，Aigner K S，Dampier B，et al. DeltaEF1 is a transcriptional repressor of E-cadherin and regulates epithelial plasticity in breast cancer cells[J]. Oncogene，2005，24（14）：2375-2385.

[36] Massagué J，Chen Y G. Controlling TGF-beta signaling[J]. Genes & Development，2000，14（6）：627.

[37] Cho H J，Baek K E，Saika S，et al. Snail is required for transforming growth factor-β-induced epithelial-mesenchymal transition by activating PI3 kinase/Akt signal pathway[J]. Biochemical & Biophysical Research Communications，2007，353（2）：337-343.

[38] Kaimori A，Potter J，Kaimori J Y，et al. Transforming Growth Factor-1 Induces an Epithelial-to-Mesenchymal Transition State in Mouse Hepatocytes in Vitro[J]. Journal of Biological Chemistry，2007，282（30）：22089-22101.

[39] Vesuna F，Diest P V，Ji H C，et al. Twist is a transcriptional repressor of E-cadherin gene expression in breast cancer[J]. Biochemical & Biophysical Research Communications，2008，367（2）：235-241.

[40] Nelson W J，Nusse R. Convergence of Wnt，beta-catenin，and cadherin pathways[J]. Science，2004，303（5663）：1483-1487.

[41] ConacciSorrell M，Simcha I，BenYedidia T，et al. Autoregulation of E-cadherin expression by cadherin-cadherin interactions：the roles of β-catenin signaling，Slug，and MAPK[J]. Journal of Cell Biology，2003，163（4）：847-857.

[42] Maralice ConacciSorrell，Inbal Simcha，Tamar Ben Yedidia，et al. Autoregulation of E-cadherin expression by cadherin-cadherin interactions：the roles of β-catenin signaling，Slug，and MAPK[J]. Journal of Cell Biology，2003，163（4）：847-857.

[43] Cano A，Pérez-Moreno M A，Rodrigo I，et al. The transcription factor snail controls epithelial-mesenchymal transitions by repressing E-cadherin expression[J]. Nature Cell Biology，2000，2（2）：76-83.

[44] Carver E A，Jiang R，Yu Lan，et al. The mouse snail gene encodes a key regulator of the epithelial-mesenchymal transition[J]. Molecular & Cellular Biology，2001，21（23）：8184-8188.

[45] Batlle E，Sancho E，Francí C，et al. The transcription factor snail is a repressor of E-cadherin gene expression in epithelial tumour cells[J]. Nature Cell Biology，2000，2（2）：84-89.

[46] Comijn J，Berx G，Vermassen P，et al. The two-handed E box binding zinc finger protein SIP1 downregulates E-cadherin and induces invasion[J]. Molecular Cell，2001，7（6）：1267-1278.

[47] Perez-Moreno M A，Locascio A，Rodrigo I，et al. A new role for E12/E47 in the repression of E-cadherin expression and

epithelial-mesenchymal transitions[J]. Journal of Biological Chemistry，2001，276（29）：27424-27431.

[48] Cheng C W，Wu P E，Yu J C，et al. Mechanisms of inactivation of E-cadherin in breast carcinoma：modification of the two-hit hypothesis of tumor suppressor gene.[J]. Oncogene，2001，20（29）：3814-3823.

[49] Morenobueno G. Correlation of Snail expression with histological grade and lymph node status in breast carcinomas[J]. Oncogene，2002，21（20）：3241.

[50] Cathew R W，Sontheimer E J. Origins and Mechanisms of miRNAs and siRNAs[J]. Cell，2009，136（4）：642-655.

[51] Gee H E，Camps C，Buffa F M，et al. MicroRNA-10b and breast cancer metastasis[J]. Nature，2008，455（7216）：1177-1179.

[52] Tavazoie SF，Alarcon C，Oskarsson T，et al. Endogenous human microRNAs that suppress breast cancer metastasis. Nature，2008，451：147-152.

[53] Valastyan S，Chang A，Benaich N，et al. Activation of miR-31 function in already-established metastases elicits metastatic regression.Genes & Development，2011，25：646-659.

[54] Gregory P A，Bert A G，Paterson E L，et al. The miR-200 family and miR-205 regulate epithelial to mesenchymal transition by targeting ZEB1 and SIP1[J]. Nature Cell Biology，2008，10（5）：593-601.

[55] Oliverasferraros C，Cufi S，Vazquezmartin A，et al. Micro（mi）RNA expression profile of breast cancer epithelial cells treated with the anti-diabetic drug metformin：induction of the tumor suppressor miRNA let-7a and suppression of the TGFβ-induced oncomiR miRNA-181a[J]. Cell Cycle，2011，10（7）：1144-1151.

[56] Cottonham C L，Kaneko S，Xu L. miR-21 and miR-31 converge on TIAM1 to regulate migration and invasion of colon carcinoma cells[J]. Journal of Biological Chemistry，2010，285（46）：35293-35302.

[57] Chen J，Wang L，Matyunina LV，et al. Overexpression of miR-429 induces mesenchymal-to-epithelial transition（MET）in metastatic covarian cancer cells. Gynecol ogic Oncology，2011，121：200-205.

[58] Deng Y，Deng H，Bi F，et al. MicroRNA-137 targets carboxyl-terminal binding protein 1 in melanoma cell lines[J]. International Journal of Biological Sciences，2011，7（1）：133-137.

[59] Reddy S D N，Pakala S B，Ohshiro K，et al. MicroRNA-661, a c/EBP alpha target, inhibits metastatic tumor antigen 1 and regulates its functions[J]. Cancer Research，2009，69（14）：5639-5642.

[60] Götte M，Mohr C，Koo C Y，et al. miR-145-dependent targeting of junctional adhesion molecule A and modulation of fascin expression are associated with reduced breast cancer cell motility and invasiveness[J]. Oncogene，2010，29（50）：6569-6580.

[61] Sachdeva M，Mo Y Y. MicroRNA-145 suppresses cell invasion and metastasis by directly targeting mucin 1[J]. Cancer Research，2010，70（1）：378-387.

[62] Jingcheng Z，Haiyan Z，Junyu L，et al. miR-30 inhibits TGF-β 1-induced epithelial-to-mesenchymal transition in hepatocyte by targeting Snail1[J]. Biochemical & Biophysical Research Communications，2012，417（3）：1100-1105.

[63] Laura P，Sandra R，Danijela V，et al. HNF1 α inhibition triggers epithelial-mesenchymal transition in human liver cancer cell lines[J]. BMC Cancer，2011，11（1）：427.

[64] Taewan K，Angelo V，Flavia P，et al. p53 regulates epithelial-mesenchymal transition through microRNAs targeting ZEB1 and ZEB2[J]. Journal of Experimental Medicine，2011，208（5）：875-883.

[65] 汤志杰，张茂娜，陈莉. 肝癌和肝纤维化发生 EMT 及相关信号通路的分子机制[J]. 实用癌症杂志，2014，29（1）113-115.

（张茂娜　季周婧　陈　莉）

Chapter 10　Epithelial Mesenchymal Transition (EMT)

According to cellular morphology, the biological organism's tissues and organs are mainly divided into two types of epithelial cells and stromal cells. They have different cell phenotypes, structures and functions.Epithelial cells have polarity. There are many connections between cells.Epithelial cells maintain the integrity of a multicellular organism, become necessary barrier for regulating the internal environment.In contrast, stromal cells don't have polarity, and lack connections between cells. It has the ability to infiltrate and migrate to adjacent tissues, take part in the formation of more complex structures and functions. The two kinds cell phenotypes are not permanent, under appropriating conditions, the reversely transformation of epithelial cells and stromal cells can occur.

Epithelial-mesenchymal transition (EMT) described in 1968 (Fig. 10-1), is a biological process, a dynamic cellular program, by which epithelial cells lose epithelial polarity, cell-cell tight contact and adhesion. They acquire a mesenchymal morphology accompanied by the secretion of extracellular matrix components increased, to become more motile andinvasive. The transition of epithelial to mesenchymal cells is not irreversible, and mesenchymal cells can return to an epithelialphenotype, a process called mesenchymal-epithelial transition (MET). Both EMT and MET all have role in physiological and pathological factors.

EMT is a highly conserved and fundamental process that governs morphogenes is inmulticellular organisms. EMT at the crossroads of multiple cellular processes (Fig. 10-2). EMT is the result of a transcriptional repression of E-cadherin gene leading to the loss of the epithelial phenotype and the remodeling of the actin cytoskeleton associated to the mesenchymal phenotype. EMT plays an important role in the emergence and progression of carcinoma by allowing carcinoma cells scattering. This cellular process is reversible; at secondary sites, solitary carcinoma cells can extravasate andform new carcinoma through a mesenchymal to epithelial transition (MET).

EMT is a complex process of cell phenotype transformation that means epithelial cells which have a polarity to translate into mesenchymal cells that can move freely in the cell matrix.Gene transcripts that switch splicing during the EMT function in complexes or pathways that define epithelial and mesenchymal cell behaviors.

The biology of EMT is a crucial trans-differentiation process, which occurs during embryogenesis and in adult tissues following wound repair and organ remodeling in response to injury, and also occurs during cancer progression. Thereby EMT plays an important role in embryonic development, wound repair, and organ fibrosis fibrotic diseases, and it contributes to tumor-invasiv ephenotypes and metastasis[1]. EMT in the context of pathophysiological conditions, such as during the repair ofinjured tissue. Tissue injury promotes the recruitment of mesenchymal stem cells (MSCs), which can secrete EMT-inducing cytokines such as TGF-β, resulting in dissolution of cell-cell contacts and accompanying morphogenetic changes. In cooperation with additional EMT inducers such as Wnt, epithelial cells transform to a fully motility mesenchymal phenotype (Fig. 10-3).

The evidence for EMT and MET is compelling in embryonic development, organ formation, wound healing, tissue regeneration, organ fibrosis, cancer progression, and metastasis. According to the biological background of how EMT occurs, it can be divided into three types (Fig. 10-4):

(1) EMT which is involved in embryonic development and organ formation.

During embryogenesis, the primitive epithelium (the epiblast) undergoes EMT forming primary mesenchyme that can migrate and undergo MET to form secondary epithelia that differentiate into new epithelial tissues.

(2) EMT which is involved in the process of tissue regeneration and organ fibrosis.

In mature or adult tissues, epithelial cells can also undergo EMT following local cellular disorganization caused by various stressors, inflammation or wounding but fail to undergo MET leading to fibroblast production and finally fibrosis.

(3) EMT which is involved in tumor progression.

Epithelial cancer cells can undergo EMT to acquire a more migratory mesenchymal phenotype that allows them to invade secondary epithelia and proliferate as secondary tumors. During the process, migrating mesenchymal cells will have to intravasate, migrate through vasculature and extravasate to invade secondary tissue, undergo MET and proliferate forming secondary tumors.

The progressive loss of the epithelial character and the acquisition of a spindle-shaped cell morphology (EMT) are major events during development and carcinogenesis[3]. In cancerous cells, EMT reflects a failure in the mechanisms that mediate cell-cell recognition and adhesion and its coupling to maintenance of cell shape and polarity. Therefore, understanding the molecular events that provoke EMT during development or cell differentiation might provide an insights into the regulatory events that play during the invasive process.

Section 1   EMT in Embryonic Development

EMT happens in early stage of embryonic development in vertebrates.The several rounds of EMT and MET are necessary for the final differentiation of specialized cell types and the acquisition of the complex three-dimensional structure of internal organs. Accordingly, these sequential rounds are referred to as primary, secondary, and tertiary EMT (Fig. 10-5). Primary EMT form gastrulation and neural crest cells; Secondary EMT: somites, palate, pancreas, liver, and reproductive tracts. From primary to tertiary EMT: heart development[4].

Section 2   EMT in Tissue Regeneration and Organ Fibrosis
1. Roles of EMT in Inflammation

Microbe-induced chronic inflammation in predisposed individuals leads to EMT. Microbe infection plays a critical role as an EMT promoter. In healthy individuals, microbe infection is contained by the innate immunity. By contrast in predisposed individuals the innate immunity is exceeded by microbe infection leading to chronic inflammation (Fig. 10-6)

The innate NFkB pathway is composed of the rapidly responding (canonical)-and the slower responding (noncanonic)pathway control the inflammatory response, and is coupled to the noncanonical pathway through a feed forward pathway by the synthesis of TRAF1 and NFKB2, two rate limiting factors in noncanonical pathway activation. Through epigenetic reprogramming and enhanced trancriptional elongation through the cyclin dependent kinase (CDK) I, the rate-limiting TRAF1/ NFKB2 translation is reduced resulting in enhanced pathway activation in EMT (Fig. 10- 7).

2. Roles of EMT in Fibrosis

Fibros is a progressive pathologic process characterized by excessive accumulation of extracellular matrix (ECM). EMT is closely related to internal organ fibrosis in chronic disease process.

(1) Hepatic Fibrogenesis

In liver fibrosis, myofibroblasts accumulate and secrete an excessive amount of collagen that is deposited as fibers, thereby injurying organ functions and leading to its failure. Fibrosis had been thought to be the pathological activative process, which fibroblasts convert to myofibroblasts to form the fibrotic collagen network in liver.

EMT in liver fibrosis is the most obvious feature, the damaged epithelial cell obtain the phenotype of motion[5]. Assumed it was an integrated escape program of liver cells growing in the adverse microenvironment, this poor microenvironments is caused by redox changes or by the effect of changed extracellular matrix complex, and related to the effect of high concentrations of growth factors and cytokines in chronic wound healing response [5]. The characters of escape program are to achieve the purpose of promoting cell survival to avoid from oxidative damage through changing cell metabolism and movement of cells. Escape program generally has two possible results: ①the moving liver epithelial cells reach a relatively good microenvironment, then redifferentiate to the original phenotype; ②the cells continuesly grow in the adverse microenvironment, losting its escape phenotype lead cells apoptosis. Compared with non-escape cells, both escape cells have obvious advantages of pathophysiology, non-escape cells cause necrosis in the adverse microenvironment, and further release the reactive oxygen and other profibrotic, proinflammatory molecules[6].Therefore, put forward a concept that generated ECM by the EMT of liver cellsthen it gains mesenchymal phenotype in hepatic fibrosis.Increasing evidence suggests that, in the process of hepatic fibrosis and chronic inflammation, EMT can induce that myofibroblasts promote the synthesis and deposition of collagen type I, that indicate liver cell lines play a role in the process of hepatic fibrosis[7].

(2) Lung Fibrogenesis

Inflammatory stimuli the EMT leading to pulmonary fibrosis in asthma (Fig. 10-8).

(3) The implications of miRNA in renal fibrosis with epithelium and endothelium cells EMT（Fig. 10-9)

EMT involving transformation of endothelial cells into mesenchymal cells is evident during cardiac and renal fibrosis. Mesothelial cells are also converted to mesenchyme in patients that receive ambulatory peritoneal dialysis and that develop peritoneal fibrosis.

(4) The key events of EMT involving the renal tubular basement membrane (TBM) and possible therapeutic interventions（Fig. 10-10).

3. Molecular Changes in EMT

(1) Molecular changes in EMT

Repression of the transcription factors Snail1, Snail2, Zeb1, and Zeb2 is important for the maintenance of epithelial morphology. Several factors that are upregulated in the context of inflammation, including NF-KB, TGF-β1, bone morphogenetic proteins (BMPs), Wnt, and Notch signaling proteins, can activate the Snail-Zeb pathway, leading to mesenchymal differentiation in epithelial cells expressed FN (fibronectin), Vim (vimentin), FSP-1(fibroblast-specific protein-1)，α-SMA(alpha smooth muscle actin) etc., diminishedE-cadherinand zonula occludens-1 (ZO-1) expression (Fig. 10-11).

(2) Molecular changes during EndMT program

The EndMT program causes decreased expression of endothelial markers VEcadherin, CD31, cytokeratins, and type 4 collagen and a gain of mesenchymal markers FSP-1, α-SMA, N-cadherin, vimentin, fibronectin,type I and type III collagen, and MMP-2 and MMP-9 (Fig. 10-12).

Section 3　EMT in Tumor Progression and Metastasis

During EMT process, the cancer epithelial cells acquire mesenchymal cell morphology through down-regulation of epithelial markers and up-regulation of mesenchymal markers, thereby leading to increased migratory capacity, invasiveness and increased resistance to chemotherapy, and with features of cancer stem cells and all of which areinvolved in cancer progression（Fig. 10-13） [7-17].

The EMT regulators transform the cancer cells from epithelial-cell like to mesenchymal-cell like with suppression of epithelial markers and expression of mesenchymal markers. The final effection cancer cells are cancer metastasis, drug resistance and with features of cancer stem cells.

1. A Critical Role of EMT in Tumor Progression

Currently a hot research is the relationship between EMT, tumor invasion and metastasis. EMT plays a critic a role during the initiation stage of metastasis. Immotile epithelial cells with the apical-basal polarity are converted to the motile, dispersed mesenchymal-like cells with spindle shape [4]. Consequently, tumor cells are detached from original sites and start to invade surrounding tissue. Enhanced motility of tumor cells is essential for the following steps of metastasis, such as invasion, intravasation and extravasation [8]. Thus, EMT is a pre-requisite step for cancer cell migration. EMT is a key step before cancer cell invasion and migration (Fig. 10-14).

In response to EMT-promoting signals, a subpopulation of epithelial cells at the invasive edge of the tumor may lose epithelial traits. As these cells detach further from the bulk of the tumor, they become less exposed to epithelial signals and acquire more mesenchymal properties in the presence of EMT signals supplied by stromal cells. The metastable mesenchymal cells are suited for invasion into surrounding tissues. A fully mesenchymal phenotype facilitates intravasation into blood capillaries or draining lymphatic vessels. In some instances, this process may be aided by macrophages. The disseminating cancer cell is also more resistant to environmental and genotoxic stresses, a characteristic that is crucial for survival in circulation. After arrival at a distant organ, the mesenchymal phenotype facilitates extravasation and invasion into the foreign tissue. Here disseminated cells are exposed to signals different from those of the primary tumor, and the mesenchymal state may confer survival advantages to single cancer cells or alternatively may support long-term dormancy. When the appropriate contextual signals become available, disseminated cells may undergo an MET and gradually reacquire epithelial properties such as rapid proliferative capabilities [16,17]. Epithelial signals are reinforced through autocrine and paracrine signals, resulting in the stabilization of an epithelial phenotype. This facilitates the outgrowth of macrometastases that are composed predominantly of epithelial cells (Fig. 10-15).

The transforming mesenchymal cells in metastasis invasion to the surrounding tissue, in which adverse microenvironment of lacking epithelial signals stimulate, continue to EMT. Once settled into the new sites, the cells regain the epithelium signals stimulation, the cells which have the characteristics of mesenchymal phonetype can be re-converted into epithelial cells, rebuild the connection of intercellular and cytoskeleton form relatively stable metastatic tumors. (Fig. 10-16). Therefore, MET have a great significance for tumor with EMT metastasis and settlement to a new sites and long-term growth.

2. EMT Related to Cancer Stem Cells (CSC)

Aberrant miRNA expression as been correlated with the formation of CSCs and the acquisition of EMT phenotype. miRNAs affect and connect CSCs through regulation of EMT. EMT cells have cancer stem cell-like features, and CSCs exhibit mesenchymal phenotype. Moreover, the cells with EMT phenotype share characteristics with cancer stem-like cell (CSLC), which confers drug resistance to these cells (Fig. 10-17) and contributes to cancer recurrence and metastasis and leads to cancer progression [9-12] (Fig. 10-18).

Summary representing the most prominent alterations of epigenetic pathways that regulate CSC/EMT features and resistance to chemotherapy (Fig. 10-19).

3. Anti-cancer Therapy Targeting EMT

Signaling by epithelial growth factor receptors (ErbBs) has been shown to stimulate epithelial to mesenchymal transition (EMT) in epithelial-like cancer cells by activating different intracellular receptor tyrosine kinases (RTK). This often results in increased activity of transcription factors, such as Snail that represses the expression of intracellular adhesion molecules like E-cadherin. As a consequence, these cells become more spindle-shaped, express mesenchyme associated molecules, such as Vimentin, N-cadherin and certain MMPs, and assume increased aggressiveness as they become more migratory and invasive. Inhibitors of ErbB signaling have been able to interfere with the EMT process in certain cancer cells. In selective cases, reversal of EMT has resulted in increased efficacy of anti-cancer therapyin otherwise EMT-associated drug resistant cancer cells (Fig. 10-20) .

Section 4   Molecule Mechanism of Regulating EMT

EMT is necessary for the progression of cancer. When stimulating with the damage, excessive growth factors and cytokines, the quality or quantity changes in extracellular matrix, as well as hypoxia or oxygen stress and other negative tumor microenvironment prompt cancer occur EMT, reprogramming the metabolism and survival of cancer cells, causing a series change of genes, molecules, and signaling pathways(Fig. 10-21).

Early stage tumor cells maintain epithelial properties similar to the neighboring normal epithelium. The accidental overexpression of master regulators of EMT, such as the transcription factors Twist, Snail and SIP1, in cancer cells leads to dramatic changes in gene expression profiles and cellular behavior. Twist,Snail and SIP1 repress the expression of E-cadherin via E boxes in its promoter and trigger expression of an entire EMT transcription program though as yet unknown mechanisms (Fig. 10-22).

1. TGF-β

An increasing number of distinct cytokines has been found to be involved in the initiation of EMT in many tissues.Among these mediators, TGF-β is considered to act as a master switch [15].Members of the TGF-β superfamily are multifunctional cytokines that play critical roles in a variety of biological pathological events [16] including embryogenesis, organogenesis, differentiation, apoptosis, immunomodulation, fibrogenesis and certain human diseases [17-18]. Such as TGF-β secretion inhibits proliferation [19], suppresses transformation [20], and induces apoptosis [21] and promote ECM deposition during carcinogenesis, disruption ofTGF-β signaling can deregulate apoptosis in many carcinomas [22]. On the other hand, EMT-derived hepatic my ofibroblasts proliferate and up-regulate their production of fibrillar collagens with a resultant increase in thedeposition of fibrotic matrix [23-25]. That activation has been associated with the progression of carcinogenesis. Indeed, human HCC strongly expresses TGF-β mRNA and protein in vivo [26], an elevated urinary TGF-β level has been related to poor survival in cirrhotic HCC [27], and constitutive expression of mature TGF-β in the liver accelerates hepatocarcinogenesis in transgenic mice [28]. Furthermore, TGF-β promotes spontaneous transformation of cultured rat liver epithelial cells [29].

There are 3 subtypes of TGF-β in mammals, respectively TGF-β1, TGF-β2 and TGF-β3. TGF-β1 is the most abundant and most expressive. While there are 3 types of transmembrane receptors on the cell membrane, the main receptors are type I and II, with serine / threonine enzyme activity. Type III receptor includes endothelial factors and β-glycan.

TGF-β has two main signaling pathways, respectively, Smads dependent signal pathway and Smads non-dependent signaling pathway.The former is a classic TGF-β signaling pathway. Smad family consists of three types which are receptor-regulated R-Smads, Co-Smads and I-Smads. R-Smads includes Smad1, 2, 3, 5, and 8; Co-Smads includes Smad4; I-Smads includes Smad6, 7. Among them Smad2 and Smad3 are associated with TGF-β signaling pathway. There are a variety of ways of Smads non-dependent signaling pathway. Complexes of TGF-β receptor can activate the MAPK（mitogen-activated protein kinase）pathways. The concurrent MAPK pathways include ERK (extracellular signal-regulated kinase) pathway, JNK (c-Jun N-turminal kinase/stress activated protein kinase) pathway and p38MAPK pathways. ERK is an important MAPK. TGF-β combined with its receptor on the cell membrane, makes receptors form dimers, its tyrosine kinase phosphorylation of residues. Tyrosine phosphorylation is combined with SH2 domain, which is Grb2 (growth factor binding protein 2) on cell membrane, however, SH3 domains of Grb2 combined with SOS (son of sevenless) of inosinic acid exchange factor. The latter makes GDP of small molecule inosinic acid-binding protein Ras dissociate and bind GTP, and then activate ras. Activated ras further combined with the amino acid serine/threonine protein kinase Raf-1, after activates Raf-1, can phosphorylate the regulated serine of MEK1/MEK2 to activate the MEKS. MEKS are dual-specificity kinase, can make serine/threonine and tyrosine phosphorylation, and ultimately result to the selective activation of ERK1 and ERK2.

(1) The EMT signaling network and transcriptome regulated by TGF-β

TGF-β is a potent EMT inducer.Increased TGF-β expression has been observed in many tumors, and is regarded as an important indicator of cancer progressionbecause it contributes to tumor invasion and metastasis through the induction of EMT [30-31]. It has become increasingly evident that both TGF-β and EMT are involved in the same various physiologic and pathologic events. Upon phosphorylation, R-Smads form complexes with a common partner (Smad4) and subsequently translocate into the nucleus to regulate the transcription of target genes responsible for EMT Smad family proteins that cooperate with other signaling molecules, such as MAPK, phosphatidylinositol 3-kinase, NF-κB, and Wnt[32] integrin，Notch, and transcriptional factors, such as Snail [33], Slug [34],Twist[35], and Zeb1/2 [36], have emerged as important factors in TGF-β induced EMT in some types of epithelial cells. TGF-β may also directly stimulate the phosphorylation of Par6 and reduce stability of intercellular tight junction and increase the expression of Snail, leding to E-cadherin reduction and the decomposition of adhesion proteins as well as activating the Rho GTP enzymes, cell cytoskeleton reorganization with loss of polarity leads to EMT.

1) The signal pathways of TGF-β (Fig. 10-23)

TGF-β triggers EMT primarily via a canonical Smad-dependent mechanism, which requires two types of receptor kinaseand a family of signal transducers called R-Smads (Smad2 and Smad3). Upon phosphorylation, R-Smads form complexes with a common partner (Smad4) and subsequently translocate into the nucleus to regulate the transcription of target genes responsible for EMT, such as Smad7, Snail, and collagen I [37-39].

2) TGF-β signaling in cancer(Fig. 10-24)

3) Pathways activated by TGF-β induce EMT (Fig. 10-25)

4) The signal pathway of integrins mediated TGF-β activation (Fig. 10-26)

Summary in the EMT signaling network and transcriptome regulated by TGF-β(Fig. 10-27)

(2) Roles of TGF-β in cancers

In normal and premalignant cells, TGF-β enforces homeostasis and suppresses tumor progression directly through cell-autonomoustumor-suppressive effects (cytostasis, differentiation, apoptosis) orindirectly through effects on the stroma (suppression of inflammation and stroma-derived mitogens). However, when cancer cells lose TGF-β tumor-suppressive responses, they can use TGF-β to their advantage to initiate immune evasion, growth factor production, differentiation into an invasive phenotype, and metastatic dissemination or to establish and expand metastatic colonie (Fig. 10-28)

1) Anti- and protumorigenic effects of TGF-β in tumor stroma (Fig. 10-29).

2) Anti- and protumorigenic effects of TGF-β in differentiation (Fig. 10-30).

3) The consequences of EMT programs induced by TGF-β

Administration of TGF-β readily elicits the formation of a metastable EMT state in normal and malignant cells. The restoration of epithelial phenotypes transpires through mesenchymal-epithelial transitions (METs), which occur normally during developmental EMTs and perhaps during metastatic outgrowth associated with oncogenic EMTs. Prolonged exposure of cells to TGF-βor other EMT-initiating factors supports the continued development and expansion of cancer stemcells, which collectively are chemoresistant and underlie disease recurrence. How, when, and where cancer stems cells undergo MET during secondary tumor outgrowth remains to be determined definitively (Fig. 10-31).

4) TGF-β and tumor progression

TGF-β induces tumor-suppressive effects that cancer cells must circumvent in order to develop into malignancies. Cancer cells can take two alternative paths to this end: (1) decapitate the pathway with receptor-inactivating mutations or (2) selectively amputate the tumor-suppressive arm of the pathway. The latter path allows cancer cells to extract additional benefits by coopting the TGF-β response for protumorigenic purposes. In both cases, cancer cells can use TGF-β to modulate the microenvironment to avert immunesurveillance or to induce the production of protumorigenic cytokines (Fig. 10-32).

2. Other Transcriptors

(1) Snail and its signal regulations

Snail is a member of the Snail superfamily, vertebrates include Snail and Slug two families. Snail gene family of mammals includes Snail1, Snail2 and Snail3. Snail genes of human are located in chromosome 20q13. Snail proteins contain the transcription factors of zinc finger type. The structure of Snail (Fig. 10-33) and the signaling pathway are associated with Snail-induced EMT (Fig. 10-34).

Transfected Snail gene to human melanoma cells the typical EMT induce the damage of regulatory T cells and dendritic cell in tumor tissuepartlythough TSP-1 (thrombospondin-1) products to inhibit the immune response. Snail-positive melanoma cells are not sensitive for immunotherapy, but when injected siRNA (small interfering RNA) targeting Snail and the TSP-1 antibodies, the tumor growth and metastasis can be inhibited by immune response, it shows that the EMT is related to immune tolerance of cancer cells.

(2) Twist

The transcription factor of Twist is binding protein composed of 202 amino acid residues, and contains highly conserved basic helix-loop-helix domain. Human Twist genes located in the chromosome 7p21, contains 2 exons and 1 introns, exon 1 with coding function, 1669 bp length of mRNA sequences and 609 bp length of open reading frame. Homology of the protein in between mice and humans is as high as 96%. It can down-regulate the expression of E-cadherin, independently, and up-regulation the expression of Fibronectin and N-cadherin to induce EMT[40-41]. Studies have shown that it is also available to induce the epithelial mesenchymal phenotype through multiple signaling pathways. Twist1 and Twist2, by inhibiting P16/ink4a and P21/CIP inhibit apoptosis in cancer cells that lead to the uncontrolled proliferation of tumor cells.

(3) Wnt

Wnt proteins are highly conservative signaling molecules that regulate the intercellular signal transduction during the period of embryo formation. The gene of wnt was firstly integrated by mouse oncogene of mammary carcinoma and the wingless gene of drosophila. Wnt proteins bind with curved volume receptors on the cell surface and LRP5/6, inhibiting the activity of GSK-3β, and then inhibiting the degradation complex regulated by ubiquit in which was formed by Axin-APC-GSK-3β[42]andβ-catenin resulting to β-catenin accumulation in cytoplasma and nucleus. β-catenin interactes with transcription factors TCF4 /LEF in the nucleus, stimulating the expression of down stream target genes cyclin D1, c-myc, Slug, Fibronectin and vimentin, letting epithelial cells to transform into mesenchymal cells. In addition, Wnt can bind with its receptor only play the roles through transcription factors, calcium-dependent kinase, calmodulin or activating the Jun-N terminal kinase (Jnk) by Dsh for regulating the activity of transcription factors p53, Elk1, DPC4, ATF2, c-Jun et al.

3. Biomarkers of Initiated EMT

(1) E-cadherin: It is the primary component of adherens junctions. During EMT, TGF-β represses E-cadherinexpression, as well as induces its internalization from the plasma membrane.It is one of the most important markers of EMT. Loss of cell adhesion and the acquisition of migratory and invasive properties are characteristic of EMT both during embryonic development and tumor progression[44-46]. As a result of the down-regulation of E-cadherin expression, a cell-cell adhesion molecule considered an invasion-suppressor gene, EMT involves the loss of the ability of cells to recognize and adhere to its neighbors. Among the transcription factors that have been implicated in the direct repression of E-cadherin transcription [45, 47-49], it is note worthy that Snail is active at the invasive front of mouse skin tumors and in human breast carcinomas [48-51]. E-cadherin transcription and degradation in normal and cancer cells is shown in Fig. 10-35 and Fig. 10-36

When the EMT occurs, cells are from the original integret into mainly scattered distribution，because the loss of E-cadherin leads to reduced cell adhesion. The morphology of cells with regular cube or flat changes into the irregular spindle cells, which affect the changes of cytoskeleton, cell polarity, and cell functions also. These changes make the cell movement and migration capabilities improve.

(2) N-cadherin, an adhesion molecule that promotes cellular migration. EMT stimulated by TGF-β is associated with increased expression of N-cadherin.

(3) Vimentin, an intermediate filament protein that is expressed in all primitive cell types, but not in differentiated epithelial cells. Vimentin may drive EMT programs, and also serves as a canonical marker for detecting transdifferentiated mesenchymal cell types

(4) Fibronectin (FN), a critical ECM component whose elevated production by cancer cellsis classically associated with EMT programs. TGF-β is a potent inducer of FN production and deposition into the ECM.

(5) α-Smooth Muscle Actin (α-SMA), a major component of contractile microfilaments and a canonical marker for detecting myofibroblasts. TGF-β stimulation of EMT elicits α-SMA expression, which strongly associates with increased tumor invasion, and with decreased patient survival.

(6) MMPs, proteolytically degrade basement membranes to allow primary tumor cells to invade the surrounding tissue and intrasvasate into tumor associated vasculature. While several MMPs are induced during EMT, MMP-9 is a well-established target of TGF-βsignaling

(7) β3 integrin, a transmembrane protein that physically links the extracellular matrix to intracellular signaling systems and the cytoskeleton via focal adhesion complexes. β3 integrin is rapidly and robustly upregulated by TGF-β and interacts physically with TβR-II via a FAK-dependent mechanism.

4. MicroRNAs Regulating EMT

MicroRNAs (miRNAs), a highly conserved group of small non-coding RNAs, regulate the expression of mRNA transcripts at post-transcriptional level [52]. Increasing evidences have proven that miRNAs take part in the regulation of many physiological and pathological processes, especially EMT and tumor metastasis [53-55]. miR-200 family and miR-205 mediated EMT through targeting ZEB1 and SIP1, which in turn regulate metastasis [56]. It has been documented that miR-21, miR-181a, miR-429, miR-137 and miR-661 were also involved in EMT [57-61]. miR-145 suppressed breastcancer cell migration via inhibiting the expression of junctional adherin molecule A (JAMA), fascin and mucin1 [62-63]. Thus, it is clear that miR145 regulates the expression of proteinsdirectly involved in cell migration. miR-145 inhibited breast cancer cell chemotaxis. During a preliminary characterization, we foundthat over-expression of miR-145 reversed the expression of EMT markers in MDA-MB-231 cells, suggesting that miR-145suppressed EMT. miR-145/Oct4 plays a balanced regulatory role in EMT (Fig. 10-37). miR-145 clearly suppresses EMT and its inhibitory role in metastasis has been well-documented.

MiR-30 can negatively regulate the expression of Snail1 through direct targeting of Snail1mRNA 3'UTR MiR-30 conserved binding sites. More importantly, transfected MiR-30b to AML12 cells significantly inhibit the EMT inducted by TGF-β[64]. By assessing changes in cell morphology, expression spectrum of Snail1, E-cadherin and other markers of fibroblast, show that liver cells with EMT by TGF-β are transfected by MiR-30b, the migration is significantly inhibited. These findings provide a new way of thinking to understand the effect of MiR-30 regulating EMT. When EMT, Snail family members (Snail1 and Snail2, Snail and Slug) elevate the expression and ZEB's family members (especially the ZEB2) are overexpression[65].

The tumor suppressor p53 is a transcription factor that induces or represses a large set of genes and miRNAs. Previous studies have shown that deletions or mutationsof p53 are frequently found in cancers, and that p53 is involved in tumor metastasis as wellas tumor progression. It is reported that the miR-200 family targets ZEB1 and ZEB2 and is significantly down-regulated in TGF-β-induced mesenchymal cells and cancer cells with mesenchymalcharacteristics. The study show first that p53 prevents EMT by repressing ZEB1 and ZEB2 expression and second, that p53-regulated miR-200 and miR-192family members are involved in p53-modulated EMT. That p53-regulated miRNAs prevent EMT by repressing ZEB1 and ZEB2 expression [66]. Lee and other researchers found that the MiR-122 had a strong tumor-suppressing effect, its expression in hepatocellular carcinoma has reduced, whereas up-regulating MiR-122 expression may be reverse the mesenchymal properties of hepatocellular carcinoma cells, reducing the invasion and metastasis of cancer cells[6]. Therefore speculated that the MiR-122 may be an important regulator in the EMT process of liver cancer.

Summary in EMT signaling pathways (Fig. 10-38)

EMT is a product of crosstalk between signaling pathways, including TGF-β, Wnt/β-catenin, Notch, FGF, STAT3 and EGF. By regulating the transcription factors (ZEBs, Snails and Twist), these signaling pathways switch the epithelial phenotype to mesenchymal phenotype. In cancer cells, KLF4 represses the EMT through interacting with TGF-β, Notch and Wnt/β-catenin signaling pathways. The degradation of KLF4 through UPS is necessary to TGF-β induced transcriptional activation. In Notch signaling pathway, KLF4 negatively regulates the expression of Notch1 and functions as a negative modulator of Notch1 target genes' transcription. KLF4 also interacts with Wnt/β-catenin by antagonizing the binding of β-catenin to tran scription factor, TCF and represses the transcriptional activity of TCF. (Fig. 10-39)

Challenges and Prospects

In summary, EMT is the process that cells undergo a switch from epithelial phenotype to mesenchymal phenotype. EMT exists not only in the embryonic development and normal physiological processes，but also plays a promoting role in tumor invasion and metastasis. Tumor cells can gain the ability of migration and movement.

EMT is central to both physiological and pathological processes, and pathological EMT can be regarded as reactivation of developmental programs in the adult. EMT is the initial stage that primary cancer cells leave the orderly site which prerequisites that cells release for dissemination or distant metastases. It is an important sign for cancer metastasis to start. Due to the EMT important role in carcinogenesis, further research will be through analyzing the validations of cellular models and in vitro experiment, through closed-related signaling pathway in live to monitor the expression of mRNA and protein of EMT related molecules, and promoter methylation levels, through reversaly transcript the regulation of genes in EMT, and so on. These studies will help to find the more molecular markers of EMT, conductive study of the molecular mechanisms and functions of EMT, conductively indepth analysis of the relationship between process of EMT and cancer progression. Because the carcinosarcoma includes malignant epithelial cells and mesenchymal cells in the tumor tissue, EMT becomes a prove for the hypothesis of epithelial carcinoma transforming sarcoma. Research results will further reveal the signal pathway inducing EMT and promoting cancer, and further awaring the role that tumor microenvironment on EMT, and further clearly starting the key factors of EMT, and further learning about the mechanism related to EMT in cancers metastasis and chemoresistance, to get more blocking EMT targets and provide a new idea and therapeutic method for the targeted treatment of cancer [67].

Consider/Questions

1. Basic concepts in this chapter

Epithelial mesenchymal transition (EMT), Mesenchymal epithelial transition (MET), TGF-β, Snail,

Twist,Wnt, E-cadherin, Vimentin, Fibronectin, α-SMA, MicroRNAs(miRNAs).

    2. Briefly descrpte the 3 types of EMT.

    3. Give an example of the relationship between EMT and fibrosis.

    4. Summarize the main steps and related genes during tumor EMT.

    5. Why are the metastases tumors composed by predominant epithelial cells?

    6. Briefly explain the significance of tumor EMT.

    7. Briefly interpret the regulation of TGF-β in cancer EMT.

本章彩图

第十一章　肿瘤侵袭与转移

　　恶性肿瘤的发展过程中可向邻近组织直接蔓延和向远处转移，称为肿瘤的扩散。肿瘤扩散是恶性肿瘤的最重要的生物学特性之一，也是恶性肿瘤难以根治的主要原因和常见的致死原因。

　　肿瘤侵袭是指恶性肿瘤的瘤细胞离开原发瘤，向周围组织直接蔓延，浸润和破坏邻近正常细胞和器官。这是肿瘤播散的第一步，其标志是肿瘤细胞突破基底膜。特别是恶性肿瘤生长迅速，压迫而且浸润和侵犯周围组织。肿瘤细胞在组织间隙内的分布，是肿瘤在局部蔓延的结果。因而浸润性肿瘤常缺乏完整的包膜和清楚的边界，使手术难以完全摘除。因此这些肿瘤的外科治疗需要切除相当多看起来似乎未受累的周边正常组织。

　　个别良性肿瘤和良性病变有时也显示浸润，如血管瘤、黏液瘤、肌间脂肪瘤、水泡状胎块、带状瘤、瘤样纤维组织增生、增殖性肌炎、结节性肌炎等。

第一节　肿瘤转移概述

　　恶性肿瘤由原发部位穿过血管和淋巴管，扩散到其他部位，远隔组织和器官继续增殖生长，形成与原发肿瘤相同性质的继发肿瘤的过程，称为肿瘤的转移（metastasis）。患者伴有广泛转移瘤时称为癌瘤病。转移瘤离原发部位距离一般较远，范围大。

一、侵袭和转移的关系

　　（1）播散肿瘤细胞与原发肿瘤的连续性。

（2）侵袭和转移是统一过程中的两个不同阶段。

（3）侵袭是转移的前奏。

（4）转移是侵袭的结果。

二、肿瘤转移途径

（一）淋巴道转移

淋巴道转移（lymphatic metastasis）是癌常见的转移途径，由近到远（与肿瘤所在淋巴管回流途径有关），如乳腺癌——同侧腋窝淋巴结；肺癌——肺门淋巴结，右锁骨上淋巴结；甲状腺癌——颈淋巴结；阴茎癌——腹股沟淋巴结，胃肠道癌——左锁骨上淋巴结（viche 淋巴结）等。有时淋巴结转移为首发症状，如鼻咽癌。肿瘤细胞侵入淋巴管，需要形成栓子进入淋巴结。肿瘤细胞首先见于淋巴结包膜下或边缘窦内，继发性肿瘤在该处生存并最终累及整个淋巴结，而后突破包膜浸润局部组织或继续延淋巴系统扩散。转移部位的淋巴结通常增大。这种增大通常是由于肿瘤细胞在淋巴结内生长所致，但有时也可能仅仅是淋巴结对肿瘤抗原的反应性增生。

前哨淋巴结（sentinel lymph node，SLN）是指原发肿瘤引流区域淋巴结发生转移必经的第一个淋巴结，然后肿瘤依次进一步转移到远处淋巴结。

根据 SLN 的情况（一般观察 SLN1~4 枚）对部分肿瘤（乳腺癌、恶性黑色素瘤、宫颈癌、胃肠癌、卵巢癌、阴茎癌、肺癌、膀胱癌、前列腺癌胰腺癌等）进行临床治疗已经取得突破性进展，临床意义获得共识。SLN 的检测方法有活性染料注射法、放射性核素标记法，前两者的联合应用或结合纳米技术的 MRI 影像技术等。

SLN 评价的局限性：①SLN 检测仅适用于早期、单发性、小肿瘤；②如有淋巴结阻塞，可出现假阴性；③如既往接受过手术或放疗等改变了局部的淋巴流向，可出现假阴性；④肿瘤偶尔可以跳跃性转移，可出现假阴性.

SLN 的应用前景：①SLN 的临床意义在于界定手术范围，确定治疗方案，进行病理分期。②SLN 价值已经肯定，但可行性、安全性还需要前瞻性随机对照，以及方法改进和大宗病例的临床研究和长期随访来验证。③提高 SLN 检出率和准确率是临床研究的重要课题，需要临床、影像、病理联合攻关。

（二）血道转移

血道转移（hematogenous metastasis）是肉瘤的典型转移方式，也是一些癌如肾癌的常见转移方式。由于静脉壁薄，所以比动脉更容易受侵犯。肝和肺是最常见的血源性转移部位，因为它们分别接受全身静脉系统和门静脉系统的血液回流。其他血源性转移的常见部位包括脑、肾上腺和骨。常见的类型有：①肺静脉型：来源于全身静脉的栓子常常进入肺。②腔静脉型：腹腔静脉内瘤栓多见。③门静脉型：进入门静脉分支的肿瘤栓子进入肝内，因此肝是肠道肿瘤转移常见的部位。④椎静脉型：通过椎旁静脉系统进入脊柱骨、肩周及骨盆。

一些肿瘤细胞可以直接进入动脉循环或穿过肺毛细血管进入体循环。肿瘤栓子停留处的组织必须能够为肿瘤组织迅速供应充足的血液和营养。有些肿瘤细胞也有可能先通过淋巴循环而后进入血流。

（三）种植性转移

种植性转移（implantation metastasis）肿瘤细胞累及质膜、黏膜后种植于腹膜、胸膜、心包膜和蛛网膜表面并形成转移瘤。

（1）质膜面种植性转移：穿透质膜，瘤细胞脱落种植于其他器官或组织，如胃肠道癌引起的卵巢转移瘤（Krukenberg 瘤）或卵巢癌穿过腹膜到达肝或腹部其他脏器表面生长。

（2）黏膜面种植性转移：呼吸道、消化道等黏膜种植，较少见。

（3）接触性种植性转移：常见于手术器械引起"医源性"种植。

三、转移的主要步骤

恶性肿瘤为什么会侵袭与转移？过程中有无标记？能否预防？问题解答最终将需从肿瘤转移的分子机制中寻找。瘤细胞侵袭转移的过程是瘤细胞与宿主细胞之间相互作用的连续过程，这个过程是复杂、多步骤的。

瘤细胞转移的主要步骤（图 11-1）如下。

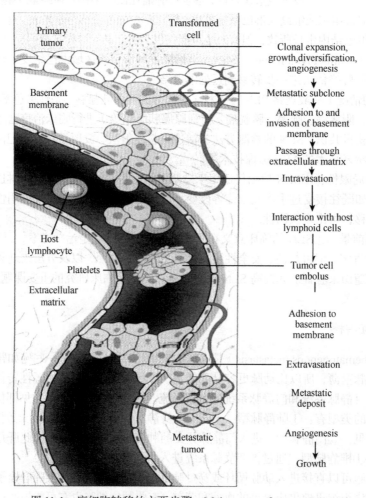

图 11-1　瘤细胞转移的主要步骤；Major steps of tumor metastasis

（1）肿瘤细胞同质型黏附降低，从原发灶脱离。

（2）肿瘤细胞与细胞外基质（ECM）发生异质型黏附增加。

（3）降解 ECM；肿瘤细胞分泌蛋白降解酶降解 ECM 成分，形成细胞移动的通道，并以此为诱导血管生成的基础。

（4）肿瘤细胞运动性增强，并穿透血管壁的基底膜进入循环。

（5）在循环中运行逃避免疫系统识别与破坏。

（6）到达继发部位后，在有新生血管形成的前提下增殖，形成转移灶。

四、转移特点

（1）不同肿瘤的转移频度、时间、途径和部位不同，有些肿瘤转移有一定的器官倾向性（前列腺癌、肺癌）。

（2）转移性肿瘤的一般特征：不连续性。多个转移瘤结节与正常组织分界较清。

淋巴道转移由近到远/血道转移-器官内分散，常位于被膜下，球形结节其表面因缺血坏死凹陷形成癌脐。

（3）多数转移瘤保留原发瘤的生物学特性。

（4）转移瘤的变异多见，转移瘤的分化程度常比原发瘤更差。

五、转移的临床意义

肿瘤转移是肿瘤临床分期的重要指标，是评估肿瘤预后的重要依据。因此必须在下列情况中鉴别肿瘤转移。

（1）区分多中心性发生的多发性肿瘤与肿瘤转移。

（2）区分容易转移肿瘤和不常发生转移的肿瘤。

（3）区分倾向于不同转移途径的不同肿瘤。

（4）区分容易发生转移的器官和不易发生转移的器官。

（5）从肿瘤的一般转移规律追溯原发性肿瘤。

（6）了解某些特殊转移规律及有关的肿瘤。

第二节　瘤细胞黏附能力改变

一、瘤细胞同质型黏附下降

同质型（Homogeneous）黏附是指同种细胞间的黏附，主要由存在于细胞表面的黏附分子（CAM）所介导。同质型黏附下降，促进肿瘤细胞从瘤体上脱落，所以 CAM 在肿瘤浸润和转移中起重要作用。

（一）钙黏蛋白（cadherin）

钙黏蛋白是钙依赖性跨膜糖蛋白，是一组依赖细胞外 Ca^{2+} 的 CAM，介导 Ca^{2+} 依赖性细胞间黏附，通过同类或同分子亲和反应相结合。例如，E-Cad 的功能（转移抑制分子）：①稳定细胞间连接；②促进细胞分化；③保持细胞特定形态；④促进细胞间信息传递。

（二）瘤细胞表面电荷增加

瘤细胞表面电荷增加时瘤细胞间的排斥力增大，促使瘤细胞从瘤体上脱落。瘤细胞表面电荷大小可以通过电泳速度表现出来。细胞电泳速度被认为是筛选不同浸润和转移潜能瘤细胞的初筛标记。

此外溶解性酶的释放、细胞间隙压力的增加，也有利于瘤细胞从瘤体上脱落下来。

（三）瘤内机械压力的作用

外部机械力通过整合素传递至细胞内或通过细胞丝状骨架蛋白施加压力。机械力是双向的（从外到内和内向外），通过相同整合素施加力到 ECM 中。然而细胞对细胞因子向受体的传递是单向的（外向内）（图 11-2）。当瘤细胞内部压力增加时，可导致瘤细胞脱离原发灶形成浸润和转移。

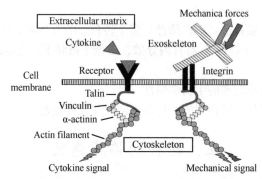

图 11-2　外部机械力是由 ECM 通过整合素传递至细胞，且该细胞可以通过相同整合素施加力到 ECM 中。外部机械力在内部传输或通过细胞骨架蛋白或细丝施加压力。因此机械力可在两个方向上（从外向内或从内向外）发送，然而细胞对细胞因子向受体的传递是单一方向的（从外向内）; External mechanical forces are transmitted to the cell by the extracellular matrix through the cell's integrins, and the cells can apply a force to the extracellular matrix through the same integrins. The external mechanical forces are internally transmitted or applied through the cell's cytoskeletal proteins or filaments. Thus mechanical forces can be transmitted in both directions（outside-in and inside-out）, while the cell's response to cytokines, transmitted through the cell's receptors, are one directional（inside-out）（From outside to inside）

二、瘤细胞异质型黏附的增加

异质型（heterogeneous）黏附是指瘤细胞与宿主细胞，或宿主基质的黏附。瘤细胞脱离瘤体，浸润到基底膜或穿过基底膜遭遇宿主基质和宿主细胞，这一过程就是异质型黏附的过程。这一过程也有利于瘤细胞穿过基质、血管壁的基底膜，有利于瘤细胞在血管内聚集。

（一）整合素

整合素（integrin）是一组介导异质黏附的细胞黏附分子。在肿瘤转移中研究整合素主要在表达增加或新增、表达减少或消失、表达构型的改变，如 $\alpha_6\beta_4$、$\alpha_v\beta_3$、$\alpha_5\beta_1$ 介导的信号通路均与肿瘤运动、转移和浸润有关。

1. $\alpha_6\beta_4$　半桥粒（hemidesmosomes，HDs）中的 $\alpha_6\beta_4$ 整合素虽无信号功能但却给上皮细胞提供结构性支撑，维持上皮细胞黏附和极性。$\alpha_6\beta_4$ 在生理上和功能上与表皮生长因子受体（EGFR，ErbB2）有关。由 SFKs（Fyn）的活化介导 ErbB2 与 $\alpha_6\beta_4$ 的联系。肿瘤中 ErbB2 表达上调增加其增殖和转移潜能。肿瘤微环境诱导 β_4 整合素胞质尾部的依赖性蛋白激酶 C-α 中关键性的丝氨酸残基的磷酸化，导致其在半桥粒中的裂解。半桥粒中 $\alpha_6\beta_4$ 动员允许 $\alpha_6\beta_4$ 与膜结构亚区中富含微丝的肌动蛋白联合，发生与 RTK 的功能性相互作用（图 11-3）。

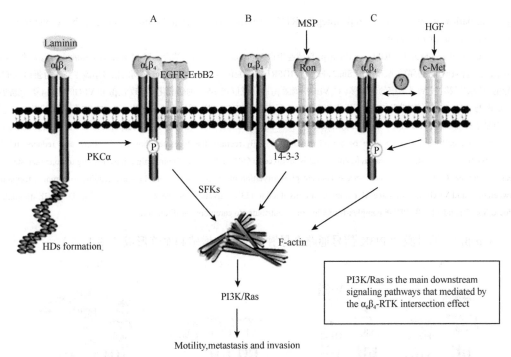

图 11-3　$\alpha_6\beta_4$ 与 RTKs 协同作用的例子；Several examples in which $\alpha_6\beta_4$ associate with RTKs are shown
A. 半桥粒中的整合素（$\alpha_6\beta_4$）虽无信号功能但却给上皮细胞提供结构性支撑。PKC-α 使胞质 β_4 尾部丝氨酸残基磷酸化，导致半桥粒的裂解。SFKs 活化介导 $\alpha_6\beta_4$ 与 ErbB2 和 EGFR 的功能。B. 作为连接分子 MSP 通过 14-3-3 诱导 $\alpha_6\beta_4$ 与 Ron 的联系。C. $\alpha_6\beta_4$ 和 c-Met 合作信号是乳腺癌浸润转移的主要原因。PI3K/Ras 是由 $\alpha_6\beta_4$-RTK 串流效应介导的主要的下游信号通路；A. The integrin（$\alpha_6\beta_4$）in HDs（hemidesmosomes），although there is no signal function，provide structural support to the epithelial cells.PKC-α makes serine residues phosphorylate which of the cytoplasmic β_4 tail，that cause Semidesmosome cracked. The functions of SFKs activation mediate $\alpha_6\beta_4$，ErbB2 and EGFR. B. MSP induces association of $\alpha_6\beta_4$ with Ron through 14-3-3，which acts as a linker molecule. C. Cooperative signaling between $\alpha_6\beta_4$ and c-Met is responsible for breast cancer invasion and metastasis. PI3K/Ras are major downstream signaling pathways mediated by $\alpha_6\beta_4$-RTK crosstalk

2. $\alpha_V\beta_3$　由 $\alpha_V\beta_3$ 整合素介导的信号通路与肿瘤迁移、骨转移、血管形成和增殖有关（图 11-4）。

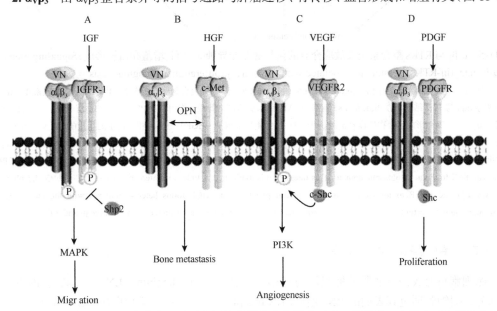

图 11-4　由 $\alpha_V\beta_3$ 与 RTKs 整合素交叉对话介导的信号通路与肿瘤迁移、骨转移、血管形成和增殖有关；

Signaling pathways mediated by α_Vβ₃ integrin-RTKs crosstalk is associated with migration，bone metastasis，angiogenesis and proliferation

A. 为了 IGF-1 反应的最大化，IGFR-1 需要 α$_V$β$_3$ 与玻连蛋白（vitronectin，VN）结合，如 MAPK 活化和肿瘤细胞运动。配体与 α$_V$β$_3$ 的结合阻碍了招募酪氨酸磷酸酶 Shp2，减少了 IGFR1 的磷酸化。B. α$_V$β$_3$ 与 c-Met 之间的信号串流参与骨桥蛋白（OPN）诱导的癌细胞迁移，导致乳腺癌的骨转移。C. VEGF 刺激 β$_3$ 胞质域依赖 c-Src 的磷酸化，导致 α$_V$β$_3$ 和 VEGFR 之间复合物的形成。α$_V$β$_3$ 与 c-Met 的复合物涉及 PI3K 的活化和血管生成反应。D. PDGF 刺激诱导依赖 Shc 的 α$_V$β$_3$-PDGF 复合物的形成，此复合物有助于肿瘤增殖；A. IGFR-1 requires vitronectin（VN）binding of α$_V$β$_3$ for maximal IGF-1 response，such as MAPK activation and carcinoma cell motility. Blockage of ligand binding to α$_V$β$_3$ recruits the tyrosine phosphatase Shp2 and reduces IGFR1 phosphorylation. B. Crosstalk between α$_V$β$_3$ and c-Met is involved in OPN-induced carcinoma migration，leading to bone metastasis of breast carcinoma. C. VEGF stimulates c-Src-dependent phosporylation of the β$_3$ cytoplasmic domain，leading to complex formation between α$_V$β$_3$ and VEGFR. α$_V$β$_3$ and c-Met complex are involved in PI3K activation and the angiogenic response. D. PDGF stimulation induces Shc-dependent α$_V$β$_3$-PDGF complex formation that contributes to carcinoma proliferation

3. α$_5$β$_1$ 通过激活 PI3K 信号通路介导肿瘤浸润、增殖和血管形成（图 11-5）。

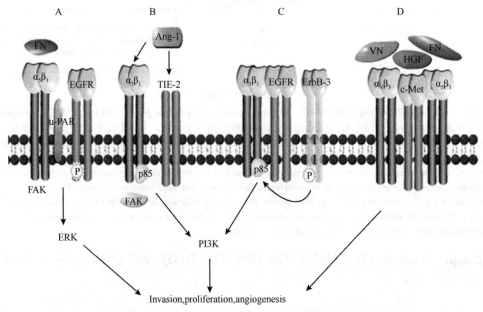

图 11-5 α$_5$β$_1$ 与 RTKs 整合素交叉效应介导的信号通路介导肿瘤浸润、增殖和血管形成；Signaling mediated by α$_5$β$_1$ integrin-RTKs crosstalk is associated withinvasion，proliferation and angiogenesis

A. 尿激酶受体（uPAR）与纤连蛋白（fibronectin，FN）和 EGFR 形成一三元复合物使 Erk 通路活化。B. 血管生成素-1（Ang-1）刺激诱导 α$_5$β$_1$ 与 Tie2 结合招募 PI3K 的 P85 亚基与 FAK 到 α$_5$ 胞质区。此相互作用涉及 PI3K 介导的血管生成。C. ErbB3 磷酸化促进 α$_5$β$_1$ 与 EGFR 形成复合物招募 p85 到 β$_1$ 上。D. 肝细胞生长因子（HGF）与 α$_5$β$_1$ 和 α$_5$β$_1$ 上的基质配体（VN 和 FN）形成异型性复合物。这些复合物促进 c-Met 和 α$_5$β$_3$ 及 α$_5$β$_1$ 的相互作用；A. uPAR, fibronectin（FN）and EGFR form a ternary complex resulting in activation of the ERK pathway. B. Ang-1 stimulation induces α$_5$β$_1$-Tie2 association, which recruits the p85 subunit of PI3K along with FAK to the α$_5$ cytoplasmic domain. This interaction is implicated in PI3K-mediated angiogenesis. C. ErbB3 phosphorylate promotes α$_5$β$_1$ and EGFR to form complexes then recruit p85 to β$_1$. D. HGF forms hetero-complexes with the matrix ligands（vitronectin and fibronectin）of α$_V$β$_3$ and α$_5$β$_1$. These hetero-complexes promote interaction of c-Met with α$_V$β$_3$ and α$_5$β$_1$

（二）整合素配体 LN 受体

癌细胞只有突破基底膜才能浸润与转移。层黏连蛋白（laminin，LN）是基底膜的重要组成部分，瘤细胞通过其表面的 LN 受体（LN receptor，LN-R）与基底膜中的 LN 结合而穿过基底膜。20 世纪 80 年代初就发现了 LN 的 67kDa 受体能识别 LN 分子的 β$_2$ 链，研究证实了 LN-R

能促进瘤细胞的黏附和移动，其高表达与许多肿瘤的浸润转移能力呈正相关。

（三）CD44 及其变体

CD44 是一种淋巴细胞表面的归巢（homing）受体，CD44 表达与肿瘤浸润、转移能力呈正相关，抗 CD44 抗体在肿瘤浸润转移的治疗中有潜力（详见第四章）。

（四）路易斯寡糖

肿瘤细胞表面唾液酸化的路易斯寡糖（louis oligosaccharides，SLEX）作为血管内皮细胞上的 E-选择素配体，是结肠癌早期诊断、癌浸润、预后不良的一个指标。结肠癌细胞表面 sLeX 抗原结构和数量的变化是导致转移的关键因素。所以检测血清或肿瘤组织中 sLeX 可以有效监测肿瘤，尤其是结肠癌的转移。

（五）免疫球蛋白超家族

大部分 Ig-SF 成员参与细胞间识别（包括那些有免疫功能的分子，如 MHA、CD4、CD8 和 T 细胞受体），参与神经发育（N-CAM、L1）、白细胞交流（ICAM-1、VCAM-1、PECAM-1）和信息传递（CSF-1 受体、PDGFR）。CEA 促进结、直肠癌细胞的转移潜能。CEA 高表达的细胞株肿瘤肝脏转移风险增加。

第三节　降解 ECM 的蛋白水解酶

细胞外基质（extracellular matrix，ECM）主要由胶原、糖蛋白、蛋白多糖和氨基葡萄糖组成。ECM 以基底膜和间质结缔组织的形式存在，胶原是 ECM 的主要成分，Ⅰ、Ⅱ、Ⅲ型胶原主要存在于间质结缔组织中，Ⅳ型胶原主要存在于基底膜。ECM 中的糖蛋白包括 LN、FN 和 ND（接触蛋白）等。ECM 是肿瘤侵袭和转移的天然屏障，肿瘤从原位增殖到浸润转移的演进过程中必须具备降解 ECM 的能力。

能降解 ECM 的酶主要是蛋白水解酶，它们的活性均与肿瘤的侵袭和转移有关。这是近年肿瘤侵袭、转移研究中的热点。蛋白水解酶有四类：基质金属蛋白酶（matrix metalloproteinase，MMP）、丝氨酸蛋白酶（serine protease，Ser protease）、半胱氨酸蛋白酶（cysteine protease）、天门冬氨酸蛋白酶（aspartic protease）。

一、基质金属蛋白酶

MMP 最早是由 Gross 和 Lapiere 在 1962 年研究蝌蚪尾巴自动吸收机制时发现[1, 2]。MMP 是由一组锌离子（Zn^{2+}）依赖性内肽酶大家族，包括间质胶原酶、明胶酶、间充质溶解素，具有降解 ECM 和 BM 及调节其他酶、化学因子、细胞受体的功能[3]。越来越多的报道指出了 MMP 与肿瘤发生密切相关，涉及肿瘤侵袭、转移等过程[4, 5]。常态下，MMP 作为合成性的惰性酶原处于非活化状态，是由一个保守的半胱氨酸在硫醇结构域和 Zn^{2+} 催化结构域之间的结合来维持这种状态[6]。溶解前肽区使该酶活化，降解胞外蛋白，如趋化因子、抗菌肽、基质成分等[7]。

（一）MMP 的结构与功能

目前为止，人们已经发现了 MMP 家族超过 23 种细胞外水解蛋白酶。典型的 MMP 由含

80 个氨基酸的前肽,含 170 个氨基酸残基的催化金属蛋白酶结构域,一个不同长度的连接肽(也称铰链区)和一个含 200 个氨基酸的血红蛋白(HPX)结构域组成,因此,又将其划分为 3 个基本结构域[8]:①前肽区,MMP 的 N 端,有一个保守的信号肽,能引导细胞内蛋白质翻译产物至内质网;②催化活性结构域,均含有 1 个结构性 Zn^{2+} 结合区、1 个催化性 Zn^{2+} 结合区和至少 1 个 Ca^{2+} 结合区,同时催化区内还含有 3 个组氨酸残基,是催化性 Zn^{2+} 结合位点;③底物结合结构域,该结构域分铰链区、类 HPX 结合区,主要与 MMP 底物特异性相关,同时在 MMP 与其抑制性结合中发挥重要作用。酶催化区和前肽区具有高度保守性。此外,膜型(MT)-MMP 还存在一个跨膜区,或称为糖基磷脂酰(glycosylphosphatidily,GPI)序列锚定区,主要起固定作用。MMPs 的结构如图 11-6 所示[9]。

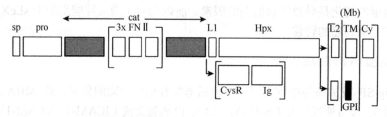

图 11-6　MMP 家族的主要结构域;Domain structures of the MMP family

sp:信号序列;pro,促结构域;cat:catalytic domain 催化结构域。FN Ⅱ:fibronectin type Ⅱ motif,纤连蛋白Ⅱ型基;L1:linker 1,连接子 1;Hpx:hemopexin domain,血红蛋白结合域;L2:linker 2,连接子 2;Mb:plasma membrane,质膜;TM:transmembrane domain,跨膜结构域;Cy:cytoplasmic tail,胞质尾区;CysR:cysteine rich,半胱氨酸富含区的结构;Ig:immunoglobulin domain,免疫球蛋白结构域;GPI:glycosyl phosphatidylinositol,糖基磷脂酰序列;sp,signal sequence;pro,pro-domain;cat,catalytic domain,FN Ⅱ,fibronectin type Ⅱ motif;L1,linker 1;Hpx,hemopexin domain;L2,linker 2;Mb,plasma membrane;TM,transmembrane domain;Cy,cytoplasmic tail;CysR,cysteine rich;Ig,immunoglobulin domain;GPI,glycosyl phosphatidylinositol anchor

根据结构域及酶作用底物的特异性,MMP 可分为胶原酶、明胶酶、间质溶素、基质溶素、MT-MMP 等。其中,①胶原酶类主要水解Ⅰ、Ⅱ和Ⅲ型胶原,包括 MMP-1、MMP-8、MMP-13 及 MMP-18。②明胶酶主要降解Ⅳ型胶原和层粘连蛋白,包括 MMP-2 及 MMP-9。③间质溶解素主要降解Ⅲ、Ⅳ型胶原和基质中的蛋白多糖、糖蛋白,包括 MMP-3、MMP-10 和 MMP-11。④MT-MMP 的主要作用是激活其他 MMP 并降解 ECM,包括四型转膜蛋白(MMP-14、MMP-15、MMP-16、MMP-24)和 GPI 锚定蛋白(MMP-17 和 MMP-25)。⑤其他分泌型 MMP,包括 MMP-7、MMP-12、MMP-19、MMP-20、MMP-22 及 MMP-23[10]。

MMP 家族中不同成员的功能及作用都不同,因此不同成员之间的组成结构域及功能区也不尽相同,如表 11-1 中列举了不同成员之间的组成成分[9]。

表 11-1　MMP 及其结构域

蛋白酶	基质金属蛋白酶	染色体定位（人）	结构域组成													
			SS	pro	CS	Px[R/K]R	Cat	FN2	LK1	Hpx	LK2	tm	GPI	Cyt	CysR-Ig
胶质酶															
	MMP-1	11q22-q23	+	+	+	−	+	−	+	+					
	MMP-8	11q21-q22	+	+	+	−	+	−	+	+					
	MMP-13	11q22.3	+	+	+	−	+	−	+	+					
	MMP-18	不存在	+	+	+	−	+	−	+	+					

续表

蛋白酶	基质金属蛋白酶	染色体定位（人）	结构域组成												
			SS	pro	CS	Px[R/K]R	Cat	FN2	LK1	Hpx	LK2	tm	GPI	Cyt	CysR-Ig
明胶酶															
明胶酶A	MMP-2	16q13	+	+	+	–	+	–	+	+					
	MMP-9	20q11.2-q13.1	+	+	+	–	+	+	+	+					
	MMP-3	11q23	+	+	+	+	+	–	+	+					
	MMP-10	11q22.3-q23	+	+	+	+	+	–	+	+					
	MMP-7	11q21-q22	+	+	+	+	+	–	–	–					
	MMP-26	11p15	+	+	+	+	+	–	–	–					
	MMP-11	22q11.2	(+)	(+)	+	+	+	–	+	+					
膜型MMPs（A）跨膜型															
MT1-MMP	MMP-14	14q11-q12	+	+	+	+	+	–	+	+	+	+	–	+	
MT2-MMP	MMP-15	15q13-q21	+	+	+	+	+	–	+	+	+	+	–	+	
MT3-MMP	MMP-16	8q21	+	+	+	+	+	–	+	+	+	+	–	+	
MT5-MMP（B）	MMP24	20q11.2	+	+	+	+	+	–	+	+	+	+	–	+	
MT4-MMP	MMP-17	12q24.3	+	+	+	+	+	–	+	+	+	–	+	–	
MT6-MMP	MMP-25	16p13.3	+	+	+	+	+	–	+	+	+	–	+	–	
其他															
Marcrophage elastase	MMP-12	11q22.2-q22.3	+	+	+	+	+	–	+	+					
–	MMP-19	12q14	+	+	+	+	+	–	+	+					
Enamelysin	MMP-20	11q22.3	+	+	+	+	+	–	+	+					
–	MMP-21		+	+	+	+	+	–	+	+					
CA-MMP	MMP-23	1p36.3	+	+	+	–	+	–	+	+	–	–	–	–	+
–	MMP-27	11q24	+	+	+	+	+	–	+	+					
Epilysin	MMP-28	17q21.1	+	+	+	+	+	–	+	+					

表11-1 显示了MMP家族的成员及其染色体定位

SS（signal peptide），单肽；pro，促结构域；CS（cysteine），半胱氨酸转换基序；RX[R/K]R（proprotein convertase recognition sequence），促蛋白转化酶的识别序列；FN2，纤连蛋白Ⅱ型；LK，连接子；TM，跨膜结构域；GPI，糖基磷脂酰；Cyt（cytoplasmic domain），胞质域；CyR-Ig（cysteine rich and Ig domain），富含半胱氨酸和Ig结构域

（二）三个水平调控 MMP 的表达和活性

（1）酶原合成：生长因子和细胞因子等活性介质（EGF，TGF-β等是酶原合成阶段最主要的调节因子）不仅能促进或抑制 MMP mRNA 的转录，而且能影响其半衰期。

（2）酶原活化：组织金属蛋白酶抑制剂（tissue inhibitor of metalloproteinase，TIMP）可以抑止 MMPs 的活性。

（3）其他抑制剂的作用：各种 MMP 之间具有一定的底物特异性，但不是绝对的。同一种 MMP 可降解多种 ECM 成分，而某一种 ECM 成分又可以被多种 MMP 降解。但不同酶的降解效率可有不同。MMP 的众多调控因素构成微妙的调节网络，正是这种精确的调控机制保证了机体内生理状态下细胞迁移的 ECM 重构；反之就成为肿瘤侵袭和转移等病理过程发生的原因。

MMP 与肿瘤侵袭转移呈正相关。

（三）MMP 家族成员

目前研究较多的是 MMP-9、MMP-7 和 MMP-2。

1. MMP-2 位于染色体 16q13，也称为 72 kDa 的明胶酶 A，主要水解Ⅳ型胶原及基底膜的主要成分[11]。其结构在前肽的 C 端不含有促蛋白转化酶识别序列（proprotein convertase recognition sequence，RX[R/K]R）。并在金属蛋白酶的结构域中含有 3 种纤连蛋白Ⅱ型重复序列，Zn^{2+}结合基序（HEXXHXXGXXH）的催化域，半胱氨酸转换器基序（PRCGXPD）的前肽区。其中含有 Zn^{2+}结合基序的 3 种组氨酸及前肽区的半胱氨酸均可与催化 Zn^{2+}基序（cys-Zn^{2+}）相互作用。这 cys-Zn^{2+}的相互协调使 MMP 前体保持无活性状态，防止催化水分子与 Zn^{2+}的结合。催化结构域还包含一个保守的甲硫氨酸（met），形成一个 "met-turn" 八残基后的 Zn^{2+}结合基序，以保证这一结构围绕在 cys-Zn^{2+}结合区周围[12]。由于 MMP-2 的三纤连蛋白Ⅱ型重复序列可以与明胶或胶原结合，因此 MMP-2 可以降解 ECM 的成分，包括Ⅳ型、Ⅴ和Ⅺ型胶原，层黏连蛋白，蛋白聚糖核心蛋白等。并以不同于 MMP-9 消化胶原酶的方式来消化Ⅰ、Ⅱ、Ⅲ型胶原[13]。

MMP-2 在多数恶性组织中高表达，如乳腺癌、结肠癌、胃癌、和肺癌[14-16]，在肿瘤细胞增殖过程中，MMP-2 作为明胶酶，以酶原的形式分泌到基质中，活化其他促进肿瘤细胞转移的细胞因子，不仅破坏了机体防御肿瘤浸润与转移的天然屏障，也与其他活化因子共同促进肿瘤的转移[17]。MMP-2 的表达量与癌细胞的侵袭及癌患者较差的预后密切相关[18]，如晚期乳腺癌高表达 MMP-2 与其整体的生存率下降有关[19]。抑制肿瘤细胞中 MMP-2 的表达能有效抑制间质干细胞的迁移，原因在于其抑制了 SDF1/CXCR4 的信号通路，因此 MMP-2 可以作为肿瘤治疗相关的一个有效靶点[20]。

2. MMP-7 属于基质溶解素类，人类 MMP-7 定位于染色体 11q22.3，其 cDNA 长 1094 bp，由 267 个氨基酸组成，是 MMP 家族中分子量最小的成员，酶原形式分子质量是 28kDa，活化形式的分子量为 19kDa。MMP-7 是由包含 Zn^{2+}活性结构域的一个 5 股 β 链和 3 种 α 螺旋及其他的 Zn^{2+}和 Ca^{2+}成分所构成，维持其结构的稳定。与其他 MMP 的结构相比，MMP-7 缺乏与 HPX 的同源序列，因此在与底物结合时并不需要特异性识别底物的结构，这一特性使其能够降解几乎所有的 ECM 成分，包括Ⅳ型胶原、明胶、弹力蛋白、黏连蛋白等，而且还可降解整合素 $β_4$，从而增加了细胞活性，促使肿瘤细胞经淋巴管和血管不断蔓延。MMP-7 也可以激活其他 MMP 前体。MMP-7 可参与和影响肿瘤细胞增殖和演进，如在 ECM 降解翻转重塑、细胞增殖与凋亡、上皮-间皮转化（EMT）等方面均起重要的作用。

研究发现 MMP-7 几乎全部由癌细胞表达，而癌间质细胞不表达。MMP-7 在良性肿瘤组织中表达高于正常组织，但低于癌组织，表明 MMP-7 在肿瘤从正常组织向恶性组织转化过程中发挥作用。MMP-7 还具有蛋白酶活性，能够促进许多生长因子的释放，包括表皮生长因子受体（EGFR）、肝素结合表皮生长因子（HB-EGF）和胞外结构域的细胞表面分子脱落，包括 Fas 配体和 E-cadherin。MMP-7 的这些特性与肿瘤进展与转移有关。过度表达的 MMP-7 可作为胃癌、食管癌、肝癌、肾癌、胰腺癌等高复发率、预后差、生存率低的一项可靠指标。在结直肠癌中血清 MMP-7 特异性高表达，已作为判断癌症患者预后的有效指标。肺癌中 MMP-7 与 TNM 分期、组织学分级与淋巴结转移相关，在Ⅲ-Ⅳ期的表达比Ⅰ-Ⅱ期高，提示 MMP-7 在肺癌进展中发挥了作用。因此 MMP-7 也作为评估肺癌增殖、分化与转移的一种潜在的生物标志物。有关研究表明 MMP-7 与口腔鳞状细胞癌、前列腺癌、胰腺癌、结肠癌、乳腺癌和非小细胞肺癌的进展相关。

3. MMP-9　又名明胶酶 B，与 MMP-2（明胶酶 A）同属明胶酶类，位于染色体 20q12-q13，基因全长为 4506bp。MMP-9 由以下几个部分组成：①氨基端单肽结构域，连接 MMP-9 分子与内质网；②富含脯氨酸的铰链区，其作用是连接催化活性区和羧基端区；③催化活性区，此区域含有 Zn^{2+}、Ca^{2+} 结合位点和保守的 met，是酶的活性中心；④前肽区，含有一个与 Zn^{2+} 作用的硫醇基，可以与半胱氨酸相结合，从而使酶以无活性的酶原形式存在，当外源性酶切割此区域后，MMP-9 被激活；⑤HPX 样区域，它通过一个铰链连接到催化区域，其中有四个重复区，间接与 TIMPs、细胞表面分子和蛋白水解底物发挥作用[21]。

MMP-9 主要由表皮细胞表达，能够降解Ⅳ、Ⅴ型胶原，凝胶蛋白和弹力蛋白等，并且能够完全破坏基底膜成分。同时，MMP-9 也是参与调节细胞生长、迁移、浸润及血管生成的关键信号分子[22]。在非小细胞肺癌中 MMP-9 高表达，与肿瘤的发生及进展有关。MMP-9 表达量和淋巴结转移、TNM 分期、肿瘤大小、组织类型有关，而与年龄、性别、是否抽烟无关；高表达 MMP-9 的肺癌患者预后较差[23]。在原发性肝癌患者血清中的 MMP-9 表达水平明显高于健康组，且与肿瘤的临床分期密切相关。在高侵袭力肝癌细胞株中 MMP-9 的表达显著上调。在动物实验中，阻断 MMP-9 的功能可以有效抑制肿瘤细胞的侵袭、转移。MMP-9 与膀胱癌的发病机制也有着密切关系[24, 25]。因此，MMP-9 可以作为这些肿瘤的主要生物学标记，可能成为肿瘤治疗的一个新靶标。

（四）在肿瘤中 MMP-2、MMP-7 和 MMP-9 启动子基因多态性的研究

多态性是指在一个生物群体中，同时和经常存在两种或多种不连续的变异型或基因型（genotype）或等位基因（allele），亦称遗传多态性（genetic polymorphism）或基因多态性。从本质上讲，多态性的产生在于基因水平上的变异，一般发生在基因序列中不编码蛋白的区域和没有重要调节功能的区域。对于个体而言，基因多态性碱基顺序终生不变，并按孟德尔定律世代相传。人类基因多态性有助于阐明人体对疾病、毒物的易感性与耐受性，疾病临床表现的多样性（clinical phenotype diversity），以及对药物治疗的反应性上差异的原因。

近年来通过人们不断地研究发现 MMP 家族的成员存在着多态性位点，尤其是在启动子区的多态性位点，这些不同的多态性位点大多能够影响其基因的表达，进而会影响肿瘤的易感性。例如，p53 抑癌基因多态性与肿瘤发生及转移的关系研究，从基因水平揭示人类发生肿瘤中不同个体间生物活性物质的功能及效应存在着差异的本质。又如，MMP-2 基因启动子包括能够与某些特定转录因子如 AP-2、p53、SP1 和 SP3 结合的序列。MMP-9 基因启动子中有两个多态性位点具有重要作用，即-90 位置存在（CA）n 微卫星多态性位点和-1562 位 C/T 单核苷酸多态性位点。MMP-7 基因启动子区单核苷酸多态性（SNP），尤其是在-181 位点（-181 A/G）（rs11568818）上 A-G 的转化，已经被证实是有功能性的。

总之 MMPs 家族成员具有降解 ECM 成分及其他细胞因子的作用，不同的成员其结构及其功能不尽相同。MMP-2、MMP-7、MMP-9 作为该家族的重要成员，在肿瘤的发生、侵袭和转移等多个环节中起着重要作用。但目前对上述过程的具体机制尚未完全明确。随着人们对基因多态性了解的不断深入，发现不同等位基因启动子的多态性会影响 MMP 基因的转录活性，从而影响其表达水平。越来越多的研究证实，MMP 启动子的多态性与癌症的易感性相关。因此，在未来的研究中，这些启动子的多态性位点将会成为癌症治疗的靶点。

二、丝氨酸蛋白酶

白细胞弹性蛋白酶和组织蛋白酶，纤溶酶原激活剂（plasminogen activator，As）可使纤溶酶原转变为纤溶酶，纤溶酶的底物较为广泛，可降解 ECM 的许多成分，包括 FN、LN 蛋白聚

糖的蛋白质核心。

（1）纤溶酶还可激活一些前 MMP 及潜伏弹性蛋白酶。已证明 As 在许多肿瘤，尤其是肝癌、乳腺癌、卵巢癌、肺癌中高度表达，它参与降解基质，促进肿瘤细胞的侵袭和转移。

（2）组织蛋白酶（cathepsin）：通过降解基底膜，间质 I、Ⅲ 型胶原，蛋白聚糖，肌动蛋白，肌球蛋白，FN，从而促进许多肿瘤细胞的侵袭和转移（图 11-7）。

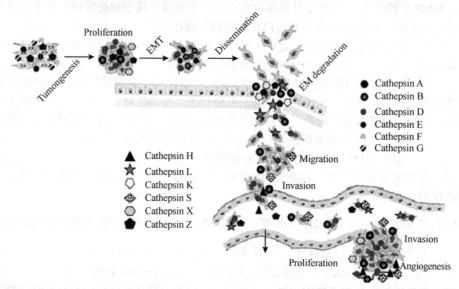

图 11-7　肿瘤转移过程中组织蛋白酶的作用；Role of cathepsins in tumor metastasis process

组织蛋白酶亚型在肿瘤发生、发展中的作用如下。

E 型、F 型、G 型、Z 型促进细胞肿瘤发生。

B 型、D 型、E 型、X 型、H 型诱导和调控肿瘤细胞的增殖。

X 型介导肿瘤细胞的上皮-间质转化。

A 型、B 型、D 型诱导肿瘤细胞的播散。

B 型、K 型、L 型、Z 型降解 ECM。

B 型、D 型、H 型、L 型、S 型、Z 型增加肿瘤细胞的运动性和浸润性，肿瘤细胞侵入周围组织、血液和淋巴管，并转移到远处；在转移部位，B 型、D 型、H 型、S 型介导血管生成和转移性肿瘤的形成。

第四节　肿瘤细胞迁移动力

一、肿瘤细胞和间质细胞对 ECM 的降解

肿瘤细胞增殖时对肿瘤和基质微环境中的细胞产生的机械力（拉伸张力和压缩力增加）将导致肿瘤间质细胞从静止状态到活化状态（如从纤维细胞转变为成纤维细胞的状态）。由于肿瘤的生长和间质的不断扩增，ECM 中机械力增加，肿瘤将重塑 ECM，以降低机械力。增加 ECM 为更多肌纤维母细胞表型转化提供合适的环境，最终合成胶原。肿瘤和间质细胞的牵引力破坏 ECM 中胶原蛋白单体和解开胶原的三重螺旋，一旦胶原蛋白三重螺旋的不稳定则将成为 MMP 作用的靶，裂解胶原蛋白 α-链，基质降解，促使肿瘤细胞浸润和迁移。

肿瘤、基质细胞如何影响肿瘤生长及通过基质扩增降解 ECM 致肿瘤细胞的侵袭和迁移见图 11-8。

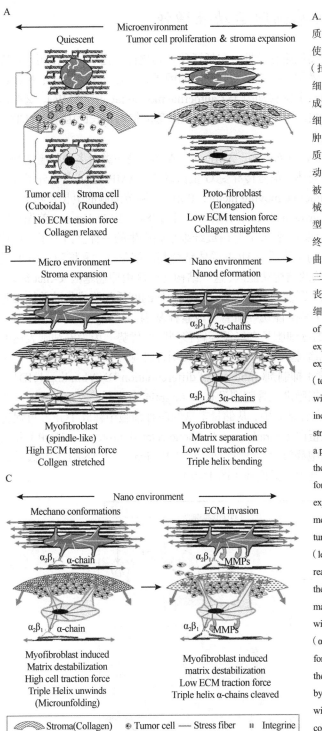

A. 静止的肿瘤细胞（左）转化成增殖细胞在瘤间质的 ECM 中扩展（右）。随着肿瘤向周围扩展，使肿瘤和基质微环境中的细胞间机械力的增加（拉伸和压缩）。机械力的增加将导致肿瘤和间质细胞从静止状态（左）到活跃的肿瘤细胞或间质成纤维细胞的状态（右）的转化。在这种状态下，细胞并没有对 ECM 产生较大的牵引力；B. 随着肿瘤在间质中不断扩展，增加了 ECM 中肿瘤和间质细胞上的机械力（张力和压缩）（左）。当内在动力达到（生物力学触发）的关键程度，信号将被发送到肿瘤和间质细胞而重塑 ECM，以降低机械力。然后细胞将转化为更多肌成纤维细胞的表型（$\alpha_2\beta_1$，3α 链）对 ECM 施加更大的牵引力，最终使胶原单体弯曲（右）。C. 肿瘤和间质细胞对弯曲作用的牵引力使胶原蛋白单体失稳并解开胶原三重螺旋（左）。一旦胶原蛋白三重螺旋的稳定性丧失将有利于 MMP 裂解胶原蛋白 α-链，促使肿瘤细胞在降解的基质中侵入和迁移（右）；A. Transition of quiescent tumor cells（left）to proliferating cells expanding the stroma ECM（right）. As the tumor expands the surrounding increased mechanical forces（tensile and compressive）will be generated in the cells within the tumor and stroma microenvironment. The increase in the mechanical forces will cause tumor and stroma cells to transition from a quiescent state（left）to a proto/mesenchymal-fibroblast state（right）. In this state the cells will have little ability to exert large traction forces on the ECM；B. As the stroma continues to expand with tumor growth, there will be increased mechanical forces（tension and compression）on the tumor and stroma cells within the extracellular matrix（left）. When a critical magnitude of intrinsic force is reached（biomechanical trigger）, a signal will be sent to the tumor and stroma cells remodel the extracellular matrix in order to lower the mechanical forces. The cells will then transition to a more myofibroblastic phenotype（$\alpha_2\beta_1$, 3α chains）with the ability to exert larger traction forces on the extracellular matrix, eventually bending the collagen monomer（right）；C. Traction forces exerted by the tumor and stroma cells on the extracellular matrix will destabilize the collagen monomer and unwind the collagen triple helix（left）. Once the collagen triple helix is destabilized it will become accessible to MMPs for cleavage of the collagen's α-chains, allowing the tumor cells to invade and migrate through the degraded stroma（right）

图 11-8　肿瘤细胞和间质细胞降解 ECM 的作用（虚拟图例）；Tumor and stroma cells degradation of ECM（hypothesized paradigm）

二、肿瘤细胞运动性增强

移动素（motogen）：可以刺激肿瘤细胞移动性，包括迁移、趋化性、化学激动作用、吞噬动力学等。移动素分为三大类：①刺激肿瘤细胞移动与浸润的因子，如移动刺激因子、单核细胞源性分散因子、胶原性移动因子和自分泌移动因子（autocrine mobile factor，AMF）。②刺激生长与移动的因子，如 HGF、EGF 和 IL-1、IL-3、IL-6。③刺激移动抑制生长的因子，如 TGF和 INF。

1. 自分泌移动因子（autocrine moving factors，AMFs） AMFs 是一类由多种肿瘤细胞产生的蛋白因子，各自有特异的糖蛋白受体，信号传导受 G 蛋白调节。AMFs 还可以旁分泌方式作用，此时称为旁分泌移动因子（paracrine moving factor，PMF），调节细胞的生长及移动。

2. 肝细胞生长因子（hepatocyte growth factor，HGF） 于 1984 年由 Nakamura 首先识别并报道，可刺激肝细胞合成 DNA，后来发现 HGF 是由成纤维细胞产生的一种蛋白因子，也称为播散因子（scatter factor）。HGF 可与细胞膜上 HGF 受体结合刺激细胞移动和增殖。HGF 是一跨膜蛋白因子，含有一个酪氨酸激酶的结构功能区，这一结构功能区由原癌基因 c-met 编码。

3. TGF-β 在（雌激素受体，ER）阴性的乳腺癌中，癌浸润处的间质细胞或骨髓前体细胞或者癌细胞本身均可表达 TGF-β。TGF-β 能诱导血管生成素样基因 4（angiopoietin-like 4，Angptl4）的表达。高表达 Angptl4 的癌细胞具有经循环转移到肺的优势。因为癌细胞表达的Angptl4 可破坏毛细血管内皮连接。癌细胞进入肺实质后，ER 阴性乳腺癌细胞还能与肺实质中的 TGF-β 反应，诱导分化/DNA 连接素 1 抑制剂（inhibitor of differentiation/DNA binding 1，ID1），后者重启肿瘤基因。而循环中的肿瘤细胞进入骨髓则没有从 Angptl4 中获利，因为骨髓毛细血管是有窗的，允许细胞不断通过。但在骨基质中，从储量丰富的破骨细胞中释放 TGF-β 可促进生长的癌细胞产生甲状旁腺激素相关蛋白（parathyroid hormone-related protein，PTHrP）和白介素-11（IL-11）。这些因子是成骨细胞释放 RANK 配体（RANK ligand，RANKL）与破骨细胞运动的其他介质维持溶骨性转移的基因激活循环（图 11-9）。

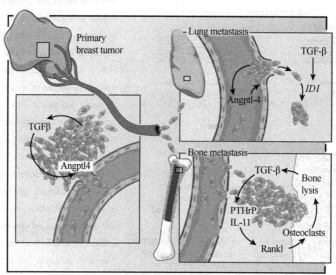

图 11-9　TGF-β 在乳腺癌迁移中的作用；Roles of TGF-β in breast cancer metastasis

褐色表示癌细胞，蓝色表示破骨细胞，绿色表示肿瘤局部间质细胞或骨髓前体细胞；cancer cells（brown），mesenchymal or myeloid precursor cells（green），osteoclasts（blue）

三、其他促进肿瘤细胞转移的因素

（一）上皮间质转化（EMT）

调节癌细胞从上皮细胞转化成间质细胞，并抑制上皮细胞标记和表达间质细胞标记，使癌细胞迁移能力增强，最终发生转移、耐药性和获得癌症干细胞（CSC）的特征。肿瘤细胞可以通过 EMT 过程转变成 CSC，即 EMT 使肿瘤细胞具有 CSC 的自我更新能力，而 CSC 也具有了 EMT 的特征（详见第 10 章）。

（二）肿瘤逃避免疫系统的识别与破坏

瘤细胞即使从瘤体脱落下来，突破基底膜或 ECM 进入血液循环或淋巴系统，也不一定能在血液或淋巴系统中存活下来，它可能会被免疫系统识别并消灭，所以逃避免疫系统的识别和攻击是肿瘤转移形成的又一关键步骤。转移瘤细胞与分化越差的瘤细胞一样人类白细胞共同抗原（HLA）的表达极弱或消失，同时主要组织相容性复合物（MHC）功能受到抑制，细胞刺激信号的作用减弱，导致了肿瘤细胞免疫逃逸（详见第 13 章）。

（三）肿瘤新生血管是转移阻力最小的通道

肿瘤长到 $1\sim2mm^3$ 时，为保证快速增殖必需新生血管支持。由肿瘤诱导产生的血管，其基底膜薄而且易断裂或不完整，肿瘤细胞很容易进入这种血管。所以新生血管的形成十分有利于肿瘤的转移，而一切有利于肿瘤新生血管形成的细胞因子也均有利于肿瘤的侵袭和转移（如 aFGF、bFGF、VEGF、EGF、TGF）。除此之外 IL-8、GM/M-GSF、IGF-1、IFN2、促血管素（angiotropin）、P 物质等能促进肿瘤新生血管形成（详见第 9 章）。

第五节　肿瘤转移的基因调控

在癌转移这个复杂的过程中，必然有许多基因在不同层次上参与调控，包括肿瘤转移基因的激活和转移抑制基因的失活。

许多与肿瘤侵袭转移有关的基因表现为多效性（pleiotropy），同一基因在不同组织类型的肿瘤中作用有异，而同一肿瘤的不同阶段又可能有不同组合的多个基因参与作用。

一、促 进 基 因

至少 10 余种癌基因可诱导或促进癌细胞的转移潜能。

（1）转移基因（MTS1）表达水平与肿瘤细胞的侵袭性明显正相关。

（2）肿瘤侵袭诱导基因（tumor invasion induced gene，TIAM-1）：TIAM-1-Ras 信号转导通路影响细胞骨架、细胞黏附和运动，促进肿瘤侵袭和转移。

二、抑 制 基 因

（1）Nm23（non-metastasis）：1988 年由美国国家癌症研究所 Steeg 等首先在 7 株具有不同转移能力的鼠 K-1735 黑色素瘤细胞系中，以消减杂交的方法从 cDNA 文库中分离到 Nm23 基因，并且是检查到的第 23 个克隆基因。这是目前分离到的唯一对肿瘤转移起着负调控作用的基因，它的出现导致了肿瘤转移基因及转移抑制基因的概念形成。

（2）KAI1/CD82 是一种高度糖基化的细胞膜蛋白，在体内分布广泛，KAI1 蛋白抑制肿瘤的转移，如抑制肝癌、直肠癌、食管癌、胰腺癌、肺癌、膀胱癌、卵巢癌、宫颈癌和乳腺癌等。

（3）Raf 激酶抑制蛋白（Raf kinase inhibitory protein，RKIP）：RKIP 可以与 Raf-MEK1/2 和 NF-κB 诱导激酶-1 结合，改变 β 生长因子激活激酶-1 的结构，从而促进肿瘤细胞的凋亡，抑制肿瘤细胞的转移、血管浸润。

（4）Kiss1：能抑制转移细胞集落形成。Kiss1 能抑制胃癌、肝癌、食管鳞状上皮癌、胰腺癌等的转移。

（5）乳腺癌转移抑制剂（breast cancer metastasis suppressor 1，BRMS 1）：BRMS1 位于 11q13，在黑色素瘤和乳腺癌肿瘤细胞中其表达能恢复细胞之间正常的缝隙连接，对生长和转移起负向调控作用。

（6）Rho GDP 分裂抑制剂（Rho GDP division inhibitor，RhoGDL）：在人类膀胱癌细胞株中鉴定出一种基因——RhoGDL，其表达的降低导致肿瘤细胞容易侵袭和转移。

（7）MAPK 激酶（MKK4/JNKK1/SEK1）：MKK4 位于人类 17 号染色体，是一种肿瘤转移抑制基因。MKK4 是有丝分裂蛋白激酶（mitogen-activated protein kinase，MAPK）的激酶，是 MAPK 信号传递级联放大反应中的一员。MKK4 广泛存在于人类和鼠各种组织中，能抑制前列腺癌、肺癌、胰腺癌、卵巢癌和胃癌等的转移。

（8）分化相关基因 1（differentiation-related gene-1，Drg-1）：Drg-1 能增加内皮细胞的分化，在人类前列腺癌细胞中 Drg-1 具有抑制肿瘤转移的作用，其表达与前列腺癌 Gleason 分级呈反相关。

第六节　肿瘤转移中的信号转导通路

信号转导（signal transduction）是 20 世纪 90 年代以来生命科学研究领域的热点与前沿。

在肿瘤侵袭转移的整个过程中，包括黏附、降解、移动都有信号转导通路的参与，细胞表面受体接受刺激将信号传入细胞内，调节细胞骨架蛋白，激发移动，激活细胞产生各种蛋白降解酶类，有利于癌细胞转移发生与过程。

一、STAT 信号通路

在 STAT 信号通路中各种配体与其同源性细胞表面受体的结合，导致磷酸化 STAT3 分子彼此在 SH2 结构域进一步二聚化及被易位至细胞核。接着该二聚 STAT3 分子结合到靶基因的启动子并激活其转录。STAT3 调控 cyclin D1，c-myc，抗凋亡蛋白 Bcl-xL、Mcd1 及 P53，从而调节细胞增殖和存活。STAT3 蛋白直接结合 MMP-2 的启动子并上调其表达。此外，STAT3 还能调节 MMP-9 和 MMP-7 活化。STAT3 通过调变 Rho 及 Rac 的活性来调控细胞的迁移。STAT3 通过上调 VEGF 和 HIF-α 的活性来调节血管生成。

二、TRP 和 ORAI1 通路

癌细胞和内皮细胞迁移的 TRP 和 ORAI1 通路如图 11-10 所示。

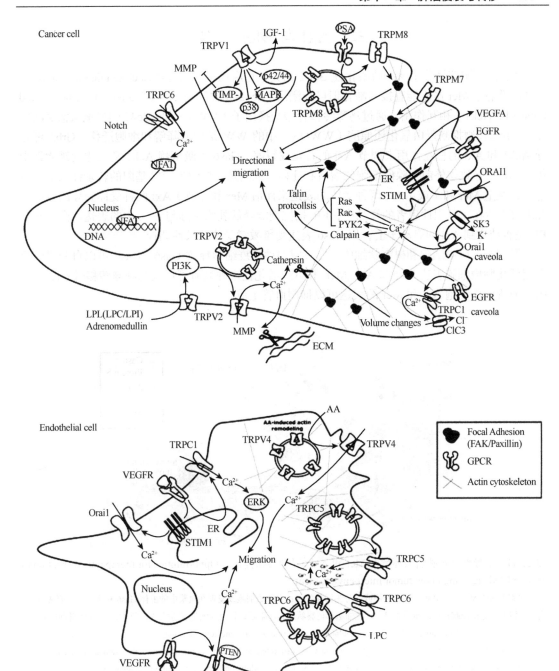

图 11-10　癌细胞和内皮细胞迁移的 TRP 和 ORAI1 通路的分子机制示意图；Schematic representation of TRP and ORAI1 channels molecular mechanisms involved in cancer cell and endothelial cell migration

AA：花生四烯酸；ClC-3：氯离子通道-3；ER：内质网；bFGF：碱性成纤维细胞生长因子；GZMA：颗粒酶 A；GPC：G-蛋白偶联受体；IGF：胰岛素样生长因子；LPL：溶血磷脂；LPC：溶血磷脂酰胆碱；LPI：溶血磷脂酰肌醇；MAPK：丝裂原活化蛋白激酶；NFAT：激活细胞的核因子；PI3K：磷脂酰肌醇 3 激酶；PTEN：磷酸酶和张力蛋白同源物；Pyk2：蛋白酪氨酸激酶；SK3：K⁺通道；TIMP1：金属肽酶抑制剂 1；AA, arachidonic acid；ClC-3, Chloride channel-3；ER, endoplasmic reticulum；bFGF, basic Fibroblast Growth Factor；GZMA, Granzyme A；GPCR, G-protein coupled receptor；IGF, insulin-like growth factor；LPL, lysophospholipids；LPC, lysophosphatidylcholine；LPI, lysophosphatidy linositol；MAPK, mitogen activated protein kinase；MMP, Matrixmetalloproteinase；NFAT, Nuclear factor of activated T-cells；PI3K, Phosphatidy linositol 3-kinase；PTEN, Phosphatase and tensin homolog；Pyk2, Protein tyrosine kinase；SK3, K⁺ channel；TIMP1, metallopeptidase inhibitor 1

三、Axl 与 Mer 通路

Axl 的下游信号分子 Akt 磷酸化使 Bcl-2 相关死亡启动子（Bcl-2-associated death promoter, BAD）失活。Mer 虽不能直接磷酸化但可与激活 Cdc42-相关激酶 1（activated Cdc42-associated kinase 1, Ack1）相互作用。通过鸟嘌呤核苷酸交换因子（VAV1）和 Cdc42 间接地激活 Ack1, Ack1 引起肿瘤抑制蛋白氧化还原酶（WWOX）中的 WW 结构域降解和细胞迁移。Grb2 可介导 Ack1 和 Axl 的相互作用来调节 Axl 的转化或裂解。Gas6 刺激依赖 Ack1 磷酸化的雄激素受体（AR），导致体外前列腺癌细胞的增殖和迁移，推测是经雄激素应答基因的转录性调节。通过对细胞上 Mer 和（或）Axl 两种受体的表达来评估 Mer 和（或）Axl 两种受体介导的效应。Axl 仅表达在 ER 阳性患者的样品中，ER 拮抗剂能降低乳腺癌细胞中 Axl 的表达。尚未确定 ER 是否结合到 Axl 的启动子上，但 Gas6 表达受雌激素受体转录性调控。

肿瘤相关巨噬细胞和树突状细胞，以及浸润性免疫细胞释放 Gas6。Gas6 可以自分泌或旁分泌活化肿瘤细胞表达 Mer 和 Axl。Mer 和 Axl 活化促进肿瘤血管形成和肿瘤转移（图 11-11）。阻断血管内皮细胞 Axl 和 Mer 的表达可以抑制血管生成。

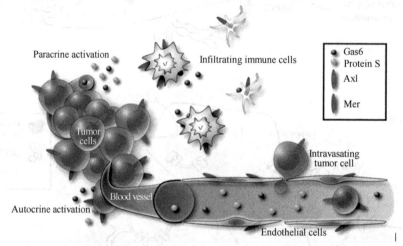

图 11-11　治疗性干预肿瘤微环境中 Mer 和 Axl 信号通路的前景；Opportunities for therapeutic disruption of Mer and Axl signaling in the tumor microenvironment

肿瘤细胞表达的 Mer 和 Axl 可能由自分泌或旁分泌活化的表达在肿瘤细胞或发现在血浆中的配体 Gas6 和蛋白 S 所刺激。Gas6 也可由浸润性免疫细胞释放，如肿瘤相关巨噬细胞和树突状细胞。阻断血管内皮细胞表达的 Axl 和 Mer 可以抑制血管生成；Axl and Mer expressed by tumor cells may be stimulated by autocrine or paracrine activation loops as the ligands Gas6 and Protein S are expressed by tumor cells and found in plasma. Gas6 is also released by infiltrating immune cells such as tumor-associated macrophages and dendritic cells. Blockade of Axl and Mer expressed by endothelial cells may inhibit angiogenesis

四、CXCL12 通路

CXCL12 与 CXCR4 和 CXCR7 的结合，作为 G 蛋白偶联受体（GPCR）可形成同源二聚体或异源二聚体。在异源二聚体中 CXCR7 改变 CXCR4/G-蛋白复合物的构象并阻断信号。由 CXCL12 活化的 CXCR4 导致 G-蛋白偶联信号通过 PI3K/Akt, IP3 和 MAPK 信号通路促进细胞生存、增殖及趋化作用。此外，GRK 激活 β-抑制蛋白通路从而内化 CXCR4。当 CXCR7 结合 CXCL12 时并不发生经典的 GPCR 钙离子调控，β-抑制蛋白通路的激活可能清除 CXCL12。在某些癌细胞（如神经胶质瘤）CXCR7 也可以通过 PLC/ MAPK 信号以增加细胞存活（图 11-12 ）。

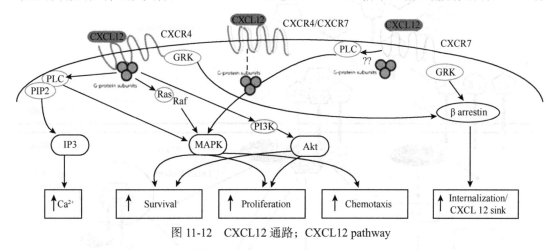

图 11-12　CXCL12 通路；CXCL12 pathway

五、TGF-β 通路

在经配体非依赖性方式的β-抑制蛋白2依赖方式的激活Cdc42中TβRⅢ介导细胞迁移。TβRⅢ通过配体依赖和非依赖方式激活 p38。TβRⅢ经胞外结构域脱落生成可溶性 TβRⅢ，后者与配体结合，抑制 TGF-β 信号（图 11-13A）。TβRⅢ提供 TβRⅡ配体，其能磷酸化 TβRⅢ及招募、磷酸化 TβRI，导致 R-Smad 蛋白磷酸化。磷酸化的 R-Smad 蛋白与共同 Smad4 的相互作用，介导 Smad 蛋白复合物的核转录活性及调控转录活性。TβRⅢ与β-抑制蛋白2相互作用导致 TβRⅢ/TβRⅡ/β-arrestin2 复合物的相互作用及随后下调 TGF-β 的信号。在 β-抑制蛋白 2 的依赖性方式中 TβRⅢ负性调控 NF-κB 信号通路。TβRⅢ与 GIPC 相互作用稳定细胞膜上的 TβRⅢ，增强TGF-β 的信号转导，介导细胞迁移和侵袭（图 11-13B）。

挑战与展望

影响肿瘤转移的因素众多，包括以下几方面。

（1）肿瘤细胞的黏附性（同质型黏附下降、异质型黏附的增加）。

（2）肿瘤细胞分泌相关蛋白酶降解 ECm。

（3）肿瘤血管形成。

（4）肿瘤转移相关基因和肿瘤转移抑制基因的信号调控。

（5）宿主局部组织的特性：肿瘤微环境、肿瘤运动性增强、CSC、EMT 等。

（6）宿主整体免疫状态和细胞因子、生长因子、激素分泌的水平。

癌转移的分子病理学研究战线很长，无论对转移各个步骤或各个有关基因的分别研究，还是从总体上探索其调控机制，都是有意义的。鉴于转移是癌细胞多基因活动和多种生物学行为特征的结果，并且受到宿主体内环境的影响，因此研究工作的重点宜放在探索那些在转移过程多个环节上起作用的分子（如黏附分子等）及关键性的调控基因。有必要在 DNA、mRNA 或蛋白产物三个水平上系统的研究，因为同样的转移表型可能是不同调控机制的结果。

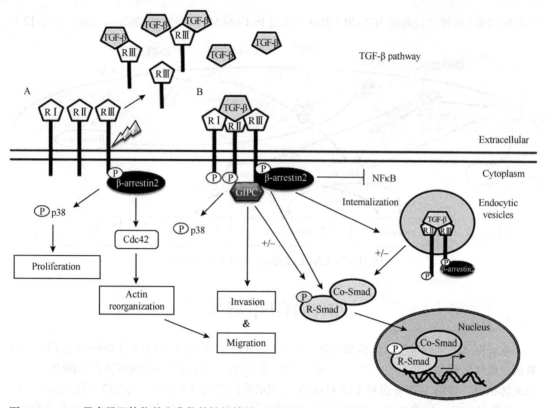

图 11-13　TβRⅢ介导配体依赖和非依赖性的效果；TβRⅢ mediates both ligand dependent and independent effects

思 考 题

1. 本章基本概念：转移（metastasis）；Krukenberg 瘤（Krukenberg's tumor）；viche 淋巴结（viche lymph node）；细胞外基质（extracellular matrix，ECM）；前哨淋巴结（sentinel lymph node，SLN）；基质金属蛋白酶（matrix metalloproteinase，MMP）；自分泌移动因子（autocrine moving factors，AMFs）；肝细胞生长因子（hepatocyte growth factor，HGF）；Nm23（non-metastasis）。

2. 解释肿瘤细胞转移主要步骤。

3. 简述肿瘤转移的特点。

4. 结合肿瘤转移病例测试分析其转移途径及可能的基因表达与信号调控。

5. 简述检测 SLN 的临床意义和可能出现的假阴性情况。

参 考 文 献

[1] Gross J, Lapiere C M. Collagenolytic activity in amphibian tissues：a tissue culture assay [J]. Proceedings of the National Academy of Sciences of the United States of America, 1962, 48（6）：1014-1022.

[2] Brinckerhoff C E, Matrisian L M. Matrix metalloproteinases：a tail of a frog that became a prince[J]. Nature Reviews Molecular Cell Biology, 2002, 3（3）：207-214.

[3] Hadler-Olsen E, Winberg J O, Uhlin-Hansen L. Matrix metalloproteinases in cancer：their value as diagnostic and prognostic markers and therapeutic targets[J]. Tumor Biology, 2013, 34（4）：2041-2051.

[4] Ra H J, Harjubaker S, Zhang F, et al. Control of promatrilysin（MMP7）activation and substrate-specific activity by sulfated

glycosaminoglycans[J]. Journal of Biological Chemistry, 2009, 284（41）: 27924-27932.

[5] Moore C S, Crocker S J. An alternate perspective on the roles of TIMPs and MMPs in pathology[J]. The American Journal of Pathology, 20 1 2, 180（1）: 12-16.

[6] Hideaki N, Robert Visse, Gillian Murphy. Structure and function of matrix metalloproteinases and TIMPs[J]. Cardiovascular Research 2006, 69: 562-573.

[7] Vu T H, Werb Z. Matrix metalloproteinases: effectors of development and normal physiology[J]. Genes & Development, 2000, 14: 2123-2133.

[8] Patterson M L, Atkinson S J, Knäuper V, et al. Specific collagenolysis by gelatinase A, MMP-2, is determined by the hemopexin domain and not the fibronectin-like domain[J]. FEBS Letters, 2001, 503（2-3）: 158-162.

[9] Huang Y C, Hung W C, Chen W T, et al. Effects of DNMT and MEK inhibitors on the expression of RECK, MMP-9, -2, uPA and VEGF in response to arsenite stimulation in human uroepithelial cells[J]. Toxicology Letters, 2011, 201（1）: 62.

[10] Bhoopathi P, Chetty C, Gogineni V R, et al. MMP-2 mediates mesenchymal stem cell tropism towards medulloblastoma tumors[J]. Gene Therapy, 2011, 18（7）: 692-701.

[11] Takeharu H, Yasukawa K, Inouye K. Thermodynamic analysis of ionizable groups involved in the catalytic mechanism of human matrix metalloproteinase 7（MMP-7）[J]. Biochimica et Biophysica Acta（BBA）- Proteins and Proteomics, 2011, 1814（12）: 1940-1946.

[12] Lin M C, Wang F Y, Kuo Y H, et al. Cancer chemopreventive effects of lycopene: suppression of MMP-7 expression and cell invasion in human colon cancer cells[J]. Journal of Agricultural & Food Chemistry, 2011, 59（20）: 11304-11318.

[13] Mäkinen L K, Häyry V, Hagström J, et al. Matrix metalloproteinase-7 and matrix metalloproteinase-25 in oral tongue squamous cell carcinoma[J]. Head & Neck, 2014, 36（12）: 1783-1788.

[14] Ulivi P, Casoni G L, Foschi G, et al. MMP-7 and fcDNA serum levels in early NSCLC and idiopathic interstitial pneumonia: preliminary study[J]. International Journal of Molecular Sciences, 2013, 14（12）: 24097-24112.

[15] Fee K, Lena N, Christoph K, et al. Serum MMP7, MMP10 and MMP12 level as negative prognostic markers in colon cancer patients[J]. BMC Cancer, 2016, 16（1）: 494.

[16] Han J C, Li X D, Du J, et al. Elevated matrix metalloproteinase-7 expression promotes metastasis in human lung carcinoma[J]. World Journal of Surgical Oncology, 2015, 13（1）: 1-10.

[17] Shin S, Oh S, An S, et al. ETS variant 1 regulates matrix metalloproteinase-7 transcription in LNCaP prostate cancer cells[J]. Oncology Reports, 2013, 29（1）: 306-314.

[18] Cheng S, Eliaz I, Lin J, et al. Triterpenes from Poria cocos suppress growth and invasiveness of pancreatic cancer cells through the downregulation of MMP-7[J]. International Journal of Oncology, 2013, 42（6）: 1869-1874.

[19] Jia Z C, Wan Y L, Tang J Q, et al. Tissue factor/activated factor VⅡa induces matrix metalloproteinase-7 expression through activation of c-Fos via ERK1/2 and p38 MAPK signaling pathways in human colon cancer cell[J]. International Journal of Colorectal Disease, 2012, 27（4）: 437-445.

[20] Yang R L, Wu C H, Wang K Y. Analysis of thrombin-antithrombin complex expressions in the plasma and the hematoma fluid of intracerebral hemorrhage patients of excess syndrome of stroke and depletion syndrome of stroke[J]. Chinese Journal of Integrated Traditional & Western Medicine, 2012, 32（3）: 338-342.

[21] Kessenbrock K, Plaks V, Werb Z. Matrix mefalloproteinases: regulators ofthe tumor microenvironment[J]. Cell, 2010, 141（1）: 52-67.

[22] Ranzato E, Martinotti S, Volante A, et al. Platelet lysate modulates MMP-2 and MMP-9 expression, matrix deposition and cell-to-matrix adhesion in keratinocytes and fibroblasts[J]. Experimental Dermatology, 2011, 20（4）: 308-313.

[23] Mehner C, Hockla A, Miller E, et al. Tumor cell-produced matrix metalloproteinase 9（MMP-9）drives malignant progression and metastasis of basal-like triple negative breast cancer[J]. Oncotarget, 2014, 5（9）: 2736-2749.

[24] Zeng F C, Cen S, Tang Z Y, et al. Elevated matrix metalloproteinase-9 expression may contribute to the pathogenesis of bladder cancer[J]. Oncology Letters, 2016, 11（3）: 2213-2222.

[25] Radisky E S, Radisky D C. Matrix metalloproteinases as breast cancer drivers and therapeutic targets[J]. Frontiers in Bioscience, 2015, 20（7）: 1144-1163.

（高小娇 陈丹艺 陈 莉）

Chapter 11 **Tumor Invasion and Metastasis**

Metastasis, the major cause of mortality among cancer patients, is a multi-step process, including detachment of tumor cells from the primary sites, invasiveness into circulation, migration along the circulation, extravasation to the secondary sites, and proliferation

In the growth and development process of cancer, it can spread directly to adjacent tissue and distant metastasis, known as the spread of cancer.

Tumor spread is one of the most important biological characteristics of malignant tumors, also the main reason for difficulty in curing cancer and a common cause of death.

Tumor invasion refers to malignant tumor cells leave the primary tumor, directly spread to the surrounding tissue, infiltrate and destruct the adjacent normal cells and organs.It is the first step of tumor spread, the mark is the tumor cells break through the basement membrane.

Tumor invasion usually occurs in malignant tumor. Malignant tumor often grow rapidly, not only by expansion but also by infiltration and invasion of surrounding tissue. Distribution of tumor cells in the tissue space is tumor spread in local. A well-defined capsule and plane of cleavage are lacking, making enucleation difficult or impossible. Surgical treatment of such tumors requires removal of a considerable margin of healthy and apparently uninvolved tissue.

Individual benign tumors showed infiltration sometimes. For instance, Hemangioma, myxoma, intermuscle lipoma, tumor-like fibrous tissue proliferation, proliferation myocarditis, nodular myositis, hydatidiform mole, ribbon tumor, etc.

Section 1　Concepts of Tumor Metastasis

The neoplastic cells from the primary site penetrate the walls of blood vessels and lymphatic channels spread to the distant tissues and organs, continue to proliferation and growth, this important process is called metastasis and the resulting secondary tumors are the same nature as the primary tumor. Patients with widespread metastases are often said to have carcinomatosis. The secondary tumor general distances far away from the primary site and have a wide range.

1. Relationship between Invasion and Metastasis

(1) Continuity of disseminated tumor cells and primary tumor

(2) Invasion and metastasis are two different stages in the unified process

(3) Invasionis a prelude to metastasis

(4) The metastasis is the result of invasion

2. Metastatic Pathways

(1) Lymphatic Metastasis

Extension by the lymphatic is the common method of spread of carcinoma depending on the location (and therefore lymphatic drainage) of the tumor.

For instance, breast cancer----ipsilateral axillary lymph node, lung cancer -hilarlymph node, right supraclavicular lymph node, thyroid cancer -necklymph nodes, penilecanceringuinal lymph nodesgastrointestinal tract cancer--left supraclavicular lymph node(Viche lymphnode), etc., Sometimes lymph node metastasis astheinitial symptom, such as nasopharyngeal carcinoma.

Tumor cells grow into lymphatic channels and are broken off and carried as emboli to a lymph node. Here, the tumor cells lodge and often can be seen initially in the subcapsular space or peripheral sinus. Thus, a secondary tumor is formed, which may eventually overwhelm the node, break through the capsule, and spread locally as well as onward in the lymphatic system.Lymph nodes that are the site of the metastases are frequently enlarged. Such enlargement usually results from the growth of tumor cells in nodes, but in some cases may result primarily from a reactive hyperplasia of the lymph nodes in response to the tumor antigens.

Sentinel lymph node (SLN) is the first lymph node that regional lymph node drainage of the primary tumor occurred metastasis must pass through and then in turn further metastasis to distant lymph nodes. It has made a breakthrough according to the situation of SLN (general observation SLN1-4 pieces) on the part of the clinical tumor therapy (breast cancer, malignant melanoma, cervical cancer, gastrointestinal cancer, ovarian cancer, penile cancer, lung cancer, bladder cancer, prostate cancer, pancreatic cancer, etc.), the clinical significance obtain consensus.

SLN detection methods include reactive dye injection method, radionuclide labeling,joint application of the first two, or a combination of nanotechnology MRI imaging technologies, etc.

Limitations Evaluating SLN:

1) SLN detection only applies to earlier, solitary, small tumors.

2) If lymph is blocked, there may be a false negative.

3) As previously received surgery or radiotherapy alters local lymph flow, there may be a false negative.

4) Tumor metastasis occasionally skips, there may be a false negative.

Application Prospect of SLN:

1) The clinical significance of SLN lies in that to define the extent of surgery, determine the treatment plan and pathological staging.

2) SLN value has been affirmed, but the feasibility and safety also needs prospective randomized controlled, improved method, the bulk of cases of clinical studies and long-term follow-up to verify.

3) Improve SLN detection rate and accuracy are an important issue in clinical research, need clinical, imaging, pathological joint research.

(2) Hematogenous Metastasis

Typical of all sarcomas but also the favored route for certain carcinoma such as those originating in the kidney. Because of their thinner walls, veins are more frequently invaded than arteries. Lung and liver are common sites of hematogenous metastases because they receive the systemic and venous outflow, respectively. Other major sites of hematogenous spread include brain and bones.

1) Type of   Pulmonary Vein Tumor emboli from systemic veins tend to lodge in the lungs

2) Type of Vena Cava

3) Type of Portal VeinTumor emboli that enter branches of the portal vein lodge in the liver, and that organ is the common site for metastasis from tumor of the intestinal tract.

4) Type of Vertebral VeinCarried by the paravertebral venous system, to reach the bones of the vertebral column, shoulder girdle, and pelvis.

Some tumor cells reach the arterial circulation directly or by passing through pulmonary capillaries. The tissue in which the emboli lodge must be capable of rapidly supplying adequate blood or nourishment for the tumor tissue. It is possible that some tumor cells enter the bloodstream after having first passed through the lymphatic circulation.

(3) Implantation Metastasis

Extension by implantation occurs when tumor cells involving a serosa or mucous membrane by seeding of surfaces in peritoneal, pleural, pericardial and subarachnoid spaces.

1) Serosa implantation metastasis: penetrate the plasma membrane, shed tumor cells to grow into other organs or tissues. For example, gastrointestinal tract cancer involves a serosal surface and seeding both side ovaries, histologically showing mucin carcinoma with multifocal lesions known as Krukenberg's tumor.Carcinoma of the ovary, for example, spreads to the surface of the liver or other abdominal viscera.

2) Mucosal surface of implantation metastasis: respiratory tract, digestive tract and so on, the mucous membrane plant is rare.

3) Contact implantation metastasis:contact tumors, surgical instruments caused "iatrogenic" to grow.

3. Major Steps of Tumor Metastasis

Why do malignant tumors occur invasion and metastasis? Whether can be prevented?

The answers will ultimately be found in molecular mechanisms of tumor metastasis.Tumor cell invasion and metastasis process is a continuous process that interact between host cells and tumor cells.This process is complex and multistep. Major steps of tumor metastasis are shown in follow (Fig. 11-1):

(1) Homogeneous adhesion of tumor cell decreased resulting in it away from the primary lesion;

(2) Heterogeneous adhesion increase in tumor cells and extracellular matrix (ECM);

(3) Degrading ECM: Tumor cells secrete protein-degrading enzyme to degrade ECM components to form a passageway for cellular mobile and as this a base to induce angiogenesis;

(4) The mobility enhancement of tumor cells, and penetrating the basement membrane of blood vessel walls into circulation;

(5) In circulation, tumor cells evade immune system identification and destruction

(6) After arriving at the secondary site, proliferation and forming metastases on the premise of angiogenesis.

4. Characteristics of Tumor Metastasis

(1) Different tumors have different metastasis frequency, time, ways and positions

Some tumor metastasis has the tendency of certain organs (prostate cancer, lung cancer)

(2) General Characteristics of Metastatic Tumor:Discontinuities, multiple metastases

Lymphatic metastasis from near to distant/blood metastasis-spread in organs, near capsule, globose tubers

(3) Most metastasis preserves the biological characteristics of the primary tumor

(4) A lot of variation of metastases Metastatic tumor differentiation degree usually is worse than the primary tumor

5. Clinical Significance of Tumor Metastasis

Whether or not, metastasis is an important indicator of tumor clinical stage and a basis for evaluating the prognosis of tumor

(1) Distinguish multi-center of multiple tumors and tumor metastases.

(2) Distinguish between easy metastasis tumor and it infrequent occurrence metastasis tumor.

(3) Distinguish the different metastasis ways in different tumors.

(4) To distinguish the organs are easy or difficult to metastasis.

(5) Retrospect primary tumor from the general metastasis law of tumors.

(6) Knowledge of certain special metastasis law and related cancers.

Section 2　Adhesion of Tumor Cells

1. Declined Homogeneous Adhesion of Tumor Cells

The Homogeneous adhesion refers to intercellular adhesion in same cells, mainly mediated by cell adhesion molecules (CAM). The homogeneous adhesion decreases which promotes the shedding of tumor cells from the tumor body,so CAM play an important role in tumor invasion and metastasis.

(1) Cadherin

Cadherin is calcium-dependent transmembrane glycoprotein, which is a group of CAM and is dependent on extracellular Ca^{2+}. It mediates Ca^{2+}-dependent cell adhesion, combination through a similar or same molecular affinity reaction. For instance, the function of E-Cad (metastasis inhibiting molecules): ①Stable intercellular junctions; ②Promoting cell differentiation; ③Maintaining cells in a specific form; ④Promoting information transmission between cells.

(2) Surface Electric Charge of Tumor Cells

When the tumor cell surface charge increases, the repulsion between tumor cells increases, promoting tumor cells fall off from tumor bodies. The size of the tumor cell surface charge can be manifested through electrophoretic velocity. The speed of cell electrophoresis is considered to be the initial screening markers for the different infiltration and metastasis of tumor cells. In addition, the release of soluble enzymes, the increases of cell gap pressure, also beneficial to tumor cells fall off from the tumor bodies.

(3) Roles of Intratumor Mechanical Forces

External mechanical forces pass to the cell through integrin or exert pressure through cytoskeleton proteins of filaments. Mechanical forces are two-way (from outside to inside and from inside to outside), impose force to the ECM by the same integrin. However, it is unidirectional that the transfer of cell to cell factor by cell receptors (From outside to inside) (Fig.11-2）. Increasing intratumor pressure may lead to tumor cells fall off from primary lesion to form invasion and metastasis.

2. Increased Heterogeneous Adhesion of Tumor Cells

Heterogeneous adhesion refers to the adhesion between tumor cells and host cells, or the tumor cells and host matrix. Tumor cells fall off from tumor bodies infiltrate into the basement membrane then encounter to the host matrix and the host cell,this process is the process of heterogeneous adhesion.This process is beneficial to tumor cells penetrate the matrix and basement membrane of blood vessel wall, also conducive to the accumulation in tumor cells in blood vessels.

(1) Integrin

It is a group of cell adhesion molecules that mediate the heterogeneous adhesion. Study on integrin in tumor metastasis focus on: ①Expression increased or newly added; ②Expressions reduces or disappears; ③Changes in expression patterns. For instance, the signal Pathways mediated by integrin $\alpha_6\beta_4$, $\alpha_v\beta_3$, $\alpha v\beta$ are responsible for cancer motility,invasion and metastasis.

1) $\alpha_6\beta_4$

$\alpha_6\beta_4$ integrin in hemidesmosomes (HDs) has no signaling functionbut does provide structural support to the epithelia. $\alpha_6\beta_4$ is physically and functionally associated with ErbB2 and EGFR. The associationof EGFR with $\alpha_6\beta_4$ is mediated by SFKs (Fyn) activation. The upregulating ErbB2 and EGFR.in tumor cells will promote its proliferation and invasion. The tumor microenvironment induces PKC-α-dependent phosphorylation of key Ser residuesin the $\beta4$ integrin cytoplasmic tail, resulting in HD disassembly. Mobilization of $\alpha_6\beta_4$ from HDs allows association of $\alpha_6\beta_4$ withactin filament-rich sub domains of membrane structures in which functional interactions with RTKs occur (Fig. 11-3).

2) $\alpha_v\beta_3$

The signal pathway mediated by integrin $\alpha_v\beta_3$ is associated with migration, bone metastasis, angiogenesis and proliferation (Fig. 11-4).

3) The signal pathway mediated by integrin $\alpha_5\beta_1$ through activating PI3K is associated with invasion, proliferation and angiogenesis (Fig. 11-5).

(2) Integrin Ligands------ LN -Receptor

Tumor cells can be produced by invasion and metastasis only through the basement membrane. LN is an important component of basement membrane, tumor cells surface LN receptor（LN-R） combination with the LN of basement membranes and then passes through the basement membrane. In the early 1980s, that 67KD LN-R could recognize β2 chain of LN molecule. Study confirms LN-R can promote the tumor cell adhesion and mobility.Its high expression was positively correlated with invasion and metastasis of many tumors.

(3) CD44 and Its Variants

CD44 is a kind of homing receptor of the lymphocyte. The expression of CD44 is positively correlated with tumor invasion and metastasis. Anti-CD44 antibodies have a potential in the treatment of tumor invasion and metastasis.

(4) Louis Oligosaccharides (SLEX)

Sialylated SLEX of the tumor cells surface as the ligand of E-selectin on vascular endothelial cell. It is an indicator for the early diagnosis of colon cancer, tumor infiltration and poor prognosis.The change of structure and amount of the SLEX antigen on colon cancer cell surface is the key factor leading to metastasis. So that detection of SLEX of serum levels or tumor tissues can effectively monitor the tumors, especially is the colon cancer metastasis.

(5) Immunoglobulin Superfamily (Ig-SF)

The most members of Ig-SF are involved in cell-to-cell recognition(including those immune function molecules, such as MHA, CD4, CD8), and T cell receptors involved in the development of neuron (N-CAM, L1), exchange of white blood cells (ICAM-1,VCAM-1,PECAM-1) and the transfer of information (the CSF-1 receptor, PDGFR). CEA promote the metastatic potential of colon and rectum cancer cells. High expression of CEA of tumor cell in the liver increases risks of metastasis.

Section 3   Proteolytic Enzymes Degrading ECM

ECM is mainly composed of collagen, glycoproteins, proteoglycan and glucosamine.ECM exist in the form of basement membrane(BM) and connective stroma. Collagen is the main component of ECM.The type I, II, III of collagen mainly exist in the interstitial connective tissues and the type IV collagen mainly exists in the BM. Glycoprotein of the ECM includes LN, FN and ND (contact protein),etc., ECM is a natural barrier to tumor invasion and metastasis, the process of tumor from in situ proliferation to infiltration and metastasis must have ability to degrade ECM

The enzymes which can degrade ECM mainly are proteolytic enzyme, their activity is associated with tumor invasion and metastasis.In recent years, it is a hot topic in the research of tumor invasion and metastasis. Four types of proteolytic enzymes include: ①Matrix metalloproteinase (MMP), ②Serine(Ser) protease, ③Cysteine proteases (Caspase family), ④Aspartic protease

1. Matrix Metalloproteinase (MMP)

MMPs was first founded in 1962 by Gross and Lapiere in studying the tadpole tail automatically absorption mechanism[2]. MMPs are a family of endogenous calcium- and zinc-dependent proteolytic enzymes, including ① Interstitial collagenase, ② gelatinase and ③Matrilysins, that are capable of degrading most ECM components and BM, as well as regulating other enzymes, chemokines and even cell receptors [3]. More and more studies have reported that the MMPs are related tumor angiogenesis, invasion and metastasis[4-5].Under normal conditions, MMP is inactive as a synthetic inactive zymogen, which is maintained by the intraction between a conserved cysteine in the thiol domain and the Zn^{2+} catalytic domain [6]. Dissolution of the peptide region can activate the enzyme, and degradate extracellular proteins, such as chemokines, antimicrobial peptides, matrix components [7].

(1) The structures and functions of MMPs

Twenty three types of MMPs have been described so far. A typical MMP consists of a propeptide of about 80 amino acids, a catalytic metalloproteinase domain of about 170 amino acids, a linkerpeptide of variable lengths (also called the F hinge region)and a hemopexin (HPX) domain of about 200 amino acids. Therefore, it can be divided into three basic domains [8]: ①the propeptide region: N-end, there is a conserved signal peptide, which can guide the translation product of intracellular proteins to the endoplasmic reticulum; ②the catalytic domain contains: one structural Zn^{2+} binding region, one catalytic Zn^{2+} binding region and at least one Ca^{2+} binding region, while catalytic region contains three   histidine residues, which is a catalytic binding site of Zn^{2+};③the substrates binding domain: That is divided into hinge region and HPX binding region, which mainly related to the substrate specificity of MMPs, and play the important role while MMPs and its inhibiting combination. The enzyme catalytic region and propeptide region are highly conserved. Additionally, The MT-MMPs have an extra domain called the transmembrane domain or GPI anchored domain, which played a role of fixation. The following Fig.11-6 shows the structure of the MMPs[9].

MMPs can be divided into subgroups according to their structure and substrate specificity. These subfamilies include collagenases, gelatinases, stromelysins, matrilysins, membrane-type(MT) MMPs, and other MMPs. ①Collagenases (MMP-1, MMP-8, MMP-13 and MMP-18) cleave fibrillar collagen types I, II, and III; ②Gelatinases (MMP-2 and MMP-9)degrade other ECM molecules including collagenstypes IV, laminin; ③Stromelysins (MMP-3, MMP-10 and MMP-11) digest a number of noncollagen ECM molecules, including collagens types III、IV, Proteoglycan and glycoprotein in stroma ; ④MT-MMPs in mammals includes four type transmembrane proteins (MMP-14, MMP-15, MMP-16, and MMP-24) and two glycosylphosphatidylinositol-anchored proteins (MMP-17 and MMP-25), which are mainly roles to activity other MMPs and degrade ECM; ⑤Other secretory MMPS including MMP-7, MMP-12, MMP-19, MMP-20, MMP-22 and MMP-23 [10].

There are different functions and roles in different members of MMPs family. Therefore, the composition domains and functional areas of the different members are different, as shown in Table 1, the composition of the different members for their domain arrangement [9]. Groups of MMPs are listed with their trivial names and chromosomal locations (Table11-1).

Table 11-1　MMPs and their domain composition

Enzyme	MMP	Chromosomal location(human)	Domain composition												
			SS	pro	CS	Px[R/K]R	Cat	FN2	LK1	Hpx	LK2	tm	GPI	Cyt	CysR-Ig
Collagcnases															
Instcrtitial collagenase; Collagenase 1	MMP-1	11q22-q23	+	+	+	−	+	−	+	+					
Ncutrophil collagenase Collagenase 2	MMP-8	11q21-q22	+	+	+	−	+	−	+	+					
Collagenase 3	MMP-13	11q22.3	+	+	+	−	+	−	+	+					
Collagenase 4 (*Xenopies*)	MMP-18	Not found in humans	+	+	+	−	+	−	+	+					
Gelatinases															
Gelatinases A	MMP-2	16q13	+	+	+	−	+	+	+	+					
Gelatinases B	MMP-9	20q11.2-q13.1	+	+	+	−	+	+	+	+					
Stromelysins															
Stromelysin 1	MMP-3	11q23	+	+	+	−	+		+	+					
Stromelysin 2	MMP-10	11q22.3-q23	+	+	+	−	+		+	+					
Matrilysins															
Matrilysin 1	MMP-7	11q21-q22	+	+		−	+								
Matrilysin 2	MMP-26	11p15	+	+	−	−	+		−	−					
Stromelysin 3	MMP-11	22q11.2	(+)	(+)	+	+	+	−	+	+					
Membrane-type MMPs (A)Transmembrane type															
MT1-MMP	MMP-14	14q11-q12	+	+	+	+	+	−	+	+		+		+	
MT2-MMP	MMP-15	15q13-q21	+	+	+	+	+	−	+	+		+		+	
MT3-MMP	MMP-16	8q21	+	+	+	+	+	−	+	+		+		+	
MT5-MMP	MMP24	20q11.2	+	+	+	+	+	−	+	+		+		+	
(B)GPI-anchored															
MT4-MMP	MMP-17	12q24.3	+	+	+	+	+	−	+	+			+		
MT6-MMP	MMP-25	16p13.3	+	+	+	+	+	−	+	+			+		
Others															
Marcrophage elastase	MMP-12	11q22.2-q22.3	+	+	+	−	+		+	+					

continued

Enzyme	MMP	Chromosomal location(human)	Domain composition												
			SS	pro	CS	Px[R/K]R	Cat	FN2	LK1	Hpx	LK2	tm	GPI	Cyt	CysR-Ig
–	MMP-19	12q14	+	+	+	–	+	–	+	+				
Enamelysin	MMP-20	11q22.3	+	+	+	–	+	–	+	+				
–	MMP-21		+	+	+	–	+	–	+	+				
CA-MMP	MMP-23	1p36.3	+	+	+	–	+	–	–	–	–	–	–	–	+
–	MMP-27	11q24	+	+	+	–	+	–	+	+				
Epilysin	MMP-28	17q21.1	+	+	+	–	+	–	+	+				

SS, signal peptide; Pro, pro-domain; CS, cysteine switch motif; RX[R/K]R, proprotein convertase recognition sequence; FN2, fibronectin type Ⅱ motif; LK, linker; TM, transmembrane domain; GPI, glycosylphophatidylinositol anchoring sequence; Cyt, cytoplasmic domain; CyR-Ig, cysteine rich and Ig domain

(2) Three levels of regulating MMP expression and activity

1) Zymogen synthesis: growth factors and cytokines (EGF, TGF-β etc.,are the most important regulators in the zymogen synthesis stage), not only promote or inhibit the transcription of MMPs mRNA, but also affect their half-life period.

2) Zymogen activation: Tissue inhibitor of metalloproteinase (TIMP) can inhibit the activity of MMPs.

3) Effects of other inhibitors

There are some certain substrate specificities among different MMPs, but no absolute. One kind of MMP can degrade many kinds of ECM components, and a kind of ECM component can be degraded by many MMPs. However, the degradation efficiency of different enzymes is different. Lots of regulatory factors of MMP constitute a subtle regulatory network, this precise regulation mechanisms ensure the ECM reconstruction of cell migration in physiological condition. On the contrary, it has become the causes of tumor invasion and metastasis. MMPs are positively correlated with tumor invasion and metastasis.

(3) MMP2, MMP7 and MMP9 have been extensively investigated recent years.

1) MMP-2

MMP-2, which is located on chromosome 16q13, is also known as the 72 kDa gelatinase A. It primarily hydrolyzes type IV collagen, the major structural component of the BM[11].MMP-2 have little a proprotein convertase recognition sequence RX[R/K]R at the C-terminus of the propeptide,but have three repeats of fibronectin type Ⅱ motif in the metalloproteinase domain. The Zn^{2+} binding motif(HEXXHXXGXXH) in the catalytic domain, and the "cysteine switch" motif(PRCGXPD) in the propeptide are common structural signatures, where three histidines in the Zn^{2+} binding motif coordinate and the cysteine in the propetide coordinate with the catalytic Zn^{2+}. This Cys- Zn^{2+} coordination keeps proMMPs inactive by preventing a water molecule essential for catalysis from binding to the zinc atom. The catalytic domain also contains conserved methionine, forming a "Met-turn" eight residues after the Zn^{2+} binding motif, which forms a base to support the structure around the catalytic Zn^{2+} [12]. Gelatinases (MMP-2 and MMP-9) readily digest gelatin with the help of their three fibronectin type Ⅱ repeats that binds to gelatin/collagen. They also digest a number of ECM molecules including type IV, V and XI collagens,laminin, aggrecan core protein, etc.MMP-2, but not MMP-9, digests collagens I, Ⅱ and Ⅲ in a similar manner to the collagenases [13].

MMP-2 is overexpressed in a variety of malignant tissues compared to normal tissues, such as cancers of the breast, colon, stomach, and lung[14-16]. In the process of tumor cell proliferation, MMP-2, gelatinase, as zymogen is secreted into stromal to activate other cytokines that promote the metastasis of tumor.It not only destroys the natural natural barrier for tumor invasion and metastasis but also promotes tumor metastasis with other factors [17]. The expression of MMP-2 is closely related to the invasion of cancer cells and poor prognosis of cancer patients [18-19]. Inhibiting the expression of MMP-2 in tumor cells can effectively inhibit the migration of mesenchymal stem cells, which is due to the inhibition of SDF1/CXCR4 signaling pathway, altogether this evidence identifies MMP-2 as an interesting target for the development of both diagnostic and therapeutic approaches[20].

2) MMP-7

MMP-7 (also known as matrilysin), which is located on chromosome 11q21-22, MMP-7 is the smallest of the MMP in size, with 28 kDa latent proform, and the mature form being 19 kDa, and its cDNA is 1094 bp, consisting of 267 amino acids[28]. MMP-7 is composed of a five-stranded β-sheet and three α-helices, with zinc containing active domain, and other zinc and calcium ions necessary for structural stability [29] Comparing with other MMPs, MMP-7 lacks the linker peptide and the Hpx domain. Therefore, the structure of the substrate is not required to be specially recognized when the substrate is combined. MMP-7 has the ability to degrade ECM components, such as elastin, type IV collagen, fibronectin, vitronectin, aggrecan and proteoglycans [30]. But it can also degrade the integrin β4, thereby increasing the activity of the cells, and promote the tumor cells to spread through the lymphatic vessels and blood vessels [31]. It is recognized that MMP7 activates other pro-MMPs [32]. MMP-7 can participate in and influence the proliferation and evolution of tumor cells, such as the transformation in the degradation of ECM flip remodeling, cell proliferation and apoptosis, epithelial-mesenchymal transition(EMT).

The study found that all MMP-7 express almost in cancer cells, not in stromal cells. The expression of MMP-7 in benign tumor tissues is higher than in normal tissue, but lower than the cancer tissue, showing that MMP-7 plays a role in normal tissues transformed to malignant. MMP-7 also exhibits proteinase activities against additional targets resulting in release of growth factors such as EGFR, heparin binding epidermal growth factor(HB-EGF) from the extracellular matrix, and in ectodomain shedding of cell surface molecules, including Fas ligand and E-cadherin. These activities of MMP-7 have important biological consequences relevant to tumor progression and metastasis. MMP-7, when overexpressed in tumor cells, plays a central role in the progression of many tumors such as gastric cancer, esophageal cancer, colorectal cancer, liver cancer, renal cancer and pancreatic cancer and is a reliable indicator for high recurrence of cancer, poor prognosis and low rate of survival[33-35]. The high expression of MMP-7 in serum has been used as an effective indicator to judge the prognosis of patients with colorectal cancer [36]. MMP-7 overexpression is reported to be associated with the TNM stage, histologic grade and LN metastasis of lung cancer. MMP-7 expression is higher in the Ⅲ-IV stage than in the I-Ⅱ stage, suggesting an important role of MMP-7 in the progression of lung cancer[37]. Thus, MMP-7 shows a great promise as a biomarker to assess lung cancer proliferation, differentiation and metastasis. Not surprisingly, a few studies have reported that MMP-7 is linked to the disease progression in oral squamous cell carcinoma, prostate cancer, pancreaticcancer, colon cancer, breast cancer and non-small cell lung cancer(Nsclc) [38-43].

3) MMP-9

MMP-9, which is located on chromosome 20q12-q13 and is also known as the 92 kDa gelatinase B with MMP-2, gelatinase B; its full length was 4 506bp.The MMP-9 consists of the following some parts: (1) single amino terminal peptide domain, linking MMP-9 molecules and endoplasmic reticulum; (2) the hinge region with rich proline, its role is to connect the catalytic region and the C-terminal region; (3) catalytic region, this region contains Zn^{2+}, Ca^{2+} and conserved met binding sites which is the active center of the enzyme; (4) the peptide, containing a thiol which has an interaction with Zn^{2+}, can be combined with cysteine, so that the enzyme exists in the inactive zymogen, when exogenous enzyme cutting in this area, MMP-9 is activated; (5) HPX like domain, through the hinge region connecting to the catalytic region, of which has four repeat, and it indirectly plays a role with TIMPs, cell surface molecules and proteolytic substrates [21].

MMP-9 is mainly expressed in epidermal cells, which can degrade collagen V, collagen IV, gelatin and elastin. At the same time, MMP-9 is a key signaling molecule involved in the regulation of cell growth, migration, invasion and angiogenesis [22]. High expression of MMP-9 in NSClc is associated with tumor progression and prognosis. The expression of MMP-9 was correlated with lymph node metastasis, TNM stage, tumor size and histological type, but not with age, gender and smoking. The prognosis of lung cancer patients with high expression of MMP-9 was poor[23]. The expression of MMP-9 was upregulated in HCC cells with high invasiveness. In animal experiments, blocking the function of MMP-9 can effectively inhibit the invasion and metastasis of tumor cells.MMP-9 is most highly expressed in tumors of the basal-like molecular subtype of breast cancer[24], notably, high MMP-9 expression was found to be significantly associated with progression to distant metastasis specifically in the subset of basal-like breast cancers[25].The present meta-analysis results markedly indicate that MMP-9 expression is associated with clinicopathological features of bladder cancer[26]. Thus, MMP-9 may be a useful biomarker in the diagnosis and clinical management of cancer, and may be a valuable therapeutic target. [27]

(4) Researching the promoter gene polymorphisms of MMP-2, MMP-7 and MMP-9 in the tumor

Polymorphism means that in a biological group, at the same time and often have two or more discontinuous variants or genotypes or alleles,also known as genetic polymorphisms. Essentially, the polymorphism is generated at the level of gene variationthat generally occurs in the unencoded protein regions of gene sequence and the regions without important regulatory functions. For individuals, the nucleotide sequence of the gene polymorphism does not change for a lifetime, according to Mendel's law. The human gene polymorphism may help to elucidate the susceptibility and tolerance of disease and poison for human, clinical phenotype diversity, and the different responses to drug treatments differences.

Furthermore, there is an increasing evidence indicating that these functional polymorphisms may contribute to interindividual differences in a wide spectrum of cancer susceptibility[44].Such as the research which is the relationship between polymorphism of tumor suppressor gene p53 and tumorigenesis and metastasis, from the level of gene, it is revealed that the function and effect of bioactive substances are different between the different individuals tumor. Such as the MMP-2 gene promoter includes a sequence that can bind to specific transcription factors such as AP-2, p53, SP1 and SP3[45]. There are two polymorphisms in the promoter of MMP-9 gene play an important role, the position of -90 exists the microsatellite polymorphism loci and the position of -1562 exists the single nucleotide polymorphism locus[53]. Single nucleotide polymorphisms (SNPs) in the promoter region of MMP-7 gene, especially the transformation of A-G in the position -181, has been proved to be functional.

In conclusion, MMPs family members have some roles in the degradation of ECM and other cytokines. The structures and functions of different members are not the same. MMP-2, MMP-7, MMP-9, as important members of the family, play an important role in the occurrence, invasion and metastasis of tumor. However, the specific mechanism of the above process is not yet fully clear. With the deep understanding of gene polymorphism, it is found that the polymorphism of the promoter of different alleles could affect the transcriptional activity of MMPs gene, which affected the expression level of these genes. More and more studies have confirmed that the polymorphism of MMPs promoter is associated with cancer susceptibility. Thus, in the future, the polymorphisms of these promoters will become the targets of cancer therapy.

2. Serine Proteases

Leukocyte elastase, cathepsin and plasminogen activator (As) can transform plasminogen into fibrinolytic enzyme (plasmin). The substrate of fibrinolytic enzyme is more extensive, and many components of the ECM can be degraded, including FN, LN, protein core of proteoglycans.

(1) Fibrinolytic enzymes also could activate MMPs and latent elastase. It has proved in many tumors, especially liver cancer, breast cancer, ovarian cancer, lung cancer, is highly expressed. It participates in the degradation of matrix and promote tumor cell invasion and metastasis.

(2) Cathepsin though degrades the Bm, stroma Ⅰ,Ⅲ collagen, proteoglycans, actin, myosin, FN, and promotes many tumor cell invasions and metastasis. The cathepsins effects in the process of tumor metastasis（Fig. 11-7）:

The substrate of cathepsins play roles in tumor progress:

E, F, G, Z:　Promoting tumorgenesis

B, D, E, X, H: Inducing and regulating the proliferation of tumor cells

X: Mediated tumor cell epithelial - mesenchymal transition (EMT)

A, B, D: Inducting tumor cells spreading

B, K, L, Z: degradating ECM

B, D, H, L, S, Z: Increasing motility and invasion of tumor cells, tumor cells invade surrounding tissue, blood and lymphatic vessels, and are metastasis into the distance; In metastatic sites, B, D, H, S mediated angiogenesis and metastatic tumor formation.

Section 4　Enhancement of Tumor Mobility

1. ECM Degradation by Tumor and Stroma Cells

The mechanical force (tension and compression Increase) generated by the cells in tumor and stroma microenvironment at the time when tumor cells proliferation will result tumor stromal cells from static state to activation state (such as the status that fibrocyte to fibroblast or desmocyte). Due to the continuous expansion of matrix and tumor growth, mechanical force (tension and compression) of ECM is increased, the tumor reshapes the ECM to reduce the mechanical force. Providing the environment for more phenotypic conversion of myofibroblasts by adding ECM then final synthesizes collagen. The traction of tumor and stroma cells to destruct collagen monomer of ECM and triple helix which unlock the collagen. Once the instable triple helix of the collagen formed, the target will be the role of MMPs broken ends of collagen α- chain, matrix degradation led invasion and migration of tumor cells.

How do tumor and stroma cells respond to tumor growth and expansion to degrade the extracellular matrix for tumor cellinvasion and migration through the stroma(Fig. 11-8).

2. Enhancement of Tumor Mobility

Motogen

Motogen can stimulate tumor cells mobility, including: migration, chemotaxis, chemical excitement effect, phagocytosis dynamics etc.

Motogen is divided into three categories: ①Factors to stimulate the movement and infiltration of tumor cells, such as migration - stimulating factor and monocyte - derived dispersion factor, collagen mobile factors and autocrine mobile factor (AMF). ②Factors to stimulate growth and movement, such as HGF, dispersing factor, EGF, and IL-1, 3, 6. ③Factors to stimulate movement but inhibit the growth, such as TGF and INF.

1) Autocrine moving factors (AMFs)

AMFs are protein factors which are produced by a variety of tumor cells.Each of which has specific glycoprotein receptors, signal transduction regulated by G proteins. Recently discovered AMFs also have paracrine action, called the latter as paracrine moving factor (PMF), which regulate the growth and movement of cells.

2) Hepatocyte growth factor (HGF)

HGF was first recognized by Nakamura in 1984. It can stimulate liver cells to synthesize DNA. Later it was that found, HGF is a protein factor produced by the fibroblasts, also known as spread factor. HGF can be combined with HGF receptor on the cell membrane to stimulate cell proliferation and move. HGF is a transmembrane protein factor, comprising a structural and functional domain of tyrosine kinase. This domain is encoded by proto-oncogene c-met.

3) TGF-β

TGF-β is derived from infiltrating mesenchymal or myeloid precursor cells or from the cancer cells themselves. In ER−breast tumors, it induces the expression of genes including Angiopoietin-like 4 (ANGPTL4). Cancer cells entering the circulation with elevated Angptl4 production have an advantage in seeding lung metastasis because of this cytokine's ability to disrupt vascular endothelial junctions when the cells lodge in lung capillaries. After entering the pulmonary parenchyma, ER-breast cancer cells may respond to local TGF-β with induction of Inhibitor of Differentiation/DNA binding 1 (ID1), which acts in this context as a tumor-reinitiating gene. The entry of circulating tumor cells into the bone marrow does not benefit from Angptl4 because these. Capillaries are naturally fenestrated to allow the constant passage of cells. However, TGF-β released by osteoclasts from rich stores in the bone matrix acts on the growing cancer cells to stimulatethe production of parathyroid hormone-related protein (PTHrP) and interleukin-11. These factors act on osteoblasts to release RANK ligand (RANKL) and other mediators of osteoclast mobilization, perpetuating the osteolytic metastasis cycle (Fig. 11-9).

3. Other Events

(1) Epithelial- mesenchymal transition (EMT) Promoting Metastasis

The EMT regulators transform the cancer cells from epithelial-cell like to mesenchymal-cell like with suppression of epithelial markers and expression of mesenchymal markers. The final effects on cancer cells are cancer metastasis, drug resistance and with features of cancer stem cells (CSCs). Cancer cells transform into CSCs by EMT. EMT makes CSCs obtain the self-renewal capacity, CSCs also have the characteristic of EMT(For details, see the chapter10 and the chapter 7).

(2) Tumor evading immune system

Even tumor cells shed down from the tumor body to break the extracellular matrix or basement membrane into the bloodstream or lymphatic system. It may not be able to survive in the blood or lymphatic system. The tumor cells in the blood or lymphatic system may be recognized and destroyed by the immune system. Therefore, that tumor cells evade to be recognized and destroyed by the immune system. This is another key step in the formation of tumor metastasis.The weak or disappearing expression of HLA antigen in metastatic tumor cells, the weak expression of HLA in tumor with poorer differentiation. When tumor metastasis, MHC function is suppressed and it weakens the effect of cell stimulation signals that leads to immune escape of tumor cells.This is an important reason for the occurrence of tumor metastasis. (For details, see the 13 chapter).

(3) Tumor angiogenesis, as a least resistance metastasis pathway

When tumor grows to 1-2mm^3, to ensure rapid proliferation it must be supported by the new vessels.Angiogenesis is induced by the tumor, its basement membrane is thin and is easy to break. Tumor cells easily enter these vessels.So angiogenesis, the formation of new blood vessels, is very beneficial to tumor metastasis. And the cytokines that benefit to tumor angiogenesis also account for the invasion and metastasis of tumor, such as α-FGF, β-FGF, VEGF, EGF, TGF. Besides, the IL-8, GM/M-GSF, IGF-1, IFN2, angiotropin and P substance all can promote tumor angiogenesis (For details, see the 9 chapter).

Section 5   Regulation of Tumor Metastasis

In this complex process of metastasis, there must be many genes involved in the regulation at different levels, including activation of promoting tumor metastasis genes and inactivation of metastasis suppressor genes. Many tumor invasion and metastasis-related genes showed pleiotropy. The same genes in different histological types of tumors the roles are different, and in different stages of the same tumor may involve in different combinations of multiple genes.

1. Promoting Genes

At least 10 kinds of oncogenes can induce or promote the metastatic potential of cancer cells.

(1) Transgene (MTS1) expression levels is positively correlated with tumor cell invasion.

(2) Tumor invasion induced gene (TIAM-1)

TIAM-1-ras signaling pathways influence the cytoskeleton, cell adhesion and motility, and promote tumor invasion and metastasis.

2. Inhibiting Genes

(1) Nm23(Non-metastasis): Nm23 gene, the first to be isolated from cDNA library by subtractive hybridization in seven different metastatic ability of K-1735 murine melanoma cell line by Steeg et al. In the US National Cancer Institute in 1988, and it (the 23rd clone genes)has been detected.This is the only gene which is currently isolated that plays a negative regulatory role in tumor metastasis, which led to form the concept of tumor metastasis genes and metastasis suppressor genes.

(2) KAI1 / CD82: KAI1 / CD82 is a highly glycosylated membrane protein and widely distributed in the human body, KAI1 protein inhibits tumor metastasis, such as liver cancer, colorectal cancer, esophageal cancer, pancreatic cancer, lung cancer, bladder cancer, ovarian cancer, cervical cancer and breast cancer etc.

(3) Raf Kinase Inhibitory Protein (RKIP): RKIP can combine with induced-kinase 1 of Raf-MEK1/2 and NF-κBto change the structure of TGF -β activate kinase-1, promotes tumor cell apoptosis and inhibits tumor cell metastasis, vascular invasion.

(4) Kiss1: Kiss1can inhibit the formation of metastatic cell colony. Kiss1 can inhibit metastasis of gastric cancer, liver cancer, esophageal squamous cell cancer, pancreatic cancer etc.

(5) Breast Cancer Metastasis Suppressor 1 (BRMS 1): BRMS1 located at 11q13, the expression of it can restore gap junctions between normal cells and in melanoma and breast cancer tumor cells, and has a negative regulation to these tumors growth and metastasis.

(6) Rho GDP Division Inhibitor 2 (RhoGDL): Rho GDL is identified in human bladder cancer cell

lines, reducing its expression can lead tumor cells to invasion and metastasis easily.

(7) MAPK Kinase(MKK4/JNKK1/SEK1): MKK4 located on human chromosome 17, is a tumor metastasis suppressor gene.MKK4 is a kinase of mitogen-activated protein kinase (MAPK), and is one member of the MAPK signaling cascade reaction.MKK4 widely exists in various tissues of humans and mice, and can inhibit metastasis of prostate cancer, lung cancer, pancreatic cancer, ovarian cancer and gastric cancer etc.

(8) Differentiation-related Gene-1 (Drg-1): Drg-1 can increase the differentiation of endothelial cells.In human prostate cancer cells, Drg-1 effectively inhibits tumor metastasis, and its expression is inversely associated with the Gleason grade of prostate cancer.

Section 6　Signal Pathways in Tumor Metastasis

Signal transduction is in the research highlights and fronts in the field of life science research since the 90's. The entire process of invasion and metastasis include adhesion, degradation, moving process. All these involve signal transduction. Cell surface receptors are stimulated to make the signal deliver to intracellular, then regulate cytoskeletal proteins, stimulate movements and activate cells to produce a variety of proteolytic enzymes.

1. STAT Signaling Pathway

In STAT signaling pathway various ligands bind to their cognate cell surface receptors, resulting in phosphorylation of STAT3 molecules that further dimerize with each other at SH2 domain and get translocation to the nucleus. Following translocation, the dimerized STAT3 molecule binds to the promoter of target genes and activates their transcription. STAT3 regulate Cyclin D1, c-Myc, Bcl-xl, Mcl1 and p53, thereby regulating cellular proliferation and survival. STAT3 directly binds to the promoter of MMP-2 and upregulates its expression. Additionally, STAT3 also regulates activity of MMP-9 and MMP-7. STAT3 regulates cellular migration by modulating the activity of Rho and Rac. Angiogenesis is required for tumor growth and metastasis. STAT3 is seen to be regulating angiogenesis by upregulating the activity of VEGF and HIF-α.

2. TRP and ORAI1 Signal Pathways

TRP and ORAI1 are involved in cancer cell and endothelial cell migration (Fig. 11-10).

3. Axl and Mer Signaling Pathways

The Pathway downstream of Axl such as inactivation of Bcl-2-associated death promoter (BAD) via phosphorylation by Akt. Mer interacts with, but does not directly phosphorylate, activated cdc42-associated kinase 1 (Ack1). Activation of Ack1 may occur indirectly through the guanine nucleotide-exchange factor Vav1 and cdc42, resulting in degradation of the tumor suppressor protein WW domain containing oxidoreductase (Wwox) and regulation of cell migration. Interestingly, Ack1 also interacts with Axl via Grb2 and may regulate Axl turnover or cleavage. Gas6 stimulates Ack1-dependent phosphorylation of androgen receptor (AR) resulting in proliferation and migration of prostate cancer cells in vitro, presumably via transcriptional regulation of androgen responsive genes. This effect could be mediated by Mer and/or Axl since the cell types evaluated express both receptors. Axl expression is only found in estrogen receptor (ER)-positive patient samples, and ER antagonists reduce Axl expression in breast cancer cells. It has not been determined whether ER binds to the Axl promoter, but Gas6 expression is transcriptionally regulated by ER.

Tumor-associated macrophages, dendritic cells and infiltrating immune cells release Gas6. Gas6 has autocrine or paracrine action on the Mer and Axl which can activate the expression of tumor cells. Activation of Mer and Axl can promote the formation of tumor blood vessels and tumor metastasis. Blockade of Axl and Mer expressed by endothelial cells may inhibit angiogenesis. (Fig. 11-11).

4. CXCL12 Signaling Pathways

CXCL12 binds to CXCR4 and CXCR7, which are G protein-coupled receptors (GPCR) that can form homodimers or heterodimers. In the latter case, CXCR7 changes the conformation of the CXCR4/G-protein complexes and abrogates signaling. Activation of CXCR4 by CXCL12 leads to G-protein coupled signaling through PI3K/Akt, IP3,and MAPK pathways, which promote cell survival, proliferation and chemotaxis. In addition, the β-arrestin pathway can be activated through GRK to internalize CXCR4. When CXCR7 binds CXCL12, the classical GPCR mobilization of Ca^{2+} does not occur, and activation of the β-arrestin pathway may lead to scavenging of CXCL12. In certain cancer cells (e.g., glioma) CXCR7 can also signal through PLC/MAPK to increase cell survival(Fig. 11-12).

5. TGF-β Signaling Pathway

TβRⅢ can mediate cell migration in a β-arrestin 2 dependent manner through the activation of Cdc42 in a ligand independent manner. TβRⅢ activates p38 in both a ligand independent and dependent manner. TβRⅢ undergoes ectodomain shedding producing soluble TβRⅢ, which can bind to and sequester ligand, inhibiting TGF-β signaling. （Fig. 11-13A）TβRⅢ presents ligand to TβR Ⅱ, which phosphorylates TβRⅢ, and recruits and phosphorylates TβRI, causing phosphorylation of the R-Smads. Phosphorylation of the R-Smads allows interaction with co-Smad4, mediating nuclear translocation of the Smad complex and regulation of transcriptional activity. Interaction of TβRⅢ with β-arrestin2 results in the internalization of the TβRⅢ/TβRⅡ/β-arrestin2 complex and subsequent down-regulation of TGF-β signaling. TβRⅢ also negatively regulates NF-κB signaling in a β-arrestin2 dependent manner. Interaction of TβRⅢ with GIPC stabilizes TβRⅢ at the cell membrane and enhances TGF-β signaling, as well as mediating effects on migration and invasion（Fig. 11-13B）.

Challenges and Prospects

1. Factors Affecting Tumor Metastasis

(1) Tumor cell adhesion (homogeneous adhesion decreased, heterogeneous adhesion increase).

(2) Tumor cells secrete the related-proteases degrading extracellular matrix.

(3) Tumor angiogenesis.

(4) The signal regulations of tumor metastasis-related genes and tumor metastasis suppressor genes.

(5) Characteristics of local organizations of the host: The tumor microenvironment, tumor motion enhanced, cancer stem cell (CSC), epithelial to mesenchymal transition (EMT), etc.

(6) Overall immunity state of the host and secreting levels of cytokines, growth factors and hormones.

Overall iwillunity state of the host and secreting levels of cytokines, groutil faeloiy and hormones.

2. Prospects

It is a long front for research the molecular pathology of cancer metastasis. There are meaningful whether to metastasis individual steps, or respectively, each about the type of research or explore the regulatory mechanisms in general. Given that metastasis is the sum of cancer activity of multiple genes and multiple biological characteristics, and is affected by host micro environment. Therefore, the research should focus on exploration of the molecules (such as adhesion molecules, etc.) that have effects on multiple aspects of the metastasis process and as well as key regulatory genes. It is necessary to systematically study DNA, mRNA, or protein product levels, because the same metastatic phenotype may be the result of different control mechanism.

Consider/Questions

1. Basic concepts in this chapter

Metastasis, Krukenberg's tumor, Viche lymphnode, extracellular matrix(ECM), Matrix metalloproteinase(MMP), autocrine moving factors(AMFs), hepatocyte growth factor(HGF), Nm23 (Nonmetastasis), sentinel lymph node(SLN).

2. Summary the main steps of tumor metastasis.

3. Briefly describe the Characteristics of tumor metastasis.

4. Contacting with a clinical tumor metastasis cases approach its metastatic patterns and analyses the possible genes expression and signal regulations.

5. Briefly describe the clinical significance and possible false-negative cases in detection of SLN.

第十二章　表观遗传学改变

现在人们已经认识到癌症的发生和发展与多年积累的遗传突变有关，从而导致细胞功能的变化。虽然遗传性或散发性突变可导致癌基因的活化或抑癌基因的失活，但是基因组特定位点的表观遗传学修饰改变不但影响相关基因表达，而且进一步影响生长、发育等生物学现象。越来越多的研究发现表观遗传学的作用范围很广，其涉及生物的生长繁殖、发育及分化、炎症、癌症等许多生理病理现象[1]。因此表观遗传学是 21 世纪以来分子生物学、遗传学及临床医学的研究热点。

第一节　表观遗传学的概念

表观遗传学是与遗传学相对应的概念。遗传学是指基于基因序列改变所致基因表达水平变化，如基因突变、基因杂合丢失等，而表观遗传学则是指基于非基因序列改变所致基因表达改变。

表观遗传学（epigenetics）是由生物学家 Waddington [2]在 1939 年首先在《现代遗传学导论》中提出的，1942 年他将表观遗传学描述为一个控制从基因型到表观型的机制。随后经过许多人的研究，到 1999 年 Wolife 把表观遗传学定义为研究没有 DNA 序列变化的可遗传的基因表达的改变，在 Allis 等的一本书中可以发现两种定义，一种是指与 DNA 突变无关的可遗传的表型变化；另一种是染色质调节的基因转录水平的变化，但这种变化不涉及 DNA 序列的改变[3]。

目前表观遗传学被定义为通过 DNA 甲基化、组蛋白共价修饰和不伴 DNA 序列变化的非编码 RNA 导致基因表达和染色体稳定性的一种可遗传改变，即改变组织中不依赖 DNA 序列变化的细胞亚群的生理学而发生的长期变化。表观遗传学是基因组 DNA 未发生变化时可以引起基因表达改变的重要化学修饰，主要包括 DNA 修饰（甲基化及羟甲基化）、组蛋白翻译后修饰（甲基化及乙酰化等）及染色质重塑；这三个部分互相交叠共同调控着基因的表达（图 12-1）。这种表达并不是依靠细胞内遗传物质 DNA 序列的变化而是在此之外的其他可遗传物质发生改变，并且这种改变能在生物的发育和增殖过程中稳定传递[3]。特别是表观遗传通路（epigenetic pathway）调控着基因组表观修饰的动态平衡，进一步与基因组学直接串联（图 12-2）。据最近的研究报道，过去认为无功能的 DNA 中有 80% 参与了表观遗传学相关的基因调控[4]。

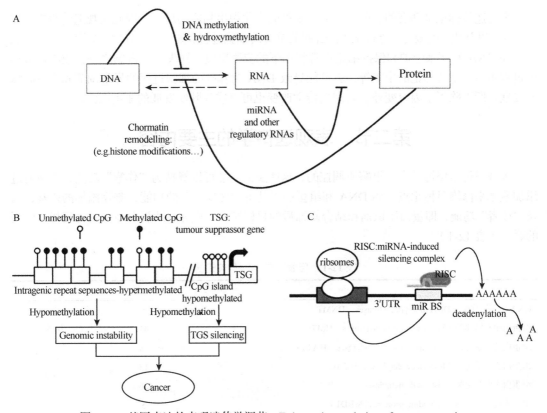

图 12-1 基因表达的表观遗传学调节；Epigenetic regulation of gene expression

A. 中心法则重新审视：由 DNA 甲基化和羟甲基化、染色质重塑和 miRNA 介导的基因表达转录和转录后表观遗传学抑制。转录和翻译的经典遗传调控途径是用实线箭头；虚线箭头则表示逆转录；B. 在肿瘤发生中 DNA 甲基化的模型。重复富集的癌基因序列低甲基化和肿瘤抑制因子超甲基化都与肿瘤发生有关；C. 经靶向 miRNA 结合位点的基因 miRNA 调节导致 mRNA 去乙酰化并抑制翻译成蛋白质；A. Central Dogma revisited：Transcriptional and post-transcriptional epigenetic repression of gene expression by DNA methylation and hydroxymethylation, chromatin remodelling and miRNA. The classical genetic regulation pathway of transcription and translation is shown by solid arrows；the dashed arrow denotes reverse transcription；B. A model of DNA methylation in tumorigenesis. Hypomethylation of the repeat-rich intragenic sequences and hypermethylation of tumour suppressor gene（TSG）are both associated with tumorigenesis；C. miRNA regulation of a gene via targeting at miRNA binding site（miR BS）leading to deadenylation of mRNA and suppressed translation into protein

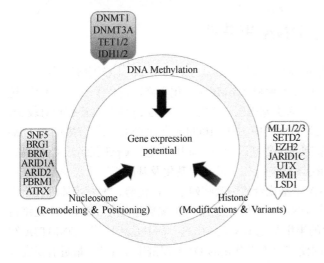

图 12-2 具体基因表达形式中表观遗传学过程的相互作用；The interaction between epigenetic processes in specifying gene expression patterns

最近全基因组测序的研究表明，在不同类型的癌症中经常观察到这三个类表观修饰的突变，进一步突出了基因组学和表观遗传学直接的串联；Recent whole exome sequencing studies show that mutations in the three classes of epigenetic modifiers is frequently observed in various types of cancers, further highlighting the crosstalk between genetics and epigenetics

表观遗传标记是动态的、可以对生理条件的变化做出相应的反应。因此表观遗传修饰（如乙酰化、甲基化、磷酸化、泛素化）精密调节重要的细胞过程，如应激、分化、基因转录、DNA修复和DNA复制来维护和保持细胞正常状态下的应激反应。缺失这些机制之一，或在调节细胞过程中表观遗传标记的串扰等，就可能导致DNA为基础的细胞过程的异常调节和导致肿瘤的发展。所以除了基因突变外，表观遗传学改变也可以成为肿瘤发展的驱动因素。

第二节　表观遗传学的主要内容

表观遗传学修饰是由一组酶所调控的，这些酶的功能可以概括为"作家"功能，即酶通过添加残基来修饰目标靶点（如DNA和组蛋白甲基）；"橡皮擦"的功能，删除添加的残基，以及"读者"功能，即蛋白质识别和结合修饰后的目标靶点，作为后续蛋白与蛋白之间相互作用的媒介（表12-1）。

表 12-1　与表观性修饰有关的酶

酶	种类	功能
DNA甲基转移酶（DNA methyltransferases，DNMT）	5	
组蛋白甲基转移酶（histone methyltransferases，HMTs）	41	作者
组蛋白乙酰基转移酶（histone acetyltransferases，HATs）	19	
组蛋白去乙酰化酶（histone deacetylases，HDACs）	13	橡皮擦
组蛋白去甲基化酶（histone demethylases，HDMS）	26	
甲基连接蛋白（methyl binding proteins，MBD1）	5	
识别和反应于特异修饰组蛋白残基的蛋白（proteins that recognize and react to specific modified histone residue）	N	读者
共计（2012年4月）	>109	

表观遗传学修饰蛋白质的数量稳定增加：2009年"只有"91种，在2012年后确定有109种以上不同的蛋白质[5]。由于在癌症中已发现介导表观遗传学（epigenetics）修饰的酶的突变，这是一个增加了肿瘤发生的间接方式，作为表观遗传学修饰的变化会影响基因表达的模式。这表明，表观遗传学修饰可以作为治疗的新靶点。具体来说HMTs和HDMS在多种组织中调控组蛋白上的四种赖氨酸残基K4、K9、K27、K36的甲基化过程中发挥重要作用。

一、DNA 甲基化

DNA甲基化是指在DNMT的作用下，将S-腺苷甲硫氨酸上的甲基转移至胞嘧啶的第5位碳原子上加一个甲基基团，使之变成5-甲基胞嘧啶（5-MC）的化学修饰过程（图12-3）[6]。这常见于基因的5'-CG-3'序列。正常情况下，人类基因组"垃圾"序列的CpG二核苷酸相对较少，并总是处于甲基化状态。与之相反，人类基因组中100~1000bp富含CpG二核苷酸的CpG岛则处于非甲基化状态，与56%的人类基因组编码基因相关。非甲基化的CpG簇组成CpG岛，位于基因启动子结构序列的核心和转录起始点。CpG岛的高甲基化及基因组广泛低甲基化是甲基化的主要内容。在CpG序列中，DNA甲基化合成胞嘧啶残基后占优势，而且当体外转染真核细胞时，甲基化启动子一般无活性[7]。DNA甲基化是被DNMT家族所催化：DNMT1是维持新的DNA链与DNA半保留复制产生的半甲基化DNA互补的一种甲基转移酶。DNMT3A和DNMT3B为新的甲基转移酶，能在体内使完全未甲基化的DNA双链甲基化[8]。最近有研究表明，5-MC 可以被 Fe^{2+} 家族氧化为 5-羟甲基胞嘧啶及 2-氧化戊二酸依赖性甲基胞嘧啶加双氧酶即为 TET 蛋白，有效地通过碱基切除修复途径来去除抑制甲基化物质的序列。此外，DNA 甲基化修饰还包括 CpG 位点以外的其他位点的甲基化及 DNA 甲酰和羧基衍生物的产生[9]。

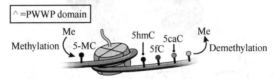

Methyltransfersae

Enzyme	Mutation	Tumor
DNMT3A^	M,F,N,S	AML,MDS,MPD

Hydroxymethlation and derivatives

Enzyme	Mutation	Tumor
TET1	T	AML
TET2	M,N,F	AML,MPD, MDS,CMML

^ =PWWP domain

Methylation 　Me　5-MC　5hmC　5fC　5caC　Me　Demethylation

图 12-3　癌突变影响 DNA 甲基化的表观遗传调节；Cancer mutations affecting epigenetic regulators of DNA methylation

胞嘧啶核苷酸的 5-C 端被 DNMTs 家族甲基化。其中 DNMT3A 在急性髓细胞白血病（ALL）、骨髓增生性疾病（MPD）和骨髓增生异常综合征（MDS）中发生突变。除了其催化活性，DNMT3A 具有染色质读取基序 PWWP 域，可辅助此酶在染色质上定位。在癌症中体细胞突变也可影响到这个区域。DNA 羟化酶的 TET 家族代谢 5-MC 成几个氧化中间体，包括 5hmC（5-hydroxymethylcytosine）、5fC（5-formylcytosine）和 5-caC（5-carboxylcytosine）。这些中间体可能参与了激活 DNA-去甲基化的过程。2/3TET 家族成员在癌症中发生突变，包括 AML、MPD、MDS 和 CMML。突变类型如下：M, missense；F, frame shift；N, nonsense；S, splice site mutation；T, translocation；The 5-carbon of cytosine nucleotides are methylated（5-MC）by a family of DNMTs. One of these, DNMT3A, is mutated in AML, myeloproliferative diseases（MPD）, and myelodysplastic syndromes（MDS）. In addition to its catalytic activity, DNMT3A has a chromatin-reader motif, the PWWP domain, which may aid in localizing this enzyme to chromatin. Somatically acquired mutations in cancer may also affect this domain. The TET family of DNA hydroxylases metabolizes 5-MC into several oxidative intermediates, including 5-hydroxymethylcytosine（5hmC）, 5-formylcytosine（5fC）, and 5-carboxylcytosine（5caC）. These intermediates are likely involved in the process of active DNA demethylation. Two of the three TET family members are mutated in cancers, including AML, MPD, MDS, and CMML. Mutation types are as follows：M, missense；F, frameshift；N, nonsense；S, splice site mutation；and T, translocation

二、组蛋白修饰

组蛋白（histones）共价修饰也是肿瘤表观遗传学调控的相关途径之一，主要的组蛋白包括 H1、H2A、H2B、H3 和 H4。不同组蛋白的不同氨基酸可以发生乙酰化、甲基化、磷酸化、泛素化等多种修饰（图 12-4）。当一个或多个组蛋白末端出现的多种修饰状态，称为组蛋白密码（histone code）[10]，可相互联合或一次被初定的蛋白酶或其他复合物识别并结合而起作用，为发动或阻遏基因转录的染色质相关蛋白提供相应的结合位点。建立和维持表观遗传学记忆的重要因素涉及上述不同的修饰方式，这些修饰方式被广泛研究，其重要性也逐步被大家所认识[11]。乙酰化和甲基化是组蛋白的重要修饰方式，乙酰化受 HATs 和 HDACs 的共同调控，通过组蛋白的乙酰化与去乙酰化使与组蛋白结合的基因准确表达，这是由 HMTs 所完成的（图 12-5）。

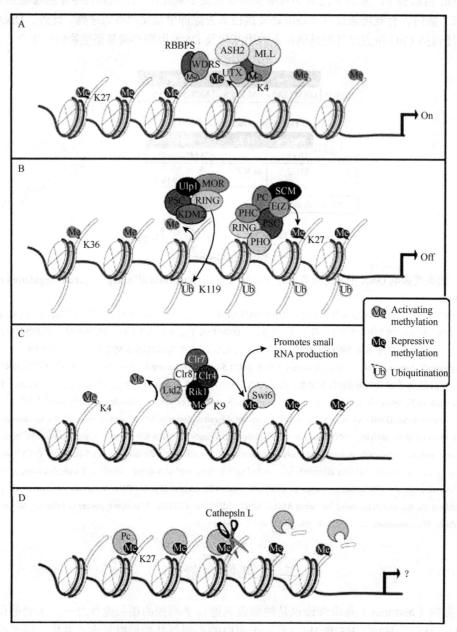

图 12-4　组蛋白修饰；Histone modification

不同组蛋白发生甲基化（A）和泛素化（B），抑制甲基化促进小 RNA 产生（C），组织蛋白酶犹如分子剪刀的作用（D）; Different histone　with activating methylation（A）, ubiquitination（B）, repressive methylation promotes small RNA production（C）, Cathepsin acts like a molecule cut （D）

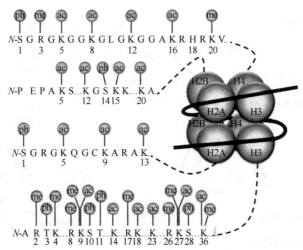

图 12-5 组蛋白尾部影响染色质修饰；Histone tails affecting chromatin modification

染色质修饰通常出现在组蛋白的 N 端尾部氨基酸（H2A、H2B、H3、H4），这为广泛的转录后修饰提供了位点。各种酶，如 HATs、HMTS、HDACs、HDMS，都参与了这些修饰，导致在标记氨基酸上的共价变化；ac：乙酰基团；me：甲基团；ph：磷酸基团；Chromatin modifications usually appear at the amino acids in the N-terminal tails of histones（H2A, H2B, H3, H4），which provide the site for a wide range of posttranslational modifications. Various enzymes, such as HATs, HMTs, HDACs, and HDMs, are involved in these modifications, which cause covalent changes at the marked amino acids; ac: acetyl group, me: methyl group, ph: phosphate group

　　甲基化修饰可以改变染色体的结构，也可以通过其他转录因子来调控基因的表达。尤其是在组蛋白特定残基上甲基化平衡对于维持基因组的完整、基因的表达及癌症的逃逸都至关重要[12]。

三、DNA 甲基化及组蛋白修饰的相互作用——"双锁原则"

　　虽然多数研究倾向于关注 DNA 或组蛋白修饰，但现已明确，一个基因的转录需要 DNA 甲基化与组蛋白修饰的相互作用。DNA 和组蛋白都应处于一个允许转录的状态，在一个开放或"解锁"的状态（图 12-6）。如果在 DNA 或组蛋白的表观遗传标记是在一个封闭的或"锁定"状态，目的基因将不被转录。这是"双锁原则"（double lock principle）概念。因为无论是 DNA 甲基化状态还是组蛋白修饰对一个基因的表达都至关重要。此外，必须有转录激活剂的存在，必须使其与双锁正确匹配。这就解释了在大量报道中基因不表达的原因，尽管可以想当然地认为它或许处于耐受状态。

四、染色体重塑

　　染色体重塑是在基因表达的复制和重塑等过程中染色质的包装状态、核小体中组蛋白及对应 DNA 分子发生改变的分子机制，包括在染色质水平发生 DNA 复制、转录、修复、重组。这些过程中，染色体重塑可导致核小体位置和结构的变化，引起染色质变化。重塑包括多种变化，一般指染色质特定区域对核酶稳定性的改变，主要涉及核小体的置换或重排，改变了核小体在基因启动序列区域的排列，增加了基因转录装置和启动序列的匹配。染色质重塑与组蛋白 N 端、C 端修饰密切相关，尤其是对组蛋白 H3 和 H4 的修饰，通过修饰直接影响核小体的结构，并为其他蛋白提供了与 DNA 作用的结合位点，染色质重塑的修饰方式主要包括两种。一

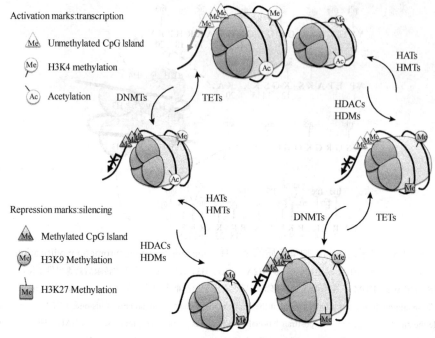

图 12-6　双锁原则；Double Lock Principle

当锁开或锁住时发生基因转录，启动子区去甲基化、组蛋白乙酰化和 H3K4me 标记。如果在锁住状态中基因沉默，DNMTs、HDACs、HMTs 和 HDMs 修饰启动子区，去除组蛋白乙酰化，修饰甲基化，基因被转录。必需的抑制标记开或未锁住状态时，通过 TETs（排除启动子甲基化）HATs 和 HMTs/HDMs。如果 DNA 存在上述的任何状态，基因仍被抑制，所以称为双锁；A gene will be transcribed when it is in the open or "unlocked" state. The promoter region is demethylated, histones acetylated and H3K4me marked. If the gene is silenced, in a closed or "locked" state, DNMTs, HDACs, HMTs and histone demethyltransferases（HDMs）have modified the promoter region, removing the histone acetylation and modifying methylation accordingly. For the gene to be transcribed, the repression marks will need to be lifted to confer the open, "unlocked" state, by the TETs（removal of methylation on the promoter）, HATs and the HMTs/HDMs. If the DNA exists in any in-between state, with only partial silencing or activation marks, the gene remains repressed, hence the term "Double Lock"

种是含有组蛋白乙酰转移酶和脱乙酰酶的化学修饰；另一种是依赖 ATP 水解释放能量解开组蛋白与 DNA 的结合，使转录得以进行。

　　虽然高度折叠的染色质结构对其包装进细胞核是必要的，但这种致密状态的染色质却阻碍了相应染色质部位的基因转录、DNA 复制及损伤修复等过程。因此，真核生物随着进化产生了一组染色质重塑酶和一些相关蛋白因子，通过调控染色质上核小体的装配、拆解和重排等来调控染色质的结构。其中就有一类蛋白质可以利用 ATP 水解产生的能量驱动核小体在 DNA 上的"滑动"，或者介导核小体中组蛋白变异体与经典组蛋白之间的"置换"，这类蛋白质就是 ATP 依赖的染色质重塑因子，通常是由多个亚基组成的一个较大分子量的染色质重塑复合物。

　　在真核细胞中，染色质重塑因子通过改变染色质上核小体的装配、拆解和重排等方式来调控染色质结构，从而在染色质 DNA 作用下、染色质结构趋于疏松时，有助于 RNA 聚合酶 II 改善转录因子对染色 DNA 的亲和性，从而启动基因的转录。反之，当染色质结构趋于致密时，RNA 聚合酶 II 和转录因子对染色质 DNA 的亲和性减弱，抑制相关基因的转录。

　　目前已经发现，一些染色质重塑复合物是组蛋白变异体置换进（或出）核小体的执行者。最典型的例子是在酵母中 Swr1 可以催化 H2AZ-H2B 异源二聚体与核小体中经典 H2A-H2B 二聚体之间的替换[13]。同样 INO80 亚家族中人源性 INO80/SRCAP/TRRAP-TIP60 复合物除了有染色质重塑功能外，还有组蛋白变异体置换功能，可以催化经典组蛋白 H2A 与组蛋白变异体 H2AZ 之间的置换[14]，具体置换机制目前尚不清楚，但有趣的是，Swr1/ SRCAP 复合物可以将 H2AZ 单向置换入核小体，而 INO80[15]则可以发挥相反作用，即将 H2AZ 从核小体中置换出来，说明不同的染色质复合物具有不同的功能特点（图 12-7）。而大部分 INO 80 则结合在转录起始位点区，发挥激活因子的作用[16]。总之，染色质重塑因子在基因转录调控中起着关键性的作用，并参与细胞内多种重要的生物学过程。

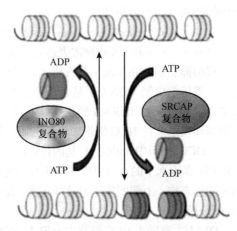

图 12-7 染色质重塑置换组蛋白变异体的模式图；Schematic of the histone exchange modulated by chromatin remodeling complexes

利用 ATP 水解酶释放能量，SWRI/SRCAP 复合物能使组蛋白变异体 H2AZ 置换入核小体内，反之 INO80 复合物则使 H2AZ 从核小体中置换出来；Using ATP hydrolyzyme to release energy, the SWRI/SRCAP complex can replace the histone mutant H2AZ into the nucleosomes, whereas the INO80 complex causes H2AZ to be displaced from the nucleosomes

五、miRNA 调控

miRNA 是一种小的、类似于 siRNA 的分子，由高等真核生物基因组编码，miRNA 通过与靶基因 miRNA 碱基配对引导沉默复合体降解 miRNA 或阻碍其翻译。miRNA 在物种进化中相当保守，在植物、动物和真菌中发现的 miRNAs 只在特定组织和发育阶段表达。miRNA 的组织特异性和时序性决定了组织和细胞的功能特异性，表明 miRNA 在细胞生长和发育过程中起多种调节作用[17]。miRNA 不编码蛋白，而是通过与靶基因序列发生特异性的相互作用，在转录后或翻译水平上表达相关基因。越来越多的证据表明，miRNA 在多种生物学过程中均发挥了重要的作用。与此同时，在多种人类疾病（包括癌症）中均发现了 miRNA 的异常表达。在肿瘤发生、发展过程中，miRNA 就像癌基因或抑癌基因一样发挥功能。最近，在 HCC 的研究中不断发现 miRNA 的异常表达，有些特异的 miRNA 与肿瘤的临床病理学特征（如转移、复发和预后）密切相关[18]。

miRNA 的合成是一个多步骤并受精细调控的生物学过程，首先 miRNA 基因在 RNA 聚合酶Ⅱ的参与下转录生成数百到数千个碱基的 Pri-miRNA，然后在细胞核内，在 RnaseⅢ作用下形成 50~80bp 的中间体 Pre-miRNA，后者因含有部分反向互补序列，可自身折叠形成颈环样结构，而后在 GTP 依赖的输出蛋白（exportin）-5 协助下主动转运入胞质[19]。再经过 Dicer 酶剪切成长度为 19~25bp 的 miRNA，随后双链解开，miRNA 则被迅速降解，而 miRNA 链以不对称的方式结合到 miRNA 诱导的基因沉默复合体（miRISC）。通过"种子序列"与靶 mRNA 3′端非翻译区的序列结合，若高度互补则降解 miRNA，若部分互补则抑制 mRNA 转录后的翻译，后者 mRNA 的水平无明显变化[20]。

越来越多的证据表明 miRNA 在肿瘤的发生发展中具有显著的作用，并可能成为对癌症诊断和预后重要的生物标志物。microRNA-122（miR-122）是肝中最丰富的 microRNA，占所有 miRNA 总数的 70%左右。一些研究表明 miR-122 对肝脏内环境稳定十分重要[21]。miR-122 在小鼠和人肝细胞中表达丰富，但在大多数 HCC 和转化细胞系中表达沉默或表达非常低。miR-122 的表达丢失与肝癌分化、分型、侵袭和肝内转移相关。最近，裸鼠体内模型证实了 miR-122 存在抑制肿瘤和增加药物敏感性的作用[22]。先前的研究发现 miR-122 能通过 p53 非依赖的细胞凋亡途径影响肝癌细胞对多柔比星（DOX）的敏感性[23]。

DNA 甲基化与 miRNA 之间存在着一些相互作用，在多种肿瘤中，他们都有着协同作用，如在肝癌中一些 miRNA 的异常表达受表观遗传学机制的调控。Datta 等[24]通过用 5-氮杂胞苷（甲基转移酶抑制剂）和（或）曲古柳菌素（组蛋白去乙酰化酶抑制剂）处理 HCC 细胞株，寻找受表观遗传学机制（DNA 甲基化）调控的 miRNA。结果发现，这些表观遗传学药物可以调节 HCC 细胞株中一些 miRNA 的表达，尤其是 miRNA-1-1。He 等[25]研究发现，miR-191 在 HCC 细胞株和人原发性 HCC 组织中表达上调，且 miR-191 基因的甲基化状态与 miR-191 表达水平有关。HCC 组织中 miR-191 基因位点的低甲基化可以引起其表达上调。在 HCC 细胞株中，miR-191 表达水平的上调可以诱导上皮细胞向间质样细胞转化，使细胞失去黏附力，下调上皮细胞的标志物。上调间质细胞的标志物，增强细胞的迁移和侵袭力：抑制 miR-191 的表达会逆转这个过程。

DNMT1 有助于 HCC 细胞中 miR-1 的沉默，从而促进靶基因 HDAC4 的富集。DNMT3 的靶标是 miR-29，在 AML 中，HDACs 下调 miR-29。同样，miR-26a 和 miR-137 被超甲基化的启动子 CpG 岛所沉默，也会引起结肠癌中靶基因 LSD1 的上调和前列腺癌中靶基因 EZH2 的上调。

不同的组蛋白调节酶，如 EZH2 和 HDACS 等，能使组蛋白甲基化和去乙酰化。myc 或 NF-κB 在 mRNA 启动子上与转录因子 YY1 或 SP1 相互作用并被假设成 mRNA 沉默的上游调节因子。在 myc 和 EZH2 之间存在一个正反馈回路。myc 通过减少 EZH2 的抑制调节因子（miR-26a 和 miR-101）来促进 EZH2 的表达，EZH2 也可以通过抑制 miR-494 来增加 myc（图 12-8）。

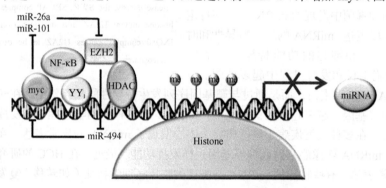

图 12-8　组蛋白修饰抑制 mRNA 的表达机制的模型；　A model depicting the mechanisms of histone modification that repress miRNA expression

六、基因印记

基因印记（genetic imprinting）：又称遗传印记，即指基因的表达取决于其在父源染色体上还是在母源染色体上，以及这些染色体上的基因是沉默还是表达。有些基因印记只表达母源染色体的基因，而有些则表达父源染色体的基因，基因印记在生物的生长发育过程中有着重要作用。基因印记遍布基因组，其内含子较小，且能在组织中特异性反映基因印记的形成和表达。这是一个复杂的调控机制，普遍认为与甲基化有关，并受多种因素的影响。正是由于基因印记是正常发育必不可少的调控机制，基因印记行为的异常必然引起多种相关疾病，特别是基因印记异常可作为一种新的致瘤机制与肿瘤的发生发展关系密切。此外，一些环境因素也会对基因印记造成影响。如果抑癌基因中有活性的等位基因失活，就会提高癌症的发病率，如 IGF2 基因印记丢失将导致多种肿瘤的发生，如 Wilims 瘤[26]。

第三节　在疾病中表观遗传学改变的意义

表观遗传学对疾病的发生、发展及预防、治疗都有着重要作用，当其控制机制发生变化时就会引起相应的病理生理变化，从而与肿瘤、免疫、心血管等多种疾病有关。

一、肿瘤中表观遗传学改变

表观遗传标记的全面重组包括 DNA 甲基化和组蛋白修饰的改变，也在癌症中表观遗传修饰的基因突变[27]。因此 DNA 和组蛋白修饰的变化（统称为表观基因）也有助于肿瘤的发生发展。

（一）基因甲基化

已知甲基化模式和组蛋白修饰是不同的，尤其是用来自它们的正常组织和肿瘤进行比较时。所有的基因表达最终是由它们的表观遗传状态所控制，因此，表观遗传学改变在肿瘤发生中起重要作用。

DNA 甲基化是导致肿瘤基因沉默常见的表观遗传学机制。

乳腺癌中，针对雌激素受体（ER）的产生可分为激素敏感型或激素不敏感型肿瘤。DNA 启动子高甲基化在肿瘤发生中起着重要作用。沉默 ESR1 产生激素不敏感型的 ER 阴性肿瘤。相反，沉默肿瘤抑制基因产生激素敏感肿瘤。抗雌激素治疗会激活肿瘤内分泌抗性的发展，从而导致启动子高甲基化和低甲基化。因此治疗可以选择伴表观遗传学改变的抗性亚群。雌激素调节基因的调节异常可能会导致 ER 信号的进一步改变。总之，肿瘤发生过程中观察到 DNA 低甲基化，在癌细胞获取内分泌抗性中，启动子低甲基化占主导地位（图 12-9）。

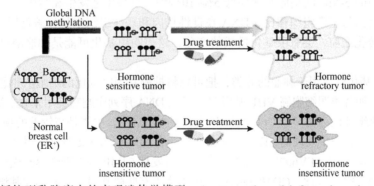

图12-9　内分泌抵抗型乳腺癌中的表观遗传学模型；A proposed model for epigenetic contribution to endocrine-resistant breast cancer

抗雌激素治疗会激活肿瘤内分泌抗性的发展，从而导致启动子高甲基化（黑色）和低甲基化（白色）。A 到 D 基因代表常见和实际的基因：A，常见肿瘤抑制因子；B，ESR1（ER）；C，常见雌激素调节基因；D，常见的上皮分化基因；Treatment with anti-estrogens may actively promote the development of endocrine resistance, resulting in promoter hypermethylation（black stalks）and hypomethylation（white stalks），Genes A through D represent generic and actual genes. A, generic tumor suppressor（e.g., CDKN2A/p16）；B，ESR1（ER）；C，generic estrogen-regulated gene（e.g., PGR/progesterone receptor）；D，generic epithelial differentiation gene（e.g., CDH1/E-cadherin）

在胶质瘤中 IDH 突变导致胶质瘤-CpG 甲基化表型（G-CIMP）和组蛋白甲基化（图 12-10）。突变的 IDH1 催化 α-KG（α-ketoglutarate）中产生 2-HG（2-hydroxyglutarate）。由于 2-HG 在结构上和 α-KG 相似，因此 2-HG 能抑制 α-KG 依赖的双氧酶。组蛋白赖氨酸脱甲基酶的 Jumonji C 家族（KDMs）和 DNA 羟化酶的 TET 组都是 α-KG 依赖的双氧酶。抑制这些酶可增加组蛋白甲基化的标记，影响 G-CIMP 的 DNA 甲基化。

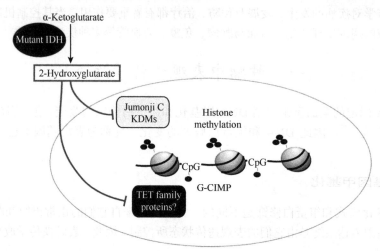

图 12-10　在胶质瘤中 IDH 突变导致 Glioma-CpG 甲基化表型（G-CIMP）和组蛋白甲基化；IDH mutations result in Glioma- CpG methylation phenotype（G-CIMP）and histone methylation in gliomas

癌细胞辐射暴露后可以减少 DNA 甲基转移酶，包括 DNMT1、DNMT3a、DNMT3b 和 MeCP2 诱导整个 DNA 低甲基化。这种现象导致了癌细胞中基因组的不稳定。辐射也能诱导组蛋白 H2AX 的磷酸化和组蛋白 H4K20 的三甲基化，影响基因表达模式，继而导致细胞死亡、细胞周期改变和基因组的不稳定性。这些事件与辐射治疗、保护或有害的反应有关。

除此之外，DNA 还存在去甲基化的行为。虽然有证据显示局部高甲基化，但与正常组织相比，肿瘤中的 5-MC 的整体水平要低 5%~10%[28]。甲基化是发生在增生与良性肿瘤之间的特定阶段，因为与正常组织相比，DNA 在良性息肉和恶性组织中是显著低甲基化[29]。因此，在病变恶性转化之前，会有甲基化模式的变化，这表明甲基化可能是肿瘤演进中的一个关键事件。

DNA 甲基化已被用于肿瘤的分类，把可以将抑癌基因甲基化的细胞从非恶性表型组织中区分出来[30]，如肾透明细胞癌 VHL 基因启动子区 DNA 序列中胞嘧啶甲基化。高水平 DNA 甲基化的肿瘤亚组被认为是一个 CpG 岛甲基化表型（CIMP），主要是与较差的预后有关。CIMP 首先是在结直肠肿瘤中发现的，其中包括大部分伴有 MMR 缺陷及 MLH1 甲基化的散发性大肠癌病例，并且其与 BRAFV600E 突变有关[31]。随后发现 CIMP 可用于确诊胶质母细胞瘤[32]、胃癌[33]及室管膜瘤[34]。因此，CIMP 肿瘤也许可以代表有些微基因改变的不同肿瘤亚群。这说明针对表观遗传机制的药物可能会提供治疗的新方法。

研究发现 HMTs 和 HDMS 的异常调控与许多类型的肿瘤有关，包括乳腺、前列腺、肺和脑的肿瘤[35]。调节细胞周期的 p16INK4A、p14ARF、p15INK4B 基因单独或联合发生甲基化后可参与口腔鳞状细胞癌的发生、发展，并且与其易复发和低生存率有关。在染色质重塑过程中，染色质重塑因子 RSF-1 的过度表达在口腔鳞状细胞癌的发生中起重要作用，并能促进肿瘤侵袭[36]。

（二）组蛋白修饰

与甲基化模式类似，组蛋白修饰模式也被用于预测多种肿瘤的预后。H3K9ac、H3K9me3 和 H4K16a 水平的降低与非小细胞肺癌的复发有关[37]。在前列腺癌中较低水平的 H3K4me2 和 H3K18ac 与较差的预后相关[38]。在急性髓细胞白血病（AML）患者的启动子核心区可发现 H3K9me3 的丢失，全部 H3K9me3 模式还能独立预测 AML 患者的预后[39]。这些癌症有扩增、缺失和体细胞突变，这一切都会导致 HMTs 和 HDMS 酶活性的变化。例如，抑制性组蛋白的标志物三甲基化的 H3K27（H3K27me3）可以被 EZH2 的催化域所调节，EZH2 是组成 PRC2（polycomb repressive complex 2）的一种蛋白。据报道，与局限性疾病或良性前列腺增生相比，EZH2 在转移性前列腺癌中表达上调，提示其有可能参与前列腺癌的进展[40]，其过度表达也与乳腺癌侵袭性和预后不良有关[41]。最近有报道称，EZH2 的两类非组蛋白底物均会影响其转录活性。GATA4 被 EZH2 甲基化，从而诱导与其辅助激活物 p300 相互作用[42]。Lee 等研究表明 EZH2 所诱导的核受体 RORα 的甲基化会导致更多的泛素化和溶酶体的降解，使转录活性下降[43]。反之，引起 RORα 肿瘤抑制活性的丢失，最终导致更多的恶性肿瘤的发展。

组蛋白修饰也与结直肠癌的发生也有关。组蛋白乙酰化是由 HAT 或 HDAC 共同介导的一个可逆性动态平衡过程。在人结直肠癌细胞系（SW1116）和人直肠癌细胞系（COLO-320）中，HDAC 抑制剂曲古抑菌素 A（TSA）和丁酸钠通过抑制 HDAC，增强乙酰化水平显著上调 p21WAF1 基因的转录，其细胞周期易被阻滞于 G_1 期[44]。除乙酰化外，组蛋白甲基化修饰也是重要的修饰机制，其甲基化修饰部位主要是组蛋白 H3 和 H4 的赖氨酸和精氨酸两类残基。组蛋白甲基化和 DNA 甲基化可联合作用共同参与抑癌基因沉默从而诱发肿瘤。

在 EGFR 表达的胶质母细胞瘤中，丙酮酸激酶 M2（pyruvate kinase M2，PKM2）催化磷酸烯醇丙酮酸盐（PEP）在糖分解的通路中转换为丙酮酸盐。EGFR 的激活导致了 PKM2 移位到细胞核，并且组蛋白 3 在苏氨酸 11 位点磷酸化（H3-T11）。这导致了去乙酰化酶从 CCND1 和 c-myc 启动位点的去除、H3K9 乙酰化和 cyclin D1 和 c-myc 转录的激活（图 12-11）。

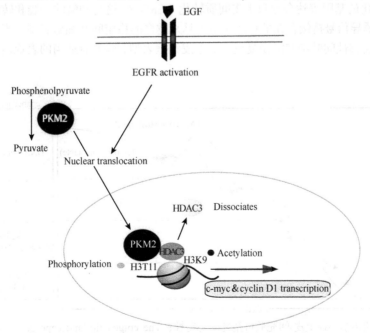

图 12-11　PKM2 调节 EGFR 表达的胶质母细胞瘤中的组蛋白修饰；PKM2 regulates histone modifications in EGFR driven glioblastoma

DNA 甲基化的状态是基因表达中"双锁"部分的关键。一般来说，DNA 甲基化的启动子往往不表达。CpG 族（甲基化的主要靶点）又被称为 CpG 岛，它常位于许多人类基因的 5′端。在组织中，大多数的 CpG 岛会发生甲基化，即使相关基因不表达[45]。然而，癌症中甲基化多发生在 CpG 岛，同样也是 DNA 低甲基化。启动子甲基化最常与基因沉默有关，提高异常甲基化可能导致沉默并使其成为转化过程的一部分。当某种已知的肿瘤抑制基因发生甲基化时，其就会以一种较强的机械性方法在肿瘤的发生过程中发挥潜在的作用。在癌变过程中会引起表观遗传学的损害，细胞周期调控基因 Rb（视网膜母细胞瘤）的高甲基化是其中一个首要表现。大约有 10%散发的单侧视网膜母细胞瘤会发生甲基化异常，这与 Rb 表达缺失有关。Rb 基因的甲基化可以作为癌症发生过程中出现异常甲基化的一个有力证据，因为在肿瘤的前体细胞中 Rb 基因常活化，并且启动子甲基化与基因的可遗传突变有着相同的作用[46]。在大肠癌的发生中，与抑癌基因 p53 相对应的染色体 17P 区域的高甲基化被证实先于等位基因的缺失，这表明，甲基化可能会非随机的标记染色体区域，这些染色体区域在特定肿瘤的发生过程中发生改变[47]。这些例子提示异常甲基化在肿瘤恶性转化过程中发挥重要作用，尤其已经证实甲基化发生在肿瘤发生的早期。肿瘤抑癌基因甲基化的细胞比其他细胞更具有选择的优势，这些细胞的增殖能力及抗凋亡能力都会增加。这些癌前细胞的克隆扩增会导致过度增生的表型，这是肿瘤发生的早期阶段的特征。在肿瘤类型中，如 Rb 基因、MLH1 和 VHL 等基因是甲基化，而且这些基因也常突变，表明在肿瘤的发生过程中 CpG 岛的高甲基化是可选择的[48]。

（三）EMT 与表观遗传学状态

较多的报告已经证明表观遗传学功能失调和遗传学的不稳定将引发肿瘤转移，即 DNA 甲基化、组蛋白乙酰化的异常导致肿瘤形成和转移[49]。上皮细胞的常态是具有上皮细胞的表型。相关信号通过介导组蛋白修饰，促进了关键性上皮基因（如 E-cadherin）的表观遗传学抑制，有助于在细胞迁移过程中特定表型的表达，这些相关信号确定了上皮细胞的可塑性和位置。改变参与细胞分化的基因表达会导致上皮间质转化（EMT），这与肿瘤的侵袭和转移密切相关。依赖于 EMT 诱导信号持续存在的作用获得了越来越多的稳定间叶细胞表型。当转移部位这些信号缺失时，转移性间叶细胞能恢复更多的上皮细胞表型，除非有适当的表观遗传学修饰的维持（图 12-12）。

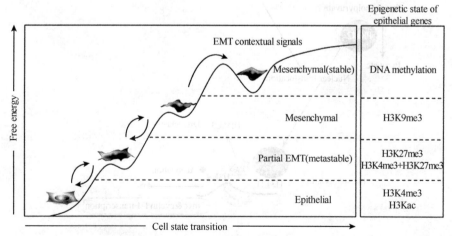

图 12-12　表观遗传学调控上皮-间充质可塑性的稳定性；The epigenetic landscape governs the stability of epithelial-mesenchymal plasticity

H3Kac 是赖氨酸乙酰化的组蛋白 H3；H3Kac，histone H3 lysine acetylation

（四）作为癌症治疗的表观遗传抑制剂

针对表观遗传学的药物开发，首先在体外恶性肿瘤细胞中检测一些待选的小分子的特异性和表型反应。评估增殖抑制、凋亡诱导和细胞周期阻滞。这些表型分析通常和基因组学、蛋白质组学方法一起识别所观察到反应的潜在分子机制。然后将体外验证的抑制剂在体内癌症动物模型中进行测试，以确定它们是否可以为生存提供治疗效果。动物研究也提供了关于该药物的毒性和药代动力学特性的有价值的信息。基于这些临床前研究，待选的小分子可以进一步临床试验。当新药通过精心设计的临床试验被证明有效时，申请监管机构如 FDA 批准用于临床常规使用。

二、糖尿病中表观遗传学改变

在当今世界中，糖尿病的高发病率已经引起了人们的广泛关注，特别是其血管病变已成为糖尿病高死亡率的主要原因。而且糖毒作用即使血糖控制在正常范围，糖尿病的血管病变依然持续进展。因此早期加强血糖控制则可产生持久的效益，这一现象被称为"代谢印记（metabolic imprinting）"或遗留效应（legacy effect）[50]。但代谢印记在分子生物学中的机制尚不明确，近年来越来越多的研究表明表观遗传学修饰不仅与糖尿病血管病变有关，而且可能是导致代谢印记的潜在机制。糖限制可以影响正常细胞和癌细胞的表观遗传学调节。在正常细胞，它导致 p16 的抑制和 hTERT 的激活，来扩展 Hayflick 界限。在癌症前期细胞中 p16 和 hTERT 具有相反的作用导致凋亡和衰老，在糖限制的细胞中有癌症抑制（图 12-13）。

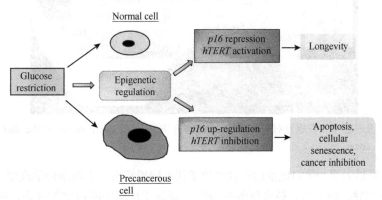

图12-13　糖限制经表观遗传学调节作用于长寿和癌症抑制；Effects of glucose restriction on longevity and cancer inhibition through epigenetic regulation

一系列研究表明 DNA 甲基化水平与糖尿病心血管病变（cardiovascular disease，CVD）和慢性肾脏损伤（chronic kidney damage，CKD）密切相关，CVD 和 CKD 患者血清中危险因子腺苷同型半胱氨酸水平增加，可抑制部分 DNA 甲基转移酶致 DNA 低甲基化[51]。与正常组相比，糖尿病大鼠肾脏和胰腺组织的 DNA 甲基化水平降低，导致很多基因处于活化状态，而胰腺组织甲基化水平升高，可能抑制了一些与胰岛素合成相关的基因[52]。从表观遗传学领域探索机制，采用甲基化特异性 PCR 技术检测大鼠主动脉各炎症因子基因启动子区的 DNA 甲基化水平显著低于正常组，并与 mRNA 和蛋白的表达水平呈负相关，一系列研究表明高糖诱导基因组 DNA 甲基化水平改变可能是糖尿病血管病变的一个潜在因素[53]。

此外组蛋白修饰也与糖尿病的血管病变密切相关，其中，糖尿病血管相关基因的表达与启动子区组蛋白乙酰化修饰密切相关。糖尿病患者单核细胞内 P300 可能与 NF-κB 相互作用促进环氧化酶 2（COX-2）和 TNF-α 基因启动子增强乙酰化过程，从而促进炎性基因表达[54]。另一项研究表明高糖环境中组蛋白 H3 的乙酰转移酶活性下降，而去乙酰化酶特别是 HDAC1、HDAC2、HDAC8 表达的增加与糖尿病性视网膜病变的进展密切相关[55]。具体的糖尿病各类血管病变中组蛋白修饰机制有待于进一步研究。

三、在其他病理情况中的表观遗传学改变

营养物质在表观遗传学的调控中也具有重要作用，人们可通过食疗、干预治疗等途径改变动物的表观遗传学[56]，如植物产物中十字花科蔬菜产生的 sulforaphane 和绿茶中 EGCG（epigallocatechin-3-gallate），修饰表观遗传学的过程，直接影响衰老和癌症。它们也可以下调与衰老和癌症有关的端粒酶（hTERT）。表观遗传学的生化机制依靠一些特定的化合物。葡萄糖限制也可以影响表观遗传学的过程，影响衰老和癌症（图 12-14）。

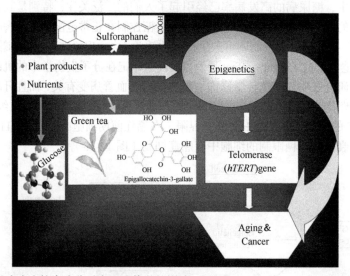

图 12-14　在衰老及癌症中饮食成分对表观遗传学的影响；Effects of components of the diet on epigenetics during aging and cancer

多项研究报道表明，孕妇低蛋白饮食可致子代不同器官出现表观遗传学改变，致子代未来成长中易发生肥胖、糖尿病、高血压等疾病[57]。暴露于环境中的毒物如砷等，可引起线粒体的破坏[58]，并且引起广泛富含 GC 区 DNA 低甲基化，也可以引起信号通路中 IGF-1、IGF 受体 2、IGF 结合蛋白 1 基因（IGF binding protein 1 gene）等表达的改变，从而引起表观遗传学的变化[59]，因此健康的饮食和良好的胎儿营养及环境可以促进胎儿早期健康发育，有利于保证胎儿出生时的正常体重，降低代谢性疾病的风险[60]。

另外，衰老与表观遗传学之间也存在着某种联系，Berdyshev 等 1967 年首次提出低等动物在衰老过程中其体内的全基因组低甲基化水平明显下降之后。通过连续 10 多年对收集的 100 多个样本 DNA 的长期研究发现随着年龄的增长全基因组低甲基化水平呈现出明显下降趋势[61]。其他调控机制如组蛋白修饰等随着衰老也会出现相应的变化，另外包括精神分裂、X 染色体失活在内的很多与衰老有关的疾病和改变都可能是表观遗传学参与调控的结果[62]。

挑战与展望

表观遗传学侧重于基因表达和细胞表型水平的研究，是在不改变 DNA 序列的情况下基因表达的可遗传变化的一门遗传学分支学科，其主要内容有 DNA 甲基化、组蛋白修饰、miRNA 调控、染色体重塑、基因印记等，这些机制与糖尿病血管病变、肿瘤、衰老等许多疾病密切相关。因此，表观遗传学机制已成为多种疾病的发生、发展及其转归研究中的一个新的领域，对其进一步的探究，不仅对疾病的预防、治疗有重要意义，而且对于一些疾病的术前诊断、鉴别诊断及预后都有着重要影响。因此，未来的研究不仅要充分了解表观遗传学与多种疾病病理变化之间的关系，更应该在明确这种关系的基础上进一步探究治疗相关疾病的策略。

思 考 题

1. 本章基本概念：表观遗传学（epigenetics），DNA 甲基化（DNA methylation），组蛋白密码（histone code），染色体重塑（chromosome remodeling），基因印记（genetic imprinting），代谢印记（metabolic imprinting）。
2. 简述组蛋白修饰的形式。
3. 简述 DNA 甲基化及组蛋白修饰的相互作用——"双锁原则"。
4. 染色体重塑包括哪些变化，存在哪些修饰方式？
5. 解释 ATP 依赖的染色质重塑复合物。

参 考 文 献

[1] Mazzio E A, Soliman K F. Basic concepts of epigenetics: impact of environmental signals on gene expression[J]. Epigenetics, 2012, 7（2）: 119-130.

[2] Waddington C H. The epigenotype[J]. International Journal of Epidemiology, 2012, 41（1）: 10-13.

[3] Mcquown S C, Wood M A. Epigenetic Regulation in Substance Use Disorders[J]. Current Psychiatry Reports, 2010, 12（2）: 145-153.

[4] The ENCOPE project consortium. An integrated encydopedia of DNA elements in the human genome[J]. Naure, 2012, 489: 57-74.

[5] Romani M, Pistillo M P, Banelli B. Environmental epigenetics: crossroad between public health, lifestyle, and cancer prevention[J]. Biomed Research International, 2015（3）: 587983.

[6] Hoque M O, Rosenbaum E, Westra W H, et al. Quantitative assessment of promoter methylation profiles in thyroid neoplasms[J]. Journal of Clinical Endocrinology & Metabolism, 2005, 90（7）: 4011-4018.

[7] Stein R, Razin A, Cedar H. In vitro methylation of the hamster adenine phosphoribosyltransferase gene inhibits Its expression in mouse L cells[J]. proceedings of the National Academy of Sciences of the United States of America, 1982, 79（11）: 3418-3422.

[8] Dodge J E, Ramsahoye B H, Wo Z G, et al. De novo methylation of MMLV provirus in embryonic stem cells: CpG versus non-CpG methylation[J]. Gene, 2002, 289（2）: 41-48.

[9] Ito S, Shen L, Dai Q, et al. Tetproteins can convert 5-methylcytosine to 5-formylcytosine and 5-carboxylcytosine[J]. Science, 2011, 333（6047）: 1300-1303.

[10] Jenuwein T, Allis C D. Translating the histone code[J]. Science, 2001, 293（5532）: 1074-1080.

[11] Santos J C, Ribeiro M L. Epigenetic regulation of DNA repair machinery inHelicobacter pylori -induced gastric carcinogenesis[J]. World Journal of Gastroenterology, 2015, 21（30）: 9021-9037.

[12] Chi P, Allis C D, Wang G G. Covalent histone modifications-miswritten, misinterpreted and mis-erased in human cancers[J]. Nature Reviews Cancer, 2010, 10（7）: 457-469.

[13] Ranjan A, Mizuguchi G, Fitzgerald P C, et al. Nucleosome-free region dominates histone acetylation in targeting SWR1 to promoters for H2A.Z replacement[J]. Cell, 2013, 154（6）: 1232-1245.

[14] Papamichos-Chronakis M, Watanabe S, Rando O J, et al. Global Regulation of H2A.Z localization by the INO80

chromatin-remodeling enzyme is essential for genome integrity[J]. Cell，2011，144（2）：200-213.

[15] Tosi A，Haas C，Herzog F，et al. Structure and subunit topology of the INO80 chromatin remodeler and its nucleosome complex[J]. Cell，2013，154（6）：1207-1219.

[16] Wang L，Du Y，Ward J M，et al. INO80 facilitates pluripotency gene activation in embryonic stem cell self-renewal，reprogramming，and blastocyst development[J]. Cell Stem Cell，2014，14（5）：575-591.

[17] Davidsonmoncada J，Papavasiliou F N，Tam W. MicroRNAs of the immune system：roles in inflammation and cancer[J]. Annals of the New York Academy of Sciences，2010，1183（1）：183-194.

[18] Huang S，He X. The role of microRNAs in liver cancer progression[J]. British Journal of Cancer，2011，104（2）：235-240.

[19] Lee Y，Ahn C，Han J，et al. The nuclear RNase Ⅲ Drosha initiates microRNA processing[J]. Nature，2003，425（6956）：415-419.

[20] Schwarz D S，Hutvágner G，Du T，et al. Asymmetry in the assembly of the RNAi enzyme complex[J]. Cell，2003，115（2）：199-208.

[21] Lagosquintana M，Rauhut R，Yalcin A，et al. Identification of tissue-specific microRNAs from mouse[J]. Current Biology，2002，12（9）：735-739.

[22] Girard M，Jacquemin E，Munnich A，et al. miR-122, a paradigm forthe role of microRNAs in the liver[J]. Journal of Hepatology，2008，48（4），648-656.

[23] Fornari F，Gramantieri L，Giovannini C，et al. miR-122/cyclin G_1 interaction modulates p53 activity and affects doxorubic insensitivity of human hepatocarcinoma cells[J].Cancer Research，2009，69（14），5761-5767.

[24] Datta J，Kutay H，Nasser M W，et al. methylation mediated silencing of microRNA-1 gene and its role in hepatocellular carcinogenesis[J]. Cancer Research，2008，68（13）：5049-5058.

[25] He Y，Cui Y，Wang W，et al. Hypomethylation of the hsa-miR-191 locus causes high expression of hsa-mir-191 and promotes the epithelial-to-mesenchymal transition in hepatocellular carcinoma[J]. Neoplasia，2011，13（9）：841-853.

[26] Feinberg A P，Tycko B. Feinberg A P，et al. The history of cancer epigenetics[J]. Nature Reviews Cancer，2004，4（2）：143-153.

[27] Han Y，Garcia B A. Combining genomic and proteomic approaches for epigenetics research[J]. Epigenomics，2013，5（4）：439-452.

[28] Feinberg A P，Gehrke C W，Kuo K C，et al. Reduced genomic 5-methylcytosinecontent in human colonic neoplasia. Cancer Research，1988，48（5）：1159-1161.

[29] Goelz S E，Vogelstein B，Hamilton S R，et al. Hypomethylation of DNA from benign and malignant human colon neoplasms[J]. Science，1985，228（4696）：187-190.

[30] Christensen B C，Marsit C J，Houseman E A，et al. Differentiation of lung adenocarcinoma，pleural mesothelioma，and nonmalignant pulmonary tissues using DNA methylation profiles[J]. Cancer Research，2009，69（15）：6315-6321.

[31] Weisenberger D J，Siegmund K D，Campan M，et al. CpG island methylator phenotype underlies sporadic microsatellite instability and is tightly associated with BRAF mutation in colorectal cancer[J]. Nature Genetics，2006，38（7）：787-793.

[32] Noushmehr H，Weisenberger D J，Diefes K，et al. Identification of a CpG island methylator phenotype that defines a distinct subgroup of glioma[J]. Cancer Cell，2010，17（5）：510-522.

[33] Figueroa M E，Abdel-Wahab O，Lu C，et al. Leukemic IDH1 and IDH2 mutations result in a hypermethylation phenotype, disrupt TET2 function，and impair hematopoietic differentiation[J]. Cancer Cell，2010，18（6）：553.

[34] Zouridis H，Deng N，Ivanova T，et al. Methylation subtypes and large-scale epigenetic alterations in gastric cancer[J]. Science Translational Medicine，2012，4（156）：156ra140.

[35] Dong C，Wu Y，Yao J，et al. G9a interacts with Snail and is critical for Snail-mediated E-cadherin repression in human breast cancer[J]. Journal of Clinical Investigation，2012，122（4）：1469-1486.

[36] Korditamandani D M，Ladies M A，Hashemi M，et al. Analysis of p15INK4b and p16INK4a gene methylation in patients with oral squamous cell carcinoma[J]. Biochemical Genetics，2012，50（5）：448-453.

[37] Song J S，Yong S K，Dong K K，et al. Global histone modification pattern associated with recurrence and disease-free survival in non - small cell lung cancer patients[J]. Pathology International，2012，62（3）：182-190.

[38] Seligson D B，Horvath S，Shi T，et al. Global histone modification patterns predict risk of prostate cancer recurrence[J]. Nature，2005，435（7046）：1262-1266.

[39] Müller-Tidow C，Klein H U，Hascher A，et al. Profiling of histone H3 lysine 9 trimethylation levels predicts transcription factor activity and survival in acute myeloid leukemia.[J]. Blood，2010，116（18）：3564-3571.

[40] Varambally S，Dhanasekaran S M，Zhou M，et al. The polycomb group protein EZH2 is involved in progression of prostate cancer[J]. Nature，2002，419（6907）：624-629.

[41] Kleer C G，Cao Q，Varambally S，et al. EZH2 Is a marker of aggressive breast cancer and promotes neoplastic transformation of breast epithelial cells[J]. Proceedings of the National Academy of Sciences of the United States of America，2003，100（20）：

11606-11611.

[42] He A，Shen X，Ma Q，et al.PRC2 directly methylates GATA4 and represses its transcriptional activity. Genes & Development，2012，26（1）：37-42.

[43] Lee J M，Lee J S，Kim H，et al. EZH2 generates a methyl degron that is recognized by the DCAF1/DDB1/CUL4 E3 ubiquitin ligase complex[J]. Molecular Cell，2012，48（4）：572-586.

[44] Mitani Y，Oue N，Hamai Y，et al. Histone H3 acetylation is associated with reduced p21（WAF1/CIP1）expression by gastric carcinoma[J]. Journal of Pathology，2005，205（1）：65-73.

[45] Bird A. DNA methylation patterns and epigenetic memory[J]. Genes & Development，2002，16（1）：6-21.

[46] Stirzaker C，Millar D S，Paul C L，et al. Extensive DNA methylation spanning the Rb promoter in retinoblastoma tumors[J]. Cancer Research，1997，57（11）：2229-2237.

[47] Makos M，Nelkin BD，Lerman MI，et al. Distinct hypermethylation patterns occur at altered chromosome loci in human lung and colon cancer[J]. Proceedings of the National Academy of Sciences of the United States of America，1992，89（5）：1929-1933.

[48] Clark SJ，Melki J. DNA methylation and gene silencing in cancer：which is the guilty party? Oncogene，2002，21：5380-5387.

[49] Tahiliani M，Koh K P，Shen Y，et al. Conversion of 5-methylcytosine to 5-hydroxymethylcytosine in mammalian DNA by MLL partner TET1[J]. Science，2009，324（5929）：930-935.

[50] Pirola L，Balcerczyk A，Okabe J，et al. Epigenetic phenomena linked to diabetic complications[J]. Nature Reviews Endocrinology，2010，6（12）：665-675.

[51] Ekström T J，Stenvinkel P. The epigenetic conductor：a genomic orchestrator in chronic kidney disease complications?[J]. Journal of Nephrology，2009，22（4）：442-449.

[52] 王萍，闫芳，何忠效，等. 糖尿病大鼠肾、胰基因组 DNA 甲基化状态的变化[J]. 北京师范大学学报自然科学版，2001，37（2）：246-249.

[53] Reddy M A，Park J T，Natarajan R. Epigenetic modifications in the pathogenesis of diabetic nephropathy[J]. Seminars in Nephrology，2013，33（4）：341-353.

[54] Sun G D，Cui W P，Guo Q Y，et al. Histone lysine methylation in diabetic nephropathy[J]. Journal of Diabetes Research，2014，2014（2014）：654148.

[55] Zhong Q，Kowluru R A. Role of histone acetylation in the development of diabetic retinopathy and the metabolic memory phenomenon[J]. Journal of Cellular Biochemistry，2010，110（6）：1306-1313.

[56] Nishida N，Kudo M. Epigenetic regulation and development of hepatocellular carcinoma[J]. Nihon Shokakibyo Gakkai zasshi（The Japanese journal of gastro-enterology），2016，113（5）：775-784.

[57] Bocock P N，Aagaard-Tillery K M. Animal models of epigenetic inheritance[J]. Seminars in Reproductive Medicine，2009，27（5）：369-379.

[58] Hyman M. Systems biology，toxins，obesity，and functional medicine[J]. Alternative Therapies in Health & Medicine，2007，13（2）：S134-139.

[59] Xie Y，Liu J，Benbrahim-Tallaa L，et al. Aberrant DNA methylation and gene expression in livers of newborn mice transplacentally exposed to a hepatocarcinogenic dose of inorganic arsenic[J]. Toxicology，2007，236（1）：7-15.

[60] Wang J，Wu Z，Li D，et al. Nutrition，epigenetics，and metabolic syndrome[J]. Antioxidants & Redox Signaling，2012，17（2）：282-301.

[61] Bjornsson H T，Sigurdsson M I，Fallin M D，et al. Intra-individual change in DNA methylation over time with familial clustering[J]. Jama the Journal of the American Medical Association，2008，299（24）：2877-2883.

[62] Benavraham D，Muzumdar R H，Atzmon G. Epigenetic genome-wide association methylation in aging and longevity[J]. Epigenomics，2012，4（5）：503-509.

（刘淑岩　王建力　陈　莉）

Chapter 12   Epigenetic Changes

Cancer initiation and progression have been recognized for many years to be secondary to the accumulation of genetic mutations which lead to changes in cellular function. While inherited or sporadic mutations may result in the activation of oncogenes or the inactivation of tumor suppressor genes, the apparent modify change of genome specific sites not only influences related genes expression, and further affects the biological phenomena, such as growth, development, and more and more studies have found that the role of epigenetics range is very wide, which involved in the growth of biological reproduction, growth and differentiation, inflammation, cancer and many other physiological and pathological phenomena [1]. Therefore epigenetics is a new century research hot point of molecular biology, genetics and clinical medicine.

Section 1   Concepts of Epigenetics

Epigenetics is corresponding to the concept of genetics. Genetics is based on the genetic sequence changes which caused by changes in the level of gene expression, such as gene mutations, gene hybrid loss, etc., while epigenetics,as genetic sequence changes, refers to the changes that caused by non-gene-sequence expression change.

Epigenetics is firstly proposed by the biologist Waddington [2] in 1939, in the book of 《An introduction to modern genetics》. In 1942, he described epigenetics as a control mechanism from genotype to apparent type. Then after many people's research, by 1999 the Wolife defined epigenetics as the study of heritable changes in gene expression which no changes in DNA sequence, as Allis etc. have had two definitions in a book, one refers to epigenetics as heritable phenotype changes that has nothing to do with the DNA mutation; Another is the change of chromatin regulation of gene transcription, but this kind of change was not involving the change of the DNA sequence [3].

Now, epigenetics is formally defined as a heritable change in gene expression or chromosomal stability by utilizing DNA methylation, covalent modification of histones or non-coding RNAs without a change in DNA sequence, it is increasingly used to define long term changes that alter the physiology of a subset of cells in a tissue independent of a change in the DNA sequence.

Epigenetics refers to under the condition of the genomic DNA not changing, it can cause changes in gene expression as the important chemical modification, which includes: DNA modification (methylation and hydroxyl methylation) and histone modification after translation (methylation and acetylation, etc.), and chromatin remodeling (Fig. 12-1). This three parts overlap each other and mutual control gene expression, which is not depending on the genetic material in the cell DNA sequence change but in the other genetic material change, and this change can be passed in the process of development and proliferation of biological stability [3]. Especially, epigenetic pathways control genome epigenetic modification of dynamic balance, further highlighting the crosstalk between genetics and epigenetics (Fig. 12-2）. According to recent research reports, 80% of DNA which used to think no function participates in the regulation of genes, and this adjustment is regulated by the epigenetics [4].

The epigenetic marks are dynamic and can respond to changes in physiological conditions and hence these epigenetic modifications(acetylation, methylation, phosphorylation, ubiquitination) tightly regulate critical cellular processes such as sternness, differentiation, transcription, DNA repair and DNA replication to safeguard and keep the cells in a normal state in response to stress. Deregulation of one of these mechanisms or crosstalk of epigenetic in the regulating cellular processes may lead to abnormal regulation of DNA based cellular processes and result in tumor development. In addition to gene mutations, epigenetic changes can be drivers of the development of the cancer.

Section 2   Main Content of Epigenetics

Epigenetic modifications are controlled by a set of enzymes whose functions can be summarized as follows: the "writers" are the enzymes that modify their target by adding residues (i.e., methyl groups to DNA or histones); the "erasers" remove the added residues and the "readers" are the proteins that recognize and bind to the modified targets and act as intermediating for subsequent protein-protein interactions (Table 12-1).

Table 12-1   Enzymes involved in epigenetic modifications.

Enzyme	N	Function
DNA methyltransferase(DNMT)	5	
Histone acethyltransferase(HAT)	19	Writer
Histone methyltransferase(HMT)	41	
Histone deacethylase(HDAC)	13	
Histone demethylase(KDM)	26	Eraser
Methyl binding proteins(MBDI)	5	
Proteins that recognize and react to specific	N	Readers
Modified histone residue		
Total(April 2012)	>109	

The number of epigenetic modifier proteins is steadily increasing: in 2009 they were "only" 91 and in 2012 more than109 different proteins were identified [5].The enzymes mediating epigenetic modifications have been found to be mutated in cancers, which adds to an indirect manner in which tumor develop as the change in the modifier can affect the gene expression patterns. This suggests also that epigenetic modifiers may act as novel targets for therapy. Specifically, the HMTs and the HDMs play important roles in multiple tissues regulating the methylation status of four lysine residues K4, K9, K27and K36 on histone H3.

1. DNA Methylation

DNA methylation refers to chemical modification process of the so-called DNA methylation transferase (DNMT), under the action of the S - adenosine methionine on methyl, transfers to cytosine 5 carbon atoms and add a methyl group, into 5 - methyl cytosine (5-MC) (Fig. 12-3)[6]. This is common in gene 5 '-CG- 3' sequence. Under normal circumstances, the human genome sequence of "junk" CPG dinucleotide is relatively scarce, and always in a state of methylation, by contrast, about 100-1000 bp in the human genome size and rich in CPG dinucleotide CPG island is in not methylation state, and is associated with 56% of the human genome encoding genes. Clusters of non-CPG methylation constitude CPG island, and they are located in the core of structure gene promoter sequences and transcription starting point. High CPG island methylation and genome widely low methylation is a major content of methylation. DNA is methylated post-synthetically on cytosine residues predominantly in the sequence CpG and in vitro methylated promoters are known to be generally inactive when transfected into eukaryotic cells [7]. DNA methylation is catalysed by a family of DNMTs. DNMT1 is the methyl transferase that maintains reciprocal methylation of the new DNA strand complementary to hemi-methylated DNA that is produced as a result of semiconservative DNA replication. DNMT3a and DNMT3b are known as de novo methyl transferases, being able to methylate the completely unmethylated DNA duplex in vivo [8]. More recently it has been shown that 5-methylcytosinecan be oxidised to 5-hydroxymethylcytosineby a family of Fe^{2+}, 2-oxoglutarate dependent methylcytosine dioxygenases known as TET proteins, effectively resulting in the subsequent removal of the repressive methyl group by a mechanism that appears to include base excision repair processes. Other DNA modifications are also described such as methylation at sites other than CpG and the generation of formyl and carboxyl derivatives of DNA [9].

2. Histone Modifications

Histone covalent modification is one of related way of the epigenetic regulation of tumor, the main histone includes H1, H2A, H2B, H3 and H4. These different amino acids can occur different modifications, such as different histone acetylation, methylation, phosphorylation, ubiquitin and other modifications (Fig. 12-4), called histone code [10], it refers to the various modified state of one or more groups of proteins at the ends, and can be identificated by a joint or be set at the beginning of protease or other complex and combined to work, and provide the corresponding binding sites for launching or repressing gene transcription of chromatin proteins. It is an important factor to establish and maintain epigenetics memory. Histone modifications involves various covalent modifications of the histones such as acetylation, phosphorylation andmethylation which have been subject to many studies and their importance is now well accepted [11] Acetylation and methylation is an important modification of histone, acetylated is commonly regulated by histone acetyl transferase and histone acetylation enzyme, and through it can make accurate and histone gene expression(Fig. 12-5).

Methylation is completed by methylation transferase, methylation modification can change the structure of the chromosome, and can regulate gene expression by other transcription factors. The histone methylation balance on specific residues in particularis crucial for maintaining genome integrity, gene expression and evasion of cancer [12].

3. Interplay between the Methylated DNA and the Modified Histones ——— Double Lock Principle

Although most studies tend to focus attention on either the DNA or histone modifications, it is clear that in order fora gene to be transcribed there is interplay between the methylated DNA and the modified histones. Both the DNA and the histones should be in an open or "unlocked" configuration, as shown in

Fig. 12-6, to be in a permissible state for transcription. If the epigenetic marks on the DNA or histones are in a closed or "locked" state, the gene of interest will not be transcribed. This is a concept that we term the "Double Lock Principle" as both the DNA methylation status and histone modifications are critical to the expression of a gene. In addition, the required transcriptional activator must be present and the necessity to have it and the "double lock" correctly aligned explains a lot of data where genes are not expressed despite what could be considered to be tolerant conditions.

4. Chromosome Remodeling

Chromosome remodeling: Packing status of chromatin during the process of the replication and remodeling of gene expression, the molecular mechanism of nucleosome histone and corresponding DNA molecules will change, the DNA replication, transcription, repair, recombination at the chromatin level, during these processes, chromatin remodeling can lead to changes in nucleosome position and structure, induced changes in chromatin. Remodeling includes a variety of changes, generally refers to changes in chromatin specific regions of ribozyme stability, mainly involved in nucleosome replacement or rearrangement, change in gene promoter regions of the nucleosome array, increased the accessibility of gene transcription and promoter sequences. Chromatin remodeling and histone modification of N C-terminal tails are closely related, especially the modification of histone H3 and H4, by modifying the direct influence of nucleosome structure, and provides the binding site for interaction with DNA for other proteins, chromatin remodeling modification mainly includes two types: one is containing histone acetyl transferase and deacetylase chemical modification; the other is the binding of DNA to the release of energy from the hydrolysis of ATP, which enables transcription to be carried out.

The highly folded chromatin structure is necessary for its packing into the nucleus, but the chromatin of this dense state prevents the process of gene transcription, DNA replication, and damage repair of the chromatin. As a result, with evolution eukaryote created a set of chromatin remodeling enzymes and related proteins that regulate chromatin structure by regulating the assembly, disassembly and rearrangement of chromatin on the chromatin. There is a kind of protein which can use the energy of ATP hydrolysis to drive the slide on the DNA, or mediated the "replacement" between the nucleosome histone variants and the classic histone, this kind of protein is chromatin remodeling factor which is ATP dependent, the chromatin remodeling complex is usually composed of a large number of subunits with a larger molecular mass.

In eukaryotic cells, chromatin remodeling factor regulate chromatin structure by altering chromatin nucleosome assembly, disassing and rearranging, thereby improving the transcription factor when the chromatin structure is loose in the presence of the chromatin DNA, increased RNA polymerase II, transcription factor on dyeing DNA accessibility, to activate gene transcription. On the contrary, when the chromatin structure tends to be dense, RNA polymerase II and transcription factors weak the accessibility of chromatin DNA, thus inhibiting the transcription of the related genes

It was found that, some chromatin remodeling complexes are the executor of histone variant replacement into (or out) nucleosome. The most typical example is that in yeast Swr1 can catalyze the replacement between the H2AZ-H2B hetero two polymer and the Classical H2A-H2B two polymer in the body[13]. Similarly, In addition to the chromatin remodeling function, human source INO80/SRCAP/TRRAP-TIP60 complex in the INO80 subfamily also has the function of replacement histone variants, can catalytic replace between catalytic classic histone H2A and histone variants H2AZ[14],the specific replacement mechanism between H2A-H2AZ is not clear at present, it is interesting that Swr1/SRCAP composite can make H2AZ one-way replacement into the nuclear, but INO80 [15] can play the opposite role, it is H2AZ is replaced from the nuclear, indicating different chromatin complexes has different function (Fig.12-7).Whereas most of the INO 80 are combined with the transcription start site region, the role of activating factor [16]. In summary, chromatin remodeling plays a key role in gene transcription regulation, and is involved in many important biological processes.

5. miRNA Regulation

miRNA is a small, similar to the siRNA molecule, encoded by the higher eukaryotic genomes, miRNA guide the silence complex to degradation the miRNA or hinder its translation by base pairing with the target gene miRNA. miRNA is quite conservative in the evolution of species, the miRNA which was found in the plant, animal and fungi expressed only in specific tissues and developmental stages, the tissue specificity and timing of miRNA, deciding the functional specificity of tissues and cells, suggest that miRNA has multiple regulatory role in cell growth and development process[17]. miRNA does not encode proteins, but through the interaction with the target gene sequence expressing the related gene in the level of post-transcription and translation. More and more evidences show that miRNA plays an important role in many biological processes. At the same time, the abnormal expression of rniRNA was found in many kinds of human diseases, including cancer. In the course of the occurrence and development of tumor. miRNA is like a cancer gene or a tumor suppressor gene and play the role. Recently, in the study of HCC, we have found that the abnormal expression of miRNA is closely related to the clinical pathological characteristics (such as metastasis, recurrence and prognosis) of tumor [18].

The synthesis of miRNA is a multi-step biological process which subject to fine control, first, the miRNA gene is involved in the RNA polymerase II to generate hundreds to thousands of base Pri-miRNA, then in the nucleus, forming the 50-80 intermediate of Pre-miRNA under the action of RNAase III, which contains part of complementary sequences, can be self-folded formed neck ring like structure, and then actively transport into the cytoplasm with the help of GTP dependent exportin-5[19]. And then through the Picer shear can create 19-25 nucleotides miRNA, then duplex melts apart, miRNA is rapidly degraded, and then miRNA chain bind to miRNA induced gene silencing complex (miRISC) by an asymmetric manner. Through the combination between "seed sequence" and target mRNA3′-UTR sequence, if highly complementary then degradating the miRNA, if the partial complementary inhibited mRNA post transcriptional translation, the latter mRNA level had no obvious change [20].

There are some increasing evidences that miRNA has a significant role in the development of cancer and may be a powerful biomarker for cancer diagnosis and prognosis.MicroRNA-122 (miR-122) is the most abundant microRNA in the liver, accounting for about 70% of the total number of all miRNA. Some studies suggest that miR-122 is important for the stability of the internal environment in the liver [21]. The expression of miR-122 is abundant in mouse and human hepatocytes, but in most HCC and transformed cell lines, the expression is very low. Loss of expression of miR-122 was associated with liver differentiation, invasion and intrahepatic metastasis [22]. Recently, the nude mouse model was confirmed that miR-122 have the effect of inhibition of tumor and increased drug sensitivity in vivo. Previous studies have found that miR-122 can affect the sensitivity of hepatocellular carcinoma cells to adriamycin (DOX) by p53 - independent apoptotic pathway [23].

There are some interactions between DNA methylation and miRNA. In many tumors, they all have a synergistic effect, such as the regulation of the abnormal expression of micRNA in HCC. Datta[24] treat the HCC cell line by 5 azacytidine (methyltransferase inhibitor) and (or) trichostatin (histone deacetylase inhibitor), by looking for miRNA which was regulated by epigenetic mechanisms (DNA methylation).The results showed that these epigenetic drugs can regulate the expression of some miRNA in HCC cells, especially miRNA-1-1. He et al [25] found that the expression of IiliR-191 is upregulated in HCC cells and primary HCC tissues, and miR-191 gene methylation status is related to the expression level. Thus, it is showed that the low methylation of miR-191 gene in HCC tissue can induce the up regulation of gene. In the HCC cell line, the upregulation of miR-191 expression can induce epithelial cells to transform into mesenchymal like cells, so that the cells can lose their adhesion and down regulated epithelial cell markers. Increase in the expression of stromal cell markers, enhanced cell migration and invasion: inhibition of miR-191 expression will reverse the process.

DNMT1 contributes to miR-1 silencing in HCC cells, thereby promoting the accumulation of its target HDAC4. The miR-29, which targets DNMT3, is down-regulated by HDACs in AML. Likewise, miR-26a and miR-137 are silenced by promoter CpG island hypermethylation, which induces the up-regulation of the target gene LSD1 in colorectal adenomas and EZH2 in prostate cancer.

Various histone modifying enzymes such as EZH2 and HDACs can be recruited to methylate and deacetylate histones. Myc or NF-κB, which interacts with transcription tors YY1 or Sp1 on miRNA promoter, is hypothesized to be the upstream regulator of miRNA silencing. A positive feedback loop exists between Myc and EZH2: Myc stimulates EZH2 expression by reducing its negative regulators, miR-26a and miR-101; EZH2 can also increase the abundance of Myc by repressing miR-494 (Fig. 12-8).

6. Genemic Imprinting

Gene imprinting: refers to gene expression depending on whether they are in the parent chromosome or maternal chromosome, and whether the genes on them are silent, so as to express. Some imprinted genes are expressed only from the maternal chromosomes, while others refer to the expression of genes from the parent chromosome, which plays an important role in the growth and development of organisms. Gene imprinting is spread across the genome, its introns are relatively small, and can express the formation and expression of imprinted genes in tissues. There is a complex regulatory mechanism, which is generally believed to be related to methylation, and is affected by many factors. It is because the imprint is the essential regulatory mechanisms of normal development, abnormal imprinting behavior must cause a variety of diseases, in particular, the imprinting anomaly can be used as a new mechanism of tumorigenesis which is closely related with the occurrence and development of tumor. In addition, some environmental factors will affect the imprinted gene. If the suppressor gene has the inactivation of an active allele is will increased the incidence rate of cancer, the loss of IGF2 gene imprinting will create lots of tumors, such as Wilim 's tumor.[26]

Section 3   Significance of Epigenetic Changes in Diseases

Epigenetics has played an important role in the occurrence and development of diseases and the prevention and treatment of diseases, when the control mechanism changes may cause the pathophysiological changes, so it is related to the occurrence and development of the tumor, immune, cardiovascular and other diseases.

1. Epigenetic Changes in Tumors

Global reprogramming of epigenetic marks, including alterations in DNA methylation and histone modifications, is known to occur in malignancy and genetic mutations in epigenetic modifiers in cancer[27]. Therefore the changes in modification of both DNA and histones (collectively the epigenome) can also contribute to the initiation and the progression of cancer.

(1) Genes Methylation

What has been found is that Methylation patterns and histone modification is different, especially from their normal tissue and tumor were compared. Eventually all of the gene expression is controlled by their epigenetic status, therefore, epigenetic changes play an important role in the tumorigenesis.

DNA methylation is a common cause of tumor gene silencing epigenetic mechanisms. During tumorigenesis, an estrogen receptor (ER)-positive progenitor can give rise to a homone-sensitive or homone-insensitive tumor. DNA promoter hyperethylation may play a role in tumorigenesis, silencing ESR1 to yield a hormone-insensitive (intrinsically resistant). ER-negative tumor, or alternatively, silencing tumor suppressors to yield a hormone-sensitive tumor. Treatment with anti-estrogens may actively promote the development of endocrine resistance, resulting in promoter hypermethylation and hypomethylation, Alternatively, treatment may select for resistant subpopulations with these epigenetic alterations. Dysregulation of estrogen-regulated genes may result in further perturbation of ER signiling. Globally DNA hypomethylation is observed during tumorigenesis, and promoter hypomethylation may predominate during acquisition of endocrine resistance. (Fig. 12-9).

IDH mutations result in Glioma- CpG methylation phenotype (G-CIMP) and histone methylation in gliomas (Fig. 12-10). Mutant IDH1 catalyzes the production of 2-hydroxyglutarate (2-HG) from α-ketoglutarate (α-KG). 2-HG is thought to inhibit α-KG dependent dioxygenase enzymes since 2-HG is structurally similar to α-KG. The Jumonji C family of histone lysine demethylases (KDMs) and the TET group of DNA hydroxylases are α-KG dependent dioxygenases. Inhibition of these enzymes may result in increasing histone methylation marks and DNA methylation contributing to G-CIMP.

When cancer exposureed in radiation, the radiation might induce global DNA hypomethylation through a decrease in DNA methylatransferases, including DNMT1, DNMT3a, DNMT3b and MeCP2. This phenomenon results in genomic instability in cancer. Radiotion also can induce phosphorylation of histone H2AX, and trimethylation of histone H4K20, which affect gene expression patterns, consequently leading to cell death, changes in cell cycle, and genomic instability. These events may be closely related to the therapeutic, protective, or detrimental response to radiation.

In addition, DNA demethylation exists. DNA demethylation has also been postulated to contribute to cancer development as despite evidence for regional hypermethylation, global levels of 5-methylcytosine have actually been found to be 5-10% less in tumors compared to normal cells [28]. The methylation changes have been suggested to occur specifically between the stages of hyperplasia and benign neoplasia as DNA was found to be significantly hypomethylated in both benign polyps and malignant tissues when compared to normal tissue [29]. Methylation patterns were therefore altered before the lesions became malignant, suggesting that they could be a key event in tumor evolution.

DNA methylation has been used in the classification of the tumor, the methylation of tumor suppressor genes can be distinguished from malignant phenotype tissues [30], such as the cytosine of the promoter region of the VHL gene DNA sequences is methylation in renal clear cell carcinoma. The tumor subgroups with DNA high methylation is considered a CpG island methylation phenotype (CIMP), is mainly associated with poor prognosis. CIMP is first found in colorectal cancer, including most sporadic colorectal cancers associated with the MMR defects and MLH1 methylation, and its associated with BRAFV600E mutation [31].Then found CIMP can be used in the diagnosis of glioblastoma [32], gastric cancer [33], and ependymoma [34].Therefore, CIMP tumor may represent different tumor subsets with slightly genetic changes. This shows the drugs targeting epigenetic mechanisms may provide a new method of treatment.

The study found that misregulation of the HMTs and the HDMs has been associated with a variety of cancer types including breast, prostate, lung and brain [35]. The gene P16INK4A, P14ARF, and P15INK4B which can regulate the cell cycle can be alone or in combination with methylation may participate in the occurrence and development of oral squamous cell carcinoma, and it has a significant relationship with its recurrence and low survival rate. During chromatin remodeling, overexpression of chromatin remodeling factor RSF-1 plays an important role in the development of oral squamous cell carcinoma, and can promote tumor invasion [36].

(2) Histone Modification

Similar to DNA methylation patterns, histone modification patterns have also been used to predict prognosis in multiple cancers. Reduced levels ofH3K9ac, H3K9me3 and H4K16ac correlated with recurrence of non-small cell lung cancer [37]. In prostate cancer, lower levels of H3K4me2 and H3K18ac were associated with poor prognosis [38]. Loss of H3K9me3 has been found in core promoter regions of genes in patients with acute myeloid leukaemia. Global H3K9me3 patterns were additionally able to independently predict patient prognosis in acute myeloid leukaemia [39]. These cancers have amplifications, deletions and somatic mutations which all lead to changes in the enzymatic activities of the HMTs and the HDMs. For example, the repressive histone mark trimethylated H3K27 (H3K27me3) is mediated by the catalytic SET domain of EZH2 (enhancer of zestehomologue 2), a protein that forms part of PRC2 (Polycomb repressive complex 2). EZH2 has been reported to be up-regulated in metastatic prostate cancer relative tolocalised disease or benign prostatic hypertrophy, suggesting a potential involvement in prostate cancer progression[40], and its over-expression also correlates with breast cancer aggressiveness and poor prognosis [41] According to recent reports, Two non-histone substrates of EZH2 have been reported recently both of which represses its transcriptional activity. GATA4 is methylated by EZH2 which reduces its interaction with its coactivator p300 [42]. Our group has shown that methylation of the nuclear receptor RORαby EZH2 results in increased polyubiquitination and proteasomal degradation leading to decreased transcriptional activity [43]. In turn this causes the loss of tumor suppressor activity of RORα, which ultimately leads to the development of more aggressive tumors.

Histone modification is also associated with the occurrence of colorectal cancer. Histone acetylation is a reversible dynamic equilibrium process mediated by histone acetyl transferase (HAT) or histone HDAC. In human colorectal cancer cell line SW1116 and human colorectal cancer cell line COLO-320, HDAC inhibitor trichostatin A (TSA) and sodium butyrate inhibited HDAC and enhanced the level of acetylation, and significantly up-regulated in the p21WAF1 gene's transcription, the cell cycle was arrested in G_1 phase [44].In addition to acetylization, histone methylation is an important mechanism of its modification, the main site of DNA methylation is the histone H3 and H4 lysine and arginine residues of two kinds. Histone methylation and DNA methylation can be combined together to participate in tumor suppressor gene silencing and induce tumor.

In EGFR driven glioblastomas Pyruvate Kinase M2 (PKM2) catalyzes the conversion of phosphoenolpyruvate (PEP) to pyruvate in the glycolytic pathway. EGFR activation results in PKM2 translocation to the nucleus and phosphorylation of histone 3 at the threonine 11 residue (H3-T11). This leads to removal of the histone deacetylase 3 (HDAC3) from the CCND1 (Cyclin D1) and c-MYC promoter regions, acetylation of H3K9 and activation of transcription of cyclin D1 and c-Myc (Fig. 12-11).

The status of DNA methylation is crucial as one part of the "double lock" of gene expression. As a generalisation, promoters with methylated DNA tend not to be expressed. Clusters of CpGs (the predominant target for DNA methylation) are known as CpG islands and are located at the 5′ ends of many human genes. In tissues, most CpG islands are unmethylated, even when the associated genes are not expressed [45]. However in cancer, DNA hypermethylation occurs at many CpG is lands, as well as global DNA hypomethylation. Promoter methylation is almost always associated with gene-silencing, raising the possibility that aberrant methylation might cause silencing and be part of the transforming process. A potential role intumorigenesis with a strong mechanistic pathway is suggested when methylation is shown to occur at known tumor suppressor genes. DNA hypermethylation of the cell cycle control gene Rb (retinoblastoma) was one of the first epigenetic lesions to be implicated in carcinogenesis. Aberrant methylation occurs in approximately10% of cases of sporadic unilateral retinoblastoma and is associated with the loss of Rb expression. The case of DNA methylation in Rb remains one of the strongest arguments in favor of a causal role for aberrant methylation in carcinogenesis as the Rb gene is usually active in the precursor cells of tumors and promoter methylation appears to have the same effect as genetic mutation of the gene [46]. In colorectal carcinogenesis hypermethylation of a region of chromosome 17p corresponding to the location of the tumor suppressor p53 has been demonstrated to precede its allelic loss, suggesting that methylation may non-randomly mark chromosome regions that are altered during the development of specific tumors [47]. Because of these examples, it has been assumed that aberrant methylation plays a role in malignant transformation, particularly when methylation has been demonstrated to occur early in the tumorigenic process. The methylation-induced silencing of tumor suppressor genes may provide cells with a selective advantage over others, either by causing their increased proliferation or resistance to apoptosis. The clonal expansion of these premalignant cells could result in the hyper proliferative phenotype that is characteristic of the early stages of tumorigenesis. Genes such as Rb, MLH1 and VHL are methylated in the tumor types in which they are also commonly mutated, suggesting that CpG island hypermethylation may be selected for during tumorigenesis [48].

(3) Epigenetic State in EMT

Increasing reports have demonstrated that epigenetic dysregulation, as well as genomic instability, contributes to tumor metastasis. Abnormalities in DNA methylation or histone acetylation induce tumorigenesis and metastasis [49]. The epithelial phenotype is a default state of epithelial cells. Contextual signals promote the epigenetic repression of key epithelial genes (for example, that encoding E-cadherin) by introducing histone modifications, which help define the plasticity of epithelial cells and the residency of cells in a given phenotypic state during the transition. Further altered expression of genes involved in cellular differentiation may lead to epithelial-mesenchymal transition, a change associated with increased tumor invasiveness and metastasis. The gain of an increasingly stable mesenchymal phenotype depends on the sustained presence of potent EMT-promoting signals. In their absence, metastable mesenchymal cells may simply revert to a more epithelial phenotype unless they are supported by the appropriate epigenetic modifications (Fig. 12-12).

(4) Epigenetic Inhibitors as Cancer Therapies

In the process for epigenetic drug development, candidate small molecules are first tested in vitro in malignant cell lines for specificity and phenotypic response. These may, in the first instance, assess the inhibition of proliferation, induction of apoptosis, or cellcycle arrest. These phenotypic assays are often coupled to genomic and proteomic methods to identify potential molecular mechanisms for the observed response. Inhibitors that demonstrate potential in vitro are then tested in vivo in animal models of cancer to ascertain whether they may provide therapeutic benefit in terms of survival. Animal studies also provide valuable information regarding the toxicity and pharmacokinetic properties of the drug. Based on these preclinical studies, candidate molecules may be taken forward into the clinical setting. When new drugs prove beneficial in well-conducted clinical trials, they are approved for routine clinical use by regulatory authorities such as the FDA.

2. Epigenetic Changes in Diabetes

In today's world, the high incidence of diabetes has aroused widespread concern, and its vascular disease has become the main cause of its high mortality. But even if the toxic effects of sugar glucose control in the normal range, diabetic vascular disease still continues to progress, and early intensive glycemic control can have a lasting effect, a phenomenon known as "metabolic imprinting" or legacy effects [50]. But the metabolic imprinting mechanism in molecular biology is unknown. In recent years, more and more studies show that genetic modification is not only related to diabetic vascular disease, and may lead to potential mechanisms of metabolic memory.

Glucose restriction can impact epigenetic regulation in both normal and cancer cells. In normal cells it leads to p16 repression and hTERT activation to extend the Hayflick limit. In precancerous cells, the opposite effects on p16 and hTERT lead to apoptosis, cellular senescence and cancer inhibition of the glucose restricted cells. (Fig 1-13)

A series of studies have shown that the levels of DNA methylation is closely related to the diabetes, cardiovascular disease (CNDS) and chronic kidney damage (CKDS), the levels of risk factors of adenosine homocysteine in the serum of CVDS and CKDS patients increase, can inhibit the partial DNA methyl transferase and induce DNA low methylation [51]. Compared with the normal group, the level of DNA methylation in kidney and pancreas tissues in the diabetic rats decreased, resulting in a lot of genes in the active state, but the level of methylation in pancreatic tissue increased, and some may inhibit insulin synthesis related genes[52]. From the field of epigenetics exploring the mechanism, by using the methylation specific PCR technique detect the level of DNA methylation in the promoter region of various inflammatory factors in rat aorta, and the level was significantly lower than the normal group, and the expression level of mRNA and protein was negatively correlated, a series of studies have indicated that high glucose induced changes in the level of methylation of genomic DNA may be a potential gene for diabetic vascular disease [53].

In addition, histone modification is closely related to the vascular lesions of diabetes, and the expression of vascular related genes in diabetic patients is closely related to the histone acetylation modification of the promoter region[54].P300 may interact with NF-KB and make COX-2 and TNF- alpha promoter enhancing the acetylation process and promote the expression of inflammatory genes in the monocytes of diabetes patients.Another study showed [55] that the decline of the activity of high glucose H3 histone acetyltransferase, but the increase of the expression of the deacetylase, especially HDAC1, HDAC2, and HDAC8,is closely related to diabetic retinopathy, and the various types of diabetic vascular disease specific histone modification mechanism still needs us to further study.

3. Epigenetic Changes in Other Pathologic Conditions

The nutrients also play an important role in the genetic control in the apparent genetics, people can change animal epigenetic through the diet and intervention treatment[56]. Plant products such as sulforaphane from cruciferous vegetables and (−)- epigallocatechin-3-gallate (EGCG) modify epigenetic processes that can have a direct impact on aging and cancer. They also lead to the down-regulation of telomerase (hTERT) which is central to both aging and cancer. The mechanisms for epigenetic modifications of the phytochemicals can vary depending on the particular compound. Glucose restriction also can impact epigenetic processes and affect aging and cancer. (Fig. 12-14)

A number of studies reported that pregnant women with low protein diet can lead to the emergence of epigenetic changes in the sub generation of different organs, the future development of the future is prone to obesity, diabetes, hypertension and other diseases [57]. Exposure to environmental poisons such as arsenic, can cause mitochondrial damage [58] and caused wide spread GC rich region of DNA hypomethylation, can also cause the gene expression changes of the IGF-1, IGF receptor 2 and IGF binding protein 1 gene in the signaling patnway, and cause the changes of epigenetic [59], so a healthy diet and good fetal nutrition and environment can promote the healthy development early, is conducive to the normal fetal birth weight, can reduce the risk of metabolic disease [60].

In addition, aging and epigenetics also exist some links, in 1967, Berdyshev first proposed that the lower animal in the aging process in the whole genome methylation level decreased significantly after in 2008, through a long-term study of 10 consecutive years and 100 samples of DNA were found with the increase of age the whole genome methylation level showed a significant downward trend [61].Other regulatory mechanisms such as histone modifications also appear to be associated with aging, including schizophrenia, X chromosome inactivation, many age-related diseases and epigenetic changes are likely to be involved in the regulation of the results of apparent genetics [62].

Challenges and Prospects

Epigenetics is focused on the level of gene expression and cell phenotype, is heritable changes in gene expression without altering the DNA sequence, as a genetics branch discipline. The main contents of epigenetics include DNA methylation, histone modification, mRNA regulation, chromosome remodeling, genes imprinting, etc., these mechanisms closely related to many diseases, such as diabetes vascular lesions, tumorgenesis senescence, and other diseases. Accordingly, epigenetics research has become a new field in variety of disease development and outcome, not only for the prevention and treatment of disease, but for some the preoperative diagnosis of the disease, differential diagnosis and prognosis. Therefore, future studies should not only fully understand the relationship between epigenetics and pathological changes in a variety of diseases, on the basis of clear the relationships it should further explore the strategy for the treatment of related diseases.

Consider/Questions

1. Basic concepts in this chapter

Epigenetics, DNA methylation, histone code, chromosome remodeling, genomic imprinting, metabolic imprinting.

2. Briefly descript the patterns of histone modifications.

3. Briefly explain that interplay between the methylated DNA and the modified histones —Double Lock Principle.

4. Are there which changes of chromosome remodeling and which patterns of its modifications?

5. Explaining the chromatin remodeling complex with ATP dependent.

第十三章　肿瘤微环境

　　早在 1889 年，Stephen Paget 提出的"种子和土壤"假说认为，某种特定类型肿瘤细胞（"种子"）经常会转移到适合其生长的部位（"土壤"），即继发性肿瘤部位与原发部位有某些相似的特点，为肿瘤微环境概念的提出奠定了基础。肿瘤微环境（tumor microenvironment，TME）不仅是一个物理空间，还是其中各种细胞及其产生的蛋白质、可溶性生长因子和细胞因子等相互作用的场所。有证据表明，癌细胞和微环境基质细胞之间的相互作用是双向和动态的。两者既相互依存，相互促进，又相互拮抗，相互斗争。例如，肿瘤细胞可以通过旁分泌的方式招募或激活基质细胞到 TME 中；而招募和激活的基质细胞又能释放刺激或抑制肿瘤生长的因子。

　　在肿瘤的八大生物学功能中有七项明显是由 TME 基质细胞所贡献（图 13-1）。

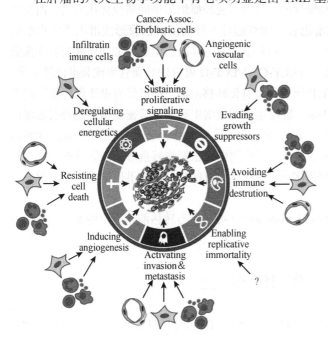

图 13-1　活化/招募的基质细胞与肿瘤的八大生物学功能，其中七项明显与 TME 中的基质细胞有关。在不同类型和不同器官的肿瘤中各种基质细胞所发挥的作用不同，受到原发性和转移性肿瘤中特定 TME 成分和具有潜在基因改变的肿瘤细胞和肿瘤干细胞调控；Multifactoral contributions of activated/recruited stromal cells to the hallmarks of cancer of the eight acquired hallmark capabilities—seven demonstrably involve contributions by stromal cells of the tumor microenvironment. The importance of each of these stromal cell classes varies with tumor type and organ, governed by parameters of the distinctive tumor microen- vironments and underlying oncogenetic altera- tions in cancer cells and cancer stem cells that arise in primary tumors, and their invasive and metastatic colonizations

第一节 TME 中血氧改变

一、血 管 成 分

血管是 TME 最重要的组成部分。无论是快速分裂的肿瘤细胞，还是微环境中的非肿瘤细胞，均需要许多营养物质和氧供其生存和生长。毛细管壁介导的气体、营养物质和代谢产物的交换可以满足这些需求，维持组织稳态。一旦细胞聚集达到营养、盐和氧气扩散极限的临界值时，细胞即进入休眠期。

但肿瘤细胞增殖过程中能启动新血管形成。新血管的形成（这个过程被称为血管生成）在正常和病变组织是由促血管生成因子或抗血管生成因子之间的平衡所调控。在正常生理状态下，这种平衡被严格限定，在需要时血管生成处于"ON"（如胚胎发育、伤口愈合、黄体形成）的状态，否则为"OFF"状态。但在肿瘤转化和肿瘤进展过程中这种平衡发生紊乱。肿瘤血管具有高渗透性特点，其间质流体压（interstitial fluid pressure，IFP）减少或缺乏，可影响治疗药物的递送。整个肿瘤 IFP 几乎是均匀的，但在肿瘤边缘 IFP 急剧下降，使得组织液从肿瘤中渗出到周围正常组织中，也带出了治疗的药物。此外，IFP 与瘤内高渗透性血管的微血管压之间的偶合消除了肿瘤血管上下游的压力差，导致肿瘤血管血流淤滞。是什么触发了新生血管的生长？这些血管与正常血管比较如何发生结构和功能作用？其异常功能对 TME 的影响是什么？

二、淋巴管生成和淋巴转运

正常的淋巴网络通过从组织中转运免疫细胞和间质体液，在发挥免疫功能和维持组织间体液平衡中发挥重要的作用。实体肿瘤受肿瘤细胞生长空间的限制产生机械应力（固体应力）压迫瘤内血管和淋巴管，导致几乎没有功能性的淋巴管，使肿瘤组织中间质流体压升高。而在肿瘤边缘和肿瘤周围组织中有功能性的淋巴管。瘤细胞可入侵周围淋巴管形成淋巴系统内的转移。大量的报道指出在 TME 中参与血管生成的分子也参与淋巴管生成，如肿瘤淋巴管和血管内皮细胞上有 VEGF 的受体（VEGFR3）VEGF-C、VEGF-D 可以诱导血管生成和淋巴管生成，与多种肿瘤淋巴道转移有关。淋巴管生长因子的具有促转移潜能。淋巴管有助于保持组织内液体平衡，流体静压力可能是一个触发因素。肿瘤边缘细胞增生和淋巴管密度增加是否引起瘤内静水压升高还不得而知。但微血管造影术、活体显微镜技术和分子靶向试剂显示，这些由 VEGF-C/D 和尚待发现的淋巴管生成因子诱导的肿瘤周围淋巴管能够携带癌细胞并介导肿瘤转移。此外，通过阻断 VEGFR3 抑制肿瘤周围淋巴管增生，可抑制早期的淋巴道转移及向淋巴结递送癌细胞。

此外，研究发现前哨淋巴结（sentinel lymph node）可能参与转移前生态位的形成。肿瘤引流淋巴结的淋巴管生成依赖于 B 细胞。

三、代 谢 环 境

缺氧和酸中毒是实体肿瘤的代谢环境特点。氧分压（PO_2）和 pH 是决定肿瘤生长、代谢、对各种疗法反应（如放疗、化疗、热疗、光动力疗法）的重要指标。

（一）缺氧

基于毛细管床的解剖及氧扩散和消耗的数学模型，近一个世纪前诺贝尔奖获得者 August Krogh 提出了 $100\sim200\mu m$ 氧扩散极限的概念，其组织单位为单一毛细血管周围 $100\sim200\mu m$ 半径。随着磷光猝灭显微镜的发展，直接测量这些血管周围梯度及同一血管的 PO_2 和血流速度已成为可能。

由于肿瘤血管中的血流量变化间歇性的，因此，肿瘤的某些区域呈周期性缺氧。这种缺氧被称为"急性缺氧"或"灌注-限制性缺氧"。间歇性血流可使血流中断后又恢复血流，由此产生的自由基会导致"再灌注性损伤"或"复氧性损伤"，给癌细胞造成了更多的选择性压力。肿瘤由于有限的动脉供应而接收氧合不充足的血液，导致远离起源小动脉的小肿瘤血管含氧量非常低。

低氧诱导因子-1（hypoxia induaible factor-1，HIF-1）其是一种异源二聚体转录因子，能增加血管生成相关基因的表达，适应缺氧、侵袭和抵抗氧化应激。在肿瘤中 HIF-1 积累可介导肿瘤生物学的四个主要方面：缺氧、血管生成、基因突变和代谢。缺氧上调多种促血管生长因子，研究最广泛的是氧稳态的主要调节剂 HIF-1。转录激活的血管生成因子，包括 VEGF、Ang2、PDGF、PIGF、TGF、IL-8 和 HGF。缺氧可能作为血管生成的开关发挥重要的作用，是肿瘤生长和扩张所必需的。

在缺氧条件下靶向肿瘤的免疫细胞不能充分发挥作用，使肿瘤逃避宿主免疫应答和以细胞为基础的治疗。此外，缺氧改变肿瘤细胞使其获得高侵袭性和转移性。最终，缺氧可能使肿瘤细胞更恶性、更活跃，基因更不稳定，更不易发生细胞凋亡，并能抵抗各种疗法。氧是影响放射治疗的重要因素。电离辐射直接和间接损害 DNA，两者的作用均依赖于氧，在实体肿瘤中缺氧将显著降低其对辐射的敏感性。肿瘤缺氧也与某些化疗药物耐药有关，会导致预后不良。因此，缺氧诱导通路中的多个分子被确定为诊断和治疗的靶标。

（二）低 pH

肿瘤微循环异常的另一个后果是细胞外的低 pH 酸中毒。肿瘤中至少有两种 H^+ 源——乳酸和碳酸。前者由无氧糖酵解产生，后者来源于碳酸酐酶转化 CO_2 和 H_2O。癌细胞内 pH 保持中性或碱性（pH 7.4），因此肿瘤细胞内外存在显著 pH 差异。应该警惕在酸化肿瘤环境中使用某些药物的疗效。如瘤细胞的跨膜 pH 梯度阻碍了细胞对弱碱性药物如[多柔比星（adriamycin）、表柔比星（epirubicin）、米托蒽醌（mitoxantrone）的摄取及其疗效。酸性 pH 也会导致免疫细胞的功能障碍，同时细胞外酸性 pH 能诱导促进侵袭和转移的蛋白酶和血管生成因子的表达。用抗血管生成剂使肿瘤血管正常化能中和肿瘤细胞外酸性环境。因此增加间质 pH 向正常值靠近可能会提高基础药物的疗效，减少肿瘤细胞的转移潜能。

第二节　TME 中的细胞成分

TME 中的非恶性细胞在肿瘤形成各个阶段均具有促癌功能。血管内皮细胞增殖和招募导致新血管形成，为肿瘤的生长和转移提供必需的营养物质；肿瘤相关的成纤维细胞可以促进血管生成，促进肿瘤的生长和浸润；TME 中的免疫细胞，特别是肿瘤相关的巨噬细胞，除了促进生长外，还能抵抗细胞毒性的攻击；并导致淋巴内皮细胞增殖，使淋巴血管密度增加，促进肿瘤转移（图 13-2）。

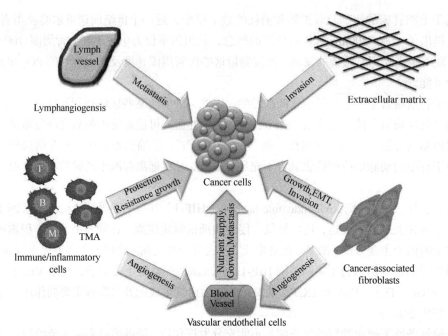

图13-2　基质支持细胞对肿瘤生长和转移的影响；Effects of stromal support cells on tumor growth and metastasis

B：B 细胞；EMT：上皮-间质转化；M：单核细胞；T：T 细胞；TAM：肿瘤相关性巨噬细胞；B, B-cell；EMT, epithelial-mesenchymal transition；M, monocyte；T, T-cell；TAM, tumor associatedmacrophage

一、反应性基质细胞

（一）肿瘤相关成纤维细胞

当组织受损，宿主成纤维细胞响应旁分泌信号分化为肌成纤维细胞。肌成纤维细胞的反应可导致器官纤维化，从而提高癌症发生的风险。在许多 TME 中含量丰富肌纤维细胞，被称为（cancer-associated fibroblasts，CAFs），常来源于间质中成纤维细胞，或来自周细胞、平滑肌细胞、间充质干细胞（MSC，通常源于骨髓），或通过上皮-间质转化（EMT）或内皮-间质转化（EndMT）而来，CAFs 密度增加，常出现在肿瘤浸润前沿。

CAFs 的功能：①支持肿瘤生长，产生更多的旁分泌生存信号，如 IGF-1 和 IGF-2，从而维持周围癌细胞的存活；②分泌 VEGF、FGFs、PDGF 和其他促血管生成信号诱导血管生成；③分泌 TGF-β参与 EMT 的癌细胞转移过程；④可产生趋化因子 CXCL12，促进恶性细胞生长和存活，并具有趋化性，刺激其他基质细胞及其前体细胞迁移到 TME；⑤与抑制细胞毒性 T 细胞和自然杀伤 T 细胞相关，有助于微环境的免疫抑制；⑥像成纤维细胞一样，分泌 ECM 成分和 ECM 重塑酶，能重塑 ECM；⑦ CAFs 也与癌细胞无氧糖酵解有关；⑧CAFs 在肿瘤中可围绕肿瘤中的纤维血管分支分布，或围绕恶性肿瘤细胞形成致密的促结缔组织增生性间质，从而限制了抗癌药物对靶细胞的毒性作用。

（二）脂肪细胞

脂肪细胞分泌的脂肪因子可招募恶性细胞，提供脂肪酸，促进癌细胞生长，如腹腔内肿瘤易转移到大网膜。

（三）脉管内皮细胞和周细胞

TME 中有许多可溶性因子均可刺激内皮细胞和周细胞，激活血管生成、淋巴管形成，从当前脉管系统中产生新生脉管。越来越多的证据表明，内皮细胞和周细胞还通过机械性调节 TME 和通过改变宿主对肿瘤的免疫反应来影响癌症的进展。例如，前哨淋巴结中的淋巴管内皮细胞（LECs）可以交叉表达肿瘤抗原 MHC Ⅰ类分子，导致 CD8$^+$ T 细胞缺失，支持 LECs 在药物耐受中的新作用。

血管周细胞为血管结构提供支持，是肿瘤血管的重要组成部分。血管周细胞覆盖率低与预后差和增加转移有关。肿瘤血管"正常"周细胞的覆盖可作为转移的一个关键性负调节因子。

二、浸润的免疫细胞

免疫系统在 TME 中具有重要作用。被募集到肿瘤局部的各种免疫效应细胞因其对肿瘤来源信号的反应不同而发挥不同作用。

（一）肿瘤相关巨噬细胞

肿瘤相关巨噬细胞（tumor-associated macrophages，TAMs）作为主要的免疫细胞，根据不同的刺激而具有分泌促炎症介质或抗炎症介质的能力。TAMs 是慢性炎症和癌症之间密切联系的一个重要成分，TAMs 被招募到肿瘤中形成癌症相关的炎症反应。与正常巨噬细胞不同，TAMs 缺乏细胞毒活性。肿瘤中有两种巨噬细胞，由 TNF-α 激活，具有抗肿瘤活性和组织破坏作用的为 M1 表型；由 IL-4 和 IL-13 等激活诱导，以组织修复、重塑和促进肿瘤为特征的为 M2 表型。由于 TME 内表达 IL-10、TGF-β、集落刺激因子-1 等多种信号分子，大多数 TAMs 为 M2 表型（图 13-3）。

TAMs 是恶性细胞迁移、浸润和转移必需的伴侣。大多数 TAMs 的表型为 IL-10 增高，IL-12 降低，且表达甘露糖受体（mannose receptor）和清道夫受体 A（SR-A，也称为 SCARA）。TAMs 聚集在肿瘤缺氧和（或）坏死区域，通过分泌 IL-10 在正常的免疫细胞监视下隐藏癌细胞；通过分泌 VEGF 和 NOS 帮助新生血管形成；通过分泌 EGF 支持肿瘤生长和重塑 ECM。TAMs 使得 NF-κB 缓慢活化，这使癌症中的炎症反应持续存在。临床前和临床证据表明，TAMs 增多与预后不良有关，抑制 M2 表型和诱导 M1 信号的策略可以恢复 TAMs 的抗肿瘤功能，有助于去除来自 M2-TAMs 的保护性信号，激活先天免疫反应，使得肿瘤体积减小。所以 TAMs 是癌症治疗的潜在靶标。

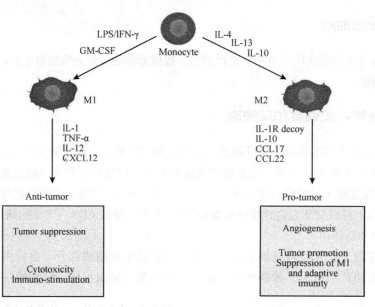

图 13-3　巨噬细胞的分化激活及其对肿瘤生长的影响；Differential activation of macrophages and their effect on tumor growth

M1：促炎；M2：抗炎；M1, proinflammatory；M2, anti-inflammatory

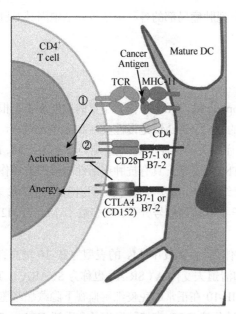

图 13-4　抗原提呈细胞和 T 细胞无能；Antigen presentation and T cell anergy

幼稚 CD4⁺淋巴细胞（活性 T 细胞或 T 辅助细胞）上的 CD4 抗原与 MHC-Ⅱ特异性结合（MHC-Ⅱ可以在任何细胞上表达），并与特异性抗原提呈细胞（APCs）-树突状细胞（DCs）相互作用是抗肿瘤免疫的关键；CD4 antigens on naive CD4⁺ lymphocytes（activated T cells and T helper cells）bind specifically to type Ⅱ MHC（MHC-Ⅱ），which can be expressed on any cell，but interactions with professional antigen presenting cells（APCs）-dendritic cells（DCs）are critical for antitumor immunity

（二）T 淋巴细胞

T 淋巴细胞激活受到双信号程序调控：①T 细胞受体必须与表面表达主要组织相容性复合体（major histocom- patibility complex，MHC）蛋白的抗原提呈细胞相结合；②CD28 必须同时与其配体 B7-1 或 B7-2 相结合。如果没有第二个信号，T 细胞不能激活（无能），适应性免疫应答被抑制，这是一种防止自身免疫反应过度活跃的保护机制的一部分，如果共抑制受体细胞毒 T 淋巴细胞相关抗原-4（cytotoxic T lymphocyte- associated antigen-4，CTLA-4）与 CD28 配体竞争性结合，或程序死亡-1（programmed death-1，PD-1）受体与其配体（PD-L1）结合，也都将导致 T 细胞无能（图 13-4）。例如，效应 T 细胞（活化 CD4⁺T 细胞或 T 辅助细胞）、CD8⁺细胞可通过其表面的 PD-1 受体与靶向肿瘤细胞上的 PD-L1 结合而"枯竭"（失活）（图 13-5）。同样，调节性 T 细胞能通过其表面的 CTLA-4 与肿瘤细胞上的 B7-1 或 B7-2 结合，使效应 T 细胞耗竭，导致这种效应的可溶性因子很可能是 TNF-β1（图 13-6）。

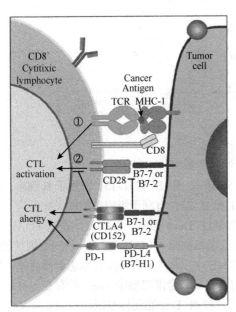

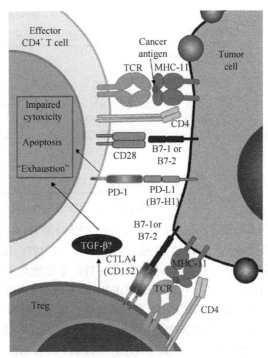

图 13-5 肿瘤细胞和 CD8⁺ 细胞无能；Tumor cells and CD8⁺T cell anergy

幼稚 CD8⁺细胞毒淋巴细胞（cytotoxic lymphocytes，CTLs）上的 CD8 抗原与 MHC- I 特异性结合（MHC- I 可以在除红细胞以外的任何细胞上表达）。肿瘤细胞可以经由 MHC-I 在其细胞表面表达自身抗原（尽管通常很少表达）。其他 APCs，如 M1 巨噬细胞或 B 细胞也可以经由 MHC- I 介导的 APC 激活 CTLs；CD8 antigens on naive CD8+cytotoxic lymphocytes（CTLs）bind specifically to type IMHC（MHC-I），which can be expressed on any cell except red blood cells. Tumor cells may present their own antigens on their cell surface via MHC-I，albeit poorly. Other antigen presenting cells，such as M1 macrophages or B cells may also activate CTLs via MHC-I-mediated APC activity

图 13-6 CTLA-4 和（或）PD-1 导致的 T 细胞耗竭；T cell "exhaustion" via CTLA-4 and/or PD-1

在 TME 中有许多不同的 T 细胞亚群，其浸润于肿瘤中或分布在肿瘤侵袭性边缘和引流淋巴器官中。①细胞毒性 CD8⁺记忆 T 细胞（CD8⁺CD45RO⁺），即 CD8⁺细胞毒性 T 细胞（CD8⁺cytotoxic lymphocytes，CTLs），有正常抗原"经验"，并能杀死肿瘤细胞，该细胞主要与细胞毒性免疫反应有关与良好的肿瘤预后密切相关。②辅助性 T 淋巴细胞均起源于同一种幼稚 T 辅助前体细胞（Th0 细胞）。根据暴露的细胞因子不同，Th0 细胞可以分化为不同表型的辅助性 T 细胞：1 型 T 辅助细胞（Th1）、2 型 T 辅助细胞（Th2）、调节性 T 细胞（regulatory T cells，Tregs）或 17 型 T 辅助细胞（Th17）。这些 T 辅助细胞中的任何类型都不会逆转回 Th0 祖细胞表型。通常认为 Th1 和 Th2 细胞是终末的永久表型。Tregs 和 Th17 细胞具有更强的可塑性，Tregs 表型可转化为 Th17 表型，而 Th17 细胞不会转化为 Tregs 表型，但可转化为 Th1 和 Th2 细胞（图 13-7）。

CD4⁺ T 辅助 1（Th1）细胞产生特征性的细胞因子 IL-2 和 IFN-γ，Th1 细胞主要为其他 T 细胞和巨噬细胞提供帮助，如激活 CD8⁺ T 细胞分化为效应杀伤 T 细胞；在 TME 中这些细胞的数

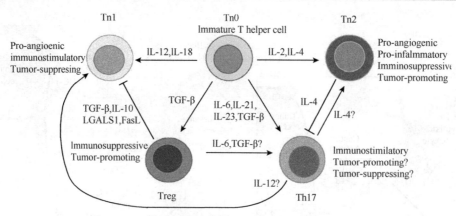

图 13-7　T 辅助细胞的分化；T-helper cell differentiation

量多与预后良好相关。CD4$^+$ Th2 细胞分泌 IL-4、IL-5、IL-6、IL-10 和 IL-13，作用于 B 细胞，调节体液免疫；Th17 细胞产生 IL-17A、IL-17F、IL-21 和 IL-22，有利于组织抗菌的炎症反应。最常被描述为具有促肿瘤作用的 CD4$^+$ T 细胞是免疫抑制性 Tregs 细胞，其特点是表达 FOXP3、CD25。通过产生 IL-10、TGF-β，以及细胞毒性 T 淋巴细胞抗原-4（CTLA-4）介导的细胞接触，抑制免疫系统识别和清除肿瘤细胞。在多种肿瘤如 TME 中出现大量 Tregs 提示患者预后差。但对于一些 B 细胞肿瘤，Tregs 则表现为肿瘤抑制作用；如霍奇金淋巴瘤中 Tregs 的存在与良好的预后密切相关，可能是通过直接抑制了肿瘤细胞生长。根据 T 细胞受体基因的结构差异又将 T 细胞分为 γδ-T 细胞和 αβ-T 细胞。其中 αβ 和 γδ 链都是由可变区和恒定区组成。由于 CD3 含有 γδε 三种链，因此 CD3 可以标记这两种细胞。αβ-T 细胞中包括了上述的 CD4$^+$和 CD8$^+$的 T 细胞。γδ-T 细胞具有与生俱来的不同于适应性免疫细胞的一些特征，其不表达 CD4 和 CD8，也不表达 CD5。γδ-T 占 T 细胞总数不到 5%。对多种恶性肿瘤细胞，包括肿瘤干细胞，具有很强的细胞毒性作用。虽然实验动物肿瘤研究表明 γδ-T 细胞具有免疫监视作用，但仍不确定是否 TME 中的 γδ-T 细胞与预后的关系。

　　在 TME 伴慢性感染的环境中，T 细胞在表型和功能上的顺序和逐步变化导致 T 细胞的耗竭，使局部抗原和（或）炎症持续存在。例如，慢性病毒性感染和荷瘤状态，耗竭的 T 细胞经过序列表型变化和效应器功能逐渐丧失（包括效应器细胞细胞因子产物、细胞毒性、细胞增殖和细胞因子介导的自我更新）；抑制受体的过表达；细胞因子受体的下调；转录因子改变；细胞内信号转导通路的改变（图 13-8）。

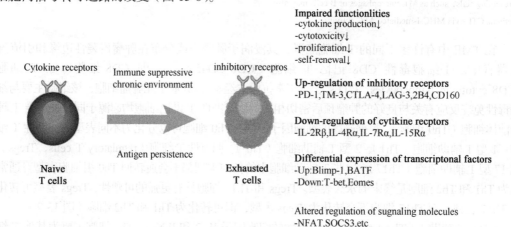

图 13-8　在伴慢性感染的 TME 中 T 细胞耗竭功能损伤；T cell exhaustion lead to impaired functionality in a TME with chronic infection

（三）B 淋巴细胞

B 细胞常见于引流淋巴结和淋巴结相邻的 TME 中，也可见于肿瘤侵袭边缘。TME 中 B 细胞的浸润与某些肿瘤的预后良好相关，如乳腺癌和卵巢癌。但在小鼠模型中，B 细胞可抑制肿瘤特异性细胞毒性 T 细胞反应。B 细胞和免疫球蛋白沉积具有促肿瘤作用。产生 IL-10 的免疫抑制 B 细胞，又称为调节性 B 细胞（Bregs）或 B10 细胞，在炎症诱导的皮肤癌中可增加肿瘤负荷，抑制肿瘤特异性免疫反应，并促进小鼠乳腺癌模型发生肺转移。在淋巴瘤小鼠模型中，Bregs 可抑制抗 CD20 抗体介导的肿瘤细胞清除作用。然而，这些影响都不是因为 TME 中有 Bregs 浸润，而是通过影响周围淋巴组织或引流淋巴结中的其他免疫细胞，并且调节骨髓细胞的活性引起。

（四）髓源性抑制细胞

髓源性抑制细胞（myeloid derived suppressor cells，MDSCs）是一群骨髓起源、具有潜在 T 细胞抑制作用的异质性细胞。MDSCs 表面的 CD40 受体与 Tregs 的 CD40 配体（CD40L）相互作用通过释放免疫抑制细胞因子，导致 Th1 活化受抑和 Th2 活化增强，使 TME 中 IFN-γ 和 IL-2 产生减少，伴 CTL 和 NK 细胞活化功能和细胞毒活性降低。MDSCs 调节创面修复和炎症，并与肿瘤中的炎症信号有关，MDSCs 在大多数恶性肿瘤中迅速扩增。人类 MDSCs 特征如同其表型多种多样，它们甚至可分化为 TAMs。小鼠和人类 MDSCs 通过激活 NOS2 和精氨酸酶（Arg1）抑制 CTL，MDSCs 还可诱导 Tregs 发育和巨噬细胞极化形成 TAMs 样表型（图 13-9）。

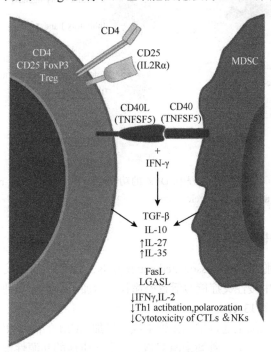

图 13-9　调节性 T 细胞和髓源性抑制细胞阻遏干扰素-γ 介导的免疫应答；Thwarting of IFN-γ-mediated immune response by Tregs and MDSCs

（五）NK 细胞和自然杀伤 T 细胞

NK 细胞和自然杀伤 T 细胞（natural killer T，NKT）也会发生肿瘤间质浸润，但未发现其与肿瘤细胞直接接触。由于 NK 细胞不具备完整的 T 细胞受体复合物，但胞质中常表达 CD3

的 ε 链，因此，对 CD3 多克隆抗体反应阳性。虽然 NK 细胞和 T 细胞在一些共同的抗原标记，如表达 CD2，CD7，CD8，CD56，CD57，与细胞毒性 T 细胞一样也可表达细胞毒性蛋白：穿孔素、粒酶 B、T 细胞内抗原（TIA-1）等，但 NK 细胞表达 CD16，而 T 细胞常不表达 CD16。在多种肿瘤中，如结肠癌、胃癌、肺癌、肾癌和肝癌，NK 细胞浸润似乎预示预后良好。大量研究显示，因受恶性细胞来源 TGF-β 的诱导，肿瘤间质 NK 细胞显示为无免疫活性的表型可能无法发挥其杀伤肿瘤的作用。

（六）树突状细胞

TME 中的树突状细胞（dendritic cells，DCs）被认为是有缺陷的，因为它们不能充分激发肿瘤相关抗原的免疫应答。TME 的缺氧和炎症微环境影响了 DCs 激活机体的免疫功能，肿瘤局部的一些 DCs 甚至能抑制 T 细胞反应。最近的两项研究表明 DCs 是一个独特的免疫细胞系统。在慢性病原体感染和癌症发展中特异性 DCs 亚群的丧失，下调 MHC 和共刺激分子配体，上调抑制配体，其分化为耐受 DCs 诱导 Tregs，通过改变 IFN-I 抑制 DCs 的发育（图 13-10）。

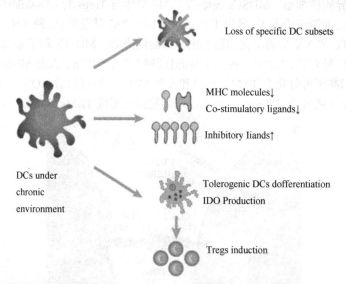

图 13-10　慢性病原体感染和癌症发生过程中 DCs 的功能性调节；Functional modulation of DCs during chronic pathogen infections and cancer development

（七）肿瘤相关中性粒细胞

肿瘤相关中性粒细胞（tumor-associated neutrophils，TANs）对原发肿瘤生长和转移的作用尚有争议。已知在肿瘤中慢性炎症能激活致癌途径，增加组织重构和肿瘤血管生成，以及激活肿瘤的免疫逃逸机制（图 13-11）。

有证据表明，中性粒细胞通过增强血管生成、增加 ECM 的降解和免疫抑制等作用促进小鼠模型肿瘤生长。此外，CD11b$^+$骨髓来源细胞，一个异质性的髓源性细胞系，与转移前肺微环境的形成及促进循环肿瘤细胞定居有关。相反，免疫或细胞因子也能激活这些细胞的抗肿瘤作用。这时中性粒细胞能主动清除或通过 TGF-β 间接抑制扩散的肿瘤细胞。

TME 中主要的间质细胞亚型及其关键性作用的概见图 13-12。

TME 中不同细胞间代谢产物的穿梭造成代谢的相互作用。效应 T 细胞、CTLs、DCs 和 TAMs M1 表型与肿瘤细胞间可能形成一种潜在的代谢拮抗。相反，TME 中 Tregs、MDSCs 和 TAMs M2

表型可能优先利用肿瘤的代谢物形成一种潜在的代谢协同现象（图 13-13）。

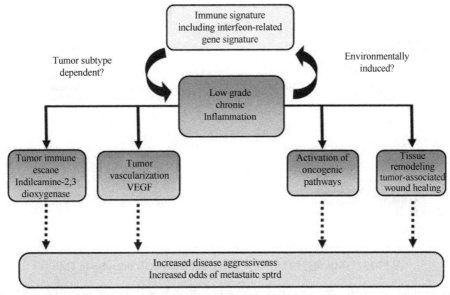

图 13-11　慢性炎症促进肿瘤进展；Chronic inflammation in tumors promote tumor progression

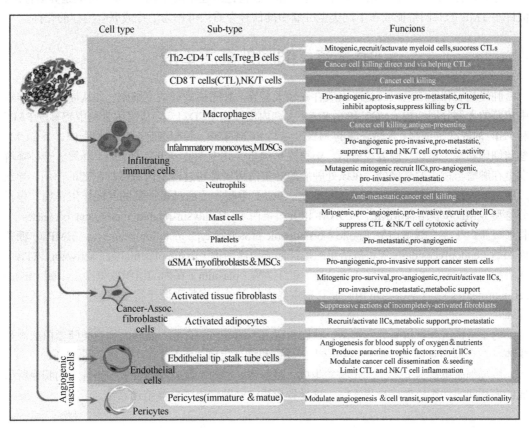

图 13-12　TME 中主要的间质细胞亚型及其关键作用的概括；Multiple stromal cell types and key functional contributions of the TME

某些亚型的拮抗作用呈灰色

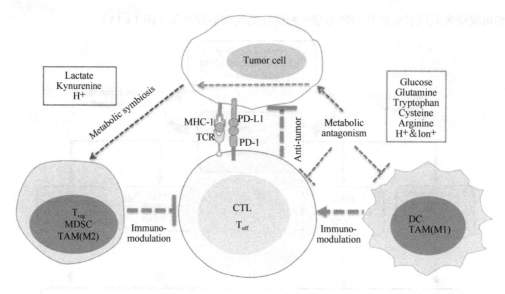

图 13-13　TME 免疫细胞的相互作用；Immunity cells interplay in TME

　　TME 的共同特征表明，靶向 TME 中的非恶性细胞或其通信的介质可应用在不同类型的肿瘤治疗中，也可以配合其他治疗方案。尽管如上述讨论所述组成 TME 的成分可能是异质性的，但许多 TME 的共同特征或在不同类型肿瘤中的信号介质均可作为治疗或联合治疗的靶标。

第三节　细胞外基质重塑

　　肿瘤基质和正常组织的基质组成存在较大差异。肿瘤招募的宿主细胞，如从局部脂肪组织中招募的大部分周细胞（NG2+和 α-SMA+）和内皮细胞（CD31+），从宿主骨髓中招募的 FAP+和 FSP+的成纤维细胞（骨髓来源的 MSC）参与 ECM 重塑。肿瘤细胞分泌多种蛋白进入 ECM，参与细胞黏附、运动、侵袭和通信。值得注意的是，其中一些分子参与 ECM 降解。这种降解发生在肿瘤与宿主的交接处，在该处肿瘤源性蛋白酶显著超过宿主内源性抑制剂的作用，导致广泛基质重建，并刺激细胞表面信号变化。ECM 重塑主要通过多种酶的共同作用实现，包括分泌型 MMP 和膜结合 MMP，ADAM-相关膜蛋白（adamalysin-related membrane proteases）、骨形成蛋白-1 型金属蛋白酶（bone morphogenic protein-1-type metalloproteinases，BMP）、糖苷内切酶（endoglycosidases）和包括组织型纤溶酶原激活剂（tissue plasminogen activator，TPA）、尿激酶（urokinase）、凝血酶（thrombin）和纤溶酶（plasmin）在内的组织丝氨酸蛋白酶（tissue serineproteases）。这些参与重构肿瘤与宿主界面的因子大多数来源于宿主细胞，而非生长中的肿瘤。

　　为了平衡这些重构酶和降解酶，肿瘤和宿主上调基质的合成。与肥大细胞类胰蛋白酶激活受体-2 结合而活化的成纤维细胞合成 I 型胶原和纤连蛋白，参与 ECM 重塑（图 13-14）。

　　巨噬细胞也参与 IL-1 和 NOS 的生成，两者均可增加 I 型胶原的合成。新合成的胶原所形成的癌周间质编织松散或排列无序，这导致形成中的肿瘤周围总体结构紊乱。

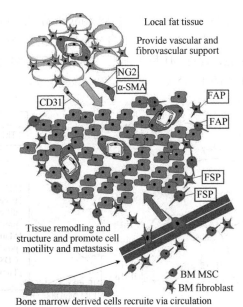

图13-14　成纤维细胞参与ECM重塑；Fibroblastes involved in ECM remodeling

肿瘤不仅由癌症细胞组成，还包括招募的宿主细胞。该模型显示，大部分周细胞（NG2$^+$和α-SMA$^+$）和内皮细胞（CD31$^+$）是从局部组织中招募的，如局部脂肪组织。参与ECM重塑的FAP$^+$和FSP$^+$的成纤维细胞是从宿主骨髓中招募的，如骨髓来源的MSC；A tumor is composed of not only cancer cells, but also recruited host-derived cells.　This model suggests that the majority of pericytes（NG2$^+$ andα-SMA$^+$）and endothelial cells（CD31$^+$）are recruited from local tissue, such as local adipose tissue. FAP$^+$ and FSP$^+$ fibroblastes involved in ECM remodeling are recruited from host bone marrow populations, such as BM MSC

第四节　肿瘤细胞和 TME 之间通信

一、TME 是一个动态的环境

　　TME 不断演进，是组织重构、肿瘤代谢变化、募集基质细胞的变化（包括多样性的免疫细胞）等共同作用的结果。TME 的另一个重要特点是 ECM 的成分和组织，其力学性质可影响肿瘤细胞的分化和侵袭，如乳腺组织中基质的硬度增加是已知的人类乳腺癌危险因素之一。在小鼠模型中通过赖氨酰氧化酶（lysyl oxidase，LOX）抑制胶原交联，可延迟和减少肿瘤的侵袭。ECM 的硬度能促进 ROCK（Rho 激酶的效应子）活化，通过与 Wnt 信号通路有关的机制增加胶原沉积，激活 STAT3，表达 CCL2 和粒细胞-巨噬细胞集落刺激因子（granulocyte macrophage colony-stimulating factor，GM-CSF）等，能招募骨髓来源细胞到 TME 的炎性区域。TME 生物力学功能的变化可影响肿瘤细胞的增殖和迁移，以及免疫调节因子的分泌。肿瘤细胞与骨髓生态位（niche）的动态相互作用影响恶变的进程。如前列腺癌患者循环造血干细胞（HSC）增多可作为骨转移的一个指标。在骨转移中，转移细胞与 HSC 竞争抢占骨髓生态位。通过甲状旁腺激素预处理或 CXCR4 抑制剂清除 HSC，可促进前列腺癌经骨髓生态位的骨转移。

　　促炎细胞因子最初来源于 Th1 淋巴细胞和 M1 巨噬细胞，它们同时也促进癌症的免疫监视和细胞毒性。Th1 淋巴细胞和 M1 巨噬细胞的作用相互促进：Th1 细胞分泌 IFN-γ 导致 M1 巨噬细胞的招募和维持其 M1 表型，进而巨噬细胞产生的 IL-12 招募、活化和维持 Th1 表型。MIG/CXCL9 和 IP-10/CXCL10 的分泌也促进 Th1 细胞和招募 CTLs，同时抑制血管生成。通过刺激 NF-κB 信号激活介导骨髓分化初反应蛋白 88（myeloid differentiation primary response protein 88，MyD88）形成 IL-1α、IL-1β 和 IL-6 的自分泌反馈回路。NF-κB 信号还可刺激 TNF-α 释放，激活 DCs 的 APC 功能，促进 M1 巨噬细胞、CD4⁺效应 T 细胞和 CD8⁺细胞的招募和细胞毒活性，并招募 NK 细胞（图 13-15）。

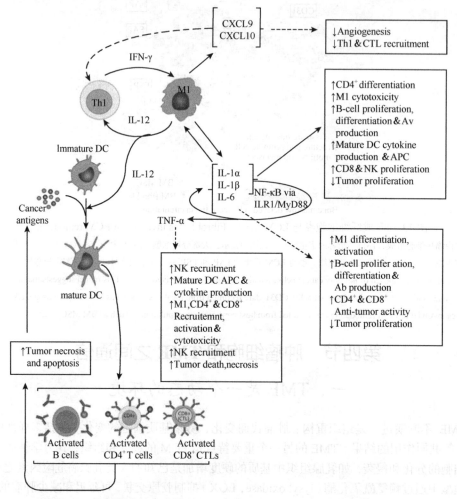

图 13-15　抑制肿瘤的炎症模型；A model of tumor-suppressing inflammation

二、TME 中免疫细胞和间质细胞的驯化作用

基质细胞和不断发展的肿瘤细胞间的相互作用是促进肿瘤进展的基础。适应性免疫和固有免疫细胞是 TME 的重要组成。免疫细胞向 Th1 型（抗肿瘤）或 Th2 型（促瘤性）发展很大程度上依赖于可溶性细胞因子和趋化因子。虽然最初用于 CD4⁺ T 细胞的描述，现已明确 Th1 型和 Th2 型因子调节几乎适用于所有免疫细胞亚型的表型和生物活性。Th2 淋巴细胞、M2 巨噬细胞和 MDSCs 相互促进增殖和分化，同时维持肿瘤性促炎和促血管生成作用。这些细胞与 Tregs 一起抑制肿瘤抑制性细胞（包括 Th1、M1、CTLs 和 NK 细胞）的活性和增殖。需要指出的是 M1 和 M2 巨噬细胞可以相互转化，但表型却是稳定的，因为 M1 和 M2 总是增强自我表型而抑制对方的表型。同样 Th1 和 Th2 淋巴细胞、Tregs 和 Th17 淋巴细胞倾向于增强自身活性而抑制其他细胞活性（图 13-16）。普通 DCs 暴露于致瘤因素后可分化为调节型 DCs（regDC），

抑制预活化 T 细胞增殖，regDC 的表型和功能不同于其前体细胞，也不同于不成熟 DCs。特别是 CD11c^{low}CD11b^{hi} 的 DCs 对植入的 3LLLewis 肺癌细胞具有免疫抑制活性，而 CD11b^{hi} 的 DCs 通过 Rho GTPase 依赖途径促进其转移。

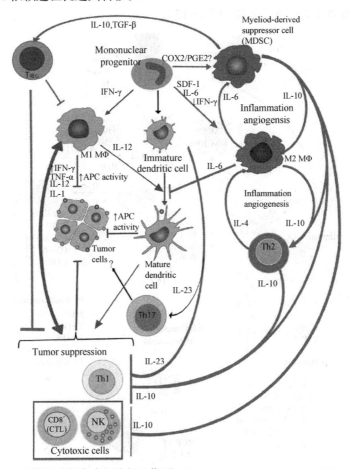

图 13-16　支持肿瘤的免疫细胞相互作用；Tumor-supporting immune cell interactions

　　巨噬细胞活化也受内源性 microRNAs 的调控。如甘露糖受体 1 基因编码的 miR-511-3p，可作为 TAMs 促瘤性极化的负调节因子，具有上调 F4/80$^+$MRC1$^+$CD11c$^+$TAMs 的功能。研究显示，巨噬细胞表型和生物学活性的关键是 NF-κB 的表达。巨噬细胞中的 NF-κB 活性对癌细胞转移的影响随空间/时间改变而变化。被循环肿瘤细胞激活的 NF-κB 具有抗肿瘤活性，相反在肿瘤进展晚期被激活的 NF-κB（如在肿瘤转移部位）对巨噬细胞的作用以促癌为主。

　　缺氧也可影响 TME 中免疫细胞的驯化，与作用于骨髓细胞的 HIF 类型有关。在低 IFN-γ 的情况下，HIF-2α 诱导 Arg1 的表达，抑制 NO 生成，促进 Th2 表型。在高 IFN-γ 的条件下，以 HIF-1α 作用为主，诱导产生 iNOS 使精氨酸转化为 NO，促进 Th1 表型。

　　肿瘤中髓源性细胞的招募也受到 B 细胞的调节。删除 B 细胞后髓系抑制细胞的扩增被阻断。Bregs 表达 IL-10 依赖于 TNF-α 的表达，因此抗 TNF-α 治疗促进抗肿瘤免疫部分是通过抑制 Bregs 表达 IL-10 而发挥作用的。

　　TME 中的 TGF-β、COX2、PGE2、Th2 相关炎症因子和促血管生成蛋白等最初是由癌细胞分泌的，新生肿瘤中的 CAFs 和其他细胞类型招募 Th2 淋巴细胞、M2 巨噬细胞（TAMs）和 N2 嗜中性粒细胞（TANs）。随后，Th2 淋巴细胞、TAMs 和 TANs 分泌更多的炎性介质和促血管生成蛋白，抑制 DCs 成熟和 CTLs 增殖活化。结果抗原提呈和细胞毒活性作用显著削弱，消除了 TME 的免疫监视作用。此外，未活化的 B 细胞增殖，可转化为肿瘤促进性 Bregs。TAMs 招募 MDSCs 至 TME，进一步增强 Th2、M2 和 N2 细胞增殖和活化的正向反馈通路，导致促肿瘤性炎症和肿瘤血管生成的持续增强（图 13-17）。

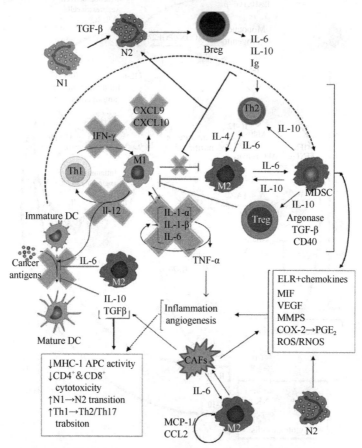

图 13-17　TME 中促肿瘤免疫细胞的协同效应；Cooperativity of cancer-promoting immune cells in the TME

　　ECM 蛋白也有助于局部免疫调节。半乳凝素（galectins），一个进化保守的糖结合蛋白家族，在驯化免疫细胞和控制血管生成中发挥重要作用。程序性死亡受体 1（programmed death-1 receptors，PD-1）是表达于 T 细胞和 B 细胞的抑制性复合受体，除外活化作用，还能导致 T 细胞耗竭，在提供 TME 免疫抑制信号中起重要作用。

　　TME 中，肿瘤细胞在"驯化"非免疫间充质细胞（如成纤维细胞、肌成纤维细胞或脂肪细胞）中发挥重要作用。通过活体显微镜和三维细胞模型的研究表明，CAFs 通过"跟随"癌细胞生成路径，局部重构 ECM，促进肿瘤细胞迁移。CAFs 介导的 ECM 重塑依赖 Rho-ROCK 信号通路，受肿瘤细胞 IL-6 的影响，CAFs 中 STAT3 活化，肌动球蛋白聚合。

　　遗传因素、表观遗传因素也有助于癌症间质的驯化。例如，结肠家族性腺瘤性息肉病（familial adenomatous polyposis coli，FAPC）影响 TME 间充质细胞，产生胶原蛋白增加。随着肿瘤从原位进展为浸润癌，恶性上皮细胞和 CAF 中 DNA 甲基化水平进一步降低。

三、肿瘤细胞与 TME 之间的交流

肿瘤细胞通过自分泌和旁分泌可溶性的信号分子介导其与宿主间质、肿瘤间质之间的交流。最常见的信号分子是 FGF、IGF、EGF、HGF、TGF-β，PDGF 家族成员。这些生长因子多数能促进肿瘤增殖和肿瘤形成。TME 细胞中表达上调其他的蛋白酶包括半胱氨酸蛋白酶家族、组织蛋白酶。组织蛋白酶 L 能加工和激活肝素酶，促进肿瘤转移、血管生成和炎症。例如，TGF-β 表现出不同特性，具有抑瘤和促瘤作用：一方面抑制上皮细胞生长，是一种肿瘤抑制基因；然而，在多种癌和肉瘤及血管增生中 TGF-β 也刺激肿瘤诱导 EMT，TGF-β 的促肿瘤作用部分由 HGF 介导。

除了这些生长因子外，细胞因子和趋化因子在 TME 中也发挥重要的信号作用。如肌上皮细胞和肌成纤维细胞表达细胞因子 CXCL14 和 CXCL12，能增加上皮细胞增殖和侵袭。

ECM 提供了肿瘤生长的周围结构；成纤维细胞和免疫细胞提供了肿瘤扩散所必需的关键信号。从这个空间发生的生理过程来看，流入的免疫细胞、间质细胞和快速分裂的肿瘤细胞大大增加对氧的需求，导致快速发展的肿瘤微环境缺氧。即使肿瘤生长仅几百个细胞，就可以启动血管生成，这就需要在上述这些分子和血管之间形成的通信。从微环境产生的生长因子和活性氧干扰新生血管内皮细胞间缝隙连接信号，可能导致更严重的缺氧和更多的异常血管生成。

因为肿瘤促进 Th2、M2、N2 和 MDSCs 活性均相互作用或自我强化，常导致炎症、血管生成及免疫抑制，所以靶向炎症和血管生成因子（如抗 VEGF 免疫球蛋白或 NSAIDs）的治疗可以协同免疫刺激治疗，如重组 IL-2、IFN-γ、TNF-α、IL-12 或 IL-18（或联合使用）。此外，靶向 TGF-β、IL-10、IL-6 和 IL-4 促进 Th2、M2、N2 和 MDSCs 细胞群的正向反馈通路（同时抑制其肿瘤抑制替代表型）、抑制 DCs 的成熟等均可成为抗肿瘤治疗的潜在靶点。靶向 Th2、M2、N2 和 MDSCs 细胞群和（或）针对有关炎症或血管生成的肿瘤促进因子的互补策略将使免疫治疗更为有效（图 13-18）。

四、肿瘤细胞与 TME 之间的交流机制

两种新的机制可能支持肿瘤细胞和 TME 之间的交流。

（一）外泌体

最初外泌体（exosomes）被认为是细胞释放有害物质的一种方式，目前已公认其具有活性，参与调节多种细胞外信号。从癌症患者血浆中分离的外泌体，其浓度和蛋白含量与肿瘤临床分期和临床预后相关。肿瘤外泌体包裹着肿瘤抗原、免疫抑制分子和 miRNA，参与动员骨髓来源细胞迁移前的生态位形成。TME 中的肿瘤细胞并非外泌体的唯一来源，CAFs 和癌症相关脂肪细胞释放含有 miR-21 的外泌体，促进肿瘤细胞迁移和侵袭。外泌体参与肿瘤细胞和基质细胞之间的双向交流。

（二）细胞融合

TAMs 和肿瘤细胞之间可发生功能性融合，诱导巨噬细胞特异性基因的表达高改变转录谱。这些巨噬细胞-癌细胞融合的杂交细胞具有模仿巨噬细胞迁移行为的能力，更容易浸润和转移。

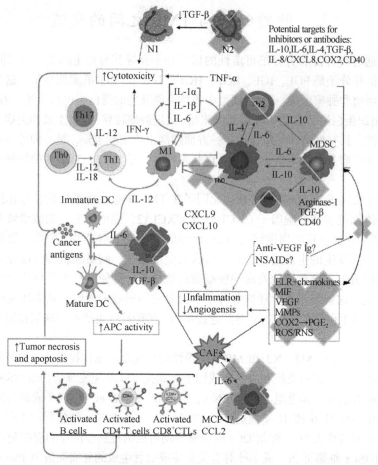

图13-18 肿瘤诱导的免疫抑制对癌症治疗的影响；Implications of tumor-induced immunosuppression for cancer therapy

五、靶向作用于 TME 的药物

靶向作用于 TME 的药物见表 13-1。

表 13-1 对 TME 进行靶向治疗的药物

靶向成分	药物归类	举例
内皮细胞/肿瘤相关的血管形成	内源性血管形成抑制剂	内皮抑素（endostatin），干扰素（IFN-α、β），白介素（IL-4、IL-12、IL-18），血栓烷素（TSP-1、TSP-2）
	合成的血管形成抑制剂	RGD 类似物，Anginex，0118
	化疗药物	5-FU 类药物（如 S-1、卡培他滨），Irofulven，美法仑，多柔比星，环磷酰胺的节律化疗，紫杉类
	抗血管的细胞因子	肿瘤坏死因子（TNF-α）
内皮细胞和树突状细胞	VEGF 信号抑制剂	贝伐单抗（bevacizumab），DC101（抗 VEGF-R2 单抗），msFLK1（可溶性 VEGF-R2）
内皮细胞、周细胞、基质细胞	小分子酪氨酸激酶抑制剂	舒尼替尼（sunitinib）、索拉非尼（sorafenib）
周细胞、成纤维细胞	PDGF 信号抑制剂	PDGFR 抑制剂（伊马替尼）
细胞外基质和血管形成	细胞外基质修饰剂	尿溶酶原激活剂/受体，基质金属蛋白酶
细胞外基质	细胞因子	IL-12 和 IL-18

续表

靶向成分	药物归类	举例
免疫细胞（淋巴细胞、NK 细胞）	细胞免疫	TIL 细胞过继输注，树突状细胞治疗，调节性 T 细胞去除
	肿瘤疫苗	细胞因子基因修饰的肿瘤疫苗
	免疫调节剂	来那度胺（lenalidomide）
免疫细胞和内皮细胞	细胞因子/趋化因子	IL-15/IL-15R, IL-2, IL-12, 分形趋化因子（fractalkine, FKN）

RGD：精氨酸-甘氨酸-天冬氨酸（arginine-glycine-aspartic acid）

挑战与展望

1. 当前面临的挑战

（1）如何评价在肿瘤启动、进展及临床前癌症模型中的 TME？

通常情况下，从整个肿瘤中提取的 DNA、RNA 对肿瘤基因组和转录因子进行分析，以及人们普遍认为的遗传和表观遗传变异及基因表达的变化对肿瘤细胞进行修饰。但情况未必如此，还必须考虑到 TME 的作用。

（2）在 TME 中免疫细胞发挥着重要的作用，但是免疫缺陷常导致肿瘤形成，此时对 TME 研究是否有价值？虽然转基因小鼠的致癌模型提供了一个理想的免疫系统，但它们代表小鼠，还没有人体癌的模型。

（3）TME 中非恶性细胞占原发肿瘤及其转移灶的 50%，但关于它们的生物学和功能仍有许多悬而未决的问题。我们对癌症进展和治疗中 TME 发展知之甚少。现在很清楚，无论是血液肿瘤还是实体瘤，都有恶性细胞的达尔文式进化，在单个肿瘤和转移的不同部位可导致异质性突变。这就提出了一个重要的问题，不同部位是否存在类似的异质性 TME 的成分？来自原发肿瘤 TME 不同于转移瘤的 TME 吗？

（4）TME 组成可以由致癌突变调节吗？的确，在乳腺癌组织中存在恶性细胞和间质细胞基因表达特征的异质性。已知不同类型的癌症之间 TME 有重要的区别。但尚不清楚相同的肿瘤发生在不同部位是否有不同的 TME 组分，此外，老化的免疫系统可以有更多的促肿瘤表型。癌症化疗和放疗不但针对肿瘤细胞，也针对 TME，这决定了治疗的成败。在设计新的癌症治疗方案中靶向 TME 重要性已显而易见。

2. 策略和展望 仅针对 TME 治疗是不可能根除癌症的，虽然该策略可能有使癌症转变成一种慢性疾病的潜力。目前努力的重点是靶向肿瘤细胞和 TME 相结合的策略。

（1）使用针对 TME 中招募和活化基质细胞信号通路的阻断剂。

（2）基于 TME 能调节肿瘤对治疗的敏感性，采用联合治疗包括靶向肿瘤细胞耐药性的通路和标准化疗和（或）靶向治疗的组合疗法。ECM 作为耐药的一个因素，也是治疗干预的目标。例如，在胰腺肿瘤中富含透明质酸基质的形成导致无灌注的血管，为肿瘤细胞提供了一个无药物作用的避难所。针对基质用透明质酸酶治疗后快速形成再灌注的血管，导致增殖下降，凋亡增加，增加对治疗的反应，改善了生存率。

（3）靶向原癌基因炎症通路，TNF、IL-6 和 CXCL12 作为肿瘤相关炎症的 3 个关键性细胞因子介导形成 TNF-α 的网络，通过旁分泌作用引起血管生成、髓衍生细胞浸润和 Notch 信号活化。采用抗人 IL-6 抗体（siltuximab）抑制肿瘤细胞中 IL-6 信号转导（STAT3 活化），已在异种移植瘤模型中显示了一定的疗效。

3. 目前关于 TME 研究主要集中在以下两方面

（1）肿瘤细胞与其 TME 中功能相关的各型细胞如何共同作用促进肿瘤侵袭和转移。

（2）在肿瘤起动和进展过程中，肿瘤细胞与其 TME 之间双向和动态的关系。

在肿瘤恶性转化的过程中，存在于 TME 中的肿瘤基质及一些除肿瘤细胞外的其他细胞分泌或表达细胞因子、蛋白酶或受体等的相互作用，可以改变组织间的渗透压，影响肿瘤组织的营养代谢环境，并发生免疫炎性作用，促进肿瘤新生血管生成等，有利于肿瘤的侵袭和转移。所以 TME 的总体作用是支持肿瘤生长和抑制免疫反应。宿主微环境通过特异因子的作用影响着肿瘤细胞的生物学特性。随着对肿瘤细胞之间、肿瘤与 TME 相互作用的信号转导和分子机制的深入研究，将为我们提供更多的信息以研究如何使肿瘤细胞恶性表型逆转及维持正常基因表型，特别是通过选择特异性化疗药物使 TME 变得更具有免疫源性，为肿瘤的诊断和治疗提供新途径。

思 考 题

1. 本章基本概念：肿瘤微环境 Tumor microenvironment（TME），肿瘤相关性纤维母细胞 Cancer-associated fibroblasts（CAFs），肿瘤相关性巨噬细胞 Tumor-associated macrophages（TAMs），髓衍生性抑制细胞 Myeloid-derived suppressor cells（MDSCs），肿瘤相关性中性白细胞 Tumor-associated neutrophils（TANs），调节性 T 细胞 Regulatory T cells(Tregcells)

2. 总结 TME 的重要元素。

3. 你怎么理解 TME 是一个动态的环境。

4. 哪些因素调节 ECM 的重塑。

5. 阅读文献，阐述某种肿瘤细胞和 TME 之间通信的机制。

6. 为什么微环境的发展需要增加氧供？

7. 简要解释肿瘤中外泌体及其作用。

参 考 文 献

[1] de Visser K E，Jonkers J. Towards understanding the role of cancer-associated inflammation in Chemoresistance [J]. Curr Pharm Des，2009，15（16）：1844-1853.

[2] Shinohara E T，Maity A. Increasing sensitivity to radiotherapy and chemotherapy by using novel biological agents that alter the tumor microenvironment [J]. Curr Mol Med，2009，9（9）：1034-1045.

[3] Hanahan D，Weinberg R A. Hallmarks of cancer：the next generation [J]. Cell，2011，4；144（5）：646-674.

[4] Onimaru M，Yonemitsu Y. Angiogenic and lymphangiogenic cascades in the tumor microenvironment [J]. Front Biosci（Schol Ed），2011，3：216-225.

[5] Räsänen K，Vaheri A. Activation of fibroblasts in cancer stroma [J]. Exp Cell Res，2010，316（17）：2713-2722.

[6] Hede K. Environmental protection：studies highlight importance of tumor microenvironment [J]. J Natl Cancer Inst，2004，96（15）：1120-1121.

[7] Fidler IJ. The pathogenesis of cancer metastasis：the 'seed and soil' hypothesis revisited [J]. Nat Rev Cancer，2003，3（6）：453-458.

[8] Lymboussaki A，Partanen T A，Olofsson B，et al. Expression of the vascular endothelial growth factor C receptor VEGFR-3 in lymphatic endothelium of the skin and in vascular tumors [J]. Am J Pathol，1998；153（2）：395-403.

[9] Minen T，Veikkola T，Mustjoki S，et al. Isolated lymphatic endothelial cells transduce growth，survival and migratory signals via the VEGF-C/D receptor VEGFR-3 [J]. EMBO J，2001，20（17）：4762-4773.

[10] Veikkola T，Jussila L，Makinen T，et al. Signalling via vascular endothelial growth factor receptor-3 is sufficient for lymphangiogenesis in transgenic mice [J]. EMBO J，2001，20（6）：1223-1231.

[11] Fukumura D，Jain R K. Tumor microenvironment abnormalities：causes，consequences，and strategies to normalize [J]. J Cell Biochem，2007，101（4）：937-949.

[12] Harris A L. Hypoxia-a key regulatory factor in tumour growth [J]. Nat Rev Cancer，2002，2（1）：38-47.

[13] Melillo G. Inhibiting hypoxia-inducible factor 1 for cancer therapy [J]. Mol Cancer Res，2006，4（9）：601-605.

[14] Taraboletti G，D'Ascenzo S，Giusti I，et al. Bioavailability of VEGF in tumor-shed vesicles depends on vesicle burst induced by acidic pH [J]. Neoplasia，2006，8（2）：96-103.

[15] Bhowmick N A，Neilson E G，Moses H L. Stromal fibroblasts in cancer initiation and progression [J]. Nature，2004，432（7015）：332-337.

[16] Cunha G R，Hayward S W，Wang Y Z，et al. Role of the stromal microenvironment in carcinogenesis of the prostate [J]. Int J Cancer，2003，107（1）：1-10.

[17] Olumi A F，Grossfeld G D，Hayward S W，et al. Carcinoma-associated fibroblasts direct tumor progression of initiated human prostatic epithelium [J]. Cancer Res，1999，59（19）：5002-5011.

[18] Tlsty T D. Stromal cells can contribute oncogenic signals [J]. Semin Cancer Biol，2001，11（2）：97-104.

[19] Tuxhorn J A，Ayala G E，Rowley D R. Reactive stroma in prostate cancer progression [J]. Urol，2001，166（6）：2472-2483.

[20] Muppalla J N，Muddana K，Dorankula S P，et al. Microenvironment-A Role in Tumour Progression and Prognosis Journal of Clinical and Diagnostic Research，2013，7（9）：2096-2099.

[21] Leyva-Illades D，McMillin M，Quinn M，et al. Cholangiocarcinoma pathogenesis：Role of the tumor microenvironment[J]. Transl Gastrointest Cancer，2012，1（1）：71-80.

[22] Hallinan N，Finn S，Cuffe S，et al. Targeting the fibroblast growth factor receptor family in cancer [J]. Cancer Treat Rev，2016，46：51-62.

[23] Manabe Y，Toda S，Miyazaki K，et al. Mature adipocytes，but notpreadipocytes，promote the growth of breast carcinoma cells in collagengel matrix culture through cancer-stromal cell interactions [J]. Pathol，2003，201（2）：221-228.

[24] Mohla S. Tumor microenvironment [J]. J Cell Biochem，2007，101（4）：801-804.

[25] Dietmar W. Siemann. Tumor Microenvironment. 2011.

[26] Sica A. Role of tumour-associated macrophages in cancer-related inflammation[J]. Exp Oncol，2010，32（3）：153-158.

[27] Mantovani A，Sozzani S，Locati M，et al. Macrophage polarization：tumor-associated macrophagesas a paradigm for polarized M2 mononuclear phagocytes [J]. Trends Immunol，2002，23（11）：549-555.

[28] Sica A，Bronte V. Altered macrophage differentiation and immune dysfunction in tumor development [J]. J Clin Invest，2007，117（5）：1155-1166.

[29] Turley S J，Cremasco V，Astarita J L. Immunological hallmarks of stromal cells in the tumour microenvironment [J]. Nat Rev Immunol，2015，15（11）：669-682.

[30] Balkwill F R，Capasso M，Hagemann T. The tumor microenvironment at a glance [J]. J Cell Sci，2012，125（Pt 23）：5591-5596.

[31] Hanahan D，Coussens L M. Accessories to the Crime：Functions of Cells Recruited to the Tumor Microenvironment [J]. Cancer Cell，2012，21（3）：309-322.

[32] Kidd S，Spaeth E，Watson K，et al. Origins of the Tumor Microenvironment：Quantitative Assessment of Adipose-Derived and Bone Marrow-Derived Stroma [J]. PLoS ONE，2012，7（2）：e30563.

[33] Brown J M. Tumor microenvironment and the response to ant icancertherapy [J]. Cancer Biol Ther，2002，1（5）：453-458.

[34] Peinado H，Lavotshkin S，Lyden D. The secreted factors responsible for pre-metastatic niche formation：old sayings and new thoughts [J]. Semin Cancer Biol，2011，21：139-146.

[35]Powell A E，Anderson E C，Davies P S，et al. Fusion between intestinal epithelial cells and macrophages in a cancer context results in nuclear reprogramming [J]. Cancer Res，2011，71：1497-1505.

[36] Kershaw M H，Devaud C，John L B，et al. Enhancing immunotherapy using chemotherapy and radiation to modify the tumor microenvironment [J]. OncoImmunology，2013，2（9）：e25962.

[37] Sun Y，Campisi J，Higano C，et al. Treatment-induced damage to the tumor microenvironment promotes prostate cancer therapy resistance through WNT16B [J]. Nat Med，2012，18（9）：1359-1368.

[38] Diresta G R，Lee J，Healey J H，et al. "Artificial lymphatic system"：a new approach to reduce interstitial hypertension and increase blood flow，pH and PO_2 in sol id tumors [J]. Ann Biomed Eng，2000，28（5）：543-555.

[39] Folkman J. Fundamental concepts of the angiogenic process [J]. Curr Mol Med，2003，3（7）：643-651.

[40] Swartz M A，Iida N，Roberts E W，et al. Tumor microenvironment complexity：emerging roles in cancer therapy [J]. Cancer Res，2012，72（10）：2473-2480.

[41] Achen M G，McColl B K，Stacker S A. Focus on lymphangiogenesis in tumor metastasis [J]. Cancer Cell，2005，7（2）：121-127.

[42] Fukumura, Jain R K. Tumor Microenvironment Abnormalities: Causes, Consequences, and Strategies to Normalize [J]. J Cell Biochem, 2007, 101 (4): 937-949.

[43] Hanahan D, Coussens L M. Accessories to the Crime: Functions of Cells Recruited to the Tumor Microenvironment [J]. Cancer Cell, 2012, 21 (3): 309-332.

（季菊玲　何　理　陈　莉）

Tumor microenvironment: the occurrence and metastasis of the tumor is closely related to the internal and external environment of the tumor cell. It includes not only the structure, function and metabolism of the tumor, but also the internal environment of the tumor cell itself (nucleus and cytoplasm). Tumor cells can improve the growth and development of tumors though altering and maintaining their own survival and development by autocretion and parecretion. Systemic and local tissues may also limit and influence the occurrence and development of tumors through changing in metabolism, secretions, immunities, structures and functions. Cancer and the environment, both of which are either interdependent and mutually reinforcing or antagonistic and fighting against each other. It is a key and central problem in modern oncology biology. In recent years, the development of cytology and molecular biology has led to more understand the interrelationship between the tumor and the environment. This is important not only to understand the occurrence, development and metastasis of tumor, and for the diagnosis, prevention and prognosis of tumor. Additionally, resistance to radiotherapy and chemotherapy is influenced by the interaction between the cancer cells and the tumor microenvironment [1-2].

Tumors do not grow in a vacuum. Instead, they are surrounded by the extracellular matrix (ECM), blood vessels, immune cells, and other supporting structures that make up human organs. Together this support system comprises a tumor microenvironment (TME).However, this is more than just a physical space. Implied within the term 'microenvironment' is a venue for these factors, including ECM, soluble growth factors and cytokines, to interact[3].There is evidence that shows that the interaction between the cancer cells and stromal cells of the microenvironment is bi-directional and dynamic. Neoplastic cells can secrete factors that recruit and activate stromal cells into the TME in a paracrine fashion. Stromal cells that have been recruited and activated can then release factors into the extracellular milieu that can stimulate or inhibit tumor growth [4-6] (Fig.13-1).

The interplay between the tumor and its microenvironment was part of Stephen Paget's 1889 "seed and soil" theory, in which he postulated that metastases of a particular type of cancer ("the seed") often metastasizes to certain sites ("the soil") based on the similarity of the original and secondary tumor sites[7]. For years cancer researchers mainly focused on a seemingly obvious target: tumor cells. While this research yielded invaluable knowledge, a comprehensive understanding of tumor behavior remains elusive. Only in recent years, cancer research experienced a paradigm shift toward trying to understand the role of the microenvironment in tumor development, growth, metastasis, and treatment.

There are two principal fields of microenvironmental research. One focuses on the physiological microenvironment. This involves the exchange of oxygen, nutrients, and waste products through tumor vasculature. The other component is cellular components, cell-cell interactions, and the matrix that makes up the tumor parenchyma in addition to tumor cells. The tumor and the surrounding microenvironment are closely related and interact constantly.

Section 1　Vascular and Metabolic Changes in TME

1. Vascular Compartment

Among the most important components of the tumor microenvironment are the growing and developing blood vessels. Both rapidly dividing tumor cells and the influx of many microenvironmental cells require oxygen and other nutrients for their survival and growth. Exchange of gas, nutrients, and metabolites over the capillary wall satisfies these requirements and maintains normal tissue homeostasis.

Likewise, cells undergoing neoplastic transformation depend on nearby capillaries for growth. Once the size of the cellular aggregate reaches the diffusion limit for critical nutrients and oxygen, however, the aggregate as a whole can become dormant. Indeed, some human tumors can remain dormant for a number of years at a stage where tumor cell proliferation and death balance. But once new blood vessel formation is initiated, which can be as early as during the hyperplastic or dysplastic phase, tumorigenesis, tumor progression, and metastasis may follow[6].New vessel formation (the process called angiogenesis) in both normal and disease tissues is governed by the net balance between pro- and anti-angiogenic factors. Under normal physiological conditions, this balance is strictly regulated so that angiogenesis is "on" when needed (e.g. embryonic development, wound healing, formation of the corpus luteum) and "off" otherwise. This balance becomes disturbed during neoplastic transformation and tumor progression. What triggers the growth of new vessels? How do these vessels compare with normal vessels with respect to structure and function? What are the consequences of their abnormal function on the tumor microenvironment?

2. Extravascular Compartment

(1) Lymphangiogenesis and Lymphatic Transport

By transporting both immune cells and interstitial fluid out of tissue, the normal lymphatic network plays an important role in immune function and in the maintenance of tissue interstitial fluid balance. Tumor cells grow in a confined space and thus create mechanical stress (solid stress), which compresses the intra-tumor blood and lymph vessels. Consequently, there are no functional lymphatic vessels inside solid tumors. Instead, functional lymphatic vessels are present in the tumor margin and the peri-tumoral tissue. Tumor cells can invade these peripheral lymphatic vessels and form metastases within the lymphatic system. Furthermore, the abnormal lymphatic valves allow retrograde flow in these lymphatic vessels and may facilitate lymphatic metastasis.

The molecules involved in angiogenesis are also involved in lymphangiogenesis. For example, VEGF-C and -D can induce both angiogenesis and lymphangiogenesis and are associated with lymphatic metastasis in a variety of tumors [8-9]. Their receptor VEGFR3 is present in both lymphatic and vascular endothelium in tumors. As is the case with vascular angiogenesis, other positive and negative regulators (e.g. angiopoietins and PDGF) are also involved in lymphangiogenesis. The mechanical and/or molecular signals that could trigger the lymphangiogenic switch are unknown. Because lymphatic vessels help maintain the balance of fluid in tissues, hydrostatic pressure is a likely trigger. Whether the hyperplasia and the increased density of lymphatic vessels seen in the tumor margins are a response to elevated hydrostatic pressure in tumors is an open question. Microlymphangiography, intravital microscopy techniques, and molecular targeting reagents revealed that these peri-tumor lymphatic vessels, which are induced by VEGF-C/D and yet-to-be-discovered lymphangiogenic factors, are able to carry cancer cells and mediate tumor metastasis. Furthermore, blockade of VEGFR3 — by inhibiting peri-tumor lymphatic hyperplasia — can inhibit early steps of lymphatic metastasis as well as the delivery of cancer cells to the lymph node [10].

(2) Interstitial Hypertension

Unlike normal tissues, in which the interstitial fluid pressure (IFP) is around 0 mmHg, both animal and human tumors exhibit interstitial hypertension (Fig.13-2). Two major mechanisms contribute to interstitial hypertension in tumors [11]. In normal tissues, the lymphatics maintain fluid homeostasis; thus, the lack of functional lymphatics in tumors is a key contributor. Indeed, the IFP reduced by placing "artificial lymphatics" in tumors. The second contributor is the high permeability of tumor vessels, endothelial cell-cell junctions are larger only in tumor vasculature with one layer. The tumor IFP begins to increase as soon as the host vessels become leaky in response to angiogenic molecules such as VEGF. Furthermore, tumor IFP goes up and down with the microvascular pressure within seconds. As a result, the hydrostatic and oncotic (colloid osmotic) pressures become almost equal between the intravascular and extravascular spaces. Reduced or lack of transmural pressure gradients decrease convection across tumor vessel walls and thus compromise the delivery of therapeutic agents. Furthermore, IFP is nearly uniform throughout a tumor and drops precipitously in the tumor margin. Thus, the interstitial fluid oozes out of the tumor into the surrounding normal tissue, carrying away the drug with it. Finally, transmural coupling between IFP and microvascular pressure due to the high permeability of tumor vessels can abolish pressure difference between up- and down-stream tumor blood vessels and lead to blood flow stasis in tumors without physically occluding the vessels.

Since IFP is a reflection of the global pathophysiology of tumors, it may be used for diagnosis and/or prognosis. The steep rise of IFP at the tumor periphery can be used to locate tumors during needle biopsy and improve diagnosis of patients. Furthermore, a study of cervical cancer has shown that elevated tumor IFP can predict a poor outcome of radiation therapy. Further studies are needed to evaluate the prognostic significance of IFP in human tumors. Decreasing vascular permeability might restore the transmural pressure gradients and potentially resume/re-establish blood flow in the nonperfused regions of tumors. Some direct and indirect anti-angiogenic therapies might "normalize" the tumor vasculature through this mechanism. In fact, IFP can be lowered by antibodies against VEGF or VEGFR2.

3. Metabolic Enviroment

Hypoxia and acidosis are hallmarks of the metabolic environment in solid tumors. Both oxygen tension (PO_2) and pH are important determinants of tumor growth, metabolism, and response to a variety of therapies such as radiation therapy, chemotherapy, hyperthermia, and photodynamic therapy.

(1) Hypoxia

A key function of the vasculature is to provide adequate levels of nutrients and oxygen to the parenchymal cells and to remove waste products. Based on the anatomy of the capillary bed and a mathematical model of oxygen diffusion and consumption, the Nobel laureate August Krogh introduced the concept of a diffusion limit for oxygen of 100~200 μm nearly a century ago. This unit of tissue—a single capillary surrounded by a 100~200 μm radius cylinder—is referred to as a "Krogh cylinder" in physiology. Fifty years ago, Thomlinson and Gray identified similar "cords" in human lung cancer and found necrotic cells beyond 180 mm away from blood vessels, presumably due to lack of oxygen. This is referred to as "chronic hypoxia" or "diffusion-limited" hypoxia. Although various hypoxia markers and microelectrodes have suggested these gradients, the first direct measurements of these perivascular gradients—along with PO_2 and blood flow rate of the same vessels— became possible only with the development of phosphorescence quenching microscopy.

Because blood flow in tumor vessels is intermittent, and thus, some regions of a tumor are starved for oxygen periodically. The resulting hypoxia is referred to as "acute hypoxia" or "perfusion-limited hypoxia". A necessary consequence of intermittent blood flow is the resumption of blood flow after shutdown, and the resulting production of free radicals can lead to "reperfusion injury" or "reoxygenation injury," applying additional selection pressure on cancer cells.

Hypoxia results from an imbalance between oxygen delivery and consumption, tissue oxygenation will fall as a result of either diminished arteriolar supply or increased oxygen consumption. First, the tumor receives an inadequate amount of oxygenated blood due to a limited arteriolar supply, which causes small tumor vessels far from the originating arterioles to contain very low levels of oxygen. Second, tumor vessels are oriented in such a way that some regions are well perfused (or even overly perfused) and others do not have enough vascularity. Also related to vessel distribution and orientation, the third feature is that the center of a tumor tends to have fewer vessels than the tumor periphery. Some tumor microvessels contain many red blood cells, whereas others contain few or none at all. Thus, the fourth feature is that tumors show wide variations in red blood cell flux, defined as the number of red blood cells that traverse a particular microvessel per unit time. All of these cause an imbalance between oxygen supply and demand, which is the fifth aspect of tumor hypoxia. Interestingly, Secomb et al. has shown that the amount of hypoxia in a tumor depends more heavily on oxygen consumption than either flow rate or arteriolar PO_2. Thus, the growing and developing microenvironment creates conditions that require increases in oxygen supply to maintain normoxia and support continued growth[12].

The oxygen tension in normal tissues generally exceeds 20mmHg. When the PO_2 dips below 10 mmHg, the hypoxic tissue begins to produce specific proteins mediated by hypoxia-inducible factor-1 (HIF-1), which has been referred to as the master regulator of oxygen homeostasis. In addition to oxygen tension, free radicals, especially oxygen containing radicals such as superoxide (O^{2-}), modulate HIF-1 levels. HIF-1 is a heterodimeric transcription factor that increases the expression of genes involved in angiogenesis, adaptation to hypoxia, invasiveness, and resistance to oxidative stress [13].

Accumulation of HIF-1 in a tumor mediates and integrates four major aspects of tumor biology: mutations and metabolism in addition to hypoxia and angiogenesis. The most notable and well study of the effects of HIF-1 are the transcriptional activation of genes involved in angiogenesis, most notably VEGF.

VEGF is a key regulator of vascular adaptation and angiogenesis. The HIF-1 complex binds to the hypoxia-responsive element upstream of the VEGF gene, directly activating VEGF transcription [14]. Other HIF-1 activated genes involved in angiogenesis include angiopoietin 1 and 2, placental growth factor, and PDGF B.

Hypoxia, HIF1, and NFkB activation help drive autophagy in the tumor microenvironment, while the upregulation of TIGAR (TP53-induced glycolysis and apoptosis regulator) in cancer cells protects the magainst apoptosis and confers autophagy resistance. TIGAR is a known inhibitor of both autophagy and apoptosis, and functionally shifts cells away from aerobic glycolysis, towards oxidative mitochondrial metabolism. This scenario allows for the vectorial and unilateral transfer of energy from the tumor stroma (catabolism) to cancer cells, thereby fueling anabolic tumor growth via oxidative mitochondrial metabolism in cancer cells (Fig.13-3).

(2) Low pH

Another consequence of the abnormal microcirculation of the tumor is low extracellular pH. There are at least two sources of H^+ ions in tumors—lactic acid and carbonic acid. The former results from anaerobic glycolysis and the latter from conversion of CO_2 and H_2O via carbonic anhydrase. The intracellular pH of cancer cells remains neutral or alkaline (pH 7.4), however, in spite of the acidic extracellular   pH. One would expect low extracellular pH and hypoxia to track each other and to co-localize with regions of low blood flow. Surprisingly, there is a lack of spatial correlation among these parameters, a discovery made possible by recent developments in optical techniques that permit the simultaneous high-resolution mapping of multiple physiological parameters. A potential explanation for this lack of concordance is that some perfused tumor vessels carry hypoxic blood. Thus, although they might not be able to deliver adequate oxygen to the surrounding cells, they may be able to carry away the waste products (e.g., lactic acid) [14].

(3) Regulation of Angiogenic Gene Expression by Metabolic Microenvironment

Generation of pro- and anti-angiogenic molecules can be triggered by metabolic stress. Hypoxia upregulates various angiogenic growth factors, including VEGF, Ang2, PDGF, placenta growth factor (PGF), transforming growth factor (TGF), IL-8, and hepatocyte growth factor (HGF). Of the various molecules involved in sensing and responding to hypoxia, Hypoxia inducible factor-1a (HIF-1a) is considered to be the master regulator of oxygen homeostasis. This transcription factor is upregulated in a number of human tumors. Hypoxia may play an important role in the angiogenic switch, which is required for tumor growth and expansion.

Low extracellular pH causes stress-induced alteration of gene expression, including the upregulation of VEGF and IL-8 in tumor cells in vitro. Despite its importance, the effect of the low and heterogeneous interstitial pH on VEGF expression in vivo, especially in relationship with hypoxia remained unknown for many years due to the lack of appropriate techniques and animal models. The combination of fluorescence ratio imaging microscopy for pH measurements, phosphorescence quenching microscopy for PO_2 measurements, and the transgenic technology for visualization of VEGF promoter activity has allowed the coordinated study of pH, PO_2, and VEGF expression in vivo. Overall, tissue PO_2 but not pH was inversely correlated with VEGF promoter activity. However, detailed analysis revealed an important insight into the regulation of VEGF by the metabolic environment. Under low pH or oxygenated conditions, tissue pH, but not PO_2, is related to VEGF promoter activity. Conversely, under hypoxic or neutral pH conditions, tissue PO_2 and not pH is correlated with VEGF expression. These results indicated that VEGF transcription in tumors is independently regulated by the tissue PO_2 and pH. In fact, subsequent analysis of the VEGF promoter region revealed that acidic pH induces VEGF expression distinct from the HIF-HRE mediated pathway. Taken together these data suggest that two major metabolic microenvironments in solid tumors regulate angiogenic factors in a complimentary manner.

Section 2   Cellular Components in TME

Cancers are not just masses of malignant cells but complex 'rogue' organs, to which many other cells are recruited and can be corrupted by the transformed cells. Interactions between malignant and non-transformed cells create the tumor microenvironment. The non-malignant cells of the TME have a dynamic and often tumor-promoting function at all stages of carcinogenesis. Intercellular communication is driven by a complex and dynamic network of cytokines, chemokines, growth factors, and inflammatory and matrix remodeling enzymes against a background of major perturbations to the physical and chemical properties of the tissue. The evolution, structure and activities of the cells in the TME have many parallels with the processes of wound healing and inflammation, but cells such as macrophages are also found in cancers that have no known association with chronic inflammatory conditions. One reason for this is that inflammatory and wound-healing processes are activated downstream of oncogenic mutations in the malignant cells. In this part we will describe the functions of major non-malignant cell types that are found in the TME of most human and experimental cancers. In stromal cells, particularly inflammatory cells, vascular endothelial cells, and fibroblasts, have been shown to actively support tumor growth in murine models of tumorigenesis [15-18]. Vascular endothelial cell proliferation and recruitment leading to the formation of new blood vessels provides the tumor with the nutrient supply necessary for its growth and metastasis. Cancer-associated fibroblasts can stimulate angiogenesis as well as promote tumor growth and invasion. The immune cells present in the TME, tumor-associated macrophages in particular, can confer resistance to toxic insults in addition to promoting growth. Finally, the proliferation of lymph endothelial cells leading to the increase in lymphatic vessel density can promote tumor metastasis (Fig. 13-4).

1. Reactive Stroma Cells

(1) Cancer-associated Fibroblasts

When tissues are injured, residential fibroblasts differentiate into myofibroblasts in response to paracrine signals. The induction of myofibroblasts can also cause organ fibrosis, which enhances the risk of cancer development. Myofibroblasts are abundant in many TMEs and are also called cancer-associated fibroblasts (CAFs) [19].

CAFs are a heterogenous group of fibroblasts whose function is pirated by cancer cells and redirected toward carcinogenesis. These cells are usually derived from the normal fibroblasts in the surrounding stroma but can also come from pericytes, smooth muscle cells, fibrocytes, mesenchymal stem cells (MSCs, often derived from bone marrow), or viaepithelial-mesenchymal transition (EMT) or endothelial-mesenchymal transition (End-MT). Unlike their normal counterparts, CAFs do not retard cancer growth *in vitro*.

CAFs perform several functions that support tumor growth, such as secreting VEGF, FGFs, PDGF, and other pro-angiogenic signals to induce angiogenesis. CAFs can also secrete TGF-β, which is associated with EMT, a process by which cancer cells can metastasize [20], and is associated with inhibiting cytotoxic T cells and natural killer T cells, and contributes to the immune-suppressive microenvironment. As fibroblasts, CAFs are able to rework the ECM to include more paracrine survival signals such as IGF-1 and IGF-2, thus promoting survival of the surrounding cancer cells. CAFs are also associated with the Reverse Warburg Effectwhere the CAFs perform aerobic glycolysis and feed lactate to the cancer cells. Such as effects of signaling molecules (HGF, hepatocyte growth factor), PDGF (platelet-derived growth factor), SDF-1 (stromal derivedfactor-1) and so on .secreted by cholangiocarcinoma-derived CAF on cholangiocarcinoma progression [21] (Fig. 13-5).

Fibroblast-produced CXCL12 chemokine can promote growth and survival of malignant cells and also has chemoat tractant properties that stimulate the migration of other stromal cell types and their progenitors into the TME. In mouse models of skin, breast and pancreatic tumors, CAFs express a proinflammatory gene signature, which contributes to the support of tumor growth by enhancing neovascularisation and the recruitment of immune cells. These tumor-promoting effects are abolished upon inhibition of the transcription factor NF-kB, suggesting that, in stromal cells, this inflammatory signaling pathway has an important function in tumor progression. Another major contribution of fibroblasts to the composition of the TME is their secretion of ECM components and of ECM remodeling enzymes.

In some cancers, CAFs are arranged in fibrovascular cores that branch throughout the tumor mass, whereas in others, they surround the malignant cells with dense desmoplastic stroma that can occupy the majority of the space and thus restrict the ability of anti-cancer drugs to reach the malignant cell target. An increased density of CAFs is often seen at the invasive front of a tumor.

A recent study investigated the impact of deleting cells that are positive for the fibroblast marker fibroblast activation protein-a (FAP) in tumor-bearing mice. Depletion of these cells induced tumor necrosis that was mediated by IFN-c and TNF-a, and the authors also showed that FAP- a positive TME cells are important mediators of immune suppression [22].

(2) Adipocytes

In some cancers, for instance intraabdominal tumors that metastasize to the omentum, adipocytes actively aid the recruitment of malignant cells through the secretion of adipokines and also promote the growth of malignant cells by providing fatty acids as fuel for the cancer cells [23].

(3) Vascular Endothelial Cells

Many soluble factors present in the TME, such as VEGFs, FGFs, PDGFs and chemokines stimulate endothelial cells and their associated pericytes during the neovascularization that is needed for cancer growth [24]. When a quiescent blood vessel senses an angiogenic signal from malignant or inflammatory cells, or owing to hypoxic conditions in the TME, angiogenesis is stimulated and new vessels sprout from the existing vasculature. The tumor vasculature is abnormal in almost every aspect of its structure and function. For example, blood vessels are heterogeneous with chaotic branching structures and an uneven vessel lumen, and are leaky. The leakiness of the vessels raises the interstitial fluid pressure causing unevenness of blood flow, oxygenation, nutrient and drug distribution in the TME. This, in turn, increases hypoxia and facilitates metastasis.

(4) Pericytes

Perivascular stromal cells, known as pericytes, are an integral component of the tumor vasculature that provide structural support to blood vessels. Clinical studies, for example in bladder and colorectal cancer, suggest that low pericyte coverage of the vasculature correlates with poor prognosis and increased metastases. An explanation for the association of pericyte coverage with poor prognosis has come from a recent study, in which pericyte depletion in mouse genetic models suppressed primary tumor growth, but increased hypoxia, EMT and MET receptor activation.

Pericyte depletion in these mouse experiments also enhanced metastasis, the authors further showed that low pericyte coverage coupled with activation of the MET receptor correlated with a poor prognosis in women with invasive breast cancer. Hence 'normal' pericyte coverage of the tumor vasculature might act as a key negative regulator of metastases.

(5) Lymphatic Endothelial Cells

Tumors drive lymphangiogenesis or lymphatic hyperplasia through the production of VEGFC or VEGFD. Although tumor cells can invade existing lymphatic vessels, if malignant cells or macrophages secrete high levels of VEGFC or VEGFD, the TME will have extensive lymphatic vessel sprouting, enlargement of collecting lymph vessels and lymph node lymphangiogenesis. Lymphatic endothelial cells in the TME and lymphatic vessels formed by them have an important function in the dissemination of malignant cells, there is emerging evidence that they also affect the progression of cancer by mechanically modulating the TME and by altering the host immune response to the tumor [25].

2. Infiltrating Immune Cells

The immune system makes an invaluable contribution to the tumor microenvironment. Inflammatory cells secrete growth factors, cytokines, and chemokines that stimulate epithelial proliferation and generate reactive oxygen species (ROS) that damage DNA, promoting tumor initiation and progression. They also release proteolytic enzymes, leading to matrix remodeling and angiogenesis.

Although various immune effector cells are recruited to the tumor site, their anti-tumor functions are downregulated, largely in response to tumor-derived signals. Infiltrates of inflammatory cells present in human tumors are chronic in nature and are enriched in regulatory T cells (Treg) as well as myeloid derived suppressor cells (MDSC). Immune cells in the tumor microenvironment not only fail to exercise antitumor effector functions, but they are co-opted to promote tumor growth. Sustained activation of the NF-κB pathway in the tumor milieu represents one mechanism that appears to favor tumor survival and drive abortive activation of immune cells. The result is tumor escape from the host immune system. Tumor escape is accomplished through the activation of one or several molecular mechanisms that lead to inhibition of immune cell functions or to apoptosis of anti-tumor effector cells. The ability to block tumor escape depends on a better understanding of cellular and molecular pathways operating in the tumor microenvironment. Novel therapeutic strategies that emerge are designed to change the protumor microenvironment to one favoring acute responses and potent anti-tumor activity.

(1) Tumor-associated Macrophages

Tumor initiation and progression are intimately related to inflammation and the immune system. A major risk factor for the development of various tumor types is chronic inflammation of the target organ. Within a tumor, tumor-associated macrophages (TAMs) are the primary immune cell found. Macrophages have the ability to secrete pro- or anti-inflammatory mediators depending on the stimuli [26]. Macrophages activated with TNF-α have anti-tumor activity and signal tissue destruction, this is known as an M1 phenotype. The M2 phenotype characterized by the initiation of tissue repair, remodeling, and tumor promotion can be induced by IL-4 activation [27]. Most TAMs are the M2 phenotype, as a result of multiple signals expressed within the TME which include IL-10, TGF-β, and colony stimulating factor-1.These immunomodulatory signals have been reported to be secreted by myeloid-derived suppressor cells, IL-10$^+$ B lymphocytes, Th2 helper T cells, and the tumors themselves [26]. Alterrnatively activated TAMs have reduced anti-tumor activities, and increase the production of angiogenic mediators that include VEGF and IL-10, in addition to M2-specificgenes known to be involved in the promotion of cell proliferation. These events are summarized in Figure13-6. Strategies that inhibit the M2 phenotype and induce M1 signals can reestablish the anti-tumor functions of TAMs and aid in the removal of protective signals that originate from the M2TAMs, perhaps activating the innate immune response thus leading to a reduced tumor size[28].

TAMs are a central component in the strong link between chronic inflammation and cancer. TAMs are recruited to the tumor as a response to cancer-associated inflammation. Unlike normal macrophages, TAMs lack cytotoxic activity. TAMs have been induced in vitro by exposing macrophage progenitors to different immune regulatory cytokines, such as IL-4 and IL-13.

TAMs are abundant in most human and experimental murine cancers and their activities are usually pro-tumorigenic. According to Condeel is and Pollard, TAMs are obligate partners for malignant cell migration, invasion and metastases. Most TAMs have an IL-10 high, IL-12 low phenotype with expression of the mannose receptor and scavenger receptor class A (SR-A, also known as SCARA). TAMs gather in necrotic regions of tumors where they are associated with hiding cancer cells from normal immune cells by secreting IL-10, aiding angiogenesis by secreting VEGF and nitricoxide synthase(NOS), supporting tumor growth by secreting EGF and remodeling the ECM. TAMs show sluggish NF-Kb activation, which allows for the smoldering inflammation seen in cancer. There is pre-clinical and clinical evidence that an increased amount of TAMs is associated with worse prognosis (TAMs represent a potential target for novel cancer therapies).

Additionally, gene array studies in follicular lymphoma demonstrate that the expression of genes that are associated with a strong 'macrophage' signature confers a poor prognosis, independent of other clinical variables. Macrophages are major contributors to tumor angiogenesis. Transcriptional profiling on high-density oligonucleotide arrays of TAMs shows that they are highly enriched in transcripts that encode angiogenic molecules. Comparison of TAM transcriptomes with available clinical databases shows that these transcriptional signatures are predictive of survival.

The bidirectional interaction between macrophages and the tumor microenvironment shapes their phenotype and response to the environmental conditions. Tumor hypoxia is important, because many TAMs accumulate in hypoxic and/or necrotic areas of tumors. It is thought that these areas attract TAMs by releasing hypoxia-induced chemoattractants, such as VEGF, endothelins and endothelial-monocyteactivating polypeptide II (EMAP2, also known as AIMP1). A distinct, hypoxia-induced pro-angiogenic human macrophage phenotype has been identified

(2) T Lymphocytes

T lymphocytes become activated via a two-signal process in which ①T-cell receptor must bind to an antigen presented on a major histocompatibility complex (MHC) protein expressed on the cell surface of another cell, and ②CD28 must concurrently bind with its ligands, B7-1 or B7-2.Without this second signal, T cell anergy (inactivation) will result, and the adaptive immune response is inhibited. As part of a fail-safe mechanism to prevent over-active autoimmune responses, T cell anergy may also result if the co-inhibitory receptor cytotoxic T lymphocyte-associate protein-4 (CTLA-4) competes to bind CD28 ligands or if programmed death-1 (PD-1) receptor binds its ligand, PD-L1 (Fig. 13-7).

There are many different T cell populations within the TME that infiltrate the tumor areas, at the invasive tumor margin and in draining lymphoid organs[29-31]. Among these, cytotoxic CD8$^+$ memory T cells (CD8$^+$ CD45RO$^+$), which are normally antigen 'experienced' and capable of killing tumor cells, which is CD8$^+$ cytotoxic lymphocytes (CTLs), are strongly associated with a good prognosis. All T helper lymphocytes are differentiated cell types derived from the same common immature T helper progenitor (Th0). Depending upon what cytokines the Th0 cells are exposed to, they may differentiate into one of several different T helper phenotypes: type 1 T helper cells (Th1), type 2 T helper cells (Th2), Treg or type 17 T helper cells (Th17). Th1 and Th2 cells are generally considered terminal, permanent phenotypes. Some in vitro evidence suggests that Treg and Th17 cells may be somewhat more plastic; However, neither reversion of any of these T helper types back to a Th0 progenitor phenotype nor conversion of Th17 cells to a Treg phenotype have been reported (Fig. 13-8）.

CD8$^+$ T cells are supported by Th1 cells, which are characterized by the production of the cytokines IL-2 and interferon gamma (IFN-γ); high numbers of these in the TME also correlate with a good prognosis. Other CD4$^+$ cell populations, such as Th2 cells producing IL-4, IL-5 IL-6, IL-10 and IL-13, which support B cell responses, or Th17 cells, producing IL-17A, IL-17F, IL-21 and IL-22 that favor antimicrobial tissue inflammation, are generally thought to promote tumor growth, although they have also been associated with a favorable outcome, as in the case of Th2 cells in breast cancer and Th17 cells in esophageal cancers. The CD4$^+$ T cells most often described as tumor promoting are the immunosuppressive Tregs, which are characterized by expression of FOXP3 and CD25. Constitutive and induced Tregs exert an immune suppressive function through the production of IL-10, TGF-β and cell-mediated contact through cytotoxic CTLA4, inhibiting recognition and clearance of tumor cells by the immune system. High numbers of Tregs in the TME correlate with worse prognosis in many types of cancer. Tregs can also be tumor suppressive as in some B cell cancers; their presence in Hodgkin's lymphoma correlates with a good prognosis, presumably through a direct suppression of tumor cell growth. γδT lymphocytes have some characteristics of innate rather than adaptive immune cells and show potent cytotoxic activity against a wide range of malignant cells, including cancer stem cells. Although experimental animal cancer studies suggest they exert immune surveillance activity, it is not yet certain whether the presence of γδT cells in the TME reflects a good or bad prognosis.

(3) B Lymphocytes

B cells can be found at the invasive margin of tumors, but are more common in draining lymph nodes and lymphoid structures adjacent to the TME. B cell infiltration into the TME is associated with good prognosis in some breast and ovarian cancers; however, this is in contrast to mouse models, in which B cells inhibit tumor-specific cytotoxic T cell responses. More recent data support a tumor-promoting role for B cells and immunoglobulin deposition in a genetic mouse model of skin cancer. An immunosuppressive population of IL-10 producing B cells, known as regulatory B cells (Bregs) or B10 cells, increases tumor burden and inhibits tumor-specific immune responses in inflammation-induced skin cancer, and also appear to favor lung metastasis in a mouse model of breast cancer. Bregs also inhibit the clearance of tumor cells by anti-CD20 antibodies in a mouse model of lymphoma. However, none of these effects are due to Bregs infiltrating the TME; instead they appear to affect other immune cells in the surrounding lymphoid tissue or in the draining lymph node, as well as modulate the activity of myeloid cells. It remains to be established if B cells and Bregs in particular have similar roles in human cancers.

(4) Myeloid-derived Suppressor Cells

Myeloid-derived suppressor cells (MDSCs) are a heterogenous population of cells of myelogenousorigin with the potential to repress T cell responses[32]. Interactions between CD40 receptors on MDSCs and CD40 ligand (CD40L) on Tregs can short-circuit this response by releasing a number of immunosuppressive cytokines. This results in decreased production of IFN-γ and IL-2 in the TME due to the suppression of Th1 activation and the promotion of Th2 polarization, as well as a concomitant decrease in the activation and cytotoxic activity of cytotoxic T lymphocytes (CTLs) and natural killer (NK) cells. Additionally, CD40 receptor expression on MDSCs is increased. (Fig. 13-9). MDSCs regulate wound repair and inflammation and are rapidly expanded in cancer, correlating with that signs of inflammation are seen in most if not all tumor sites. Tumors can produce exosomes that stimulate inflammation via MDSCs. The characterization of human MDSCs is difficult as their phenotype is quite variable. Indeed, they can even differentiate into TAMs. Murine and human MDSCs inhibit CD8+ T cell activation through the expression of nitric oxide synthase 2 (NOS2) and arginase (ARG1). They also induce the development of Tregs and the polarization of macrophages to a TAM-like phenotype.

(5) NK and NKT Cells

Innate cytotoxic lymphocytes, natural killer (NK) cells and natural killer T (NKT) cells, also infiltrate the tumor stroma, but are not found in contact with tumor cells. For many cancers, such as colorectal, gastric, lung, renal and liver, they appear to predict a good prognosis. However, although they are present in the TME, NK cells might not be able to exert their tumor-killing function. A number of studies reported that NK cells in the tumor stroma have an anergic phenotype that is induced by malignant cell-derived transforming growth factor beta (TGF-β).

(6) Dendritic Cells

Dendritic cells (DCs) have important functions in antigen processing and presentation. The DCs that are found in the TME are thought to be defective, that is, they cannot adequately stimulate an immune response to tumor-associated antigens[29-31]. The hypoxic and inflammatory microenvironment of the TME further impairs DC function to activate immune function, and some DCs have been found to suppress T cell responses at the tumor site. Two recent studies designate ZBTB46 as a new transcription factor that is specifically expressed in all classical human and murine DCs. This work suggests that DCs are a unique immune cell lineage and will help in our understanding of DCs in the TME(Fig 13-10).

(7) Tumor-associated Neutrophils

The contribution of tumor-associated neutrophils (TANs) to primary tumor growth and metastasis is somewhat controversial[29-31]. There is evidence that neutrophils promote primary tumor growth in mouse cancer models and have a pro-tumorigenic effects by enhancing angiogenesis increasing degradation of the ECM and immune suppression(Fig.13-11). Furthermore, CD11b$^+$ bone-marrow-derived cells, a heterogeneous myeloid cell population, have been associated with priming of the premetastatic lung and enhanced seeding of circulating tumor cells. By contrast, an antitumor function of these cells has been observed following immunological or cytokine activation. Under these conditions, neutrophils can actively eliminate disseminated tumor cells, as well as indirectly through inhibition of TGF-β.

(8) Metabolic interplay through shuttling of metabolites among different cell compartments in TME serves as a form of intercellular communication and intercellular coordination. T effector cells (T_{eff}), CTL, DCs, and TAM-M1 may form a potential metabolic antagonism (Fig. 13-12red color makerd) with tumor cells. On the contrary, T_{regs}, MDSC and TAM-M2 may preferentially utilize metabolic products of tumor to form a potential metabolic symbiosis (Fig. 13-12, blue color marked) in TME.

Multiple stromal cell types and subcell types of the TME can variably contribute to different tumor types and subtypes, and stages of progression (Fig. 13-13). In Fig. 13-13, the lists of subtypes and of their key functions are not comprehensive, but rather prominent examples. Not listed are molecular regulatory signals for, and effector agents of, the noted functions. Both lists will certainly be refined in coming years [31]. Also not shown are the crucial cancer cells and cancer stem cells, with which these stromal cells dynamically interact to manifest cancer phenotypes.

Section 3   Extracellular Matrix Remodeling

Within a carcinoma, epithelial cells are supported by a three-dimensional structure known as the ECM. The proteins that make up the ECM are produced by fibroblasts. The stroma is separated from the epithelium and endothelium by the base mentmembrane, a specialized type of ECM composed of collagen IV, laminin, and heparan sulfate proteoglycans.

There are considerable differences in matrix composition between tumor stroma and the stroma associated with normal tissue. Cells from the tumor secrete a variety of proteins into the ECM that are involved in cell adhesion, motility, communication, and invasion. Notably, some of these molecules are involved in degrading the ECM. This degradation occurs near the tumor-host interface, where the tumor-derived proteases overwhelm the host' sendogenous inhibitors leading to extensive remodeling and stimulating alternative signals from the cell surface. Remodeling is achieved by combined efforts of secreted and membrane-anchored matrixmetalloproteinases (MMPs), adamalysin-related membrane proteases, bone morphogenicprotein-1-type metalloproteinases, endoglycosidases, and tissue serine proteases including tissue plasminogen activator, urokinase, thrombin, and plasmin. Interestingly, most of these factors involved in remodeling the tumor-host interface originate from host cells, not from the growing carcinoma.

Infiltrating inflammatory cells release MMP-9, MMP-12, and MMP-8 from intracellular stores, but they also release cytokines including IL-1β and tumor necrosis factor-α (TNF-α) that stimulate fibroblasts to produce more MMPs. In addition to fibroblasts and inflammatory cells, paracrine signal stimulate other stromal cells to be the predominant source of microenvironmental MMPs during tumorigenesis.

Secreted MMPs degrade both ECM and other proteins in the microenvironment, including growth factors, cytokines, and receptors. Therefore, the effects of individual MMPs on the microenvironment are diverse, but they are critical players in establishing the environment surrounding tumor cells. One potent example is MMP-7, which is expressed by malignant breast epithelial cells. MMP-7 degrades the ECM, disrupts the basement membrane, and cleaves E-cadherin, weakening the connection between breast epithelial cells.

MMPs are found in the microenvironment in zymogen form, and they require activation by other MMPs and related molecules. MMP overexpression alone, which has often been reported in tumors, does not explain MMP activity in the microenvironment, since immunohistochemistry often does not distinguish between the zymogen and active forms. Under normal conditions MMPs are also regulated by endogenous tissue inhibitors of metalloproteinases (TIMPs), so the balance between TIMPs and MMPs critically affects the microenvironment.

To balance these remodeling and degradative enzymes, synthesis of matrix components is upregulated by both the tumor and host. Activated fibroblasts synthesize collagen type I and fibronectin in response to the binding of mast cell tryptase toprotease-activated receptor-2 involved in ECM remodeling (Fig. 13-14).

Macrophages also contribute IL-1β and NOS, both of which augment type I collagen synthesis. The newly synthesized collagen that forms the peri-tumoral stroma is loosely woven and disorganized, contributing to the overall disorder surrounding a developing tumor.

Section 4　Communication between Tumor Cells and TME

1. TME is a Dynamic Milieu

The TME is in constant evolution as a result of tissue remodeling, metabolic alterations in the tumor, and changes in the recruitment of stromal cells including a diversity of immune cells. Tissue remodeling that occurs in the post-partum breast during mammary gland involution, for example, perpetuates an increased risk of breast cancer. Pepper Schedin (University of Colorado, Aurora, CO) described how such remodeling creates a tumor-promoting inflammatory environment similar to the environment of a wound, characterized by an influx of Th 2-type macrophages, abundant fibrillar collagen, and increased COX-2 activity. Human mammary tumor cells implanted into mouse mammary fat pads formed tumors more readily, with increased metastatic potential, when implanted in involuting (postlactation) mammary glands, rather than during pregnancy, whereas COX-2 inhibition during weaning slowed tumor growth and limited metastasis. These results raise the intriguing possibility that short-term anti-inflammatory treatment during the postpartum period may decrease breast cancer risk, similar to results in colon cancer.

Another important feature of the TME is the content and organization of the ECM, whose mechanical properties affect neoplastic cell differentiation and invasiveness. Increased stromal stiffness in breast tissue is a known risk factor of breast cancer in humans, as described how inhibition of collagen cross-linking by lysyl oxidase (LOX) in murine models delayed and decreased tumor invasion. ECM stiffening promoted activation of ROCK, a Rho kinase effector, which increased collagen deposition by mechanisms associated with increased Wnt signaling, activation of STAT3, and expression of inflammatory cytokines, including CCL2 and granulocyte macrophage colony-stimulating factor (GM-CSF), that recruited bone marrow (BM)-derived cells into the TME. These compelling data indicate that changes in the biomechanical function of the TME impact neoplastic cell proliferation and migration, as well as secretion of immunomodulatory factors. Using second harmonic generation microscopy showed that altering the alignment of collagen fibers in solid tumors impacted malignant cell invasion and their metastatic properties, in part, via regulation of TNF-α and macrophages. Thus, the involuting mammary gland not only the amount of stromal collagen but also its organization are drivers of the malignant process.

Dynamic interactions between tumor cells and cells of the bone marrow niche (Fig. 13-15) affect malignant evolution. It has been appreciated for some time that in patients with prostate cancer, increased presence of circulating hematopoietic stem cells (HSC) is an indicator of bone metastasis. Russell Taichman showed that prostate carcinomas seeded into BM remained dormant and insensitive to drug treatment. During bone metastasis, these cells competed with HSCs for occupation of the bone marrow niche. Similarly, altering the bone marrow niche in mice by pretreatment with parathormone or by clearing HSCs with a CXCR4 inhibitor promoted prostatic bone metastasis.

Anticancer therapies alter the TME in ways that either promote or inhibit tumorigenicity, depending on a diverse array of heterotypic mechanisms[33]. This concept was elegantly illustrated for the case of anti-VEGF therapy by Gabriele Bergers (University of California San Francisco) who showed that glioblastoma-bearing mice treated with Avastin exhibited a transient beneficial therapeutic response that was followed by tumor revascularization and enhanced invasiveness associated with increased c-Met expression and epithelial-to-mesenchymal transformation (EMT). This is explained by the observation that VEGFR2 and c-Met were antagonistically associated, where c-Met signaling became dominant in the presence of VEGFR2 signaling blockade and vice versa. Thus, combined therapy targeting both signaling pathways may be required for efficient, durable antitumor responses.

2. Significance of Immune and Stromal Cell Education in the TME

Emerging studies indicate that reciprocal interactions between the diverse assemblages of stromal cells and evolving neoplastic cells fundamentally regulate tumor progression. Adaptive and innate immune cells represent a significant component of the TME. Largely dependent on soluble cytokines and chemokines, immune cells become variably polarized toward TH1- (generally antitumor) or Th2-type (generally protumor) phenotypes. While initially described for CD4$^+$T cells, it is now clear that Th1- and Th2-type factors regulate the phenotype and bioactivity of essentially all immune cells subtypes. Th2 lymphocytes, M2 macrophages and MDSCs mutually reinforce the proliferation and phenotypes of one another, as well as maintaining tumor-promoting inflammation and angiogenesis. These cells, along with Tregs suppress the activity and proliferation of tumor-suppressing cells, including Th1, M1 and CTLs and NK cells. It should be noted that M1 & M2 macrophages can interconvert, but these phenotypes are stable as the M1 and M2 expression profiles reinforce their own macrophage phenotypes, while suppressing the other. Similarly, Th1 & Th2 lymphocytes, as well as Tregs & Th17 lymphocytes tend to self-reinforce their own activation profiles and inhibit the other (Fig. 13-16). Michael Shurin (University of Pittsburgh, Pittsburgh, PA) showed that conventional dendritic cells (DCs) exposed to tumor-derived factors polarize into regulatory DCs (regDC) that suppressed the proliferation of preactivated T cells and were phenotypically and functionally different from their precursors and from immature conventional DCs. In particular, CD11clow CD11b high DCs exhibited immunosuppressive activity toward implanted 3LL Lewis lung carcinoma, whereas CD11c high DCs instead promoted their metastasis dependent on RhoGTPase. In the presence of Clostridium difficile toxin, DCs failed to polarize and exhibited altered activity and effector functions. Related to DCs, the significance of macrophage Th2 polarization was reported by Lisa Coussens. Th2-type TAM are common constituents of many solid tumor types and not only provide proangiogenic and proinvasive factors to growing tumors but also suppress CTL mediated antitumor immunity. Accordingly, blocking recruitment of macrophages into mammary tumors by treating mice with agents that blocked CSF1R signaling not only diminished tumor vascularity and slowed primary tumor development but also reduced formation of pulmonary metastases and improved survival, when given in combination with chemotherapy, by CD8$^+$T-cell-dependent mechanisms. These preclinical data highlight the multifunctional role of macrophages in solid tumors and importantly reveal that TAMs blunt cell killing by $CD8^+$T cells as well as by various forms of chemotherapy suggesting a novel combinatorial anticancer approach. A therapeutic CSF1R kinase inhibitor, PLX3397, is currently being tested with eribulin in a phase Ib / II clinical trial in patients with metastatic triple-negative breast cancer.

Macrophage polarization is also modulated by endogenous microRNAs (miR). Michele de Palma presented data identifying miR-511-3p, an miRNA encoded by the mannose receptor*Mrc1*gene that was specifically upregulated in $F4/80^+MRC1^+CD11c^+$ TAMs and functioned as a negative regulator of TAM protumoral polarization. Also, critical for macrophage phenotype and bioactivity is the expression of the NF-κB. Fiona Yull reported that NF-κB activation in macrophages variably affected carcinoma cell metastasis dependent on spatial/temporal features. When activated in the presence of circulating tumor cells, NF-κB exerted antitumorigenic activities whereas when activated later in tumor progression, for example, in secondary sites of metastasis, protumorigenic activities on macrophages predominated.

Hypoxia can also affect immune cell education in the TME depending on the type of HIF involved in myeloid cells. That whereas HIF-1α fostered Th1 polarization, HIF-2α instead favored Th2 polarization of immune cells. Experimentally, when HIF-2α was either inhibited via acriflavine or genetically deleted, $CD68^+$macrophage infiltration into colons of mice challenged with dextran sodium sulphate (DSS) was decreased, and carcinogenesis was reduced. Randall Johnson presented complementary data showing that HIF regulated inducible nitric oxide synthase (iNOS) and arginase 1 (Arg1) expression. In the presence of low IFN-γ, HIF-2α induced the expression of Arg1, reducing the production of NO and fostering a T_H2 phenotype. Under conditions of high IFN-γ, HIF-1α dominated and iNOS was induced converting arginine into NO and promoting a T_H1 phenotype.

Tumor recruitment of myelocytic cells is also regulated by B cells. Using a mouse model of squamous cell carcinoma induced by K-Ras expression in basal keratinocytes，the K-ras activation led to cutaneous inflammation, including expansion of immunosuppressive myeloid cells. However, when B cells were deleted, myeloid suppressor cells were ablated, indicating the requirement of B cells to stimulate the recruitment and suppressive activity of these myeloid cells. Notably, Breg expression of IL-10 was critically dependent on TNFα expression, suggesting that anti-TNFα therapy promotes antitumor immunity by suppressing B regulatory expression of IL-10.

In the TME, first, TGF-β, COX2, PGE2, Th2-associated inflammatory factors and proangiogenic proteins are secreted by cancer cells, CAFs and other cell types in the nascent tumor recruit Th2 lymphocytes, M2 macrophages (TAMs) and N2 neutrophils (TANs). Then, Th2 lymphocytes, TAMs and TANs secrete additional inflammatory and proangiogenic proteins that suppress maturation of DCs and proliferation and activation of CTLs. As a result, antigen presentation and cytotoxic activities plummet, practically eliminating immunosurveillance in the tumor milieu. Additionally, B cells proliferate, but are not activated, turning the minto tumor-promoting Bregs. M2 macrophages recruit MDSCs to the TME, further reinforcing the positive feedback loop of Th2, M2, and N2 proliferation and activation, resulting in substantial increases in tumor-promoting inflammation and concomitant angiogenesis (Fig. 13-17).

ECM proteins also contribute to local immunoregulation. Sabina Sangaletti showed that the matricellular secreted protein acidic rich in cysteine (SPARC) with profibrotic actions was expressed in remodeling tissues and in tumors and promoted Th1-type polarization by regulating expression and activation of TGF-β1 and in turn modulating macrophage production of TNFα. In the absence of SPARC, macrophages did not down modulate TNFα in response to TGF-β1, and thus fostered fibrosis. SPARC could thus be a potential therapeutic target to render the TME unsuitable for cancer cell proliferation.

Galectins, a family of evolutionarily conserved glycan-binding proteins, play an important function in educating immune cells and controlling angiogenesis. Gabriel Rabinovich discussed how galectin-1 associated with VEGFR2 in tumor-associated endothelial cell stimulated VEGFR2-mediated signaling and angiogenesis in the absence of VEGF. Accordingly, a monoclonal antibody (mAb) against galectin-1 inhibited growth of Kaposi sarcoma and B16 melanomas in mice with increased recruitment of Th17-type lymphocytes and decreased tumor vascularization.

In addition to polarization, programmed death-1 (PD-1), an inhibitory coreceptor expressed on T and B cells, exhaust T cells, plays an important role in providing immune-inhibitory signals in the TME. Effector T cells (activated CD4$^+$T cells or T helper cells) may be "exhausted" (inactivated) by PD-1 on their surface binding to PD-L1 ligands on target tumor cells. Also, Tregs can exhaust effector T cells by CTLA-4 on their cell surface binding to B7-1or B7-2 on tumor cells, which releases a soluble factor that causes effector T cell "exhaustion"; a likely suspect for this effect is TGF-β1. Drew Pardoll (Johns Hopkins University, Baltimore, MD) showed that PD-1 was expressed by activated T and B cells and monocytes and interacted with the ligand B7-H1 expressed by DCs and many tumor cells, providing them with adaptive resistance and an immune escape mechanism. Accordingly, a therapeutic mAb against B7H1 is currently being tested in a phase I clinical trial in patients with advanced solid tumors and preliminary data suggest clinical activity against melanoma and non-small cell lung cancer(NSCLC).

Nonimmune mesenchymal cells, such as fibroblasts, myofibroblasts, or adipocytes, play an important role in TMEs where they are "educated" by neoplastic cells. Frank Marini used mice transplanted with EGFP-labeled BM cells to show that BM-derived mesenchymal progenitor cells (MPC) were recruited into primary tumors where they differentiated into CAF, expressing fibroblast activation protein (FAP) and fibroblast-specific protein (FSP). The presence of these cells in the tumor affected growth and promoted immune escape. Deletion of CD44 led to a loss of FAP/FSP-producing cells in the tumor, suggesting that CD44 was critical for their recruitment. When in the TME, MPCs and CAFs interact with tumor cells by a variety of mechanisms. One mechanism is activation of the hedgehog (HH) pathway. MPCs and CAFs are a source of multiple growth factors and chemokines/cytokines including IL-6 and FAP. Yves DeClerck (University of Southern California, Los Angeles, CA) reported that IL-6 expression in MPCs was increased in the presence of tumor (neuroblastoma) cells and that it activated STAT3, which by upregulating expression of survivin, Mcl-1, and Bcl-xL in neoplastic cells, increased their resistance to cytotoxic drugs. Interestingly, TAMs collaborated with MPCs by being a source of the agonistic soluble IL-6 receptor enhancing STAT3 activation. Targeting CAFs may be an attractive therapeutic target; however, it may have a toxic effect as these cells are present in normal tissue. Using intravital microscopy and 3-dimensional cell-based models, Eric Sahai (London Research Institute, London, United Kingdom) showed that CAFs contributed to tumor cell migration by locally remodeling the ECM to generate routes used by "following" carcinoma cells. ECM remodeling by CAFs depended on Rho-Rock signaling that occurred under the influence of neoplastic cells via IL-6 that induced actomyosin polymerization in CAFs by STAT3 activation.

Genetic factors can also contribute to education of the stroma in cancer. Germ line mutations that affect formation of carcinomas such as in the case of familial adenomatous polyposis coli (FAPC) affect mesenchymal cells in the TME. For example, Monica Bertagnolli (Harvard Medical College, Boston, MA) presented data showing that in$Apc^{Min/+}$mice, Wnt signaling was also deregulated in mesenchymal cells and desmoid tumors formed as the result of a COX-2-dependent activation of the mesenchyme associated with an increased production of collagens. Furthermore, epigenetic factors may contribute. Benjamin Tycko (Columbia University, New York, NY) showed that in pancreatic intraepithelial neoplasia, there was a decrease in global methylation not only in malignant epithelial cells but also in CAFs. DNA methylation further decreased as lesions progressed from *in situ* to invasive carcinoma. Interestingly, in transgenic mice prone to develop pancreatic cancers, treatment with the hypomethylating agent 5-azacytidine led to a hypomethylation crisis associated with reduction in tumor growth and upregulation of a subset of IFN target genes affecting cell proliferation.

3. Communication Between the Tumor Cells and TME

It is clear that many components go into making up a heterogeneous tumor that is capable of surviving, growing, and invading other tissues. However, this complex system requires organization. Communication between the tumor cells, host stroma, and tumor stroma is mediated by soluble autocrine and paracrine signaling molecules. The most common of these factors are members of the FGF, insulin-like growth factor (IGF), EGF, hepatocyte growth factor (HGF), TGF-β, and PDGF families. The majority of these fibroblast-derived factor senhance proliferation and tumorigenesis. Other proteases that are upregulated in the cells of the TME include a large family of cysteine proteases, the cathepsins. Cathepsin L, for instance, processes and activates heparanase, thereby aiding metastasis, angiogenesis and inflammation.

However, TGF-β exhibits different properties. Secretion of TGF-β regulates cell proliferation and normal fibroblast transformation. Early studies showed that TGF-β inhibits the growth of epithelial cells, and subsequent transgenic mouse experiments reinforced the hypothesis that TGF-β is a tumor suppressor. However, TGF-β is also known to both stimulate tumor progression by inducing epithelial-tomesenchymaltransition (EMT) in a variety of carcinomas and sarcomas and promote angiogenesis. Therefore, TGF-β exhibits both tumor suppressive and tumor promoting behavior. At least some of the protumor effects of TGF-β appear to be mediated by HGF.

In addition to these growth factors, cytokines and chemokines play an essential signaling role in the microenviron mental milieu. Analysis of the gene-expression profiles of cells from normal breast and breast carcinomas showed that expression of the cytokines CXCL14 and CXCL12 by myoepithelial cells and myofibroblasts augments epithelial cell proliferation and invasion. CXCL12, in addition to promoting proliferation, enhances recruitment of endothelial progenitor cells (EPCs), thereby supporting angiogenesis. The proangiogenic effects of CXCL12 may be mediated by MMP-9, since the cytokine is known to activate MMP-9 in bone marrow cells and MMP-9 knockout mice are unable to respond to CXCL12-triggered EPC recruitment. CXCL12 also affects inflammatory cells in the tumor microenvironment, and these effects are likely synergistic with those of TGF-β.

While cancer cells are critical components of a malignant tumor, they develop in acomplicated milieu that makes up the tumor's microenvironment. The ECM provides a structure around which a tumor grows. Fibroblasts and immune cells contribute key signals necessary for tumor propagation. But the physical microenvironment does not exist in isolation from the physiological processes occurring within this space. The influx of immune and stromal cells and rapid division of tumor cells greatly increases the demand for oxygen, causing regions of hypoxia in the rapidly evolving microenvironment. To grow beyond even a few hundred cells, tumors initiate angiogenesis, which requires communication between all of these elements and the developing vessels. Seemingly, growth factors and ROS from the microenvironment interfere with gap junction communication between endothelial cells in the neovasculature, which likely induces more hypoxia and aberrant angiogenesis. Only by understanding tumors in the context of the complex interactions between these components can we hope to find effective ways to kill tumors and treat human malignancies.

4. The Mechanisms of Communication between Tumor Cells and TME

Two novel mechanisms potentially supporting the communication between tumor cells and stromal cells.

(1) Exosomes

Initially considered to be primarily responsible for release of unwanted material by cells, exosomes are now recognized as active entities involved in regulating a variety of extracellular signals. Exosomes have been isolated from the plasma of patients with cancer, and their concentration and protein content correlated with tumor stage and clinical outcome. David Lyden (Cornell University Weill Medical College, New York, NY) presented data suggesting that tumor exosomes, which package not only tumor antigens and immunosuppressive molecules but also miRs, were involved in mobilizing BM-derived cells to premetastatic niches. Preconditioning of BM cells with exosomes purified from metastatic melanoma cells, transplanted into lethally irradiated recipient mice significantly increased metastasis. Tumor cells within the TME are not the sole source of exosomes, and Ngai-Na Chloe Co (University of Texas MD Anderson Cancer Center, Houston, TX) from Samuel Mok's laboratory presented work showing that CAFs and cancer-associated adipocytes from ovarian tumors released miR-21 containing exosomes that in co-culture, transferred miR21 to tumor cells promoting migration and invasion. Exosomes thus appear to be involved in a 2-way communication between tumor cells and stromal cells[34].

(2) Cell Fusion

Melissa Wong (Oregon Health and Science University) presented *in vitro* and *in vivo* data showing that functional fusion between TAMs and neoplastic cells occurred and altered the transcriptome by introducing the expression of macrophage-specific genes. These macrophage-carcinoma cell fusion hybrid cells may be more prone to migrate and metastasize due to their ability to mimic migratory behaviors of macrophages[35].

Section 5 Clinical Implications

Although there might be heterogeneity in the composition of the TME as discussed above, the common features of many TMEs suggest that targeting the cells that are present, or mediators of their communication have applications across different tumor types and could also complement other treatment options.High throughput cancer therapeutics screens are performed *in vitro* without the accompanying microenvironment. However, studies also investigate the effects of supportive stroma cells and their resistance to therapy. The latter studies revealed interesting therapeutic targets in the microenvironment including integrinsandchemokines.

1. Enhancing Immunotherapy Using Chemotherapy and Radiation to Modify TME

TME is a complex assortment of cells that includes a variety of leukocytes. The overall effect of the microenvironment is to support the growth of tumors and suppress immune responses. Immunotherapy is a highly promising form of cancer treatment, but its efficacy can be severely compromised by an immunosuppressive TME. Chemotherapy and radiation treatment can mediate tumor reduction through cytotoxic effects, but it is becoming increasingly clear that these forms of treatment can be used to modify TME to liberate tumor antigen sand decrease immunosuppression. Chemotherapy and radiotherapy can be used to modulate TME to enhance immunotherapy.

Targeted therapies using small molecules that inhibit signaling pathways represent alternative drug treatments for some malignancies with less toxic profiles, and these are also able to lead to changes in the TME. However, some molecular pathways targeted by small molecule inhibitors can be important in the survival and function of immune system cells, and some targeted therapies can be detrimental to immune responses. A greater understanding of the impact of these drugs on immune system components and the TME will enable the design of more effective combination treatments for cancer. Thus, the TME can be rendered more immunogenic by choosing particular types of chemotherapeutic agent [36].

The treatment of TME components as a new target can overcome many of the current limitations of traditional treatments. Targeted therapy for the tumor matrix will not be too toxic because of the specificity of the target. Unlike tumor cells, the genes of endothelial cells are stable and therefore unlikely to be mutated. In addition, in view of the multiple components of targeted therapy in tumor microenvironment of the joint application, can avoid the single target tumor by compensatory remedy when needed by the survival environment. In addition, the combination would reduce the amount of the individual dose, thereby reducing the toxic side effects associated with treatment. The ultimate goal of this treatment is to improve the effectiveness of the treatment and extend the survival of the patient. Targeted drugs of ME are seen in Table 13-1.

Table 13-1　A drug targeted to the TME

Targeted ingredients	Drug classification	For example
Endothelial cells/neoplastic vessels formed	Endogenous angiogenesis inhibitors	Endostatin, IFN-α,β,IL-4, IL-12 ,IL-18, TSP-1, TSP-2
	Synthetic angiogenesis inhibitors	RGDanalogue, Anginex, 0118
	Chemotherapy drugs	5-FU (S-1, capecitabine), Irofulven, Marfarlane, azithromycin, cyclophosphamide and chemoradiotherapy, yew
	The cytokines that resist blood vessels	TNFα
Endothelial cells and dendritic cells	VEGF signal inhibitors	Bevacizumab, DC101, msFLK1 (VEGF-R2)
Endothelial cells, pericytes, and stromal cells	Small molecule tyrosine kinase inhibitors	Sunitinib、Sorafenib
pericytes, fibroblasts	PDGF signal inhibitors	PDGFR inhibitors
ECM and angiogenesis	ECM modifier	lysozyme/receptor, MMP
ECM	Cytokines	IL-12, IL-18
Immune cells (lymphocytes, NK cells)	Cellular Immune	TIL cell relay infusion, dendritic cell therapy, Treg removal
	Tumor vaccine	A tumor vaccine that is genetically modified by cytokines
	Immune modulators	Lenalidomide
Immune cellsandEndothelial cells	Cytokines/chemokines	IL-15/IL-15R，IL-2，IL-12,Fractalkine(FKN)

RGD：arginine-glycine-aspartic acid

2. Correcting Hypoxia

Oxygen is an important component of radiation therapy. Ionized radiation directly and indirectly damages DNA, and the effect of both is dependent on oxygen. Therefore, hypoxia in solid tumors significantly reduces their radiation sensitivity. Tumor hypoxia correlated with poor outcome. Tumor hypoxia is also associated with resistance to some chemotherapeutics such as bleomycin and neocarzinostatin.

Hypoxia induces apoptosis via p53 and HIF-1- dependent mechanisms. On the other hand, tumor cells develop many mechanisms to survive under hypoxic conditions including HIF-HRE mediated inductions of the genes for angiogenesis, vasodilation, glycolysis, and hematopoiesis. Mutations in p53 make tumor cells resistant to apoptosis and more prone to further mutations. The balance between hypoxia-induced apoptosis/ necrosis and the increased resistance to cell death mediated by various hypoxia-induced pathways determines whether a tumor can survive and even grow under hypoxic conditions. Immune cells targeting tumor cells cannot be fully functional under hypoxic conditions and thus, allow tumors to evade the host immune response and cell based therapies. Furthermore, exposure to hypoxia alters tumor cells to be highly invasive and metastatic. Ultimately, hypoxia might select for tumor cells that are more malignant, more aggressive, and genetically unstable, and less susceptible to apoptosis, thus rendering them resistant to various therapies. Therefore, several molecules in the hypoxia-induced pathways are now being targeted in the development of diagnostic and therapeutic agents.

For nearly half a century, considerable preclinical and clinical efforts have been focused on alleviating hypoxia. These efforts include improving tumor perfusion with mild hyperthermia or drugs; increasing oxygen content of the blood (via hyperbaric oxygenation, for example); or increasing hemoglobin/ hematocrit (via erythropoeitin, for example). Unfortunately, these strategies have not shown much success in the clinic. One reason for the failure is abnormal structure and function of tumor vasculature causing uneven perfusion. This makes it difficult to increase PO_2 in all regions of tumors to optimal levels and/or to deliver radiation sensitizers or chemotherapeutic drugs to all regions of a tumor at therapeutically effective levels. Alternatively, one can exploit tumor hypoxia by using cytotoxic agents which are specifically activated under hypoxia. Although this approach would allow high therapeutic index (ratio between effect on tumors and normal tissues), the physiological barrier in solid tumors may not permit the delivery of these drugs to all hypoxic cells.

3. Correcting Low Extracellular pH

Low extracellular pH can also affect the outcome of therapeutics adversely or in some case favorably. Despite the low extracellular pH, the intracellular pH in tumor cells in vivo remains neutral. As a consequence, significant intracellular-extracellular pH difference exists in tumors [38]. This trans-membrane pH gradient hinders the cellular uptake of weak base drugs such as adriamycin, doxorubicin, and mitoxantrone and thus, their efficacy. Acidic pH also causes dysfunction of immune cells. On the other hand, it may be exploitable for the treatment of cancer by weak acid drugs such as chlorambucil that are membrane permeable in their uncharged state. In an acidic extracellular environment, the non-ionized fraction of a weak acid increases, allowing more drugs to diffuse through the cell membrane into the relatively basic intracellular compartment where the ionized fraction increases, resulting in an increased intracellular drug concentration. Systemic injection of glucose could further acidify extracellular pH without changing intracellular pH and enhance tumor growth delay by a weak acid drug (chlorambucil), whereas worsen the effect of a basic drug (doxorubicin).

There is, however, a caveat in acidifying tumor to enhance the efficacy of certain drugs. Exposure of tumor cells to acidic extracellular pH induces expression of proteinases which facilitates invasion and metastasis. As discussed earlier, acidic pH induces expression of angiogenic factors and thus contributes to growth of metastatic tumors. Normalization of tumor vasculature by antiangiogenic agents may neutralize the acidic extracellular pH in tumors. Increasing interstitial pH toward normal values may enhance efficacy of base drugs and reduce the metastatic potential of tumor cells.

4. Anti-angiogenic Agents

The balance of endogenous pro- and antiangiogenic factors is well maintained in normal tissues [39]. Excess production of pro-angiogenic molecules and/or diminished production of anti-angiogenic molecules may cause abnormalities in vessels and microenvironment in tumors resulting in insufficient drug delivery and therapeutic efficacy. Thus, if one were to judiciously downregulate angiogenic signaling such as VEGF, which is overexpressed in the majority of solid tumors, then the vasculature might revert back to a more "normal" state. Indeed, neutralizing antibody against VEGF receptor 2 pruned the immature and leaky vessels of transplanted tumors in mice and actively remodeled the remaining vasculature so that it more closely resembled the normal vasculature. This "normalized" vasculature had less leaky, less dilated, and less tortuous vessels with a more normal basement membrane and greater coverage by perivascular cells. These changes in tumor vasculature were accompanied by normalization of the tumor microenvironment—decreased IFP, increased tumor oxygenation, and presumably neutralized pH. As a result, penetration of drugs in these tumors and efficacy of radiation treatments were improved.

Anti-VEGFR2 antibody-induced vascular normalization may be transient. The combination of anti-angiogenic treatment and radiation therapy delayed tumor growth synergistically only when ionizing radiation was given during this "normalization window". Therefore, prolongation of the normalization window would make the normalization strategy more clinically beneficial. Understanding of cellular and molecular mechanisms of vascular normalization would help such a development. Along that line, we found that perivascular cell recruitment via Tie2 signaling and normalization of basement membrane by balancing its synthesis and degradation appear to be involved in the vascular normalization induced by anti-VEGFR2 treatment. Finding and validating reliable surrogate markers is also urgently needed not only for clinical translation of the vascular normalization strategy, but also for antiangiogenic treatment in general. Circulating endothelial cells appear to be a useful candidate. Furthermore, it is critical to determine the presence and extent of vascular normalization with different clinically available anti-angiogenic agents in different type of orthotopic tumors. Our current goal is to exploit this knowledge to improve the therapeutic outcome and to prolong the overall survival of patients beyond the 2-5 months which is currently achievable with bevacizumab. To this end, we and others have initiated a number of preclinical studies and corresponding clinical trials in cholangiocarcinoma, glioblastoma multiforme, head and neck, breast and ovarian cancers, and sarcoma patients using antibodies or tyrosine kinase inhibitors that target VEGF and / or PDGF pathways.

5. Other Immunotherapies and Kinase Inhibitors

Since tumor-promoting Th2, M2, N2 and MDSC activities are all mutually self-reinforcing and generally promote inflammation and angiogenesis as well as immunosuppression, therapies that target inflammatory and angiogenic factors (such as anti-VEGF immunoglobulin or NSAIDs) may be synergistic with immunostimulatory treatments, such as recombinant IL-2, IFN-γ, TNF-α,IL-12 or IL-18 (or combinations thereof). Additionally, the central roles of TGF-β, IL-10, IL-6 and IL-4 in the positive feedback loop supporting Th2, M2, N2 and MDSC populations (and inhibiting their tumor-suppressing alternative phenotypes) and inhibition of DCs maturation make these potential targets for antitumor therapies. Overall, this model suggests that any successful cancer therapy will likely improve antitumor immune response and that immunotherapies may benefit from complementary strategies for targeting Th2, M2, N2 and MDSC populations and/or their tumor promoting effects on inflammation and angiogenesis.[40] (Fig. 13-18)

Antibodyies targeting immunoregulatory membrane receptors succeeded in some patients with melanoma, MSCLC, urothelial bladder cancer and renal cell cancer. In mice, anti-CTLA-4 therapy leads to clearance from the tumor of Foxp3$^+$ Treg whose presence may impair effector T cell function. Similarly anti-PD-1/anti-PD-L1 therapy blocks the inhibitory PD-1 receptor. Other, potentially more fundamental TME inhibitory reactions (as in microsatellite stabl colorectal cancer, ovarian cancer, prostate cancer, and PDA) have yet to be overcome. The TME appears to aid in excluding killer T cells from the vicinity of cancer cells.

Many other small molecule kinase inhibitors block the receptors for the growth factors released, thus making the cancer cell deaf to much of the paracrinensignaling produced by CAFs and TAMs. These inhibitors include Sunitinib, Pazopanib, Sorafenib and Axitinib, all of which inhibit platelet derived growth factor receptors (PDGF-Rs) and VEGFRs. Cannabidiol (acannabisderivate without psychoactive effects) has also been shown to inhibit the expression of VEGF in Kaposi's sarcoma. Natalizumabis amonoclonal antibodythat targets a molecule responsible for cell adhesion (integrin VLA-4) and has promising in vitroactivity in B cell lymphomas and leukemias. Trabectedinhas immunomodulatory effects that inhibit TAMs. An antitumor mAb (cetuximab) in treating B cells lymphoma that binds to TA (EGFR) on tumor cell surface, whereas Fc region of mAb binds to FcγR on immune cells (NK cells). This event activates NK cells leading to the lysis of tumor cells that generates TA and TA: mAb complex. The tumor antigenic materials are engulfed by immature DC and TA are processed and presented by mature DC to generate TA-specific T cells via MHCI through cross-presentation. Mature DC may furthermore activate NK cell reciprocally. Moreover, cytokines secreted by mAb-activated NK cells during ADCC may provide additional maturation inducing signals to DC（Fig. 13-20）.

6. The sentinel lymph node

Many tumors metastasize first to the sentinel lymph node after entering lymphatic vessels around the tumor. Although tumor-associated lymphatic vessels were previously considered passive transporters of fluid, molecules, and cells, the last decade has seen numerous reports correlating lymphatic growth factors in the TME with metastatic potential. Furthermore, observations that sentinel lymph nodes undergo lymphangiogenesis before metastasis led to the notion that lymph node lymphangiogenesis may be involved in the premetastatic niche[41]. Some presentations illustrated how tumor-associated lymphatic vessels, lymph flow, and the sentinel lymph nodes promote immune tolerance and distant metastasis.

Michael Detmar discussed how podoplanin, expressed by lymph node stromal cells in the T-cell zone, can be present in the tumor stroma and how its presence correlated with tumor lymphangiogenesis. One mechanism by which podoplanin-induced lymphangiogenesis occurred is via endothelin-1 upregulation. In vitro, podoplanin increased tumor cell motility as well as lymphatic endothelial cell (LEC) migration and tubulogenesis. Podoplanin upregulation may be induced by increased lymph flow to the draining lymph nodes, which occurs in lymphangiogenic tumors unless metastasis is extensive enough to be obstructive. Interestingly, both increased lymph flow from the tumor as well as lymph node metastasis appear to depend on tumor-draining lymph node lymphangiogenesis, according to new evidence presented by Alanna Ruddell (Fred Hutchison Cancer Research Center, Seattle, WA). She showed that lymphangiogenesis in the tumor-draining lymph nodes was dependent on B cells and that normally metastatic tumors grown in B-cell-deficient mice failed to provoke lymph node lymphangiogenesis, to increase flow or metastasis. Furthermore, in Eμ-c-Myc mice with B-cell expansion in the lymph node, melanoma and lymphoma metastasis to the sentinel lymph node was increased and more rapid, and hematogeneous metastasis also increased. However, metastatic colonization of the same tumors after intravenous injection was unchanged in these mice, supporting the hypothesis that B-cell-driven lymph node lymphangiogenesis affects lymphatic spread of lymphoma and melanoma and that hematogeneous spread occurs after lymphatic spread.

Why does sentinel lymph node lymphangiogenesis promote metastasis? Melody Swartz (Swiss Federal Institute of Technology, Lausanne, Switzerland) presented data suggesting that lymphatic involvement by tumors and lymph node lymphangiogenesis promoted tolerance from host immunity. B16 melanoma expression of VEGF-C protected tumors against preexisting, vaccine-induced immunity. VEGF-C upregulated CCL21 in the tumor stroma, which attracted naive T cells and promoted their education in the regulatory chemokine environment. In addition, LEC in the sentinel lymph node could cross-present tumor antigen MHC class I molecules leading to CD8$^+$T-cell deletion, supporting a new role for LECs in tolerance. On the other hand, CCL21 in tumors and lymphoid stroma drove antitumor as well as protumor effects by attracting naive and regulatory T cells along with antigen-presenting cells. David Peske (University of Virginia, Charlottesville, VA) from the laboratory of Victor Engelhart showed that CCL21 expression in the stroma of ovalbumin-expressing melanomas could attract adoptively transferred naive ovalbumin-specific CD8$^+$T cells after adoptive transfer from T-cell receptor transgenic mice and activated them in the TMEs. In contrast, naturally arising host CD8$^+$T cells proliferated from a rare population of naive CD8$^+$T cells and existed in balance with regulatory T cells. These studies highlight the importance of context and timing for both antitumor immune responses and tumor tolerance to develop.

The session closed with Dontscho Kerjaschki (University of Vienna, Wien, Austria) describing new work on mammary carcinomas, whose lymph node metastasis correlated with lymphangiogenesis in the sentinel lymph nodes and with metastatic tumors but not with the primary tumor. Histopathology of invasive mammary tumors revealed large gaps in lymphatic vessels where tumor cells entered, and this was consistent with *in vitro* data showing tumor spheroids forming gaps in LEC monolayers. Invasive but not benign tumors induced this gap formation, and only in lymphatic but not blood endothelial cells, in a lipoxygenase-dependent manner. In mice with lipoxygenase knockdown, metastasis was prevented, even in VEGF-C-overexpressing tumors. These exciting new data identify lipoxygenase as a potential new drug target to prevent lymphatic spread of mammary carcinomas.

7. Significance of Chronic Infection in TME

A chronic inflammation in tumors has been linked to activation of oncogenic pathways, increased tissue remodeling and tumor vascularization and the development of tumor immune escape mechanisms (Fig. 13-21) .

(1) The microbial floracan be friend or foe of cancer

The recent possibility of examining the entire microbiome in the gut is shedding new light on the role of commensal/pathogenic bacteria in cancer initiation and progression. One of the burning questions is how the microbiota regulates the inflammatory components of the TME and affects inflammation-associated carcinogenesis. The protumorigenic role of gut*Helicobacter hepaticus*in extra-intestinal carcinogenesis was discussed by Susan Erdman (Massachusetts Institute of Technology, Cambridge, MA) who reported that introduction of *H. hepaticus*to Apc$^{Min/+}$ Rag2$^{-/-}$ mice led to development of colitis and intestinal tumors but also to mammary gland tumors heavily infiltrated with macrophages. Systemic anti-TNFα treatment or adoptive transfer of IL-10 producing CD4$^+$T regulatory cells abolished both intestinal and mammary tumorigenesis. Because Rag2$^{-/-}$mice lack both T and B cells, inflammation-associated carcinogenesis found in Apc$^{Min/+}$Rag2$^{-/-}$mice was mediated by cells of the innate immune system. The presence of mammary tumors in these mice suggest that *H. hepaticus*inhabiting the gut elicits a systemic inflammatory reaction driven by innate immune cells that is also carcinogenic in tissues not directly in contact with the pathogens. Noriho Iida (NCI, Frederick, MD) explored the potential ability of intestinal commensal bacteria to augment antitumor immune responses in treatment-induced acute inflammation. They used a model in which mice subcutaneously implanted with melanoma cells and treated with an anti-IL-10R antibody and intratumoral injection of CpG oligonucleotides developed an intratumoral hemorrhagic necrosis due to production of TNFα by macrophages and exhibited prolonged survival. He showed that depletion of gut commensal bacteria by administration of antibiotics impaired production of TNFα in the tumor and decreased survival in treated colon carcinoma and melanoma-bearing mice. Thus, proper activation of innate myeloid cells by CpG nucleotides requires an intact intestinal microbiota. These two presentations illustrate the opposite roles that the microbial flora may have on cancer initiation and progression as a function of the type of inflammation present.

During chronic pathogen infections and cancer development, DCs are modulated by different mechanisms as follows: Loss of DC subset, down-regulation of MHC and co-stimulatory molecules, up-regulation of inhibitory molecules, differentiation into tolerogenic DCs followed by induction of Tregs, and inhibition of DC development by altered production of IFN-I.

(2) Chronicviral Infection

Chronic environment negatively regulating immune responses during chronic viral infection and tumor growth. Dysfunctional or suppressive APCs can negatively modulate T cell responses. Increase of multiple inhibitory receptors on T cells can limit T cell functions and control of disease. Tregs including traditional Foxp3$^+$ CD4$^+$ T cells can modulate T cell responses. Immunosuppressive cytokines such as IL-10 and TGF-β produced in a chronic environment.

Sequential and progressive changes of T cells in phenotype and functionality lead to T cell exhaustion in a TME with chronic infection, in which antigen and/or inflammation persist. During persistent antigen stimulation, such as chronic viral infections and the tumor bearing state, exhausted T cells undergo sequential phenotypic changes and a progressive loss of effector functions: including effector cytokines production, cytotoxicity, proliferation, and cytokine mediated self-renewal; overexpression of inhibitory receptors; down-regulation of cytokine receptors; changes in transcription factors; alteration of intracellular Signaling.

(3) The roles of tumor-suppressing inflammation.

Th1 lymphocytes and M1 macrophages are the primary sources of pro-inflammatory cytokines that also promote cancer immunosurveillance and cytotoxicity. Their interactions are mutually reinforcing: Secretion IFN-γ by Th1 cells results in the recruitment of M1 macrophages and maintenance of M1 phenotype, while IL-12 produced by M1 macrophages recruits, activates and maintains a Th1 phenotype. Secretion of MIG /CXCL9 and IP-10/CXCL10 also promotes the recruitment of Th1 cells and CTLs and inhibits angiogenesis. IL-1α, IL-1β and IL-6 for man autocrine feedback loop by stimulation of myeloid differentiation primary response gene 88 (MyD88)-mediated activation of NF-κB signaling. TNF-α, also released by the activation of NF-κB signaling, which activates APC functions of DCs and the recruitment and cytotoxic activation ofM1 macrophages, effector CD4$^+$ T cells, and CD8$^+$ T cells, as well as the recruitment of NK cells.

Challenges and Perspectives

Normal cells may become nascent tumors by evading tumor suppression after carcinogenicmutation and/or apoptosis that would normally result from gross chromosomal changes. Pro-inflammatory and pro-angiogenic factors can help to establish blood supply for the growing nascent tumor. Activation of the adaptiveor native immune response can eliminate the nascent tumor, the tumor may remain in equilibrium as an occult tumor, or the tumor may escape immunosurveillance to create a viable tumor-supportive microenvironment. Innate and adaptive immune responses may still work to eliminate the tumor via immunosurveillance. Tumors may also metastasize to move to another location; this may be an additional mechanism of avoiding immunosurveillance by evacuation of the "hostile" TME. So it is very important of TME in tumorgenesis and progressions[40].

1. Questions and Challenge

(1) How should we include the TME in the initial evaluation of a tumor and in preclinical cancer models? Typically, genomic and transcriptomic analyses of tumors are conducted on DNA and RNA

extracted from entire tumors and it is generally assumed that genetic and epigenetic alterations and changes in gene expression observed reflect modifications in the tumor cells. This may not necessarily be the case.

(2) Another important question is the development of preclinical cancer mouse models that take the TME into consideration. The important role played by immune cells in the TME indicates that xenotransplanted tumor models in immunodeficient mice are of limited value in the study of TME. Genetically engineered mice have the advantage to recapitulate an oncogenic event within the context of a competent immune system but they represent murine and not human cancer models.

(3) The non-malignant cells of the TME can comprise 50% of the mass of primary tumors and their metastases, but there are still many unanswered questions regarding their biology and function. We know little about evolution of the TME during cancer progression and treatment. It is now clear that in both hematological cancers and solid tumors there is Darwinian evolution of malignant cells, leading to heterogeneous mutations within single tumors and at different sites of metastasis. This raises important questions, such as is there a similar heterogeneity in the other TME constituents? Is the TME of metastases different from that of matched primary tumors?

(4) Can the composition of the TME be modulated by oncogenic mutations? Certainly in breast cancers there is heterogeneity in both malignant and stromal gene-expression signatures. It is also still not clear whether tumors at different sites in the body have a different TME composition, but we do know that there are important differences in the TME between different cancers. In addition, an aging immune system could have a more tumor-promoting phenotype. Although VEGF inhibitors, such as bevacizumab, extend disease-free interval in a variety of advanced human cancers, it has been difficult to determine their impact on overall survival, mainly because the hypoxia that is induced by VEGF blockade switches on a more invasive and metastatic program in the malignant cells. In addition, the TME might also evolve to produce other angiogenic factors. Hence, targeting the TME could also stimulate further evolution of the cancer and its resistance to treatment. We now recognize that cancer chemotherapy and radiotherapy do not just target malignant cells, but that their actions on the TME contribute to success or failure of the treatment. In mouse cancers and clinical trials, there is evidence that chemotherapy is most successful when it causes a form of cell death that stimulates an anti-tumor immune response.

Conversely, chemotherapy stimulates a rapid increase in the infiltration of innate cells into the damaged TME. The addition of chemokine and cytokine receptor antagonists, or of MMPs inhibitors might therefore increase the effectiveness and toxicity profile of traditional chemotherapy. The importance of the TME in designing new cancer treatment regimes is now apparent. Targeting several different aspects of the TME during cancer treatment might allow us to reach a 'tipping point' where its tumor-promoting and suppressive immune system is disabled or reprogrammed, its chaotic blood supply is normalized or destroyed, and as malignant cells are destroyed, new antigens are uncovered that are recognized by the reawakened immune system.

2. Strategies and Perspectives

Therapies solely targeted at the TME are unlikely to eradicate cancer, although they could have the potential to convert cancer into a chronic disease. The major focus of ongoing efforts have thus been on strategies that combine targeting tumor cells and the microenvironment [42].

(1) The use of agents blocking pathways responsible for the recruitment and activation of stromal cells in the TME as first shown for Avastin, that is now part of the armamentarium to combat colon cancer and glioblastoma. William Dougall (Amgen, Seattle, WA) presented data illustrating the efficacy of targeting receptor activator of NF-κB ligand (RANKL) in bone metastasis with denosumab, a fully human mAb against RANKL. Three phase III clinical studies with denosumab recently completed in patients with

bone metastasis from breast cancer, castration-resistant prostate cancer (CRPC), and other advanced malignancies showed effective inhibition of bone remodeling and the superiority of denosumab over Zometa (zoledronic acid) in decreasing the number of skeletal-related events in these patients. Denosumab was also effective in delaying the development of bone metastasis in men with CRPC, showing that targeting the TME can also have a preventive effect on metastasis. RANKL is also a mediator of the mitogenic activity of progesterone in mouse mammary epithelium and pharmacologic inhibition of RANKL in progesterone-dependent mouse mammary tumors attenuated tumorigenesis.

(2) Based on the concept that the TME modulates tumor susceptibility to therapy. Combination therapies that include agents targeting pathways affecting tumor cell resistance to drugs with standard chemotherapy or targeted therapy have garnered renewed excitement. William Dalton (H. Lee Moffitt Cancer Center and Research Institute, Tampa, FL) discussed environment-mediated drug resistance (EMDR) as a mechanism where the interaction between tumor cells and the BM environment allows for discrete tumor populations to survive as minimal residual disease and emerge as drug-resistant clones. Interfering with these mechanisms may increase cancer response to therapy and prevent resistance. In myeloma, in which such resistance has been extensively studied, the mechanisms involve activation of specific pathways such as IL-6/STAT3, SDF1/CXCR4, Notch, or TRAIL and miR that provide tumor cells with a survival advantage. Several inhibitors of such pathways are currently in clinical trials. The ECM can also be a factor of therapeutic resistance and thus a target for therapeutic intervention. Sunil Hingorani (Fred Hutchinson Cancer Research Center) showed that the formation of a hyaluronic acid-rich stroma in pancreatic tumors resulted in unperfused blood vessels that provided a drug-free sanctuary for tumor cells. Treatment of the stroma with hyaluronidase in transgenic mice prone to develop pancreatic cancer was followed by a rapid reperfusion of the blood vessels that led to decreased proliferation, increased apoptosis, increased response to therapy, and improved survival.

(3)Targeting protumorigenic inflammatory pathways, an approach taken by Frances Balkwill's (Barts Cancer Institute) laboratory. She identified TNF, IL-6, and CXCL12 as a TNF network of 3 key cytokine mediators of cancer-related inflammation, having a paracrine action on angiogenesis, infiltration with myeloid cells, and Notch signaling. She reported that siltuximab, an anti-human IL-6 antibody inhibited IL-6 signaling (STAT3 activation) in cancer cells and had therapeutic effects in xenograft models. A phase II clinical trial of siltuximab as single agent in platinum-resistant ovarian cancer indicated that it was well-tolerated and had some therapeutic effects.

3. At Present, the Research on TME is Mainly Focused on the Following 3 Aspects:

(1) How the tumor cells and various types of cells related to function in their surrounding tissue to promote tumor invasion and metastasis;

(2) The relationship between tumor cells and TME;

(3) In the process of tumor initiation and progression, the interaction between tumor cells and their ECM

The above 3 aspects are both different and related. But we believe that in the process of malignant transformation of the tumor, is the interaction of cytokines and other components of tumor stroma in TME and tumor extracellular secretion or expression of cytekins, proteases or receptors changed the osmotic pressure between the organization, effected the nutrition metabolic environment of tumor tissue, and play immune inflammation role to promote tumor angiogenesis, which is conducive to tumor invasion and metastasis. In conclusion, the host microenvironment influences the biological characteristics of tumor cells through the actions of specific factors. Study of signal transduction and the molecular mechanism of interaction between tumor cells, tumor and microenvironment will provide us more information to reversalthe malignant phenotype of tumor cells and maintain the normal gene phenotype, provide a new ways for the diagnosis and treatment of tumor [43].

Consider/Questions

1. Basic concepts in this chapter

Tumor Microenvironment (TME), cancer-associated fibroblasts (CAFs), Tumor-associated macrophages (TAMs), Myeloid-derived suppressor cells (MDSCs), tumor-associated neutrophils (TANs), Treg cells.

2. Summarize the important elements of TME.

3. How do you understand the TME is a dynamic milieu?

4. Which factors regulate the extracellular matrix remodeling?

5. Read the literqture and explain the mechanism of communication between the some tumor cells and TME.

6. Why do the developing microenvironment require increases in oxygen supply?

7. Briefly explain exosomes and its roles in tumor.

第十四章 肿瘤的靶向性治疗

随着肿瘤分子生物学的发展，分子靶向治疗（molecular targeted therapy）和精准医疗作为肿瘤治疗的新手段逐渐成为热点。分子靶向治疗又被称为"生物导弹"，其治疗靶点可以是细胞表面的生长因子受体或是胞内信号转导通路中的重要酶或蛋白。广义的分子靶点则包括参与肿瘤细胞分化、分裂、凋亡、迁移、浸润、淋巴结及全身转移过程，从 DNA 到蛋白水平的任何亚细胞分子，即是针对肿瘤发生、发展过程中的关键分子，通过特异性阻断肿瘤细胞的信号转导，来控制其基因表达和改变生物学行为，或是通过阻止肿瘤血管生成，抑制肿瘤细胞的生长和增殖，靶向杀死肿瘤细胞，并不会波及肿瘤周围的正常细胞，达到治疗目的。因此只有特定基因突变的肿瘤患者，才适用于靶向性药物治疗。

第一节 分子病理学在肿瘤靶向治疗中的作用

目前对肿瘤的治疗措施不断改进，除传统的手术、化疗、放疗、免疫治疗和中医中药等，分子靶向治疗正在成为一种新的疗法。

一、分子靶向治疗的优势

分子靶向治疗与传统的化疗相比，表现在靶向治疗具有特异性强、疗效明显、对正常组织损伤较小等优点，具有明显优势。

（1）分子靶向治疗是个体化治疗、精准医疗的主要内容。例如，对于存在表皮生长因子受体（epidermal growth factor receptor，EGFR）突变的非小细胞肺癌（non small cell lung cancer，NSCLC）用靶向 EGFR 突变的酪氨酸激酶抑制剂（EGFR-TKI）治疗，其有效率在 90% 以上，因此通过组织 EGFR 检测可以预测治疗效果。

（2）根据药物的性质和作用靶点的不同，分子靶向治疗的靶点专一、毒副反应轻。与细胞毒作用的化疗不同，靶向药物往往是针对异常的突变位点发生作用，能够瞄准肿瘤细胞上特有的靶点，准确打击肿瘤细胞而又不伤害正常细胞，因而胃肠道反应和血液学毒性较轻，并能迅速改善患者症状，患者容易耐受。相反，用细胞毒性作用的药物治疗晚期肿瘤患者虽然能使部分患者延长生存期，但副作用大，使患者对治疗产生恐惧，生活质量下降。

（3）分子靶向治疗的方法简便易行。目前很多靶向药物通过口服给药，患者依从性和耐受性良好，可在门诊和家庭治疗，患者很容易接受。

（4）分子靶向药物与化疗联合使用能提高疗效，并且毒副作用无明显增加。

二、肿瘤靶向治疗中分子病理学的作用

开展分子靶向治疗中首先需要明确诊断，判断其肿瘤组织和细胞上是否有适合的靶点，然后进行针对性的靶向治疗，并可预知靶向药物是否会奏效。因此分子靶向治疗必须依靠分子病理学的研究手段。分子病理学是在蛋白质和核酸等生物大分子水平上，应用分子生物学理论、技术及方法研究疾病发生、发展的过程。分子病理学常用的相关技术有原位杂交、荧光原位杂交（fluorescence in situ hybridization，FISH）、多聚酶链式反应技术（polymerase chain reaction technique，PCR）、原位 PCR 显微切割技术（micro-dissection）、基因测序技术、生物芯片技术、Southern 印迹杂交法、免疫组织化学（immunohistochemistry，IHC）等。由于分子病理学的应用，使得我们能更全面地认识疾病本质，特别是在肿瘤的诊断和治疗中已取得了很大的进展。其主要表现在以下几个方面。

（1）肿瘤易感基因的检测：检测肿瘤遗传相关的易感基因对于肿瘤高危人群的筛检具有实用价值，已明确的肿瘤易感基因及其相关肿瘤有 Rb（视网膜母细胞瘤）、WT1（肾母细胞瘤）等。除了检测高危人群的易感基因外，有些方法也应用于正常人群肿瘤易感性检测，如检测 Ret 基因突变用于诊断 II 型多发性内分泌肿瘤，或通过分析 GST 基因型以判断个体暴露于致癌物时的致癌危险性等。

（2）肿瘤相关病毒的检测：如高危型 HPV（16、18、31 型等）感染与宫颈癌的发生密切相关，通过检测 HPV 可对宫颈癌起到预防和早诊、早治的作用。而当前国际上诊断 HPV 感染以 DNA 检测为主。

（3）肿瘤的早期诊断：K-ras 基因突变在结肠癌、胰腺癌和肺癌等肿瘤中发生率较高，如应用细针穿刺活检材料检测胰腺癌的第 12 密码子变突。应用 PCR-RFLP 方法检测结肠癌患者粪便中的 Ras 基因突变，其检出率与瘤组织中的检出率相似，可用于高危人群的筛选。

（4）疑难肿瘤的诊断和分类：传统的病理学诊断主要通过形态学和免疫表型来判断淋巴细胞增生与淋巴瘤，这对医生的经验要求较高，且难度较大。应用 RFLP 分析免疫球蛋白或 T 细胞受体基因重排，具有鉴别诊断作用，这种分子病理分型比免疫学分型更为准确。

（5）肿瘤预后的监测：利用癌症患者的全基因序列开发出的个性化血液检测方法有助于医生调整癌症患者的治疗方案，可以监测癌症治疗后的情况及发现是否复发。

（6）为肿瘤个体化和前瞻性治疗提供依据：肿瘤在发生、发展的不同时期，可能涉及不同基因的变化形式，而这种变化与肿瘤临床治疗的敏感性密切相关，如能在分子水平提供肿瘤基因变化的情况，就能对肿瘤的分子靶向性的精准治疗具有指导意义。

（7）肿瘤预后的判断：肿瘤基因的突变、扩增及过表达等改变常与肿瘤的预后密切相关。如 HER-2 基因扩增与乳腺癌发生发展及临床预后密切相关，乳腺癌 HER-2 阳性表达提示预后不良，可通过 FISH 技术进行检测，配合术后治疗，指导临床用药。

第二节 常用的分子靶点及靶向药物

分子靶向治疗的出现在癌症的治疗中令人鼓舞。近年来 40 多种分子靶向治疗方法已经被验证，其中 10 多种分子靶向治疗方法提高了在 NSCLC、乳腺癌（HER2 阳性）、淋巴瘤（CD20阳性）、大肠癌、肝细胞癌（hepatocellular carcinoma, HCC）、胃肠间质瘤（CD117/CD34 阳性）、肾癌、头颈部肿瘤和隆突性皮肤纤维瘤患者的生存率。

一、抗 EGFR 单克隆抗体

EGFR 也称为 HER1 或 ErbB1，是 ErbB 受体酪氨酸激酶家族的四个成员之一。HER-2 是一种跨膜酪氨酸激酶受体，是具有蛋白酪氨酸激酶（protein tyrosine kinase, TPK）活性的蛋白，人类 EGFR 家族成员之一。HER-2 在控制上皮细胞生长、分化、黏附和激活等细胞信号转导通路的活化上起重要作用。目前抗 EGFR 单克隆抗体主要有西妥昔单抗（cetuximab）、马妥珠单抗（matuzumab）及帕尼单抗（panitumumab）。其中，西妥昔单抗已被批准用于临床。

（1）曲妥珠单抗（trastuzu-mab）（赫赛汀，herceptin）是一种重组 DNA 衍生的人源化单克隆抗体，能与 HER-2 受体结合，干扰其自身磷酸化，下调 HER-2 基因表达，拮抗 HER-2家族的促生长作用，介导抗体依赖的细胞毒性作用（antibody dependent cytotoxicity，ADCC），增强化疗所致的细胞毒性等，达到遏止肿瘤细胞生长、转移或攻击和杀伤肿瘤靶细胞的效果。而且对 HER-2 阴性的肿瘤细胞或正常细胞没有影响。因此，在使用曲妥珠单抗治疗前，必须检测肿瘤组织 HER-2 的表达[1]。但曲妥珠单抗可导致某些患者的心脏毒性反应，2007 年美国临床肿瘤学会/美国病理医师学院（ASCO/CAP）在相关指南中对 HER-2 阳性乳腺癌病例的靶点检测和阳性标准进行了细致和严格的规范[2]。近年来曲妥珠单抗已广泛应用于乳腺癌、胃癌的治疗中。

（2）帕尼单抗是靶向 HER-2 分子的单克隆抗体，与 HER-2 靶点结合后可以形成二聚体有效抑制靶点的作用。小分子的 TPK 抑制剂（tyrosine kinase inhibitor, TKI）通过对 HER-2 靶点分子内的 TPK 的活性进行可逆或不可逆的抑制。例如，neratinib，一种新型的 TKI，可同时作用于 HER-2 和 HER-4，并且其临床疗效也较佳。

二、靶向 EGFR 基因突变的小分子 TKI

EGFR 在多种肿瘤中过表达和（或）突变，突变的 EGFR 能够选择性激活 Akt 信号转导蛋白和转录激活物（STAT）信号转导途径，从而延长细胞存活，导致肿瘤细胞生长失控和恶性演进。小分子 TKI 主要抑制以下信号通路。

（1）抑制 TPK 的磷酸化相关的信号转导：主要有吉非替尼（gifitinib）、厄洛替尼（erlotinib）和拉帕替尼（lapatinib）等。其中吉非替尼主要用于治疗晚期 NSCLC、头颈部肿瘤、前列腺癌及乳腺癌等。吉非替尼通过阻断癌细胞信号转导通路的机制抵抗肿瘤增殖、抑制血管生长和抗细胞迁移等作用实现治疗效果。并且临床证实其对亚洲人种的治疗效果更好，值得今后研究确认。厄罗替尼主要用于治疗晚期和转移性 NSCLC。

由于 85% 的促癌基因和癌基因均是 TPK 的产物，并在癌组织中 TPK 活性增加，所以通过靶向 TPK 以抑制其催化活性可以抑制癌细胞增殖。目前研究相对集中在抑制 TPK 介导的信号转导通路（特别是受体型 TPK-Ras-MAPK 信号通路），如单抗能阻断 TPK 配体与受体的结合。

（2）舒尼替尼（sunitinib）是一种口服的多靶点小分子 TKI，其作用机制是抑制 VEGF 以及血小板源生长因子受体-β（platelet-derived growth factor receptor-β，PDGFR-β）、KIT、KLT-3和 RET 的 TPK 活性，通过特异性阻断这些信号转导，达到抗肿瘤效应。

（3）索拉非尼（sorafenib）是口服多靶点 TKI，作用于肿瘤细胞和肿瘤血管上的丝氨酸、苏氨酸及受体 TPK，既可抑制 Raf-MEK-ERK 信号转导通路直接抑制肿瘤生长，又可抑制 VEGF 和 PDGFR 间接抑制肿瘤细胞的生长。

第二代不可逆 EGFR TKI，如 dacomitinib 和阿法替尼（afatinib），是泛 ErbB 抑制剂，具有体外活性对抗激活 EGFR 突变和 T790M 抗性突变的作用。

第三代 EGFR TKI（rociletinib 和 AZD9291）比目前的 EGFR TKI 具有更多的 T790M 选择性，临床更有效，毒性更低。rociletinib 和 AZD929 已有的研究结果明确提示该药将能改善耐受性和提高临床疗效。

三、靶向 *K-ras* 基因突变的 EGFR 单抗

K-ras 蛋白是鸟苷三磷酸酶 Ras 家族的成员。原癌基因 K-ras 在多种肿瘤的发展中发挥关键性的作用。K-ras 蛋白又称 P21 蛋白，为膜结合型的 GTP/GDP 结合蛋白，通过 GTP 和 GDP 的相互转化可以调节 P21 对信号系统的开启和关闭，完成生长、分化等信号传入细胞内的过程。当 K-ras 基因发生突变后，即不受上游 EGFR 基因状态的影响，始终处于活化状态，持续刺激细胞生长，导致肿瘤发生。K-ras 突变增加肿瘤复发和转移的风险，预后较差[3]。BRAF 基因是 Raf 家族成员之一，其编码蛋白为一种丝氨酸-苏氨酸蛋白激酶，是 MEK/ERK 信号通路中最关键的激活因子。研究者发现 EZH2 和 MEK-ERK 或 PI3K/Akt 结合能抑制细胞与特定 K-ras 基因突变的敏感性，可用于针对癌细胞中 MEK-ERK 和 PI3K/Akt 通路激活的靶向性治疗[3]。通过不同 K-ras 基因突变调节肺癌中 MEK-ERK 或 PI3K-Akt 信号途径中 EZH2 的表达。Ras 是介导 TPK 信号转导通路的关键分子，抑制 Ras 的转膜作用可以抑制 Ras 的活性，或使 Ras 失活突变可阻断 Ras 的信号转导过程。西妥昔单抗和帕尼单抗是针对 EGFR 细胞外结构域的人鼠嵌合 IgG 单抗，可与细胞表面受体结合而产生 ADCC 活性，与细胞是否存在 EGFR 突变无关。目前西妥昔单抗已成为晚期转移性结肠直肠癌的一线治疗药物。

四、抗 VEGF 分子的靶向药物

抗 VEGF 的分子靶向药物包括贝伐珠单抗（bevacizumab），又称阿瓦斯汀（avastin），是一种人源化的 VEGF 单抗，可与 VEGF 特异性结合，阻断其与受体相互作用，产生抗肿瘤血管的多种效应。抗血管内皮细胞制剂——人血管内皮细胞抑制素国产的恩度（endostar），以及美罗华（利妥昔单抗，rituximab）、格列卫（伊马替尼，imatinib，治疗 CD117/CD34 阳性胃肠间质瘤）等。

五、其他靶向性药物

（1）ADP 核糖核酸聚合酶 I（ADP RNA polymerase I，PARP-1）抑制剂 PARP-1 酶是一种重要的修复 DNA 与细胞增殖的酶类，目前此药物如 olaparib、veliparib（ABT-888）等都已经显示出令人满意的疗效。

（2）mTOR 抑制剂，主要有依维莫司（everolimus）、坦西莫司（temsirolimus），可用于在

曲妥珠单抗失败时进行治疗，并且在对于曲妥珠单抗耐药患者的治疗中被寄予厚望。目前也已开展多项关于依维莫司的研究。有研究者发现新的抗肿瘤药物 ABTL0812 通过上调 tribbles-3 假性激酶[4]抑制 Akt/mTORC1 激活，具有抗肿瘤细胞增殖作用。

（3）c-Met 抑制剂、胰岛素样生长因子受体 1（IGFR1）抑制剂及 Wnt 抑制剂。

第三节 常见肿瘤的分子靶向治疗

分子病理学检测为肿瘤的早期诊断和开发新的治疗方法提供了机会。采用 IHC、原位杂交和基因测序等多种手段进行肿瘤的分子病理学评估，以明确癌分类，确定肿瘤侵袭范围和外科手术切缘的受累程度（如阳性或阴性切缘），区分原发肿瘤及转移性肿瘤，还可用于分子诊断性研究，确定是否存在特定基因表达异常或突变，对肿瘤预后及疗效进行预测，并据此进行个体化的分子靶向治疗[1]。

一、靶向性治疗肺癌

肺癌仍然是全世界癌症死亡的首要原因。有研究者将 2014 年，确诊 224 210 例新肺癌患者，其中大多数是进展期 NSCLC，不管什么组织学亚型的进展期 NSCLC 患者均接受顺铂（platinum）化疗。实行化疗患者与最佳支持治疗的患者相比，总体生存（overall survival，OS）有所改善，但已经达到治疗平台，反应率（response rate）约为 20%，中位存活仅 8～10 个月[5]。

随着分子遗传学研究的进展通过识别不同的分子区分 NSCLC 亚群，将引导合理的分子靶向治疗的发展，改进临床结果。在肺癌中发现和开发了许多基于基因组的生物标志物，包括 DNA、分子网络或染色体定位的表达、测序或表观遗传学的标志[6]。

肺癌是基因组医学中最早研究的疾病之一，并且较早开发了许多用于靶向治疗的特异性药物。

通过对 NSCLC 分子遗传学的研究已经可以鉴定出 NSCLC 中关键性的遗传变异。这些遗传变异（驱动突变）发生在编码对细胞增殖和存活至关重要的信号蛋白的癌基因中。"癌基因成瘾"（oncogene addiction）的概念基于肿瘤细胞的存活极大依赖于单一致癌基因的表达而提出[7]。在 NSCLC 中已经鉴定出癌基因成瘾的肿瘤，并且开发了特异性分子靶向药物。

（一）针对肺腺癌靶向性治疗

肺腺癌是 NSCLC 最常见的组织学亚型，占所有 NSCLC 的 50%以上。随机试验显示，在该组晚期患者中顺铂-培美曲塞的治疗结果优于顺铂-吉西他滨[8]。最近，肺腺癌进一步被分为临床相关的分子亚型，包括 EGFR、K-ras、HER-2、PIK3CA、BRAF、Met 基因的突变和 ALK、ROS1 和 RET 基因的重排。

常用的肺癌分子靶向药物有针对肿瘤血管的，包括抗 VGFR 的单克隆抗体（贝伐单抗）和恩度。作用于肿瘤细胞信号转导通路的小分子 EGFR-TKI，如吉非替尼（易瑞沙）、厄洛替尼（特罗凯）等。其中吉非替尼临床主要用于治疗晚期伴有 EGFR 基因突变的 NSCLC。

EGFR 是 NSCLC 中重要的靶标，因为在该型肿瘤中经常过表达，其活化引起重要信号转导途径的下游激活，导致增加了细胞增殖、存活、血管生成和转移[9]。吉非替尼和厄洛替尼最初用于未接受过化疗的 NSCLC 患者。其后开发的其他 EGFR-TKI 包括阿法替尼和 dacomitinib。吉非替尼是市场上首个口服 EGFR 抑制剂。2003 年 5 月 5 日，美国 FDA 批准用于对多烯紫杉醇（taxotere）和铂无效的 NSCLC 患者。虽然吉非替尼没有总体生存优势；但吉非替尼在治疗亚裔患者和从不吸烟者的这两个特定 NSCLC 亚组中的存活时间更长。

由于 EGFR 基因的突变在女性、非吸烟者、腺癌、亚裔人群中发生频率较高,因此吉非替尼对于东方女性、非吸烟、腺癌这一亚组特别有效[9]。随后确定了对 EGFR-TKI 敏感性增加的分子基础是由于 EGFR 的外显子 18-21(通常是外显子 19 缺失和外显子 21 中的 L858R 点突变)中的体细胞激活突变,其编码 EGFR 的 TPK 结构域[9]。已知外显子 18 的突变赋予 EGFR-TKI 敏感性;然而,外显子 20 的插入很大程度上与对 TKI 治疗的原发性抗性相关。EGFR 突变在具有前述临床特征的患者中更频繁。高达 15% 的白种人和 30%~50% 的东方亚洲人肺腺癌携带 EGFR 突变[10]。在东亚地区,NSCLC 中患有肺腺癌,从不吸烟,发病率高达 50%~60%。

在具有致敏 EGFR 突变的未治疗 NSCLC 患者中,多项研究显示 EGFR TKI 在总反应率(overall response rate,ORR)、无进展生存期(progression-free survival,PFS)和生活质量方面均优于化疗[11]。

肺未分化腺癌、腺鳞癌、小细胞癌(尤其是与腺癌的复合型)等患者中也经常可以检测到 EGFR 基因的突变,用吉非替尼治疗也有一定的疗效。临床统计表明,该类人群治疗的有效率在 30%,疾病控制率在腺癌中达到 60%,但对鳞癌的疗效不如化疗。

证据表明,厄洛替尼可能比吉非替尼更有效。厄洛替尼似乎延长了大多数其他亚组患者的存活期。这种明显的功效部分归因于厄洛替尼以其最大耐受剂量(maximum-tolerated dose,MTD)(150mg/d)给药,而吉非替尼的给药剂量为其 MTD 的 1/3 左右[12]。

以前吸烟者或从未吸烟的患者血浆厄洛替尼浓度大约是当前吸烟者的两倍。非吸烟者的较高生存获益可能是某些基因突变率较低,如 K-ras 的发生率,以及由香烟烟雾导致的细胞色素 P450(CYP)1A 同种型的缺乏,吸烟者中厄洛替尼的血浆清除快。

这些研究提供了在治疗晚期 NSCLC 患者中基于分子检测的结果合理选择性治疗。因此,用 EGFR-TKI 对晚期 NSCLC 患者进行一线治疗应根据 EGFR 突变状态,所以肺癌诊断中应常规地进行 EGFR 突变检测。

EML4-ALK 基因重排是染色体 2p 内倒位的结果,是肺腺癌中新鉴定的驱动致癌基因。EML4 和 ALK 之间的融合产生嵌合蛋白持续活化,并通过 PI3K-Akt、MAPK 和 JAK-STAT 途径[13]促进肿瘤发生。EML4-ALK 重排在很大程度上与 NSCLC 中的其他驱动突变相互排斥。42EML4-ALK 基因重排常通过荧光原位杂交(FISH)或免疫组织化学检测。

ALK 基因重排不常见,占所有 NSCLC 的 4%~7%,除去 EGFR 和 K-ras 突变的 NSCLC 患者有 33%,多见于年轻的、从未或轻吸烟者,伴有印戒细胞或腺泡样组织学特征的腺癌[14]。ALK 抑制剂包括克唑替尼(crizotinib)、ceritinib 和 alectinib。

已经报道了对克唑替尼的获得性耐药有多种机制,包括 ALK 中 TPK 结构域的次级突变(最常见的是 L1196M 突变),ALK 拷贝数增加和新癌基因驱动如 EGFR 和 K-ras 突变的出现[15]。获得性抗药的不同机制可能影响随后的治疗策略。针对 ALK 的治疗,如第二代 ALK TKI 可以直接干预 ALK 突变或拷贝数增加的肿瘤,相反继发于新的驱动癌基因的耐受性肿瘤可以从化疗中获益。

BRaf 是丝氨酸/苏氨酸蛋白激酶的 Raf 激酶家族的成员,其通过 MEK 的磷酸化和 ERK 信号传导途径的下游激活来介导肿瘤发生[16]。在 1%~3% 的 NSCLC 中观察到 BRaf 突变,并且约 50% 的 BRaf 突变是 BRaf V600E 突变[17]。NSCLC 中的 BRaf 突变在腺癌中发生的可触性更大,并且 BRaf V600E 突变在不吸烟女性患者中发生的频率更高[17]。BRaf 抑制剂达拉非尼(dabrafenib)和 vemurafenib 对含有 BRaf V600E 突变的 NSCLC 具有积极的治疗作用。

Met 是 TPK 受体,其在活化时诱导细胞增殖、运动、扩散、浸润、转移、血管生成和上皮间质转化。最近提供的初步数据表明由 FISH 评估的携带 Met 扩增的 NSCLC 患者可用克唑替尼治疗。

K-ras 与腺癌亚型和吸烟相关，在白种人中比在东亚患者中更常见[18]。口服 MEK 抑制剂 selumetinib 与化疗联合能增加疗效。

与 EGFR 相似，HER-2（ErbB-2）是酪氨酸激酶 ErbB 家族的成员。HER-2，一种主要的增殖驱动因子，通过扩增、过表达或突变在 NSCLC 中失调。在 NSCLC 中 HER-2 扩增和蛋白过表达分别为 20% 和 6%～35%，只有 1%～2% NSCLC 中发现 HER-2 突变。大多数患有 HER-2 突变的患者是女性、从不吸烟者和腺癌患者[19]。

在具有 HER-2 突变的 NSCLC 患者的回顾性研究中已经报道了曲妥珠单抗或阿法替尼是有希望的药物[20]，然而，IHC 检测过表达 HER-2 的 NSCLC 患者用曲妥珠单抗联合化疗显示阴性结果[20]。

肺腺癌患者有 1% 可以检测 RET 基因及其各种融合伴侣 CCDC6、KIF5B、NCOA4 和 TRIM33 之间的易位，而且在年轻不吸烟的肺腺癌患者中有 7%～17% 的检测频率[21]。TKI，如卡博他尼（cabozantinib）、凡德他尼（vandetanib）、舒尼替尼和帕纳替尼（ponatinib），这些是已知的抑制 RET 的靶向性药物已被批准用于其他恶性肿瘤和目前正在 RET 重排的 NSCLC 中研究。其他 RET 抑制剂包括 regorafenib 和 lenvatinib。

（二）针对肺鳞状细胞癌的靶向性治疗

肺鳞状细胞癌（SQLC）是 NSCLC 中第二常见的组织学类型，包括高达 20%～30% 的病例。虽然 EGFR 突变在 SQLC 中并不常见，但最近在 SQLC 中发现的具有癌基因作用的包括成纤维细胞生长因子受体-1（fibroblast growth factor receptor-1，FGFR1）基因扩增，盘状蛋白死亡受体 2（discoidin death receptor 2，DDR2）基因突变和 PI3KCA 基因扩增和突变。

FGFR1 是通过 MAPK 和 PI3K 途径介导肿瘤发生的受体 TPK，并在 13%～25% 的 SQLC 中检测到[22]。据报道 FGFR1 扩增与吸烟有关，但在腺癌亚型中不常见。针对 SQLC 的 FGFR 抑制剂正在开发，如 BGJ398[23]。

DDR2 是跨膜受体 TPK，其在被胶原激活时促进细胞迁移、增殖和存活。DDR2 的激活突变具有致癌性，在 4%～5% 的 SQLC 中可检测到[24]。DDR2 驱动转化对 DDR2 抑制剂达沙替尼（dasatinib）敏感，该药原用于治疗慢性粒细胞白血病的 TKI[25]。在具有 DDR2 激酶结构域突变的 SQLC 和同步慢性骨髓性白血病中已经有对达沙替尼反应的报道。目前正在对具有 DDR2 突变的 SQLC 患者进行达沙替尼的临床应用研究。

PI3K 信号通路是癌细胞存活和增殖的核心。由于 PIK3CA 和 Akt1 基因功能突变的扩增或增加或由于 PTEN 功能的丧失而产生信号通路的改变。在 NSCLC 中 PI3KCA 扩增或突变分别为 37% 和 9%。PI3KCA 的扩增和突变是 SQLC 的不良预后因素[26]。正在进行 PIK3CA 抑制剂作为单一疗法或与化疗联合应用的研究。

（三）针对肺癌异质性的靶向治疗

在肺癌靶向性治疗中应更多地关注癌的同质性和异质性，这在发展耐药性、遗传复杂性，以及在早期诊断和治疗的困惑和不理想疗效中发挥重要作用。染色体重定位可能是肺癌细胞同质性和异质性对药物不敏感性和抗性发展的关键机制。异质性与药物抗性和肺癌发生机制相关。

作为染色体组成的一部分，在异源二倍体基因组的稳定性和干细胞的分化中单倍体/二倍体基因组起关键作用。单倍体或二倍体的改变可能是 X 染色体失活的重要调节机制之一，并且用于定义活化基因的调节表型差异。循环肿瘤细胞（circulating tumor cells，CTCs）的数量与肺中转移性结节的数量，原发瘤的生长，与正常组织交界的肿瘤组织切缘及患者的预后相关。此外，通过细胞角蛋白（cytokeratin，CK）18 的表型和染色体 8 的核型分析反映了 CTCs 中的染色体重定位可能涉及可以改变癌细胞对治疗敏感性的机制。CK18 阴性的二倍体 CTCs 和多数 CK18 阳性的二倍体 CTCs 亚型对化疗敏感，而 CK18 阳性多倍体 CTCs 亚型对顺铂不敏感。

已经发现并开发了许多靶向治疗用于肺癌，以提高治疗的准确性和效率，减小化疗药物的毒性、克服对化疗的不敏感性和副作用。临床试验证明具有某些遗传特征的肺癌细胞亚型，如基因突变对靶向治疗敏感。根据靶基因突变数和拷贝数的不同来选择靶向治疗肺癌的敏感人群。靶向治疗后产生的抗药性仍然是提高靶向药物效果的挑战。

二、靶向性治疗乳腺癌

（1）以 HER-2 为靶点的靶向性治疗：基因扩增检测发现 HER-2 在约 20%的乳腺癌患者中过表达，并提示预后不良。曲妥珠单抗是目前临床针对 HER-2 靶点的最重要药物之一，曲妥珠单抗的使用标志着乳腺癌进入分子靶向治疗的新时代。该药可以与多种化疗药物如多烯紫杉醇、卡培他滨等联合治疗，有效增加患者的生存率。对有淋巴结转移的 HER-2 阳性的乳腺癌病例已广泛采用曲妥珠单抗单独治疗或与其他化疗药物联合治疗[27]，明显提高患者的生存率。曲妥珠单抗和 pertuzumab 联合治疗在抑制乳腺癌细胞的生长中有明显的协同作用。小分子 TKIs 可同时作用于 HER-2 和 HER-4，显示了较好的临床疗效。

（2）以 EGFG 为靶点的靶向性治疗：PARP-1 抑制剂 olaparib、veliparib（ABT-888）特别对 ER、PR、ErbB2 均阴性的三阴乳腺癌（triple negative breast cancer）等有更佳疗效。吉非替尼、厄洛替尼和拉帕替尼等也可用于乳腺癌的治疗。有研究者发现在三阴性乳腺癌中 miR-34a 使 C-SRC 沉默可衰减肿瘤的生长[28]。在人类肿瘤标本中 miR-34a 和 SRC 水平呈负相关。根据体内外显示的 miR-34a 的有效抗肿瘤作用提出了 miR-34a 的替代疗法，有希望成为三阴乳腺癌的治疗策略。

（3）多种因子可以阻断癌细胞膜上 TKRs，使用单克隆抗体拮抗 EGFR（西妥昔单抗），或者 ErbB2/HER-2/neu（曲妥珠单抗）可以有效阻止 EGFR 通路。西妥昔单抗经美国 FDA 批准，用于头颈部癌症及大肠癌的治疗；曲妥珠单抗可用于治疗 HER-2 阳性表达的转移性乳腺癌。此外，一些小分子也可以成功抑制通路活性，如拉帕替尼可以拮抗 EGRF 和 HER-2 用于治疗乳腺癌。在乳腺癌中 HER-2 过表达或基因扩增与对 HER-2 抑制剂如曲妥珠单抗、帕妥珠单抗和拉帕替尼的敏感性相关。

三、靶向性治疗肝癌

HCC 发病的分子机制是复杂的。该肿瘤可以发生于正常的肝组织、异常但非硬化的肝组织或肝硬化组织。80%的病例是不同环境危险因子共同作用的结果。以上每种情况都涉及不同遗传和表型的改变、染色体畸变、基因突变和分子路径的改变。

HCC 治疗中针对分子变异的主要靶点是蛋白激酶[29]。在 HCC 的发病机制中，关键性的信号转导通路有 Wnt-β-catenin 通路、EGFR-RAS-MAPKK 通路、c-Met 通路、IGF 信号、Akt/mTOR 信号，以及 VEGF 和 PDGFR 信号级联。HCC 发生中其他通路如 JAK-STAT，TGF-β 等的关联性和潜在性的治疗价值需进一步研究。基于对全基因组的研究确定出 HCC 的分子分类，并根据患者对药物的反应，开发更加个性化的药物。

（一）索拉菲尼

索拉菲尼是一种多激酶抑制剂，研究显示除了具有抑制 TPK 和丝氨酸/苏氨酸作用外还具有抑制 Raf-1、B-Raf、VEGFR-2、PDGFR-β、c-Kit 受体的作用。索拉菲尼是目前唯一被批准用于 HCC 治疗的药物。它具有吸引人的临床前和早期临床试验数据。临床前研究表明在体外实验中索拉菲尼具有降低 HCC 细胞活性和诱导凋亡的潜力。在异种移植模型中具有抗肿瘤活性。虽然药物可观的临床前研究结果已经在临床Ⅱ期研究中得到证实。但是临床前模型与临床结果仍有分歧，这可能是由于人类 HCC 与细胞株之间的异质性、选用的细胞系表达的分子不同、肿瘤异位与原位的不同、药物应用的剂量和时间不同及选择观察点的不同等引起。然而，最大的不同可能是由于炎症和纤维化引起的肿瘤微环境的差别[33]。通过检测磷酸化细胞外信号相关激酶（p-ERK）阳性的 Ras/MAPK 通路激活的患者生存期更长。与单纯放疗比较，索拉菲尼有明显的优势，索拉菲尼的疗效与其他已经证实的药物疗效相当。例如，曲妥珠单抗治疗乳腺癌、贝伐珠单抗治疗结直肠癌、厄洛替尼治疗 NSCLC，死亡危险减少 25%～35%。总的来说，索拉菲尼最常见的副作用为腹泻、疲劳、体重丧失、手足皮肤反应。但药物相关的不良反应是可控的，并无毒性死亡相关的报道。

多激酶抑制剂索拉菲尼在晚期 HCC 中显示有良好效果，这是 HCC 治疗的一项突破，证明了分子疗法在 HCC 治疗中是有效的。

（二）Ras/MAPK 途径

在 HCC 中，Ras/MAPK 通路激活或是因信号的异常上调（EGFR 信号、IGF 信号），或是因异常甲基化导致的肿瘤抑癌基因的失活[13]。Raf 和 Ras 的突变较为少见。索拉菲尼可以在纳摩尔浓度阻断 B-Raf。其他阻断 Ras/MAPK 信号的药物仍在探索中[29]。

（三）c-Met 途径

肝细胞生长因子（hepatocyte growth factor，HGF）是肝细胞损伤后再生的关键分子。它由肝星状细胞分泌并与 c-Met 受体结合。在人类肿瘤中由于 Met 扩增使间质上皮转化因子异常活化、胚系或体细胞突变、转录、上调 HGF 依赖的自分泌循环。c-Met 和 HGF 的失调在 HCC 中较为常见[29, 30]。已经研究出一些靶向 Met 通路的抑制剂，包括抗 HGF 或者 Met 受体的抗体，选择性的小分子 Met 阻断剂，但是这些抑制剂还未用于进展期 HCC 的研究。

（四）PI3K/Akt/mTOR 途径

PI3K/Akt/mTOR 通路在肿瘤发生中起着关键作用。Akt 可以通过 TPK 受体激活（EGF 或 IGF 信号）、PI3K 的持续激活、由表观遗传沉默而导致的肿瘤中抑癌基因 PTEN 功能的丧失或体细胞突变。PTEN 的突变可能使肿瘤对 EGFR 小分子产生抵抗。虽然 pAkt 在 HCC 中的作用还需进一步的研究，最近研究表明 HCC 伴 Akt 活性的患者预后更差[31]。

PI3K-Akt 信号通路中的一个重要介质是 mTOR，mTOR 通过感知细胞营养状况和允许细胞从 G_1 期进入到 S 期在细胞生长和增殖中起到调节中心作用。在某种 HCCs 亚型中 mTOR 通路被激活，用西罗莫司或依维莫司阻断此通路可以抑制 HCC 细胞系的生长，在试验模型中结果亦是如此。依维莫司（西罗莫司类似物）和 Termsirolimus 已经被批准用于肾癌的治疗。目前新型化合物已经处于早期临床试验测试阶段。这些分子（西罗莫司类似物）用于肝移植术后的免疫抑制治疗。

（五）其他途径

1/3 的 HCCs 患者中 Wnt 信号级联反应被激活，尤其多见于由 HCV 诱导的 HCCs。抑癌基因 APC（adenomatous polyposis coli）的异常甲基化和增加自分泌/旁分泌 Wnt 配体激活 E-钙黏素均可激活 Wnt 经典信号通路。靶向作用于这一信号通路的新药物正处于早期临床开发阶段。

凋亡逃避是肿瘤发生的标志之一。目前正在研究靶向作用于外源性凋亡途径的促凋亡受体激动剂，如配体重组体人 Apo2L/ TRAIL（tumor necrosis factor-related apoptosis inducing ligand）。靶向内源性凋亡途径如反义 Bcl-2。在实验模型中联合小分子药物和 Apo2L/TRAIL 途径激动剂的治疗具有协同作用，如索拉菲尼能增加 TRAIL 诱导癌细胞死亡的敏感性，这为联合治疗提供理论依据[32]。

虽然近年随着诊断水平的提高可以诊断出可疑的小癌结节，但只有 30%～40%的 HCC 患者可以接受根治疗法。在精心挑选的患者中，手术切除和肝移植患者的 5 年生存率为 70%，而局部切除后再接受放疗患者的 5 年生存率为 50%。可能是这些治疗方法改变了疾病的自然病程。第 3 年时约一半的患者肿瘤复发。

蛋白激酶是肿瘤发生过程中的主要药物靶点。根据主要的靶点药物分为①抗内皮生长因子受体如厄洛替尼、吉非替尼、拉帕替尼和西妥昔单抗；②抗血管生成的药物：贝伐珠单抗、索拉菲尼、舒尼替尼及联合药；③mTOR 抑制剂：依维莫司、坦西莫司；④其他药物：c-Met 抑制剂、胰岛素样生长因子受体 1 抑制剂及 Wnt 抑制剂。这些药物已显示了较好的效果。

四、靶向性治疗结直肠癌

结直肠癌是常见的发生于肠道的消化道恶性肿瘤，发病率占胃肠道肿瘤的第 3 位。随着结直肠癌病例发病率增高，全球每年新发病例超过 100 万例。

2004 年 2 月美国 FDA 批准贝伐珠单抗联合 5-FU 为基础的化疗方案作为转移结直肠癌的一线治疗。Ⅲ期临床试验、HORIZON Ⅱ和 HORIZON Ⅲ试验评估了西地尼布（cediranib）对晚期结直肠癌的疗效，结果显示基于联合草酸铂的方案，能显著提高中位 PFS（8.6 个月和 8.2 个月，P=0.012），但没有提高中位 OS，其不良反应如腹泻、高血压、白细胞减少等发生率较高，在安全性和生活质量评估中不如贝伐珠单抗联合化疗组[34]。目前西妥昔单抗已成为晚期转移性结肠直肠癌的一线治疗药物。在常规化疗药物基础上加入西妥昔单抗后，患者的客观缓解率明显提高，生存期延长。西妥昔单抗联合 FOLFIRI 方案一线治疗还能使 K-ras 野生型转移结直肠癌患者的疾病进展风险降低 30%，并显著延长患者的无进展生存时间，从 8.4 个月延长至 9.9 个月[35]。帕尼单抗在多中心随机对照Ⅲ期临床试验的 PRIME 研究[36]中，帕尼单抗联合 FOLFOX4 方案能显著提高野生型基因。PRIME 研究结果也成为美国国家综合癌网络（NCCN）指南将帕尼单抗联合 FOLFOX4//FOLFIRI 作为晚期结直肠癌一线方案的重要依据。新版的《NCCN 结直肠癌临床诊疗指南》指出，所有转移结直肠癌患者均应检测 K-ras 及 BRAF 基因突变情况，只推荐 K-ras 和 BRAF 野生型患者接受西妥昔单抗治疗。

五、靶向性治疗胃癌

胃癌在我国各种恶性肿瘤中居首位，其防治形势严峻，迫切需要新的治疗方法提高疗效。继肺癌、乳腺癌、结肠癌和食管癌等肿瘤治疗中取得了良好的疗效后，分子靶向药物单药或与常规化疗药物联合应用治疗胃癌的临床研究也取得了理想的进展。

（1）抗 VEGF 单克隆抗体贝伐珠单抗（bevacizumab）联合多烯紫杉醇、顺铂及氟尿嘧啶对胃癌有一定的疗效，患者中位无进展生存期为 12 个月，中位总生存期为 16.2 个月。一项临床试验显示，增加贝伐珠单抗后，晚期胃癌患者的中位无进展生存期和总缓解率有显著改善。有些生物标志物可评估贝伐珠单抗的疗效，贝伐珠单抗联合化疗治疗胃癌有良好的前景，不良反应主要包括血栓形成、高血压及穿孔，进一步的疗效和安全性有待观察。

（2）Ⅱ期临床研究[37]显示，小分子 TKI 舒尼替尼联合多烯紫杉醇治疗转移性胃癌患者可提高客观缓解率（41.1% vs 14.3%）。Ⅱ期临床研究结果显示，索拉非尼联合多烯紫杉醇、顺铂治疗进展期胃癌及胃食管交界癌的缓解率为 38.6%，中位无进展生存期为 5.8 个月，中位总生存期为 14.9 个月[38]。

（3）EGFR-2 抑制剂近年来，曲妥珠单抗在胃癌治疗中的研究成为热点。10%~55% 的胃癌中有 HER-2 过表达，约 20% 预后不良的胃癌患者中 HER-2 表达阳性。前瞻性国际多中心随机对照Ⅲ期临床实验 ToGA 研究已证明靶向治疗能延长晚期胃癌生存时间。

六、靶向性治疗淋巴瘤

淋巴瘤是最常见的造血系统的恶性肿瘤，可以分为霍奇金淋巴瘤（Hodgkin lymphoma，HL）和非霍奇金淋巴瘤（non-Hodgkin lymphoma，NHL）。大约 85% 的淋巴瘤起源于 B 细胞，其余起源于 T 细胞或 NK 细胞。不同的亚型中有明显的异质性使临床表现不尽相同，这种复杂的异质性表明需要发展更加具有针对性的治疗策略。

（一）以细胞周期异常为靶点

（1）Bcl-6：Bcl-6 在淋巴结生发中心（germinal center，GC）表达以调节 B 细胞受体（B-cell receptor，BCR）介导的淋巴细胞活性和免疫球蛋白（immunoglobulins，Ig）亲和力成熟的生理学水平。通过 IHC 鉴别高表达 Bcl-6 的淋巴瘤，用以蒽环类药物（anthracycline）为基础化疗可以提高 Bcl-6 阳性淋巴瘤的无病生存期（disease-free survival，DFS）和无进展生存期（progression-free survival，PFS）。相反，用利妥昔单抗（抗 CD-20 抗体）治疗 Bcl-6 阴性淋巴瘤有效，而在 Bcl-6 阳性淋巴瘤的效果不理想，尤其在弥漫性大 B 细胞淋巴瘤（diffuse large B-cell lymphoma，DLBCL）的治疗中[39]。因此，以 Bcl-6 为靶点的靶向疗法可以克服淋巴瘤中的转录抑制和分化障碍。

（2）85% 的滤泡淋巴瘤（follicular lymphoma，FL）中存在 Bcl-2 染色体 t（14：18）（q32；q21）易位，而在其他淋巴瘤中罕见。这一染色体易位使位于 14 号染色体长臂的 Ig 重链基因和位于 18 号染色体的 Bcl-2 基因的转录活性位点拼接，造成 Bcl-2 基因的过度表达，导致 Bcl-2 蛋白转录增加，使 B 淋巴细胞免于凋亡而长期存活，产生化疗耐受，因此 Bcl-2 阳性的肿瘤要比 Bcl-2 阴性的肿瘤预后更差。目前临床研究比较活跃的是利用反义寡核苷酸（antisense oligonucleotides，ASO）和小分子 Bcl-2 抑制剂抑制 Bcl-2 介导的化疗耐受，在复发/难治（relapsed/refractory，r/r）型 NHL 临床试验中，ASO（oblimersin）联合利妥昔单抗疗法显示总缓解率（overall response rate，ORR）超过 40%[40]。一些 Bcl-2 小分子抑制剂，如 ABT-263、ABT-737、特别是 ABT-199 也纳入临床试验的研究范围。

（3）CDK 抑制剂：可以引起线粒体损伤减少细胞的增殖和减少 DNA 合成。Ⅱ期临床试验评估 CDK 抑制剂 flavopiridol 治疗套细胞淋巴瘤（mantle cell lymphoma，MCL）的疗效，结果显示 11% 的患者发生部分缓解（partial response，PR），71% 的患者病情稳定[41]。这种药物在治疗复发/难治 r/r 型慢性淋巴细胞白血病（CLL）中显示 ORR 为 53%，中位 PFS 为 10~12 个月。该药物还可以使高危组（如 del17p，del11）的患者发生缓解，这一发现促进了其他新型 CDK 抑制剂的开发与应用[42]。

（4）c-myc：myc 位点位于 8 号染色体，当与染色体 lg 基因发生 t（14；2）或 t（14；22）易位时，可导致具有淋巴细胞增殖能力的融合蛋白的产生。这种改变通常是伯基特淋巴瘤的特点，也可以在其他类型的淋巴瘤中观察到。在 Bcl-2 或 Bcl-6 共表达存在的情况下，将放大 c-myc 促进肿瘤侵袭的能力。最近，一种新的化合物结构域蛋白抑制剂（bromodomain protein inhibitor）JQ1 以核染色质依赖的信号转导 RNA 聚合酶为靶点，这是理想的 c-myc 抑制剂，正在进行对 r/r 型淋巴瘤的 I 期研究[43]。

（二）以调节免疫系统为靶点

由于利妥昔单抗作为单药或联合放射性同位素的疗法，即放射免疫治疗（radio-immunotherapy）治疗淋巴瘤的较好效果，推动了对淋巴瘤表面抗原的鉴定，针对不同表面抗原开发更多的抗体。已有很多商业性地针对不同淋巴瘤抗原（如 CD2、CD19、CD22、CD23、CD30、CD40、CD52、CD80 和 HLA-DR）的有效抗体处于不同阶段的临床试验中。过去集中研究了针对 B 细胞淋巴瘤的单克隆抗体，今后将重点研究与创制免疫调节药物和这一领域中其他以 APC 为靶点的药物。

1. 免疫调节药物 已知免疫调节药物（immunomodulatory drugs），如沙利度胺（thalidomide）和来那度胺（lenalidomide）是治疗淋巴瘤的有效药物。免疫调节药物作用机制多种多样，包括减少血管生成、促进免疫监视、抑制 Akt/MAPK/STAT3 通路、下调 NF-κB 通路和促进肿瘤细胞凋亡。在 DLBCL 中，免疫调节药物的效果优于非 GCB 亚型，可能是由于产生 1 型 IFN 继发产生 IL-β。单药来那度胺（CTLA-4 antibody）治疗 r/r 型淋巴瘤的总缓解率为 34%，CR 率为 12%，中位 PFS 为 4 个月。进一步的研究在于探索肿瘤复发情况下，来那度胺治疗 B 细胞和 T 细胞淋巴瘤的疗效，包括少数高危亚型，如在高危亚型 r/r 型 CLL（11q or 17p 缺失）中来那度胺作为单药治疗显示 ORR 为 38%，19% 的患者达到 CR。随后美国 FDA 批准来那度胺治疗复发性 MCL。比较只用来那度胺治疗和接受过两种或两种以上的药物治疗，其中一种药物为硼替佐米（bortezomib）治疗的患者，结果表明来那度胺的治疗优于或等于两种或两种以上药物的疗效。近期的报道表明来那度胺联合 R-CHOP 方案可以作为一线药物治疗老年 DLBCL，ORR 和 2 年 OS 超过 90%[44]。这些研究表明免疫调节药物是一种治疗高危淋巴瘤（常规单药化疗疗效不佳的淋巴瘤）的有效新药。进一步应考虑该药适当地联合用药将改善淋巴瘤的预后。

2. 趋化因子（CCL3、CCL4、CXCR5、CXCR4 和 CXCL12） 趋化因子（chemokines）有助于白细胞向损伤、炎症和增殖的组织游走。在许多淋巴瘤中，趋化因子可以激活抗凋亡途径，增加血管生成，并使淋巴瘤细胞产生耐药性。由于趋化因子作用的多重性，使其对淋巴瘤预后有复杂的影响。例如，趋化因子 CCL3 和 CCL4 高表达的 DLBCL 患者，其 PFS 和 OS 均低于其低表达者。有些患者在被诊断为淋巴瘤前数年中，其趋化因子水平就较高，这可能与某种慢性免疫激活促进高危患者（如 HIV 阳性患者）发展成淋巴瘤有关。同样，趋化因子水平升高也是 T 细胞淋巴瘤预后不良的标志，并且是该病一个潜在的治疗靶点。临床前研究表明，组蛋白去乙酰化酶抑制剂（histone decetylase inhibitor）和组蛋白抑制剂（BTK inhibitor）具有抑制趋化因子活性的作用[45]。针对 CC 受体-4 的人源化单克隆抗体（kw-0761），在治疗复发性 T 细胞淋巴瘤的 I 期临床研究中获得了较好的疗效[46]。在 II 期研究中显示，kw-0761 治疗复发性 T 细胞白血病/淋巴瘤的 ORR 为 35%，PFS 为 3 个月。在这些研究的基础上促成 III 期临床的随机研究（目前正在进行中），以比较伏立诺他（vorinostat）与 kw-0761 治疗皮肤 T 细胞淋巴瘤（cutaneous T-cell lymphoma，CTCL）中的优劣。这些临床研究的结果将提供更多的趋化因子抑制剂治疗 T 细胞淋巴瘤的有效信息。

（三）以信号转导通路为靶点

1. 针对淋巴瘤中 NF-κB 通路异常的分子治疗 NF-κB 家族调控和介导淋巴细胞中细胞增殖和存活的蛋白转录。持续性激活 NF-κB 通路可以通过抑制细胞凋亡和产生抵抗化疗的细胞克隆来增加恶性细胞的生存[47]。一些 B 细胞和 T 细胞淋巴瘤中可出现 NF-κB 高表达。来那度胺、姜黄素（curcumin）和蛋白酶体抑制剂硼替佐米等，在体内、外具有靶向 NF-κB 的活性。在正常情况下，NF-κB 蛋白绑定 I-κBα（nuclear factor of kappa light polypeptide gene enhancer in B cells inhibitor，α），通过蛋白酶复合体使其免于降解。在淋巴瘤中，由于泛素-蛋白酶体降解使 I-κBα 降解，使 NF-κB 通路持续活化。I-κBα 降解导致胞质释放游离 NF-κB 进入细胞核，诱导细胞抗凋亡基因的产生[48]。硼替佐米是一种泛素-蛋白酶体抑制剂，通过蛋白酶复合体抑制 I-κBα 降解和维持 NF-κB 绑定 I-κBα，从而防止细胞抗凋亡蛋白的转录。基于这一原理，硼替佐米在治疗 r/r 型 B 细胞淋巴瘤时显示出良好的效果，尤其在 MCL 患者中。硼替佐米单药治疗 r/r 型 MCL 患者中显示 ORR 33%；中位进展期 6.2 个月，促使 FDA 批准该药用于 r/r 型 MCL 患者的治疗。其他研究探索了细胞毒素或其他生物药物联合硼替佐米治疗惰性和侵袭性淋巴瘤的疗效，这种联合疗法对淋巴浆细胞性淋巴瘤/华氏巨球蛋白血症（lymphoplasmacytic lymphoma /Waldenstrom's macroglobulinemia，LPL/WM）和 T 细胞淋巴瘤疗效尤其显著。目前许多临床试验正在探索蛋白酶体抑制剂和化疗药物的最佳组合。

2. 针对淋巴瘤中 JAK-STAT 通路异常的分子治疗 JAK-STAT 通路由 JAK 家族（JAK1-3，TPK-2）和 STAT 家族（STAT1-6）信号转导蛋白组成，能够调节正常细胞周期。常在 HL、活化 B 细胞（activated B-cell，ABC）变异的 DLBCL、原发性纵隔 B 细胞淋巴瘤（primary mediastinal large B-cell lymphoma，PMLBCL）、T 细胞淋巴瘤及多种 NHL 异常表达[49]。某些抗凋亡蛋白如 Bcl-xL 和 Bcl-2，为 STAT 家族的下游蛋白，这些蛋白参与了淋巴瘤的生长。在 HL 和 PMLBCL 细胞株中，JAK2 与 JMJD2c 基因相互作用，改变表观基因组的表达，促进 myc 基因的表达，从而促进淋巴瘤的增殖。同时，淋巴瘤细胞中，JAK2 蛋白还能与程序性死亡蛋白（programmed death ligands，PDL）1 和 2 共表达。而 PDL 表达增高也是 PMLBCL 常见的遗传学异常，这类异常使淋巴瘤细胞逃避细胞毒性 T 细胞的免疫监视[50]。STAT 家族基因的多态性也妨碍正常淋巴细胞成熟，其过表达影响淋巴瘤的预后，如 IHC 检测发现 HL 中 RS（Reed-Stenberg）细胞磷酸化 STAT5 阳性的患者，其预后优于 STAT5 阴性患者[51]。在 DLBCL，尤其是非生发中心 B 细胞型淋巴瘤中，即使是应用免疫治疗，STAT3 的表达也与预后呈负相关。研制针对 JAK-STAT 通路的靶向药物，将可以消除其对预后的消极影响。

3. 淋巴瘤中 JAK2 抑制剂的作用 体内外研究证实，JAK-STAT 抑制剂可导致淋巴瘤细胞死亡。JAK2 抑制剂能促进细胞凋亡，抑制细胞增殖和炎症因子、趋化因子和 PDL1 的表达，并抑制 Bcl-2 合成[52]。在 I 期临床研究中，应用 JAK2-FLT3 抑制剂 SB1518 对 34 名复发性 HL 和 NHL 患者进行治疗，15 名患者病情稳定。病情稳定的患者肿瘤体积缩小 50%，标准差为 4%~46%。34 名患者中，3 名患者达到部分缓解，并对药物的耐受性较好[53]。这些结果促进了 JAK2 抑制剂在淋巴瘤治疗中的研究。

4. PKC 抑制剂治疗淋巴瘤 蛋白激酶 C（protein kinase C，PKC）是 BCR 信号通路的下游蛋白。这些蛋白通过活化 NF-κB 通路，使得恶性淋巴细胞获得生存优势。IHC 和基因检测分别发现，PKC-β 高表达的 DLBCL 患者，即使是应用化疗和免疫疗法，其生存率仍很低[54]。研发的 PKC 抑制剂，如 enzastaurin 和 sotrastaurin 等正在进行临床试验。enzastaurin 能抑制淋巴瘤细胞的增殖和生长，并能降低血管新生。在对 r/r 型 MCL 的 II 期研究中发现，enzastaurin 可以使 27% 患者的无进展生存期（PFS）大于 6 个月。在另一项 II 期研究中，对病理确诊为 1 级或 2 级的滤泡淋巴瘤（follicular lymphoma，FL）III/IV 期患者使用为期≤3 年的 enzastaurin 治疗，每天剂量 500 mg。在进行治疗的 58 名患者中，25.9% 的患者部分缓解（partial response，PR），3.4% 的患者完全缓解（complete response，CR）。相关分析表明，PKC-β_2 低表达与缓解率（response rate，RR）和 PFS 相关，因此认为 PKC-β_2 可以作为预测患者对 enzastaurin 反应的生物学标志。但对已经使用 R-CHOP 方案治疗获得完全缓解的高危组 DLBCL 的 III 期临床研究显示，给予 enzastaurin 作为维持疗法，并不能给患者带来任何好处，其治疗效果与安慰剂无异。enzastaurin 维持疗法不能改善患者的无病生存期（DFS）、PFS 和总生存期（OS）。因此，仍需进行更多的研究，以确定该药在淋巴瘤治疗中的最佳使用时机。

挑战与展望

分子靶向治疗肿瘤已经取得了很大进步，对肿瘤发生机制有了较深入的认识，可实现选择性杀伤肿瘤细胞，减小毒副作用，但仍存在许多问题。目前大部分靶向治疗药物的有效率比较低，疗效不甚理想。加上现有的靶向药物对肿瘤治疗靶点选择性不够特异，存在"非靶向作用"，如过敏、心脏毒性等不良反应，有时十分严重。此外靶向药物在使用过程中也出现耐药现象，且其价格较高，在一段时间内难以广泛应用。因而在一定程度上导致了目前靶向药物的治疗效果与人们的期望值存在一定距离。随着临床试验的开展，发现有些靶向药物在使用过程中也经历了由敏感到耐药的过程，进一步反映出肿瘤生长的复杂性。随着对肿瘤发病机制研究的不断深入，新的靶向药物不断出现，一方面可通过靶向药物的联合应用来增强疗效，降低药物耐药性；另一方面可通过研发多靶点的分子靶向药物，来达到增强疗效的作用，如 mTOR 抑制剂西罗莫司对胃癌及肝癌等消化系统肿瘤具有一定效果，多靶点激酶抑制剂（RAF、VEGF、PDGF 抑制剂）索拉非尼已经用于肝癌的治疗。多靶点药物由于其靶点多，作用范围较广，必然也带来较多副作用，同时，在众多的靶点之中，如何预测其有效性也有一定的困难。相信随着对肿瘤本质的进一步认识，如对肿瘤干细胞的认识，必将有更多、更有效的分子靶向药物进入临床，为肿瘤患者的个体化治疗带来希望，从而为肿瘤患者带来福音。

通过分子靶向性治疗和肿瘤免疫治疗使患者的预后得到了显著改善，特别是高通量的基因芯片筛查技术对肿瘤细胞凋亡、血管生成、细胞运动周期等细胞重要生物学事件中的基因调控信号通路的认识和分子机制的阐明，发现了很多靶向特定突变和（或）解除对转录调控的基因与分子，其中有些具有引发肿瘤细胞进程并代表了潜在治疗靶点的基因分子。通过深入分析肿瘤的病理学来寻找更有效的靶点将有助于治疗的进展。分子靶向治疗和肿瘤免疫治疗是基因组医学、精准医疗、个体化治疗和转化医学的一个新的里程碑。

基因组医学进入"单细胞"生物学的时代，单细胞基因测序作为基因组医学的一部分，在肿瘤研究中受到特别关注，以了解单个肿瘤细胞的机械表型、单细胞生物学、异质性和染色体定位和功能，强调指出单细胞生物学是在多维、多层、多交叉和立体单细胞水平上识别和验证疾病特异性生物标志物的一种新方法[55]。但是，将来还面临许多问题。例如，如何将单细胞测量应用于临床实践？如何将单细胞系统生物学的信息翻译成临床表型？如何解释单细胞基因测序的改变和患者治疗反应效果的关系？单个癌细胞、相应组织中的细胞或循环细胞的 RNA 和 DNA 测序将有利于对癌细胞之间、癌和正常细胞之间、起源组织和位置之间的同质性和异质性的深入理解。单细胞生物学允许我们在癌亚型中鉴定和开发疾病特异性生物标志物、网络生物标志物、动态网络生物标志物和基于治疗的靶标[56]。

有人提出开发人类细胞的智能单细胞机器人（intelligent single-cell robot，ISCT），将分子、基因、蛋白质、细胞器、膜、结构、信号和功能的系统信息整合在一起。它可以是一个强大的自动系统，以协助临床医生的决策，促进在分子水平上的理解，以及风险分析和预后预测。

思 考 题

1. 本章基本概念：分子靶向治疗，分子病理学，癌基因成瘾。
2. 与化疗比较分子靶向治疗的优势有哪些？
3. 分子病理学常用的相关技术有哪些？
4. 根据文献结合自己的专业报道分子靶向治疗临床研究进展。

参 考 文 献

[1] Nakhleh R E，Grimm E E，Idowu M O，et al. Laboratory compliance with the American Society of Clinical Oncology/college of American Pathologists guidelines for human epidermal growth factor receptor 2 testing：a College of American Pathologists survey of 757 laboratories[J]. Archives of Pathology & Laboratory Medicine，2010，134（5）：728-734.

[2] Wolff A C，Hammond M E，Schwarlz J N，et al. American Society of Clinical Oncology/college of American Pathologists guideline recommendations for human epidermal growth factor receptor 2 testing in breast cancer[J].Journal of Clinical Oncology，2007，25（1）：118-145.

[3] Riquelme E，Behrens C，Lin H Y，et al. Modulation of EZH2 expression by MEK-ERK or PI3K-AKT signaling in lung cancer is dictated by different KRAS oncogene mutations[J]. Cancer Research，2016，76（3）：675-685.

[4] Erazo T，Lorente M，López-Plana A，et al. The new antitumor drug ABTL0812 inhibits the Akt/mTORC1 axis by upregulating tribbles-3 pseudokinase[J]. Clinical Cancer Research An Official Journal of the American Association for Cancer Research，2016，22（10）：2508-2519.

[5] Group M A C. Chemotherapy in addition to supportive care improves survival in advanced non-small-cell lung cancer：a systematic review and meta-analysis of individual patient data from 16 randomized controlled trials[J]. Journal of Clinical Oncology，2008，26（28）：4617-4625.

[6] Gu J，Wang X，New future of cell biology and toxicology：thinking deeper[J]. Cell Biology and Toxicology，2016，32（1）1-3.

[7] Weinstein I B. Cancer. Addiction to oncogenes—the Achilles heal of cancer. Science 2002，297：63-64.

[8] Scagliotti G V，Parikh P，Von Pawel J，et al. Phase Ⅲ study comparing cisplatin plus gemcitabine with cisplatin plus pemetrexed in chemotherapynaive patients with advancedstage non-smallcell lung cacer[J]. Journal of Clinical Oncology，2008，26（21）：3543-3551.

[9] Sharma S V，Bell D W，Settleman J，et al. Epidermal growth factor receptor mutations in lung cancer[J]. Nature Reviews. Cancer 2007，7：169-181.

[10] Shi Y，Au S K，Thongprasert S，et al. A prospective，molecular epidemiology study of EGFR，mutations in Asian patients with advanced non-small-cell lung cancer of adenocarcinoma histology（PIONEER）[J]. Journal of Thoracic Oncology Official Publication of the International Association for the Study of Lung Cancer，2014，9（2）：154-162.

[11] Wu Y L，Zhou C，Hu C P，et al. Afatinib versus cisplatin plus gemcitabine for first-line treatment of Asian patients with advanced non-small-cell lung cancer harbouring EGFR mutations（LUX-Lung 6）：an open-label，randomised phase 3 trial[J]. Lancet Oncology，2014，15（2）：213-222.

[12] Shepherd F A，Pereira J，Ciuleanu T E，et al. A randomized placebo-controlled trial of erlotinib in patients with advanced non-small cell lung cancer（NSCLC）following failure of 1st line or 2nd line chemotherapy. A National Cancer Institute of Canada Clinical Trials Group（NCIC CTG）trial[J]. Amercan society Clinical Oncology，2004，22：7022.

[13] Lindeman N I，Cagle P T，Beasley M B，et al. Molecular testing guideline for selection of lung cancerpatients for EGFR and ALK tyrosine kinase inhibitors：guideline from the College of American Pathologists，International Asso-ciation for the Study of Lung Cancer，and Association for Molecu-lar Pathology. The Journal of Molecular Diognostics. 2013，15（4）：415-453.

[14] Takahashi T，Sonobe M，Kobayashi M，et al. Clinicopathologic features of non-small-cell lung cancer with EML4-ALK fusion

gene[J]. Annals of Surgical Oncology, 2010, 17 (3): 889-897.

[15] Doebele R C, Pilling A B, Aisner DL, et al. Mechanisms of resistance to crizotinib in patients with ALK gene rearranged non-small cell lung cancer[J]. Clincal Cancer Research. 2012, 18: 1472-1482.

[16] Paik P K, Arcila M E, Fara M, et al. Clinical characteristics of patients with lung adenocarcinomas harboring BRAF mutations[J]. Journal of Clinical Oncology, 2011, 29 (15): 2046-2051.

[17] Brustugun O T, Khattak A M, Trømborg A K, et al. BRAF-mutations in non-small cell lung cancer[J]. Lung Cancer, 2014, 84 (1): 36-38.

[18] Li S, Li L, Zhu Y, et al. Coexistence of EGFR with KRAS, or BRAF, or PIK3CA somatic mutations in lung cancer: a comprehensive mutation profiling from 5125 Chinese cohorts[J]. British Journal of Cancer, 2014, 110 (11): 2812-2820.

[19] Mazières J, Peters S, Lepage B, et al. Lung cancer that harbors an HER2 mutation: epidemiologic characteristics and therapeutic perspectives[J]. Journal of Clinical Oncology 2013, 31 (16): 1997-2003.

[20] De G J, Teugels E, Geers C, et al. Clinical activity of afatinib(BIBW 2992)in patients with lung adenocarcinoma with mutations in the kinase domain of HER2/neu[J]. Lung Cancer, 2012, 76 (1): 123-127.

[21] Drilon A E, Hellmann M D, Wang L, et al. Clinicopathologic features of advanced RET fusion-positive lung cancers and outcomes in comparison to other fusion-positive lung cancers[J]. Journal of Clinical Oncology, 2014.

[22] Kim H R, Kim D J, Kang D R, et al. Fibroblast growth factor receptor 1 gene amplification is associated with poor survival and cigarette smoking dosage in patients with resected squamous cell lung cancer[J]. J. Clin. Oncol. 2013, 31: 731-737.

[23] Nogova L, Sequist L V, Cassier P A, et al. Targeting FGFR1-amplified lung squamous cell carcinoma with the selective pan-FGFR inhibitor BGJ398[J]. 2014.

[24] Miao L, Wang Y, Zhu S, et al. Identification of novel driver mutations of the discoidin domain receptor 2 (DDR2) gene in squamous cell lung cancer of Chinese patients[J]. BMC Cancer, 2014, 14 (1): 369.

[25] Pitini V, Arrigo C, Mirto C D, et al. Response to dasatinib in a patient with SQCC of the lung harboring a discoid-receptor-2 and synchronous chronic myelogenous leukemia[J]. Lung Cancer, 2013, 82 (1): 171-172.

[26] Wang L, Hu H, Pan Y, et al. PIK3CA Mutations Frequently Coexist with EGFR/KRAS Mutations in Non-Small Cell Lung Cancer and Suggest Poor Prognosis in EGFR/KRAS Wildtype Subgroup[J]. PloS One, 2014, 9 (2): e88291.

[27] Wolff A C, Hammond M E, Schwarlz J N, et al. American Society of Clinical Oncology/college of American Pathologists guideline recommendations for human epidermal growth factor receptor 2 testing in breast cancer[J]. J Clin Oncol, 2007, 25 :(1): 118-145.

[28] Adams B D, Wali V B, Cheng C J, et al. miR-34a silences c-SRC to attenuate tumor growth in triple negative breast cancer[J]. Cancer Research, 2016, 76 (4): 927-939.

[29] Villanueva A, Newell P, Chiang D, et al. Genomics and signaling pathways in hepatocellular carcinoma[J]. Semin ars in Liver Diseases, 2007, 27: 55-76.

[30] Comoglio P M, Giordano S, Trusolino L. Drug development of MET inhibitors: targeting oncogene addiction and expedience[J]. Nature Reviews Drug Discovery, 2008, 7 (6): 504-516.

[31] Schmitz K J, Wohlschlaeger J, Lang H, et al. Activation of the ERK and AKT signalling pathway predicts poor prognosis in hepatocellular carcinoma and ERK activation in cancer tissue is associated with hepatitis C virus infection[J]. Journal of Hepatology, 2008, 48 (1): 83-90.

[32] Ashkenazi A, Herbst R S. Ashkenazi A, et al. To kill a tumor cell: the potential of proapoptotic receptor agonists[J]. Journal of Clinical Investigation, 2008, 118 (6): 1979-1990.

[33] Farazi P A, Depinho R A. Hepatocellular carcinoma pathogenesis: from genes to environment[J]. Nature Reviews Cancer, 2006, 6 (9): 674-687.

[34] Peeters M, Van Cutsem E, Siena S, et al. A phase 3, multicenter, randomized controlled trial of panitumumab plus best supportive care (BSC) vs BSC alone in patients with metastatic colorectal cancer[C]. Program and Abstracts of the 97th Annual Meeting of the American Association for Cancer Research, April 1-5, 2006, Washington DC.

[35] Van C E, Köhne C H, Láng I, et al. Cetuximab plus irinotecan, fluorouracil, and leucovorin as first-line treatment for metastatic colorectal cancer: updated analysis of overall survival according to tumor KRAS and BRAF mutation status[J]. Journal of Clinical Oncology, 2011, 29 (15): 2011-2019.

[36] Douillard J, Siena S. infusional fluorouracil, leucovorin, and oxaliplatin (FOLFOX4) versus FOLFOX4 alone as first-line treatment in patients with previously untreated metastatic colorectal[J]. Journal of Clinical Oncology, 2010, 28(31): 4697-4705.

[37] Van C E, De H S, Kang Y K, et al. Bevacizumab in combination with chemotherapy as first-line therapy in advanced gastric cancer: a biomarker evaluation from the AVAGAST randomized phase III trial[J]. Journal of Clinical Oncology, 2012, 30(17): 2119-2127.

[38] Yi J H, Lee J, Lee J, et al. Randomised phase Ⅱ trial of docetaxel and sunitinib in patients with metastatic gastric cancer who were previously treated with fluoropyrimidine and platinum[J]. British Journal of Cancer, 2012, 106（9）: 1469-1474.

[39] Shustik J, Han G, Farinha P, et al. Correlations between BCL6 rearrangement and outcome in patients with diffuse large B-cell lymphoma treated with CHOP or R-CHOP[J]. Haematologica, 2010, 95（1）: 96-101.

[40] Pro B, Leber B, Smith M, et al. Phase Ⅱ multicenter study of oblimersen sodium, a Bcl-2 antisense oligonucleotide, in combination with rituximab in patients with recurrent B-cell non-Hodgkin lymphoma[J]. British Journal of Haematology, 2008, 143（3）: 355-360.

[41] Kouroukis C T, Belch A, Crump M, et al. Flavopiridol in untreated or relapsed mantle-cell lymphoma: results of a phase Ⅱ study of the National Cancer Institute of Canada Clinical Trials Group[J]. Journal of Clinical Oncology, 2003, 21（9）: 1740-1745.

[42] Lin T S, Ruppert A A. Phase Ⅱ study of flavopiridol in relapsed chronic lymphocytic leukemia demonstrating high response rates in genetically high-risk disease.[J]. Journal of Clinical Oncology, 2009, 27（35）: 6012-6018.

[43] Delmore J E, Issa G C, Lemieux M E, et al. BET bromodomain inhibition as a therapeutic strategy to target c-Myc[J]. Cell, 2011, 146（6）: 904-917.

[44] Goy A, Sinha R, Williams M E, et al. Single-Agent Lenalidomide in Patients With Mantle-Cell Lymphoma Who Relapsed or Progressed After or Were Refractory to Bortezomib: Phase Ⅱ MCL-001（EMERGE）Study[J]. Journal of Clinical Oncology, 2013, 31（29）: 3688-3695.

[45] de Rooij M F, Kuil A, Geest C R, et al. The clinically active BTK inhibitor PCI-32765 targets B-cell receptor- and chemokine-controlled adhesion and migration in chronic lymphocytic leukemia[J]. Blood, 2012, 119（11）: 2590-2594.

[46] Yamamoto K, Utsunomiya A, Tobinai K, et al. Phase I study of KW-0761, a defucosylated humanized anti-CCR4 antibody, in relapsed patients with adult T-cell leukemia-lymphoma and peripheral T-cell lymphoma[J]. Journal of Clinical Oncology, 2010, 28（9）: 1591-1598.

[47] Ersing I, Bernhardt K, Gewurz B E. NF-kappaB and IRF7 pathway activation by Epstein-Barr virus latent membrane protein 1[J]. Viruses, 2013, 5（6）: 1587-1606.

[48] Juvekar A, Manna S, Ramaswami S, et al. Bortezomib induces nuclear translocation of IkappaBalpha resulting in gene-specific suppression of NF-kappaB--dependent transcription and induction of apoptosis in CTCL[J]. Molecular Cancer Research, 2011, 9（2）: 183-194.

[49] Kleppe M, Tousseyn T, Geissinger E, et al. Mutation analysis of the tyrosine phosphatase PTPN2 in Hodgkin's lymphoma and T-cell non-Hodgkin's lymphoma[J]. Haematologica, 2011, 96（11）: 1723-1727.

[50] Twa D D, Chan F C, Ben-Neriah S, et al. Genomic rearrangements involving programmed death ligands are recurrent in primary mediastinal large B-cell lymphoma[J]. Blood, 2014, 123（13）: 2062-2065.

[51] Martini M, Hohaus S, Petrucci G, et al. Phosphorylated STAT5 represents a new possible prognostic marker in Hodgkin lymphoma[J]. American Journal of Clinical Pathology, 2008, 129（3）: 472-477.

[52] Kirk R. Haematological cancer: Hit the lymphoma, JAK[J]. Nature Reviews Clinical Oncology, 2012, 9（11）: 608.

[53] Younes A, Romaguera J, Fanale M, et al. Phase I study of a novel oral Janus kinase 2 inhibitor, SB1518, in patients with relapsed lymphoma: evidence of clinical and biologic activity in multiple lymphoma subtypes[J]. Journal of Clinical Oncology, 2012, 30（33）: 4161-4167.

[54] Li S, Phong M, Lahn M, et al. Retrospective analysis of protein kinase C-beta（PKC-β）expression in lymphoid malignancies and its association with survival in diffuse large B-cell lymphomas[J]. Biology Direct, 2007, 2（1）: 1-13.

[55] Niu F, Wang D C, Lu J, et al. Potentials of single - cell biology in identification and validation of disease biomarkers[J]. Journal of Cellular & Molecular Medicine, 2016, 20（9）: 1789-1795.

[56] Wu D, Wang X. Application of clinical bioinformatics in lung cancer-specific biomarkers[J]. Cancer and Metastasis Reviews, 2015, 34（2）: 209-216.

（付鲁渝 王建力 陈 莉）

Chapter 14 Targeted Therapy for Tumor

With the development of tumor molecular biology, molecular targeted therapy and precision medicine are the new methods for tumor therapy that have gradually become a hot topic. The molecular targeted therapy is the key molecule to the tumor process and development, through blocking tumor cells signal transduction specifically, controlling its gene expression and the biological behavior changes, or through blocking tumor angiogenesis, thus inhibiting the growth and reproduction of tumor cells, thereby inhibiting or killing the tumor cells without affecting normal tissue around the tumor cells and playing an anti tumor role. Therefore only the specific gene mutation is suitable for targeted drug therapy. Molecular targeted therapy is also known as "biological missile". Iits target is the growth factor receptor on the cell surface or an important enzyme or protein in intracellular signal transduction pathway. Molecular targets are generally involved in tumor cell differentiation, apoptosis, migration, division, infiltration, lymph node and whole body metastasis from DNA to any subcellular protein levels.

Section 1 Roles of Molecular Pathology in Targeted Therapy of Tumors

The tumor treatment measure is in continuous improvement. In contrast to traditional surgery, chemotherapy, radiotherapy, immunotherapy and traditional chinese medicine, molecular targeted therapy is a new therapy.

1. Advantages of Molecular Targeting Therapy

Compared with traditional chemotherapy, molecular targeted therapy has the advantages of strong specificity, obvious curative effect, less damage to normal tissue and so on, which has obvious advantages:

(1) The molecular targeted therapy is a major content of personality treatment and precision medicine. For example, in the presence of epidermal growth factor receptor (EGFR), mutations in non-small cell lung cancer (NSCLC) are treated by the use EGFR tyrosine kinase inhibitors (EGFR-TKIs). Its effective rate is more than 90%. So through the EGFR detection of organization it can predict the therapeutic effect.

(2) Because the drugs nature and target functions are different, the molecular targeted therapeutic has target specificity, mild toxicity. Unlike cytotoxic chemotherapy, targeted drugs are often for abnormal mutations site make effect, can be aimed at a specific target on the tumor cells, can accuratly strike tumor cells and don't damage normal cells, Therefore, gastrointestinal tract reactions and blood toxicity is mild and can improve the patients symptoms rapidly. Patients can easily tolerate. In contrast to the use of cytotoxic drugs in the treatment of patients with advanced cancer some patients have prolonged survival period because those patients have fear of treatment and so they have side effects.

(3) The molecular targeted therapy is a simple and easy way. At present, a lot of targeted drugs are given through oral administration, Patients have good compliance and tolerance. They can be treated by clinic or family therapy, the patients are very easy to accept.

(4) The molecular targeted drugs combind with chemotherapy can improve the efficacy, and the side effects are not increased significantly.

2. Roles of Molecular Pathology in Targeted Therapy of Tumors

To do molecular targeted therapy, we first need to determine the diagnosis, determine the tumor tissues and cells whether they meet the conditions target or not, and then carry out targeted therapy, and in this way we can predict whether the target drug is effective or not. Therefore, molecular targeted therapy must be dependent on the methods of molecular pathology research. The molecular pathology in biological macromolecules such as protein and nucleic acid level, uses the theory, technology and methods of molecular biology to research the development and progression of disease. The researching techniques of molecular pathology are commonly used to include in situ hybridization, fluorescence in situ hybridization (FISH), polymerase chain reaction technique (PCR), in situ PCR microdissection (micro-dissection), gene sequencing technology, biochip technology, southern blotting method and so on. Due to the application of molecular pathology, we are enable to deeply understand the nature of the disease. We have made great progress in the diagnosis and treatment of cancer, mainly in the following aspects:

(1) Detection of tumor susceptibility genes: Cancer genetic susceptibility gene detection is useful for screening the high-risk population of cancer. It is clear that the tumor susceptibility genes and its related tumors have Rb1 (retinoblastoma), WT1 (renal cell tumor) and so on. In addition to detect susceptible genes in high-risk population, these methods are also applied to screening tumor susceptibility genes in the normal population, such as detection of Ret gene mutation for the diagnosis of type II multiple endocrine neoplasia, or analysis of the GST gene type to determine individual exposure to carcinogens and carcinogenic risk.

(2) Detection of tumor related viruses: Such as HPV infection and cervical cancer have a great relationship. Through detecting and analysing the types of HPV, we can prevent and treat the early stage of cancers. The current international diagnosis of HPV infection is mainly based on the DNA detection.

(3) Early diagnosis of cancer: Such as the mutation rate of K-ras gene is high in colon cancer, pancreatic cancer and lung cancer. Detection of the twelfth codon mutation of the pancreatic cancer in fine needle aspiration biopsy material. Detection of Ras gene mutations in stool of colorectal cancer patients with PCR-RFLP method, in which detection rate is similar to the tumor tissue, which can be used for screening the high-risk groups.

(4) The classification and diagnosis of difficult tumors: Such as the traditional pathological diagnosis

is mainly based on morphology and immunity phenotype to judge the lymphocyte proliferation and lymphoma, it has the higher requirement of doctor's experience. Application of RFLP analysis for immunoglobulin or T cell receptor gene rearrangement can play differential diagnosis effect. The molecular type is more accurate than the immunophenotype.

(5) Monitoring tumors prognosis: Develops the individual blood testing methods using the full gene sequence of cancer patients and helps doctors to adjust the treatment options, monitor the effects of treatment and find the recurrence in cancer patients.

(6) Providing a basis for the cancer personality and predictable treatment: The tumor development in different period may involve the different forms of different genes, which is closely related to the sensitivity of clinical therapy of tumor. If it can provide that indicators of tumor gene changes at the molecular level, which has guiding significance for tumor molecular targeted therapy and precision medicine.

(7) Judging tumor prognosis: The mutations, amplification and overexpression of the oncogenes are often associated with the prognosis of the tumor. Such as HER-2 gene amplification is closely related with the development of breast cancer and clinical prognosis, the positive expression of HER-2 indicates a poor prognosis, by FISH, combined with postoperative treatment, to guide the clinical medication.

Section 2 Common Used Molecular Targets and Targeted Drugs

At present the clinical molecular targeted therapy is divided into (1) Anti-EGFR, (2) Anti- angiogenic agents and (3) mTOR inhibitors, etc.

1. Anti EGFR Monoclonal Antibody

EGFR also known as HER1 or ErbB1 is one of the four members of the ErbB receptor tyrosine kinase family. HER-2 is a transmembrane tyrosine kinase receptor, with activity of receptor tyrosine kinase protein, a member of the human EGFR family .HER-2 plays an important role in the control of cell growth, differentiation, adhesion and activation in cell signaling pathways. At present the main anti EGFR monoclonal antibody have cetuximab, Malaysia trastuzumab (matuzumab) and panitumumab. Among them, cetuximab has been approved for clinical.

1) Trastuzu-mab (Hessaitin) is a humanized monoclonal antibody from the derivative of recombinant DNA, it binds to HER-2 receptor to disrupt its auto-phosphorylation, down-regulating the expression of HER-2 gene and antagonisting the promoting growth effect of the HER-2 family, mediating the antibody dependent cytotoxicity (ADCC) function, enhancing the chemotherapy-induced cytotoxicity, to curb the growth of tumor cells or attack and kill tumor cells, restrain tumor metastasis effect. And it has no effect on HER-2 negative tumor cells or normal cells. Therefore, detecting the HER-2 expression of tumor tissue is required before use trastuzumab treatment   But trastuzumab can cause cardiac toxicity for some patients, 2007 ASCO/CAP carried out detailed and strict specifications for target detection and positive standards of HER-2 positive breast cancer cases in the relevant guidelines. In recent years, trastuzumab has been widely used in the treatment of breast cancer, gastric cancer.

2) Panitumu-mab is a monoclonal antibody of HER-2 molecules, and bind HER-2 target forms two dimers can inhibit target function effectively. The small molecules TKIs can reversible or irreversible inhibit the tyrosine kinase activity within HER-2 target molecules. Such as Neratinib is a new type of TKI, can also act on HER-2 and HER-4 at the same time, and its clinical effect is also better.

2. Small Molecule Tyrosine Kinase Inhibitors Targeting EGFR Mutation (EGFR-TKIs)

EGFR is over expression and (or) mutation in a variety of tumors, mutant EGFR can activate AKt signal transducer protein and   transcription activator (STAT) signal transduction pathway selectively, so as to prolong cell survival, lead to tumor cell uncontrolled growth and malignant development. The small molecule tyrosine kinase inhibitors (TKI) is mainly inhibit this signal pathway:

1) By inhibiting the phosphorylation of tyrosine kinase, thereby inhibiting the associated signal transduction; mainly involved gefitinib, erlotinib and lapatinib. gefitinib is mainly used for treat advanced NSCLC, head and neck cancer, prostate cancer and breast cancer. It should be noted that gefitinib play the roles of anti proliferation, angiogenesis and cell migration through blocking the signaling pathway of cancer cells to obtain the clinical therapeutic effect. The Asian race confirmed that the treatment effect is better, worthy of future research to confirm. Erlotinib is mainly used for the treatment of advanced and metastatic NSCLC patients.

Due to 85% of protocarcinogenic gene and cancer gene products are tyrosine protein kinase （TPK） and TPK activity increases in tumor, so cell proliferation can be blocked by targeting TPK to inhibit TPK catalytic activity. The present study is relatively concentrating on inhibiting cell signal transduction pathways mediated by TPK (receptor type TPK-Ras-MAPK pathway). Such as monoantibody can block the combination of ligand and receptor TPK.

2) Sunitinib is an oral multitargeted TKI and its action   mechanism is to inhibit the tyrosine kinase activity of VEGF and platelet-derived growth factor receptor -β(PDGFR--β), KIT, KLT-3 and RET though specificity blocking the signal transduction to achieve antitumor effect.

3) Sorafenib is an oral multitargeted TKI, effects serine, threonine and receptor tyrosine kinase on tumor cells and tumor blood vessels ,it can directly inhibit tumor growth by inhibiting the Raf-MEK-ERK signal transduction pathway as well as   indirectly inhibit the tumor cells growth by inhibiting VEGF and PDGFR.

The second-generation irreversible EGFR TKI, such as dacomitinib and afatinib, is pan-ErbB inhibitors with in vitro activity against both activating EGFR mutations and the T790M resistance mutation.

Third-generation EGFR TKI (CO-1686 and AZD9291) are more T790M selective, clinically more potent and less toxic than the current EGFR TKI. Preliminary results of both CO-1686 and AZD929 are highly promising given their improved to lerability and clinical activity.

3. EGFR Monoclonal Anibody Targeted K-ras Mutation （Cetuxi-mab）

The KRAS protein is a member of the RAS family of guanosine triphosphatases. KRAS mutations result in a constitutively active KRAS, resulting in oncogenesis. KRAS mutations portend a worse outcome with increased risk of recurrence in early-stage disease and poorer survival in metastatic stage.

The proto oncogene K-ras play a key role in the development of a variety of tumors. K-ras protein is also called P21 protein, as a membrane-bound GTP/GDP binding protein, moderate regulate P21 is opened and closed to signal system , completed by growth of conversion between GTP and GDP, the differentiation of signals into cellular processes. When the K-ras gene mutation, which is not affected by the EGFR gene upstream state, always in the active state, continued to stimulate cell growth and tumorigenesis. BRAF gene is a member of the RAF family, its encoding protein is a serine / threonine protein kinase, which is the key factor in the MEK/ERK signaling pathway. The researchers found that combination of EZH2 and MEK-ERK or PI3K/AKT binding can inhibit sensitivity in the cell and specific K-ras gene mutations, which can be used for targeted therapy of MEK-ERK and PI3K/AKT pathway activation in cancer cells. The expression of EZH2 in MEK-ERK or PI3K-AKT signaling pathway was regulated by different K-ras gene mutations in lung cancer. Ras is the key molecules in mediating TPK signal transduction pathways. Inhibiting Ras transfering to membrane can to block its activation, or using inactive mutated Ras block the Ras signal transduction process. Cetuximab and panitumumab are against the extracellular domain of EGFR cell chimeric human mouse IgG monoclonal antibody, can be produced ADCC activity by binding to cell surface receptors, which is independent of the presence of EGFR mutations. At present, Cetuximab has become a first-line therapy drug for metastatic colorectal cancer.

4. Anti VEGF Molecular Targeted Drugs

Bevacizumab(Avastin) is a kind of anti VEGF humanized monoclonal antibody that can specifically bind to VEGF, blocking its interaction with receptors and produce a variety of effects of anti angiogenesis. Endostar anti endothelial cell preparations -- human endostatin (En-dostar), domestic and rituximab, Gleevec (treating gastrointestinal stromal tumor with CD117/CD34 positive), etc.

5. Other Targeted Drugs

1) ADP RNA polymerase I (PARP-1) inhibitor，PARP-1 enzyme is an important enzyme about DNA repair and cell proliferation, the drugs such as olaparib, ABT 888, has shown efficacy in exciting.

2) mTOR inhibitors: Everolimus, mainly used for the failure of trastuzumab for treatment, and in treatment of Hesse Ding resistant patients were high hopes. The current study has also been carried out on a number of everolimus. Recently, some researchers have found that the new anti tumor drugs A BTL0812 by up regulating the tri-bbles-3 pseudo kinase inhibits AKT/mTORC1 axis, with anti-tumor cell proliferation.

3) c-Met inhibitors, IGFR1 inhibitors and Wnt inhibitors.

Section 3　Molecular Targeted Therapy in Common Tumors

Molecular targeted therapies have created an encouraging trend in the management of cancer. More than 40 molecular targeted therapies have been tested during recent years , and more than 10 of them have improved the survival of patients with NSCLC, breast cancer (HER-2 positive), lymphoma (CD20 positive), gastrointestinal stromal tumor (CD117/CD34 positive),colorectal cancer, hepatocellular Caicinoma (HCC), renal, head and neck cancers and dermatofibroma protuberans.

1. Molecular Targeted Therapy for Lung Cancer

Lung cancer remains the number one cause of cancer deaths worldwide. In 2014, an estimated 224 210 new cases of lung cancer will be diagnosed, of which the majority of patients are NSCLC and in the advanced stage. Historically, patients with advanced stage NSCLC were treated with platinum chemotherapy regardless of histological subtype. Despite an improvement in overall survival (OS) when compared with best supportive care, 3a therapeutic plateau has been reached with a response rate of about 20% and a median survival of $8\sim10$ months. Molecular pathological examination provides an opportunity for the early diagnosis and development of lung cancer. Evaluating the molecular pathology By immunohistochemistry, in situ hybridization and gene sequencing and other methods to clear the classification of lung cancer, to determine the range of tumor invasion and the extent of surgical resection margins (e.g., positive or negative margins), to distinguish primary lung cancer and metastatic tumor, it can also be used in molecular diagnosis research, to determine whether there are specific abnormal gene expression or mutation, to predict lung cancer prognosis and curative effect, and according to the individual molecular targeted therapy.

Advances in the understanding of molecular genetics have led to the recognition of multiple molecularly distinct subsets of NSCLC. This has led to the development of rationally directed molecular targeted therapy, leading to improve clinical out-comes.

A number of genome-based biomarkers were discovered and developed in lung cancer, including the expression, sequencing, or epigenetics of DNA, element networks, or chromosome positioning.

Lung cancer is one of the most explored diseases in genome medicine and was early considered for precision medicine with a number of developed targeted therapies.

Advances in the understanding of molecular genetics in NSCLC have led to the identification of key genetic aberrations in NSCLC. These genetic aberrations (driver mutations) occur in oncogenes that encode signaling proteins that are crucial for cellular proliferation and survival. The concept of oncogene addiction is based on the notion that tumors become greatly dependent on the expression of single oncogenes for survival oncogene-addicted tumors have been identified in NSCLC and exploited with specific molecular targeted agents.

(1) Targeting Lung adenocarinoma therapy

Lung adenocarcinoma is the most common histological subtype of NSCLC, comprising of more than 50% of all NSCLC. When a randomized trial showed superior outcomes for platinum-pemetrexed than for platinum-gemcitabine in patients with advanced stage non-squamous NSCLC. More recently, lung adenocarcinoma can be subdivided into clinically relevant molecular subsets, include mutations in the EGFR, KRAS, HER2, PIK3CA, BRAF, MET genes, andgene rearrangement in ALK, ROS1 and RET.

Tumor angiogenesis, including anti VGFR monoclonal antibodies (bevacizumab) and endostatin (domestic Endostar). Small molecules substance acting on tumor cell signal transduction pathway of tumor EGFR-TKI gefitinib (Iressa), erlotinib (Tarceva) etc. Among them, the gefitinib clinical mainly for the treatment of advanced stage NSCLC with EGFR genes mutations.

EGFR is an attractive target in NSCLC as it is frequently overexpressed, and its activation results in the downstream activation of important signaling pathways, leading to increased cell proliferation, survival, angiogenesis and metastasis. [18-19] Small-molecule EGFR tyrosine kinase inhibitors (TKI), such as gefitinib and erlotinib, were initially introduced in unselected NSCLC patients previously treated with chemotherapy. Other EGFR TKI developed since then includes afatinib and dacomitinib. Gefitinib (Iressa®; AstraZeneca, London, UK, http://www. astrazeneca.com) was the first oral EGFR inhibitor to come on the market. On May 5, 2003, it was granted Subpart H approval by the U.S. Food and Drug Administration (FDA) on the basis of response rate in patients with NSCLC refractory to both docetaxel (Taxotere®; Sanofi-Aventis, Paris, http://en.sanofi-aventis.com) and platinum. However, gefitinib-treated patients survived longer than placebo treated patients in two specific patient subsets: patients of Asian origin and never-smokers.

Due to the high frequency of mutations in the EGFR gene in women, non smokers, adenocarcinoma, and Asian populations, therefore, gefitinib is particularly effective for Oriental women, non smoking, adenocarcinoma subgroup. The molecular basis for increased sensitivity to EGFR TKI was subsequently identified to be due to somatic activating mutations in exon 18-21 of EGFR (commonly exon 19 deletions and L858R point mutation in exon 21) that encode the tyrosine kinase domain of the EGFR. Mutations in exon 18 are known to confer sensitivity to EGFR TKI; however, exon 20 inframe insertions are largely associated with primary resistance to treatment with TKI. EGFR mutations are more frequent in patients with the clinical features described previously. Up to 15% of Caucasians and 30%~50% of East Asians with lung adenocarcinoma harbour EGFR mutations. The incidence is as high as 50%~60% in East Asians, who have lung adenocarcinoma and are never smokers.

In patients with untreated NSCLC with sensitizing EGFR mutations, multiple studies have shown EGFRTKI to be superior to chemotherapy in terms of overall response rate (ORR), progression-free survival (PFS) and quality of life.

The EGFR gene mutations can be detected in patients with undifferentiated adenocarcinoma, squamous cell carcinoma, small cell carcinoma (especially compound with adenocarcinoma) and so on. with gefitinib therapy has certain curative effect. The clinical statistics show that the treatment efficiency 30% in the crowd, the disease control rate reached 60% in adenocarcinoma, but the effect is not as chemotherapy for squamous cell carcinoma.

The evidence suggests, therefore, that erlotinib may be a more efficacious agent than gefitinib erlotinib appears to prolong survival for most of the other patient subsets.This apparent efficacy may be in part attributable to the fact that erlotinib was dosed at its maximum-tolerated dose (MTD) 150mg daily, while gefitinib was dosed at about one third of its MTD.

Former smokers or patients who had never smoked, however, had median erlotinib plasma concentrations that were approximately twice that of the patients who were current smoking. Greater survival benefit in nonsmokers may involve a lower incidence of certain gene mutation effects, such as those involving K-ras, and also the lack of induction of cytochrome P450 (CYP) 1A isoforms by cigarette smoke, which results in faster plasma clearance of erlotinib in smokers.

These studies have provided the basis for the rational selection of treatment based on molecularly defined criteria in the treatment of patients with advanced stage NSCLC. Thus, the selection of patients with advanced stage NSCLC for the first-line treatment with EGFR TKI should be based on EGFR mutation status, and EGFR mutation testing should be performed routinely at the time of diagnosis.

The EML4-ALK gene rearrangement, a result from an inversion within chromosome 2p, is a newly identified driver oncogene in lung adenocarcinoma. The fusion between EML4 and ALK results in a chimeric protein that is constitutively active and promotes tumourigenesis via the PI3K-AKT, MAPK and JAK-STAT pathways. EML4-ALK rearrangements are largely mutually exclusive from other driver mutations in NSCLC. The EML4-ALK gene rearrangement is usually detected by fluorescence in situ hybridization (FISH) or immunohistochemistry.

ALK gene rearrangements are uncommon, occur-ring in about 4%~7% of all NSCLC, and it is seen in up to 33% in patients with NSCLC after exclusion of EGFR and Kras mutants, and more likely in younger patients, never or light smokers, adenocarcinomas with signet ring, or acinar histology. ALK inhibitors include crizotinib, and more recently ceritinib and alectinib.

Multiple mechanisms of acquired resistance to crizotinib have been reported, including a secondary mutation in the ALK tyrosine kinase domain (most commonly the L1196M mutation), ALK copy number gain, and the appearance of new oncogene drivers such as EGFR and Kras mutations. Knowledge of the different mechanisms of acquired resistance may impact on subsequent treatment strategies. ALK-directed treatment, such as second-generation ALK TKI, may be directed towards tumors with ALK mutations or copy number gain, whereas resistant tumors secondary to new driver oncogenes may benefit more from chemotherapy.

BRAF is a member of the RAF kinase family of serine/ threonine protein kinases that mediates tumouri-genesis by phosphorylation of MEK and downstream activation of the ERK signaling pathway. BRAF mutations are observed in 1%~3% of NSCLC, and about 50% of BRAF mutations are BRAF V600E mutations. BRAF mutations in NSCLC are more likely in adenocarcinoma, and BRAF V600E mutations are more frequent in women and non-smokers. The BRAF inhibitors dabrafenib and vemurafenib are active in NSCLC harbouring BRAF V600E muta-tions.

Met is a tyrosine kinase receptor, which upon activation induces cell proliferation, motility, scattering, invasion, metastasis, angiogenesis and epithelial to mesenchyme transition. In preliminary data presented recently, in patients with NSCLC harbouring Met amplifications are assessed by FISH treated with crizotinib.

K-ras is associated with adenocarcinoma subtype and smoking, and is more common in Caucasian than East Asian patients. The oral MEK inhibitor selumetinib has shown activity in combination with chemotherapy

Similar to EGFR, HER-2 (ErbB-2) is a member of the ErbB family of tyrosine kinases. HER-2, a major prolif-erative driver, is dysregulated in NSCLC through amplification, overexpression or mutation. HER-2 amplification and HER-2 protein overexpressions occurs in about 20% and in 6%~35%, respectively, in NSCLC, whereas HER-2 mutations are seen in 1%~2%. The majority of patients who harbour HER-2 mutations are female, never smokers and adenocarcinoma.

Promising activity with trastuzumab or afatinib has been reported in retrospective studies of patients with NSCLC with HER-2 mutations. However, studies of trastuzumab combined with chemotherapy in patients with NSCLC overexpressing HER-2 on IHC were negative.

Translocations between the RET gene and its various fusion partners, CCDC6, KIF5B, NCOA4 and TRIM33, have been detected in 1% of patients with lung adenocarcinoma, but it can be as frequent as 7%~17% in an enriched population of younger patients and never smokers. TKI, such as cabozantinib, vandetanib, sunitinib and ponatinib, which are already approved for other malignancies are known to inhibit RET and are currently being studied in RET-rearranged NSCLC. Other RET inhibitors include regorafenib and lenvatinib.

(2) Targeting lung squamous cell carcinoma therapy

Squamous cell lung carcinoma (SQLC) is the second most common histological variant of NSCLC, comprising up to 20%~30% cases. While EGFR mutations are uncommon in squamous cell lung cancer, actionable oncogenes discovered recently in SQLC include fibroblast growth factor receptor-1 (FGFR1) gene amplification, discoidin death receptor 2 (DDR2) gene mutation, and PI3KCA gene amplifications and mutations.

FGFR1 is a receptor tyrosine kinase that mediates tumorigenesis via the MAPK and PI3K pathways, and has been detected in 13%~25% of squamous cell lung cancers.

FGFR1 amplification has been reported to be associated with smoking and is uncommon in adenocarcinoma subtype. FGFR inhibitors are being developed in squamous cell lung cancer, as BGJ398.

The DDR2 is a transmembrane receptor tyrosine kinase that upon activation by collagen promotes cell migration, proliferation and survival. Activating mutations in DDR2 are oncogenic and are detected in about 4%~5% of SQLC.

DDR2-driven transformation is sensitive to the DDR2 inhibitor dasatinib, a TKI used in the treatment of chronic myeloid leukaemia. Response to dasatinib has been described in a patient with SQLC of the lung harbouring a DDR2 kinase domain mutation and synchronous chronic myelogenous leukaemia. Dasatinib is currently being investigated in SQLC patients with DDR2 mutations.

The PI3K signaling pathway is central to cancer cell survival and proliferation. Alterations in the signaling pathway may arise due to amplification or gain of function mutations in the PIK3CA and AKT1 genes or from loss of PTEN function. PI3KCA amplifications and mutations in NSCLC have been reported in 37% and 9%, respectively. Both amplifications and mutations of PI3KCA are poor prognostic factors in SQLC. Studies of PIK3CA inhibitors as monotherapy or in combination with chemotherapy are ongoing.

(3) Targeting therapy for the heterogeneity of lung cancer

In lung cancer should focus more on the homogeneity and heterogeneity of lung cancer which play an important role in the development of drug resistance, genetic complexity, as well as confusion and difficulty of early diagnosis and therapy. The chromosome repositioning may be a critical mechanism of lung cancer cell homogeneity and heterogeneity responsible for the development of drug insensitivity and resistance. The heterogeneity associated with drug resistance, and the mechanism of lung carcinogenesis.

The haploid/diploid genome, as part of chromosome compositions, was found to play a critical role in the stability of allodiploid genome and the differentiation of stem cells [65]. The alterations of haploid or diploid may be one of important regulatory mechanisms of X chromosome inactivation and are used to define regulating phenotypic differences of activated genes. The number of circulating tumor cells (CTC) correlated with the number of metastatic nodules in lung, the growth of primary cancer, the cutting edge of removed tumor from the normal tissue, and the prognosis of patients with cancer. The chromosome repositioning in CTCs reflected by phenotyping of cytokeratin 18 and karyotyping of chromosome 8 was furthermore noticed to be involved in the mechanism by which the cancer cell sensitivity can be changed. The cytokeratin 18-negative diploid and majority of cytokeratin 18-potive diploid CTC subtypes were sensitive to chemotherapy, while the cytokeratin 18-positive multiploid CTC subtype were insensitive to Cisplatin.

Single-cell gene sequencing, as part of genome medicine, was paid special attention in lung cancer to understand mechanical phenotypes, single-cell biology, heterogeneity, and chromosome positioning and function of single lung cancer cells. Some one proposes to develop an intelligent single-cell robot of human cells to integrate together systems information of molecules, genes, proteins, organelles, membranes, architectures, signals, and functions. It can be a powerful automatic system to assist clinicians in the decision-making, molecular understanding, risk analyzing, and prognosis predicting.

A number of targeted therapies have been discovered and developed for lung cancer to increase the accuracy and efficacy of therapy, minimize the toxicity of drugs, and overcome insensitivities and side effects of chemotherapy. Clinical trials demonstrate that subtypes or subgroups of lung cancer cells with certain genetic characters, e.g. gene mutations are sensitive to targeted therapy. The mutation number and copy number variations of targeted genes were applied to select the sensitive population of patients with lung cancer for targeted therapy. The drug resistance developed after targeted therapy is a rising challenge to improve the efficacy of targeting drugs.

2. Molecular Targeted Therapy for Breast Cancer

(1) Targeted therapy for taget HER-2   Gene amplification detecte found that HER-2 was overexpressed in approximately 20% of breast cancer patients, and often suggests poor prognosis. Trastuzumab is currently in clinical use one of the most important drug for HER-2 target point, use of trastuzumab marking breast cancer a new era to molecular targeted therapy. The drug with a variety of chemotherapy drugs such as docetaxel, capecitabine combined treatment can increase the patients survival rate effectively. The lymph node metastasis of HER-2 positive breast cancer cases have been widely used trastuzumab treatment alone or in combination with other drugs chemotherapy can improve the survival rate of patients. Trastuzumab combined with Pertuzumab treatment can inhibit the growth of breast cancer cells have obvious synergistic effect. Small molecule TKIs also showed good clinical effect on HER-2 and HER-4.

(2) Targeted therapy for target EGFG   ADP polymerase I(PARP-1) inhibitor ABT, olaparib 888, especially for the Triple Negative Breast Cancer（ER,PR,ErbB2 all are negative) have a better curative

effect. Gefitinib, erlotinib and La Patini can also be used for the treatment of breast cancer .Some researchers found that miR-34a in three negative breast cancer silencing C-SRC can attenuate tumor growth. It was found that miR-34a and SRC levels were negatively correlated with human tumor specimens. In vitro and in vivo miR-34a anti-tumor effect effectively, and proposed a miR-34a alternative therapy, which is a promising treatment strategy for three female breast cancer.

(3) Most of the agents under investigation block membranous TKRs. Effective blockade of the EGFR signaling pathway can be achieved by the use of monoclonal antibodies against EGFR (cetuximab) or ErbB2/Her-2/neu (trastuzumab). Cetuximab is approved by the U.S. Food and Drug Administration for the treatment of head and neck cancer and colorectal cancer, and trastuzumab for overexpressing-HER-2 metastatic breast cancer. Alternatively, pathway activation can also be successfully inhibited by small molecules such as Erlotinib, which acts against the catalytic domain of EGFR active in advanced stages of NSCLC, or lapatinib, which acts against EGFR and HER-2 and is effective in the treatment of breast cancer.

In breast cancer, HER-2 overexpression or gene amplification is associated with sensitivity to HER-2 inhibitors, such as trastuzumab, pertuzumab and lapatinib.

3. Molecular Targeted Therapy for Hepatocellalar Carcinoma

The molecular pathogenesis of HCC is complex. This neoplasm arises in norma livers, abnormal but noncirrhotic livers, and in cirrhotic livers in 80% of cases as a result of different environmental risk factors.4,5 Each of these scenarios involves different genetic and epigenetic alterations, chromosomal aberrations, gene mutations, and altered molecular pathways. The molecular aberrations described harbor the main targets for liver cancer therapy: protein kinases. Description of the whole kinome a few years ago has facilitated the discovery of new oncology drugs. The key signal transduction pathways implicated in the pathogenesis of HCC are Wnt-β catenin pathway, EGFR-RAS-MAPKK pathway, c-Met pathway, IGF signaling, Akt/mTOR signaling, and VEGF and PDGFR signaling cascades .Other pathways involved in hepatocarcinogenesis such as JAK-STAT, TGF-β, and Hedgehog need further attention to define their relevance and potential therapeutic interest. Ultimately, a molecular classification of HCC based on genomewide investigations and identification of patient subclasses according to drug responsiveness will lead to a more personalized medicine.

(1) Sorafenib is a multikinase inhibitor with reported activity gainst Raf-1, B-Raf, VEGFR2, PDGFR, c-Kit receptors, among other receptor tyrosine kinases and serine threonine kinases. Sorafenib, the only drug approved for treatment of HCC so far, showed appealing preclinical and early clinical trial data. Preclinical studies show potent activity in decreasing HCC cell viability and inducing apoptosis in vitro, and antitumoral activity in xenograft models. Although drugs showing appealing preclinical results have been validated in early phase II studies. Divergent results between preclinical models and clinical outcomes can be due to the heterogeneity of tumors in humans versus in cell lines, the molecular aberrations of the cell line chosen, ectopic versus orthotopic location of tumor, dosage and scheduling of the compounds, and variability in selected end points. However, the greatest discrepancies are likely due to critical differences in the microenvironment. This is particularly relevant to HCC, which arises in an environment of inflammation and fibrosis. patients with activation of RAS/MAPK pathway assessed by positive staining for phosphorylated extracellular signalrelated kinase (p-ERK) had a longer time to progression sorafenib showed a significant benefit to progression .That the effect of sorafenib compares well with other well-established treatments, such as trastuzumab in breast cancer, bevacizumab in colorectal cancer, or erlotinib in NSCLC, where the decrease in the hazard of death is about 25%~35%. Overall, the most frequent adverse events were diarrhea, fatigue, weight loss, and hand-foot skin reaction.

But drug-related adverse events were considered manageable, and no death related with toxicity was described. Recently a multikinase inhibitor, sorafenib, has shown survival benefits in patients with advanced HCC. This advancement represents a breakthrough in the treatment of this complex disease and proves that molecular therapies can be effective in HCC.

(2) Ras/MAPK pathway In HCC, Ras/MAPK pathway activation might result from aberrant upstream signals (EGFR signaling, IGF signaling) or inactivation of tumor suppressor genes by aberrant methylation, as NORE1A.32 Mutations of Raf and Ras are rare findings in HCC. Potent drugs blocking Ras/MAPK signaling are still at the exploratory phase, except for sorafenib, which has activity inhibiting B-Raf at nanomolar concentrations.

(3) c-Met Signaling

Hepatocyte growth factor（HGF） is a critical molecule for hepatocyte regeneration after injury. It is secreted by stellate cells and binds to the c-Met receptor. Aberrant activity of mesenchymal-epithelial transition factor (Met) has been described in human cancers as a result of Met amplification, germline or somatic mutations, transcriptional up-regulation, or HGF-dependent autocrine loops. Dysregulation of c-Met and HGF are common in HCC, although the exact role of this pathway in the pathogenesis of HCC is not established. Several compounds have been developed that target the Met pathway, including antibodies against HGF or Met receptor, or selective small-molecule Met inhibitors,but none of them are yet in an advanced stage of research in HCC.

(4) PI3K/Akt/mTOR Pathway. The PI3K/Akt/mTOR pathway plays a critical role in carcinogenesis. Akt can be activated through a tyrosine kinase receptor (EGF or IGF signaling) or through constitutive activation of PI3K or loss of function of the tumor suppressor gene PTEN by epigenetic silencing or somatic mutations. Mutations of PTEN might confer resistance to small molecules against EGFR. Although the role of pAkt in HCC needs further investigation, recent studies have suggested a worse prognosis for HCC with activated Akt.

An important mediator of the PI3K-Akt pathway is mTOR, which acts as a central regulator of cell growth and proliferation, by sensing nutritional status and allowing progression from G_1 to S phase. The mTOR pathway is activated in a subset of HCCs, and its blockade with rapamycin or everolimus inhibits growth in HCC cell lines, and in experimental models. Everolimus (a rapamycin analog) and termsirolimus are approved for the treatment of renal cancer. Novel compounds are currently being tested in early clinical trials. These molecules (rapamycin and analogs) are already approved as immunosuppressive treatments after liver transplantation.

(5) Other Pathways

Activation of the Wnt cascade has been shown in one third of HCCs, particularly in HCV-induced HCCs.Wnt canonical pathways can also be activated by aberrant methylation of the tumor supressors APC (adenomatous polyposis coli) and E-cadherin or by increase of autocrine/paracrine secretion of Wnt ligands. New drugs targeting this pathway are under early clinical development.

Evasion of this mechanism is one of the hallmarks of cancer. Several proapoptotic receptor agonists targeting the extrinsic apoptosis pathway (including the ligand recombinant human Apo2L/tumor necrosis factor-related apoptosis inducing ligand [TRAIL]) and the intrinsic apoptotic pathway (Bcl-2 antisense) are in development. Synergistic effects have been described with the combination of small molecules and agonists of Apo2L/TRAIL pathway in experimental models. For instance, sorafenib has been shown to sensitize resistant human cancer cells to TRAIL-induced death, providing the rationale for testing these combinations.

Despite recent improvements in surveillance programs and diagnostic tools allowing identification of small suspicious nodules, only 30%～40% of patients with HCC are eligible for curative treatments. In well-selected patients, resection and liver transplantation provide 5-year survival rates of 70% whereas local ablation with radio frequency reaches 50%. It is assumed that these treatments change the natural history of the disease. Tumor relapse complicates half of the patients at 3 years.

Protein kinases are the major drug targets in oncology. Agents are grouped according to the main targets: (1) Anti-EGFR: erlotinib, gefitinib, lapatinib and cetuximab; (2) Anti-angiogenic agents: bevacizumab, sorafenib, sunitinib, vatalanib, cediranib, and combinations; (3) mTOR inhibitors: everolimus, termsirolimus; (4) Other agents: cmet inhibitors, IGFR1 inhibitors and Wnt inhibitors. These agents showed very promising efficacy.

4. Molecular Targeted Therapy for Colorectal Cancer

Colon cancer is a common malignant tumor in the colon digestive tract, the incidence of gastrointestinal cancer is third. With the incidence of colorectal cancer cases increased, the global new cases each year more than 1 million cases.

In February 2004 FDA approved bevacizumab combined with 5-FU based chemotherapy as the first-line treatment for metastatic colorectal cancer (mCRC). phase III clinical trial HORIZON II and HORIZON III trial to assess the efficacy of Cediranib for treatment of advanced colorectal cancer. The results show that oxaliplatin based scheme can significantly increase in PFS (8.6 months vs. 8.2 months P=0.012), but no increase in median OS (19.7 months vs. 18.9 months, P > 0.05), the adverse reactions such as diarrhea, hypertension, leucopenia occurred at a higher rate, the safety and life quality assessment not as good as bevacizumab combined with chemotherapy group. Currently cetuximab has become a first-line therapy for metastatic colorectal cancer (colorectal cancer metastatic, mCRC). The objective remission rate of patients was increased significantly and the survival time was prolonged after based the conventional chemotherapy drugs were added cetuximab. cetuximab combined with FOLFIRI regimen in the treatment can reduce the progression risk of K-ras wild type patients with mCRC disease, it can make progress risk in K-ras wild type patients with mCRC disease reduced 30%, and significantly prolonged free progression survival time of patients, from 8.4 months to 9.9 months. Panitumumab in PRIME of multicenter randomized phase III clinical trial, panitumumab added FOLFOX4 regimen can improve the wild type significantly.The results of PRIME will also become NCCN guide, it make panitumumab combined with FOLFOX4/ /FOLFIRI as an first-line therapy important basis for advanced colorectal cancer chemotherapy. The new version of the (NCCN colorectal cancer clinical diagnosis and treatment guidelines) pointed out that all patients with mCRC should be detected K-ras and BRAF gene mutation, only recommended K-ras and BRAF wild-type patients receiving West rituximab treatment.

5. Molecular Targeted Therapy for Gastric Cancer

Gastric cancer ranks first among all kinds of malignant tumors in China, its prevention and treatment situation is severe, so it is urgent need new treatment methods to improve the curative effect. After lung cancer, breast cancer, colon cancer and esophageal cancerachieved good efficacy, molecular targeted drugs alone or combined with conventional chemotherapy drugs in clinical research on the treatment of gastric cancer has also made considerable progress.

1) Anti VEGF monoclonal antibody bevacizumab (bevacizumab) combined with docetaxel, cisplatin and 5-fluorouracil has certain curative effect on gastric cancer patients, the median progression free survival was 12 months, median overall survival was 16.2 months in patients. A clinical trial showed that the increase bevacizumab in patients with advanced gastric cancer, the median progression free survival and overall remission rate was significantly improved. Some biomarkers can evaluate the efficacy of bevacizumab, bevacizumab combined with chemotherapy in the treatment of gastric cancer has good

prospects, the main adverse reactions including thrombosis, hypertension and perforation, efficacy and safety remain to be further observed.

2) II clinical research showed that small molecule tyrosine kinase inhibitors sunitinib combined with docetaxel in the treatment of patients with metastatic gastric cancer can improve the objective response rate (41.1% vs 14.3%). Phase II clinical trial results showed that sorafenib combined with docetaxel and cisplatin in the treatment of advanced gastric cancer and esophagogastric junction cancer remission rate 38.6%, the median progression free survival was 5.8 months, median overall survival was 14.9 months.

3) The human epidermal growth factor receptor-2 inhibitor. In recent years, the research of trastuzumab treat gastric cancer has become a hot spot. 10%~55% in gastric cancer has HER-2 over expression, about 20% of patients with poor prognosis in patients with gastric cancer, the HER-2 express is positive. Prospective international multicenter randomized phase III clinical trial To GA study, it is proved that targeted therapy can prolong the survival time of advanced gastric cancer.

6. Molecular Targeted Therapy for Lymphoma

Lymphoma is the most common haematopoietic system malignant tumors, which can be divided into Hodgkin's lymphoma (tll, HL) and non Hodgkin lymphoma (NHL). Approximately 85% of the lymphomas originate in B cells, and the rest originated in T or NK cells. In different subgroups, there are significant heterogeneity in clinical manifestations, make clinical manifestations are not the same, this complex heterogeneity indicates that the need to develop more targeted therapeutic strategies.

(1) Targeting Abnormal Cell Cycle

1) BCL-6   In the lymph node germinal center (GC) Bcl-6 express to regulate B cell receptor（BCR) mediated physiological level of lymphocyte and immunoglobulin (LG) affinity maturation. Immunohistochemistry (IHC) can be identified with high expression of Bcl-6 lymphoma, use of anthracycline based chemotherapy (anthracycline) can improve disease-free survival of Bcl-6 positive lymphoma (disease-free survival, DFS) and free progression survival (PFS). In contrast with rituximab monoclonal antibody (anti CD-20 antibody) in the treatment of Bcl-6 negative lymphoma, while Bcl-6 positive lymphoma effect is not ideal, especially in the treatment of DLBCL. Therefore, Bcl-6 targeting therapy can overcome the transcriptional repression and impaired differentiation of lymphoma.

2) 85% follicular lymphomas (FL) have Bcl-2 chromosome t in (14:18) (q32; q21) translocation, as compared to other lymphomas. This rare chromosomal translocation, which is located in the long arm of chromosome 14 of the immunoglobulin heavy chain gene, is located on chromosome 18 and Bcl-2 gene transcription active site splicing, caused by overexpression of the Bcl-2 gene, guide Bcl-2 induced protein transcription, make B lymphocyte apoptosis and immunity from long-term survival, tolerance to chemotherapy, make Bcl-2 positive tumors poor prognosis than Bcl-2 negative tumors. The clinical study more active is use antisense oligonucleotide (ASO) and small molecule Bcl-2 inhibitor Bcl-2 mediated chemoresistance and in relapsed / refractory （r/r) NHL clinical trials, ASO (Oblimersin) combined with rituximab therapy showed the total remission rate (overall response rate, ORR) more than 40%. Some Bcl-2 small molecule inhibitors, such as ABT-263, ABT-737, ABT-199 in particular is also included in the study of clinical trials.

3) CDK inhibitors   CDK inhibitors can cause mitochondrial damage to reduced cell proliferation, and reduce DNA synthesis. Phase II clinical trials evaluating CDK inhibitor flavopiridol (flavopiridol) curative effect in the treatment of man the cell lymphome(MCL), the results showed that 11% of patients with partial remission (partial response, PR), 71% of patients in stable condition. This drug showed ORR was 53% in the treatment of r/r CLL, the median PFS was 10~12 months. The drug can also make the

high risk group (del17p, del11) of patients with remission, this discovery to promote the development and application of other new CDK inhibitors.

4) C-myc   Myc locus is located on chromosome 8,   when t (14; 2) or T (14; 22) translocation with chromosome LG gene can lead to the production of the fusion protein with the ability of lymphocyte proliferation. This change is usually characteristic of Burkitt's lymphoma, it can also be observed in other types of lymphomas. In the presence of Bcl-2 or Bcl-6 co-expression, it will enlarge the ability of c-myc to promote tumor invasion. Recently, a new domain of compound protein inhibitor JQ1 (bromodomain protein inhibitor) by nuclear chromatin dependent signal transduction RNA polymerase as a target is the ideal c-myc inhibitor, which is being carried out in the I phase of the r/r type lymphoma.

(2) To Regulate Immune System as a Target

The efficacy of rituximab as monotherapy or in combination with radioactive isotopes, namely radioimmunotherapy have superior efficacy in the treatment of lymphoma, promote the identification of lymphoma surface antigens, antibodies against the development of more different surface antigens. There are many commercially available antibodies against different lymphoma antigens (e.g., CD2, CD19, CD22, CD30, CD40, CD52, CD23, CD80, and HLA-DR) in clinical trials at various stages. In the past, focusing on the study of monoclonal antibodies against B cell lymphoma ,In the future, it will focus on the study of immune regulatory drugs and other drugs in this field to create APC targets.

1) Immunoregulatory drugs

Known immunomodulatory drugs such as thalidomide and lenalidomide are effective drugs for the treatment of lymphoma. The mechanisms of immune regulation drugs are diverse, including to reduce angiogenesis, promote immune surveillance, inhibit the AKT/MAPK/STAT3 pathway, down regulate NF-kappa B pathway and promote tumor cell apoptosis. In DLBCL, the effect of immune modulating drugs is better than non GCB subtypes, may be due to type 1 IFN secondary that produce IL-β. Single Yaolai lenalidomide (CTLA-4 antibody) for the treatment of r/r type lymphoma ORR is 34%, CR rate was 12%, the median PFS was 4 months. The further study is to explore the tumor recurrence, the curative effect of lenalidomide treatment of lymphoma B cells and T cells, including a few high-risk subtypes, such as lenalidomide in type r/r (CLL 11q or 17p deletion) as monotherapy showed ORR was 38%, 19% patients achieved CR. then FDA approved lenalidomide treat for recurrent MCL. Only lenalidomide treatment and received two or more than two kinds drugs, one of the drugs treatment for patients with bortezomib, the results indicate that the lenalidomide is better or equal than the treatment of two or more than two kinds drug efficacy. Recent reports suggest that lenalidomide combined with R-CHOP scheme can be used as the first-line drug treatment of elderly DLBCL, ORR and 2 years OS more than 90%. These studies suggest that immunomodulatory drug is an new effective drug for the treatment with a high risk of lymphoma. (conventional single drug therapy for lymphoma with poor efficacy). Further consideration should be given to the appropriate combination of the drug that will improve the prognosis of lymphoma.

2) Chemokines (CCL3, CCL4, CXCR5, CXCR4 and CXCL12)

Chemokine contributes to white blood cells that migrate to the tissue of injury, inflammation, and proliferation. In many lymphomas, chemokines can activate the anti apoptosis pathway, increased angiogenesis, and make lymphoma cell resistant to the drug. Because of multiplicity of chemotactic factors, which have complicated effects on the prognosis of lymphoma. For example, chemokine CCL3 and CCL4 are highly expressed in DLBCL patients, whose PFS and OS are lower than those low expressions. A few years ago, some patients were diagnosed with lymphoma with higher chemokine level, which may be related to chronic immune activation promote high-risk patients (e.g. HIV positive patients) developed into lymphoma. Similarly, the elevation of chemokines is a marker for poor prognosis in T cell lymphoma, and the disease is a potential therapeutic target point. Preclinical studies have indicated that histone deacetylase inhibitors and histone inhibitors (inhibitors BTK) have a role in inhibiting chemokine activity. Be aimed at CC receptor -4 humanized monoclonal antibody (kw-0761), achieved a good effect in phase I clinical study on the treatment of recurrent T cell lymphoma. In the phase II study, kw-0761 treats recurrent T cell leukemia / lymphoma with a ORR for 35%, and PFS for 3 months. To study randomized phase III in clinic on the basis of these studies (ongoing), to compare the vorinostat and kw-0761 in the treatment of cutaneous T cell lymphoma (CTCL)in quality. The results of these clinical studies will provide more effective information for the chemokine inhibitors treating T cell lymphoma.

(3) Signal Transduction Pathway as Target

1) Targeting NF-κB Pathway in Lymphomas

The NF-κB family regulates the transcription of proteins mediating cell proliferation and surival in lymphocytes. Constitutively activated NF-κB pathway enhances the survival of malignant cells by inhibiting apoptosis and creating a clone of cells resistant to chemotherapy. High NF-κB expression is noted in several B-cell and T-cell lymphomas. Various agents, including lenalidomide, curcumin and proteasome inhibitors such as bortezomib, have demonstrated the ability to target NF-κB in vivo and in vitro.

Under normal circumstances, NF-κB proteins are bound to Ikβα (nuclear factor of kappa light polypeptide gene enhancer in B cells inhibitor, α) and are protected from degradation by the proteasomal complex. In lymphomas, there is constitutive activation of the NF-κB pathway, due to breakdown of IKβα by ubiquitination-associated proteasomal degradation. Ikβα breakdown leads to the release of free NF-κB in the cytoplasm which then enters the cell nucleus and induces the production of antiapoptotic genes. Bortezomib is a ubiquitin-proteasomal inhibitor and exerts its action by inhibiting Ikβα degradation by the proteasomal complex and keeping NF-κB bound to Ikβα, thereby preventing the transcription of antiapoptotic proteins. Based on this rationale, bortezomib has been used to treat relapsed/refractory (r/r) B-cell lymphomas and showed encouraging activity specifically in cohort of patients with MCL. The excellent single agent activity of bortezomib in patients with r/r MCL was further confirmed in a subsequent study [overall response rate (ORR) 33%; median time to progression 6.2 months] and led to its FDA approval for this indication. Other studies have explored combinations of cytotoxic or other biological agents with bortezomib in indolent and aggressive lymphomas, with the most promising activity seen in lymphoplasmacytic lymphoma/Waldenstrom's macroglobulinemia (LPL/WM) and T-cell NHL Many other ongoing clinical trials are also exploring the optimal combination of proteasome inhibitors with chemotherapy drugs.

2) Targeting JAK-STAT Pathway in Lymphomas

The JAK-STAT pathway is a conglomerate of the JAK family (JAK1-3, tyrosine kinase-2) and STAT family (STAT 1-6) signal transduction proteins, that regulate the normal cell cycle. Deregulated JAK-STAT is seen in HD, ABC (activated B-cell) variant DLBCL(diffuse large B-cell lymphoma), PMLBCL (primary mediastinal large B-cell lymphoma) , T-cell lymphoma and numerous other NHL. Some antiapoptotic proteins like Bcl-Xl and Bcl-2 are downstream targets of the STAT family of proteins and help in STAT mediated growth of lymphomas. In HL and PMLBCL cell lines, JAK2 in cooperation with JMJD2 cgenes alter the epigenome and trigger myc expression assisted proliferation of lymphocytes. Also, JAK2 expression on lymphoma cells leads to co-expression of programmed death ligands (PDL-1 and 2). Increased PDL transcripts on PMLBCL samples are recurrent genetic event that help lymphoma cells overcome the immune surveillance by cytotoxic T cells Polymorphisms of the STAT family of genes perturb normal lymphocyte maturation, are overexpressed in lymphomas and impact prognosis. For example, the phosphorylated STAT5 (pSTAT5+: activated form that initiates nuclear transcription) status detected by IHC on the neoplastic Reed-Stenberg (RS) cells in HL is associated with superior freedom from treatment failure in comparison to pSTAT5-negative status. A similar negative prognostic significance with reduced OS for STAT3 expression is noted in DLBCL, especially in the non-GCB (germinal center B-cell) variants despite immune-chemotherapy. These findings highlight the need to develop targeted therapy against the JAK-STAT pathway and reverse its negative prognostic significance in lymphoid malignancies.

3) Jak2 Inhibitors in Lymphoma

Targeting the JAK-STAT pathway in vivo or in vitro causes cell death in lymphomas. JAK2 inhibitors promote apoptosis and exert inhibitory effect on proliferation, inflammatory cytokines and chemokines, PD-L1 expression and Bcl-2 synthesis. In a Phase I study of the oral JAK2-FLT3 inhibitor SB1518 (pacritinib), which included patients with relapsed HL and NHL, 15 out of 34 patients had SD. Tumor size reduction was achieved in approximately 50% of patients with SD and varied between 4 and 46%. Three of 34 patients achieved PR and the drug was well tolerated. This encouraging result prompted ongoing studies of JAK2 inhibitors in lymphomas.

4) Protein Kinase C Inhibitors

As mentioned above, the protein kinase C (PKC) group of proteins is an integral part the downstream BCR (B cell receptor) signaling pathway. If activated, they confer a survival advantage to malignant lymphocytes by activating the NF-κB pathway. High PKC-β expression in DLBCL, as identified by IHC staining or gene expression studies has been associated with poor survival, despite therapy with chemoimmunotherapy. This has encouraged the development of PKC inhibitors like enzastaurin and sotrastaurin which is tested in clinical trials. Enzastaurin suppresses proliferation, decreases angiogenesis and inhibits growth in lymphoma cell lines. In a Phase II study in r/r MCL, enzastaurin showed freedom from progression of greater than 6 months in approximately 27% of patients and a favorable hematologic profile. In another Phase II study, patients with histologically confirmed grade 1 or 2 follicular lymphoma(FL) and stage III/IV were treated with enzastaurin 500 mg daily for less than or equal to 3 years or until disease progression or toxicity. Out of the 58 patients who received greater than equal to one dose of enzastaurin, 25.9% had a PR (partial response) and 3.4% had a CR (complete response). Correlative studies confirmed low PKC-β2 expression to be associated with increased RR (response rate) and PFS (progression-free survival), thereby allowing its use as a biomarker predictive of response to this agent. Despite encouraging results in Phase II studies, when enzaustarin was used in a Phase III study (PRELUDE) as maintenance therapy for patients with high-risk DLBCL who had achieved CR following R-CHOP, no benefit was observed when compared with placebo. There was no improvement in DFS(disease-free survival), EFS or OS (overall survival) with enzaustarin maintenance. More research is necessary to determin the optimal use of this agent in lymphomas.

Challenges and Prospects

Molecular targeted therapy has made great progress in the treatment of cancer. It has a deeper understanding of the mechanism of the tumor, which can selectively kill tumor cells and reduce the side effects, but there are still many problems. At present, most of targeted therapy drugs have low efficiency relatively , the curative effect is not ideal. In addition to the existing targeted drug not highly selective for tumor treatment targets , there is a "non targeting", such as allergies, heart toxicity and other adverse reactions, sometimes very serious. In addition, targeted drugs also have drug resistance phenomenon in the use process , and the price is high. It is difficult to widely apply it in a period of time. So in a certain extent it caused a certain distance between the therapeutic effect of current targeted drugs and people's expected value. Along with the developed sub targeted drugs in use process also experienced from sensitive to resistant phenomenon in clinical trials, to further reflect the complexity of tumor growth.With the continuous development of the research on the cancer pathogenesis, new targeted drugs continue to emerge, on the one hand, through the combination of targeted drugs to enhance the efficacy and reduce drug resistance; on the other hand, through develop molecular target drugs of multiple targets, in order to enhance the curative effect, such as mTOR inhibitor rapamycin has a certain effect on gastric cancer and liver cancer and other digestive system tumors, multitargeted kinase inhibitor (RAF, VEGF, PDGF inhibitor) Sola Fini has been used for the treatment of liver cancer. Multiple target drugs, because of its targets, has a wide range of effects, but it also brings more side effects inevitably, at the same time, in a number of targets. Therefore, how to predict its effectiveness is also a problem. I believe that with the further understanding of the tumor nature. As for tumor stem cells or cancer stem cells, there will be more and more effect to molecular target drugs in clinic, hope for the individualized treatment of tumor patients, so as to bring the gospel for cancer patients.

The prognosis of patients was improved significantly by molecular targeted therapy and tumor immunotherapy, especially clarify the understanding of gene regulation pathway and molecular mechanism of tumor cells apoptosis, angiogenesis, cell movement cycle and other cell important biological events by the high-throughput gene chip screening technology, found a lot of target specific mutation and / or release the transcriptional regulated genes and molecules, some of which have potential to trigger tumor cell progression and represents a potential therapeutic target gene. Through tumor pathology with an in-depth analysis to find a more effective therapy will be help the progress of treatment. The molecular targeted therapy and tumor immunotherapy should be a new milestone for genome medicine, precision medicine, personalized medicine, and translational medicine.

Genome medicine enters an era of the "single-cell" biology where single-cell gene sequencing, single-cell systems biology, whole cell models, single molecule imaging, and single-cell biological functions have been investigated to understand mechanical phenotypes, single-cell biology, heterogeneity, and chromosome positioning and function. It was highly emphasized that single-cell biology should be considered as a new approach to identify and validate disease-specific biomarkers at multi-dimensional, multi-layer, multi-crossing, and stereoscopic single-cell levels. A number of questions have been raised, e.g. how to apply single-cell measurements to clinical practice, translate the message of single-cell systems biology into clinical phenotype, or how to explain alterations of single-cell gene sequencing and function in patients' response to therapies. The RNA and DNA sequencing of single cancer cell, correspondent its tissue cell, or circulating cell will benefit from deeper understanding of homogeneity and heterogeneity between cancer cells, cancer and normality, origins, and locations. The single-cell biology allows us to identify and develop disease-specific biomarkers, network biomarkers, dynamic network biomarkers, and therapy-based targets in cancer subtypes.

Consider/Questions

1. Basic concepts in this chapter

Molecular targeted therapy, Molecular pathology, Oncogene addiction.

2. Which advantages of molecular targeted therapy compared with conventional chemotherapy?

3. Which relevant techniques used in molecular pathology?

4. According to the literature, combining with your professional reports that the clinical research progress in molecular targeted therapy.